BASIC GYNECOLOGY AND OBSTETRICS

First Edition

Edited by:

Norman F. Gant, M.D.
Professor, Department of Obstetrics & Gynecology
The University of Texas Southwestern Medical Center at Dallas
Attending Staff, Parkland Memorial Hospital
Executive Director, American Board of Obstetrics & Gynecology

F. Gary Cunningham, M.D.
Professor and Chairman, Department of Obstetrics & Gynecology
Jack A. Pritchard Professor of Obstetrics & Gynecology
The University of Texas Southwestern Medical Center at Dallas
Chief of Obstetrics & Gynecology, Parkland Memorial Hospital

Contributors

Karen D. Bradshaw, M.D.
Assistant Professor, Departments of Obstetrics & Gynecology and Surgery
Associate Director of Ob/Gyn Residency Education
The University of Texas Southwestern Medical Center at Dallas
Attending Staff, Parkland Memorial Hospital

Bruce R. Carr, M.D.
Paul C. MacDonald Professor of Obstetrics & Gynecology
Director of Reproductive Endocrinology
The University of Texas Southwestern Medical Center at Dallas
Attending Staff, Parkland Memorial Hospital

Larry C. Gilstrap, III, M.D.
Professor, Department of Obstetrics & Gynecology
Director of Maternal-Fetal Medicine Fellowship and Clinical Genetics
The University of Texas Southwestern Medical Center at Dallas
Attending Staff, Parkland Memorial Hospital

David L. Hemsell, M.D.
Professor, Department of Obstetrics & Gynecology
Director of Gynecology
The University of Texas Southwestern Medical Center at Dallas
Attending Staff, Parkland Memorial Hospital

Paul C. MacDonald, M.D.
Professor, Departments of Obstetrics & Gynecology and Biochemistry
Cecil H. and Ida Green, Distinguished Chair in Reproductive Biology
The University of Texas Southwestern Medical Center at Dallas
Attending Staff, Parkland Memorial Hospital

Alan K. Munoz, M.D.
Clinical Associate Professor, Department of Obstetrics & Gynecology
The University of Texas Southwestern Medical Center at Dallas

Barry E. Schwarz, M.D.
Associate Professor and Vice Chairman,
Department of Obstetrics and Gynecology
The University of Texas Southwestern Medical Center at Dallas
Attending Staff, Parkland Memorial Hospital

Roberto Yazigi, M.D.
Fellow, American College of Obstetricians and Gynecologists
Gynecologic Oncology
Santiago, Chile

APPLETON & LANGE
Norwalk, Connecticut/San Mateo, California

0-8385-9633-9

Notice: The authors and the publisher of this volume have taken care to
make certain that the doses of drugs and schedules of treatment are correct
and compatible with the standards generally accepted at the time of
publication. Nevertheless, as new information becomes available, changes in
treatment and in the use of drugs become necessary. The reader is advised to
carefully consult the instruction and information material included in the
package insert of each drug or therapeutic agent before administration.
This advice is especially important when using new or infrequently used drugs.
The publisher disclaims any liability, loss, injury, or damage incurred as
a consequence, directly or indirectly, of the use and application of any of
the contents of this volume.

93 94 95 96 97 / 10 9 8 7 6 5 4 3 2 1

Prentice Hall International (UK) Limited, *London*
Prentice Hall of Australia Pty. Limited, *Sydney*
Prentice Hall Canada, Inc., *Toronto*
Prentice Hall Hispanoamericana, S.A., *Mexico*
Prentice Hall of India Private Limited, *New Delhi*
Prentice Hall of Japan, Inc., *Tokyo*
Simon & Schuster Asia Pte., Ltd., *Singapore*
Editora Prentice Hall do Brasil Ltda., *Rio de Janeiro*
Prentice Hall, *Englewood Cliffs, New Jersey*

ISBN: 0–8385–9633–9
ISSN: 1069–8841

Production Editor: Christine Langan
Designer: Janice Bielawa

PRINTED IN THE UNITED STATES OF AMERICA

Contents

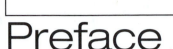

Preface

Basic Gynecology and Obstetrics was designed to combine rather than artificially separate a discussion of women's health care. Moreover, an attempt was made to provide this information in a compact form which would be affordable to medical and nursing students, house officers, nurses, midwives and other health care professionals who provide health care maintenance and care for women. Our intent in writing this text was to present obstetrics and gynecology in a concise and easily readable format. The obstetrics section is based on information presented in *Williams Obstetrics*, the standard work in obstetrics since its publication in 1902, now in its 19th edition. The gynecology section is new, but contains portions of *Williams Obstetrics*, including discussions of abortion, ectopic pregnancy, trophoblastic disease, uterine anomalies, normal anatomy, contraception, and reproductive endocrinology. Whenever possible, redundant sections between gynecology and obstetrics were deleted. When such deletions were impossible or reduced the effectiveness of specific chapters, all of the information was repeated.

Basic Gynecology and Obstetrics is designed for all medical and nursing disciplines, not just for obstetricians. We emphasize that this book does not provide "the plan" or the "answer" to all questions. There is no such tome. The "Parkland way" often is presented because of its success in our major teaching facility, Parkland Memorial Hospital. We stress, however, that methods presented in this book have served us well in the care of more than 300,000 women delivering their babies at Parkland Hospital and in providing women with more than 100,000 gynecologic operative procedures. We have, however, presented different approaches to management in controversial areas. One such area in obstetrics is the management of postterm pregnancies. An example in gynecology is the diagnosis and management of ectopic pregnancies.

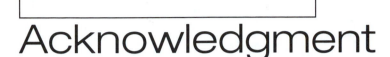

Acknowledgment

The development of any textbook is demanding and extracts a toll from its authors, their families, and their colleagues. Our families saw even less of us than usual; this means that our children and pets began to wonder who we were. Equally important, our colleagues wondered where we were. To our families, we wish to express our extreme gratitude for allowing us to practice our profession, demanding enough, but made even more so by our choices to share our own, and others, views of obstetrics and gynecology. To our colleagues, fellows and house officers, thank you and keep a light in the window. We will be back.

We wish to express our thanks to Drs. Charles Brown, Kenneth Leveno, Michael Lucas, Mark Maberry, Paul Marshburn, Mark Peters, Susan Ramin, Rigoberto Santos, and George Wendel, all of whom proofread the manuscript and added their own views to many of the chapters. This was a departmental effort, not just the effort reflected under the author's names and titles.

Planning and development of the book was provided by our colleagues at Appleton & Lange. We wish to acknowledge their guidance and counsel. Nancy Evans, Anne-Marie Zwierzyna, Becky Hainz-Baxter, and Jim Ransom were the heart of the project, but we also want to thank the following key members of the team: Jane Licht and Chris Langan for their help and attention to detail.

In our department, Rosemary Bell, Laurie Daniels, Terry Daniels, Lynne McDonnell, Sandy Nance, Julie Thompson, Ann Whisenand, and Helen Wirkler spent days revising manuscript and served as occasional psychiatrists. Marsha Congleton provided her experience as production coordinator, as she had with the 18th and 19th editions of *Williams Obstetrics*. To all of these people, we are grateful.

Introduction: The Woman as a Patient

For three decades, women have been able to demand explanations from their physicians about their illnesses and their general health and to participate in decisions about management and care. This has been the occasion for significant changes in attitude on the part of all who hold themselves out as deliverers of health care to women. For example—35 years ago a woman had to have ten living children, her husband's consent, and the approval of the hospital administrator in order to have a tubal sterilization procedure at Parkland Memorial Hospital, in Dallas, Texas. Twenty years ago, at the same institution, a woman wanting the same procedure had to have four living children, her husband's consent if married, and the approval of the hospital administrator. Today, a woman wanting a tubal sterilization must be able to give informed consent and be able to convince one or more physicians that she understands the impact of the procedure on her future fertility. What this means is that a woman's reproductive function is no longer the property of her husband or the subject matter of bureaucratic authority. Decisions about a woman's reproductive function are made by her in consultation as an equal with her physician. Many would argue that this change in attitude was the result of the legalization of abortion in the United States. Most contend that these changes were the result of the commercial availability of reliable oral contraceptives and the willingness by our patients to accept responsibility for their own reproductive function. Women in the United States and Canada have demonstrated this by making "the pill" enormously popular. Not only has the practice of obstetrics and gynecology changed dramatically, but the practice of medicine in general has changed with this change in patient attitude.

It follows that if a woman has responsibility for her reproductive function, she has personal responsibility regarding her health care generally. Just as a woman's responsibility for her health care is not limited to her reproductive function, the responsibility of the obstetrician-gynecologist is not confined to the patient's pelvis. Screening for cardiovascular disease and for malignant tumors is as important in the practice of modern gynecology as the diagnosis of pregnancy or uterine infection.

The demand by women for more information about and more participation in health care decisions has not simplified the practice of obstetrics and gynecology. Some patients do not want to help make health care decisions. Others think they are more informed than their physicians, and occasionally they may be right. The modern practitioner, and thus the student of modern practice, must individualize this aspect of patient care as artfully and scientifically as the choice of surgical approach or dosage of potent medication. Patients must be appropriately informed and allowed to participate in health care decisions. How much information is appropriate and how much patient participation is desirable is probably different in each instance. In any case, a very important piece of information needed by the patient to make a reasonable decision is the summation of the physician's knowledge and experience and, finally, the physician's recommendation. The physician's responsibility is not lessened by the patients' demand for participation—if anything, it is enhanced.

Medical students in their haste and zeal to assimilate the science of medicine occasionally lose sight of the art of medicine and even of their own humanity. Most patients in obstetrics and gynecology are women. To refer to our patients as "females" implies an uncertainty of species that does not exist. All of our patients have names. That many of them have diagnoses, hospital room numbers, and bed numbers is irrelevant to an individual's identity and dignity. To refer to a patient as "the diagnosis in room such-and-such" is needlessly impersonal. All doctors who practice the art of medicine should refer to patients by name, and failure to do so dehumanizes both the patient and the doctor. Students must realize that patients are special people—people asking for help, or guidance, or information, or reassurance.

General Gynecology

1

Anatomy of the Female Reproductive Tract & Normal Menstruation

I. ANATOMY

The dorsal lithotomy position is not the normal anatomical position. Nevertheless, physicians frequently refer to anatomical landmarks based upon the patient being examined from this position. This practice has resulted in the common use of "upward" and "above" for anterior and "downward" and "below" for posterior.

EXTERNAL GENERATIVE ORGANS

The **female pudendum,** or the external organs of generation, also called the **vulva,** comprises all the structures visible externally from the pubis to the perineum, ie, the mons pubis, the labia majora and minora, the clitoris, the hymen, the vestibule, the urethral opening, and various glandular and vascular structures (Figure 1–1).

THE PERINEUM

Most of the support of the perineum is provided by the pelvic and urogenital diaphragms. The **pelvic diaphragm** consists of the levator ani muscles plus the coccygeus muscles posteriorly and the fascial coverings of these muscles. The levator ani muscles form a broad muscular sling that originates from the posterior surface of the superior rami of the pubis, from the inner surface of the ischial spine, and—between these two sites—from the fascia of the obturator muscle. The median raphe of the levator ani,

which is positioned between the anus and the vagina, is reinforced by the central tendon of the perineum, on which converge the bulbocavernosus muscles, the superficial transverse perineal muscles, and the external anal sphincter. These structures, which contribute to the perineal body and provide much of the support for the perineum, often are lacerated during delivery unless an adequate episiotomy is made at an appropriate time.

MONS PUBIS

The **mons pubis** is the fatty cushion that lies over the anterior surface of the symphysis pubis. After puberty, the skin of the mons pubis is covered by curly hair that forms the **female escutcheon.**

LABIA MAJORA

The **labia majora** are two rounded folds of adipose tissue, covered with skin, that extend downward and backward from the mons pubis. In adult women, these structures vary in appearance depending mainly upon the amount of fat present. Embryologically, the labia majora are homologous with the male scrotum. The round ligaments terminate at the upper borders of the labia majora. After repeated deliveries, the labia majora are less prominent, and after menopause they usually begin to atrophy.

LABIA MINORA

The **labia minora** are two flat, reddish folds of tissue, visible when the labia majora are separated, that join at the upper extremity of the vulva. They vary greatly in size and shape. In nulliparous women, the labia minora usually are not visible behind the nonseparated labia majora, whereas

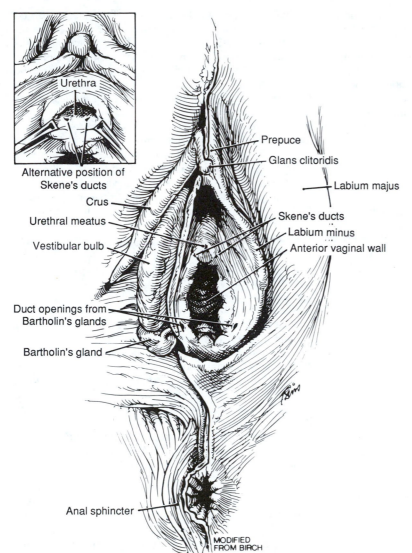

Urethra

Alternative position of
Skene's ducts

Crus

Urethral meatus

Vestibular bulb

Duct openings from
Bartholin's glands

Bartholin's gland

Anal sphincter

Prepuce

Glans clitoridis

Labium majus

Skene's ducts

Labium minus

Anterior vaginal wall

MODIFIED
FROM BIRCH

Figure 1–1. The external genitalia with the skin and subcutaneous tissue removed from the right side.

in multiparous women, it is common for the labia minora to project beyond the labia majora. There are no hair follicles in the labia minora, but there are many sebaceous follicles and occasionally a few sweat glands. The interior of the labial folds is composed of connective tissue in which there are many vessels and some smooth muscular fibers, as is the case in typical erectile structures. These structures are extremely sensitive and are supplied with a variety of nerve endings.

CLITORIS

The **clitoris,** the homologue of the penis, is a small cylindric, erectile body located near the superior extremity of the vulva. It projects downward between the branched extremities of the labia minora, which converge to form

the prepuce and frenulum of the clitoris. The clitoris is composed of a glans, a body (corpus), and two crura. The glans, which rarely exceeds 0.5 cm in diameter, is covered by stratified squamous epithelium richly supplied with nerve endings and is, therefore, extremely sensitive to touch. The vessels of the erectile clitoris are connected with the vestibular bulbs; the clitoris is the principal erogenous organ of women.

VAGINAL VESTIBULE

The **vaginal vestibule** is an almond-shaped area enclosed by the labia minora laterally and extending from the clitoris above to the fourchette below. It usually is perforated by six openings: the urethra, the vagina, the ducts of the two Bartholin glands, and, at times, the ducts of the two paraurethral glands, also called Skene's ducts and glands (Figure 1–1). Related to the vestibule are the **major vestibular glands,** ie, **Bartholin's glands** (Figure 1–1), a pair of small compound glands about 0.5–1 cm in diameter, each of which is situated beneath the vestibule on either side of the vaginal opening. The Bartholin glands lie under the constrictor muscle of the vagina and sometimes are partially covered by the vestibular bulbs. During sexual arousal, mucoid material is secreted from these glands.

URETHRA

The lower two-thirds of the **urethra** lies immediately above the anterior vaginal wall and terminates externally at the urethral meatus. The urethral meatus is in the midline of the vestibule, 1–1.5 cm below the pubic arch and a short distance above the vaginal opening; usually it is puckered in appearance.

VAGINAL OPENING

The **vaginal opening** is in the lower portion of the vestibule and varies considerably in size and shape. In virginal women, it most often is hidden entirely by the overlapping labia minora, and when exposed it usually appears almost completely closed by the membranous **hymen.**

INTERNAL GENERATIVE ORGANS

VAGINA

The vagina is a tubular musculomembranous structure that extends from the vulva to the uterus; the vagina is interposed anteriorly and posteriorly between the urethra and the urinary bladder and the rectum (Figure 1–2). The vagina is an organ of many functions, serving as the excretory organ of the uterus, through which uterine secretions and menstrual flow escape; as the female organ of copulation; and as part of the birth canal at vaginal delivery. The upper portion of the vagina arises from the müllerian ducts; the lower portion is formed from the urogenital sinus. Anteriorly, the vagina is in contact with the bladder and urethra, from which it is separated by connective tissue that often is referred to as the vesicovaginal septum. Posteriorly—ie, between the lower portion of the vagina and the rectum—there are similar tissues that together form the rectovaginal septum. The upper one-fourth of the vagina is usually separated from the rectum by the **rectouterine pouch,** or, as it is sometimes called, the **cul-de-sac of Douglas.**

The upper end of the vagina is the termination of a vault into which projects the lower portion of the uterine cervix. The vaginal vault is subdivided into the anterior, posterior, and two lateral fornices. The lateral fornices are intermediate in depth. The fornices are of considerable clinical importance, since the internal pelvic organs usually can be palpated through the thin walls of the fornices. Moreover, the posterior fornix usually provides ready surgical access to the peritoneal cavity.

Prominent longitudinal ridges project into the vaginal lumen from the midlines of both the anterior and the posterior walls. In nulliparous women, these numerous transverse ridges, or **rugae,** extend outward from—and almost at right angles to—the longitudinal vaginal ridges. The mucosa of the vagina is composed of noncornified stratified squamous epithelium. Beneath the epithelium there is a thin fibromuscular coat; an inner circular layer and an outer longitudinal layer of smooth muscle can usually be identified. A thin layer of connective tissue overlying the mucosa and muscularis is rich in blood vessels and harbors a few small lymphoid nodules. Normally, glands are not present in the vagina.

There is an abundant vascular supply to the vagina; the upper third is supplied by the cervicovaginal branches of the uterine arteries, the middle third by the inferior vesical arteries, and the lower third by the middle hemorrhoidal (rectal) and internal pudendal arteries. An extensive venous plexus immediately surrounds the vagina, vessels that follow the course of the arteries; eventually, these veins empty into the internal iliac veins. For the most part, the lymphatics from the lower third of the vagina, along with those of the vulva, drain into the inguinal lymph nodes; those from the middle third into the hypogastric nodes; and those from the upper third into the iliac nodes.

UTERUS

The uterus is a muscular organ partially covered by peritoneum, or serosa. The cavity of the uterus is lined by the endometrium. During pregnancy, the uterus serves for reception, implantation, retention, and nutrition of the conceptus, which it then expels during labor. The uterus of the nonpregnant woman is situated in the pelvic cavity between the bladder anteriorly and the rectum posteriorly (Figure 1–2). The inferior portion—ie, the cervix—projects into the vagina. Almost the entire posterior wall of the uterus is covered by serosa, or peritoneum, the lower portion of which forms the anterior boundary of the **rectouterine cul-de-sac,** or pouch of Douglas. Only the upper portion of the anterior wall of the uterus is so covered.

The uterus resembles a flattened pear in shape and consists of two major but unequal parts: an upper triangular portion, the **body** (or **corpus**) and a lower, cylindric, or fusiform portion, the **cervix.**

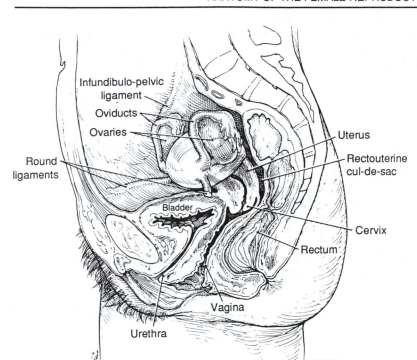

Figure 1–2. Sagittal section of the pelvis of an adult woman that is illustrative of relations of pelvic viscera.

1. UTERINE CERVIX

The cervix is the specialized portion of the uterus that is below the isthmus. Anteriorly, the upper boundary of the cervix, the internal os, corresponds approximately to the level at which the peritoneum is reflected upon the bladder. Laterally, it is attached to the cardinal ligaments, and anteriorly it is separated from the overlying bladder by loose connective tissue. The external os is located at the lower extremity of the vaginal portion of the cervix, the **portio vaginalis.** The cervix is composed of some smooth muscle fibers but predominantly of collagenous tissue plus elastic tissue and blood vessels. The transition from the primarily collagenous tissue of the cervix to the primarily muscular tissue of the body of the uterus, although generally abrupt, may be gradual and may extend over as much as 10 mm.

Characteristically, the mucosa of the cervical canal, although embryologically a direct continuation of the endometrium, is differentiated in such a way that the appearance of sections through the canal is reminiscent of a honeycomb. The mucosa is composed of a single layer of very high, columnar epithelium that rests upon a thin basement membrane. Numerous cervical glands extend from the surface of the endocervical mucosa directly into the subjacent connective tissue; since there is no submucosa as such, these glands furnish the thick, tenacious secretion of the cervical canal. If the ducts of the cervical glands are occluded, retention cysts may form, which are a few millimeters in diameter, the so-called **nabothian cysts.**

Normally, the squamous epithelium of the vaginal portion of the cervix and the columnar epithelium of the cervical canal form a sharp line of division very near the external os, ie, the squamocolumnar junction in nulliparous women.

2. BODY OF THE UTERUS

The anterior surface of the body of the uterus is almost flat, whereas the posterior surface is distinctly convex. The **uterine tubes** (oviducts, fallopian tubes) emerge from the **cornua** of the uterus at the junction of the superior and lateral margins. The convex upper segment between the points of insertion of the uterine tubes is called the **fundus.** The great bulk of the body of the uterus—but not the cervix—is composed of muscle. The inner surfaces of the anterior and posterior walls of the uterus lie almost in contact; the cavity between these walls forms a mere slit. The cervical canal is fusiform and opens at each end at the **internal os** and **external os.**

The wall of the body of the uterus is composed of three layers: serosa, muscularis, and mucosa. The serosal layer is formed by the peritoneum that covers the uterus and to which it is firmly adherent except at sites just above the bladder and at the lateral margins, where the peritoneum is deflected so as to form the broad ligaments.

The innermost portion of the uterus—the mucosal layer, which lines the uterine cavity in nonpregnant women—is the **endometrium.** The endometrium is a thin, pink, velvety membrane that on close examination is seen to be perforated by a large number of minute openings, the ostia of the uterine glands. Because of the repetitive cyclic changes that occur during the reproductive years of a woman's life, the endometrium normally varies greatly in thickness and measures between 0.5 and 5 mm. The endometrium is composed of surface epithelium, glands, and interglandular mesenchymal tissue in which there are numerous blood vessels.

The epithelium of the endometrial surface is composed of a single layer of closely packed, high columnar, usually ciliated cells. During much of the endometrial cycle, the oval nuclei are situated in the lower portions of the cells but not so near the base as in the endocervix.

The vascular architecture of the endometrium has great significance in the phenomena of menstruation and pregnancy. Arterial blood is transported to the uterus by the uterine and ovarian arteries. As the arterial branches penetrate the uterine wall obliquely inward and reach its middle third, these vessels ramify in a plane that is parallel to the surface—thus the name **arcuate arteries.** Radial branches extend from the arcuate arteries at right angles toward the endometrium. The endometrial arteries are composed of **coiled** or **spiral arteries,** which are a continuation of the radial arteries, and **basal arteries,** which branch from the radial arteries at a sharp angle.

The tissue that makes up the major portion of the uterus—the myometrium—is composed of bundles of smooth muscle that are united by connective tissue in which there are many elastic fibers. The number of muscle fibers of the uterus progressively diminishes caudally, until in the cervix, muscle comprises only 10% of the tissue mass. In the inner wall of the body of the uterus, there is relatively more muscle than in the outer layers, and in the anterior and posterior walls there is more muscle than in the lateral walls. During pregnancy, the myometrium—chiefly through hypertrophy—increases greatly, but there is no significant change in the muscle content of the cervix.

3. LIGAMENTS OF THE UTERUS

The broad, the round, and the uterosacral ligaments extend from either side of the uterus. The **broad ligaments** are specialized folds of peritoneum composed of two winglike structures that extend from the lateral margins of the uterus to the pelvic walls and thus divide the pelvic cavity into anterior and posterior compartments. Each broad ligament consists of a fold of peritoneum enclosing various structures and which has superior, lateral, inferior, and medial margins. The inner two-thirds of the superior margin form the **mesosalpinx,** to which the uterine tubes are attached. The outer third of the superior margin of the broad ligament, which extends from the fimbriated end of the uterine tube to the pelvic wall, forms the **infundibulopelvic ligament** (suspensory ligament of the ovary), which is traversed by the ovarian vessels.

At the lateral margin of each broad ligament, the peritoneum is reflected onto the side of the pelvis. The base of the broad ligament, which is quite thick, is continuous

with the connective tissue of the pelvic floor. The densest portion—called the **cardinal ligament,** or transverse cervical ligament—is composed of connective tissue that medially is united firmly with the supravaginal portion of the cervix. The uterine vessels and the lower portion of the ureter are enclosed in the base of the broad ligament.

A vertical section through the uterine end of the broad ligament is triangular; the uterine vessels are found within its broad base (Figure 1–3). In its lower part, it is widely attached to the connective tissues that are adjacent to the cervix, ie, the **parametrium.** The upper part is composed of three folds that, in turn, nearly cover the uterine tube, the utero-ovarian ligament, and the round ligament.

The **round ligaments** extend outward on either side from the lateral portion of the uterus; these ligaments arise somewhat below and anterior to the origin of the oviducts. Each round ligament is located in a fold of peritoneum that is continuous with the broad ligament and extends outward and downward to the inguinal canal, through which it passes to terminate in the upper portion of the labium majus.

Each uterosacral ligament extends posterolaterally from an attachment to the supravaginal portion of the cervix to encircle the rectum and thence insert into the fascia over the second and third sacral vertebrae. The uterosacral ligaments are composed of connective tissue and some smooth muscle and are covered by peritoneum.

The vascular supply of the uterus is derived principally from the uterine and ovarian arteries. The uterine artery—a main branch of the anterior division of the internal iliac or hypogastric artery—descends for a short distance, enters the base of the broad ligament, and makes its way medially to the side of the uterus. The **ovarian artery**—a direct branch of the aorta—enters the broad ligament through the infundibulopelvic ligament, or suspensory ligament, of the ovary.

The **lymphatics** from the various segments of the uterus drain into several sets of lymph nodes. Those from the cervix terminate mainly in the external iliac nodes, which are situated near the bifurcation of the common iliac vessels between the external and internal iliac arteries. The lymphatics from the body of the uterus are distributed to two groups of nodes. One set drains into the superficial inguinal, then the femoral, and then the external iliac nodes; the other set, after joining certain lymphatics from the ovarian region, terminates in the periaortic lumbar lymph nodes.

The **nerve supply** of the uterus is derived chiefly from the sympathetic nervous system but also partly from the cerebrospinal and parasympathetic systems. The parasympathetic system is represented on either side by the pelvic nerve, which is composed of a few fibers derived from the second, third, and fourth sacral nerves. In the 11th and 12th thoracic nerve roots, there are sensory fibers from the uterus that transmit the painful stimuli of uterine contractions to the central nervous system. The sensory nerves from the cervix and upper part of the birth canal pass through the pelvic nerves to the second, third, and fourth

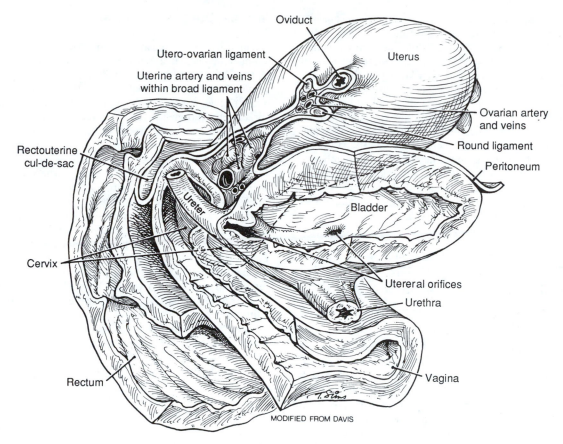

Figure 1–3. Vertical section through uterine end of the right broad ligament.

sacral nerves, whereas those from the lower portion of the birth canal pass primarily through the pudendal nerve.

UTERINE TUBES

The uterine tubes (oviducts, fallopian tubes) extend from the uterine cornua to a site near the ovaries and provide access for the ova to the uterine cavity. The uterine tubes vary from 8 to 14 cm in length, are covered by peritoneum, and the lumen is lined by mucous membrane. Each uterine tube is divided into an **interstitial portion, isthmus, ampulla,** and **infundibulum.** The uterine tube varies considerably in thickness; the narrowest portion of the isthmus measures from 2–3 mm in diameter and the widest portion of the ampulla measures between 5 and 8 mm. The uterine tube is surrounded completely by peritoneum except at the attachment of the mesosalpinx. The musculature of the uterine tube is arranged, in general, in two layers—an inner circular and an outer longitudinal layer.

The uterine tube is lined by a mucous membrane, the epithelium of which is composed of a single layer of columnar cells, some of them ciliated and others secretory. The current produced by the tubal cilia is such that the

direction of flow is toward the uterine cavity; indeed, minute foreign bodies introduced into the abdominal cavities of animals may eventually appear in the vagina after they are transported through the tubes and the cavity of the uterus. Tubal peristalsis is believed to be an important factor in transport of the ovum.

OVARIES

The ovaries are almond-shaped organs, the functions of which are the development and extrusion of ova and the synthesis and secretion of steroid hormones. The ovaries vary considerably in size. During the childbearing years, the ovaries are 2.5–5 cm in length, 1.5–3 cm in width, and 0.6–1.5 cm in thickness. After menopause, the size of the ovary is diminished remarkably.

The ovary is attached to the broad ligament by the **mesovarium.** The **utero-ovarian ligament,** also called the **ovarian ligament,** extends from the lateral and posterior portions of the uterus, just beneath the tubal insertion, to the uterine (lower) pole of the ovary. The **infundibulopelvic (suspensory) ligament of the ovary** extends from the upper (tubal) pole to the pelvic wall; through it course the ovarian vessels and nerves.

The general structure of the ovary can be studied best in cross sections, in which two portions may be distinguished, the **cortex** and the **medulla.** The cortex, or outer layer, varies in thickness with age and becomes thinner with advancing years. It is in this layer that the ova and **graafian follicles** are located. The outermost portion of the cortex, which is dull and whitish, is called the **tunica albuginea;** on its surface, there is a single layer of cuboidal epithelium. The medulla, or central portion, of the ovary, is composed of loose connective tissue continuous with that of the mesovarium. There are a large number of arteries and veins in the medulla and a small number of smooth muscle fibers continuous with those in the suspensory ligament; the muscle fibers may have functional significance in movements of the ovary.

II. NORMAL MENSTRUATION

In response to the changes evoked by hormonal actions in the ovary during each ovulatory cycle, there are morphologic changes in the endometrium that evolve with such precise regularity that the histologic features of the endometrium can be used by an experienced morphologist to estimate the day of the ovarian cycle on which the endometrium was removed. The endocrine changes during the ovarian cycle can be summarized as follows: (1) During the preovulatory (follicular) phase of the ovarian cycle, estradiol-17β is secreted principally by the dominant follicle in increasing quantities. (2) During the postovulatory (luteal) phase, progesterone—in addition to estradiol-17β—is secreted by the corpus luteum. (3) During the premenstrual phase, the corpus luteum regresses and the rates of secretion of both estradiol-17β and progesterone diminish.

In response to these changes in sex steroid hormones that are secreted during the ovarian cycle, there are four main stages of the endometrial cycle: (1) postmenstrual reorganization and thus **proliferation** in response to stimulation (directly or indirectly) by estradiol-17β; (2) abundant glandular **secretion,** which results from the combined action of estrogen and progesterone; (3) **premenstrual ischemia** and involution; and (4) **menstruation,** which is accompanied by collapse and desquamation of all but the deepest layer of the endometrium. Ultimately, menstruation is the consequence of progesterone withdrawal. The follicular (preovulatory, or proliferative) phase and the postovulatory (luteal, secretory) phase customarily are divided into early and late stages. The normal secretory phase may be subdivided rather finely (almost day by day), based on histologic criteria, from shortly after ovulation until the onset of menstruation.

THE MENARCHE & PUBERTY

Historically, the age at which menstruation begins—the **menarche**—has declined steadily until recent years. This decline has ceased in the United States. The average time at which menstruation begins is now between 12 and 13 years of age, but in a small number of apparently normal girls, menarche may occur as early as the tenth or as late as the 16th year. The term "menarche" specifically denotes the first menstruation, whereas "puberty" is a broader term that denotes the entire transitional stage between childhood and sexual maturity. The menarche is therefore just one sign of puberty, but if it is the consequence of ovulation (and attendant hormonal secretion), it is indicative of completion of the fundamental physiologic event of puberty, namely, release of an ovum.

Although the **modal interval** at which menstruation occurs is considered to be 28 days, there is considerable variation among women generally as well as in the cycle lengths of a given individual. Marked variations in the lengths of menstrual cycles do not necessarily imply infertility.

The duration of menstrual flow also is variable; the usual duration is 4–6 days, but lengths between 2 and 8 days may be considered normal. In any individual woman, however, the duration of flow is usually similar from cycle to cycle.

The menstrual discharge consists of shed fragments of endometrium mixed with a variable quantity of blood. Usually the blood is liquid, but if the rate of blood flow is excessive, clots of various sizes may be present. The amount of blood lost averages about 25–60 mL per cycle.

CERVICAL CHANGES DURING MENSTRUATION

Cyclic changes occur in the endocervical glands, especially during the follicular phase of the cycle. During the early follicular phase, the glands are only slightly tortuous and the secretory cells are not very tall. Secretion of mucus is meager. The late follicular phase, however, is characterized by pronounced tortuosity of the glands, deep invagination, tumescence of the epithelium, high columnar cells, and abundant secretion. The connective tissue acquires a looser texture and more extensive vascularization. After ovulation, these characteristics regress.

The secretory activity of the endocervical glands is maximal at about the time of ovulation and is the result of estrogenic stimulation. Only at that time, in most women, is the quality of the cervical mucus such as to permit penetration by spermatozoa.

THE MENOPAUSE & CLIMACTERIC

Menopause is the cessation of menses. There are wide variations in the age at which menopause occurs. About half of all women cease menstruating between the ages of 45 and 50, about one-quarter before age 45, and another one-quarter continue to menstruate until past 50 years of age. The term **climacteric** is derived from a Greek word that means "rung of a ladder" and bears the same relation to menopause as the term "puberty" bears to menarche. The climacteric is the time in a woman's life known to the laity as the "change of life."

SUGGESTED READINGS

Cunningham FG, MacDonald PC, Gant NF: Anatomy of the Reproductive Tract in Women. In Cunningham FG, MacDonald PC, Gant NF, Leveno KJ, Gilstrap LG, (eds): *Williams Obstetrics,* 19th ed. Appleton & Lange, 1993.

2

Gynecologic History & Physical Examination

HISTORY

In the absence of symptoms, sexual activity, or menstrual problems, it is generally unnecessary for a woman to have a pelvic examination before the age of 18–22 years. Many pediatricians see females through the mid to late teen years in adolescent clinics; pelvic examinations are not routinely performed. When sexual activity begins, annual pelvic examinations with cervical cytology and sexually transmitted disease screening should be performed; a complete physical examination at the same time is appropriate—and this includes the years after the menopause. If the uterus, tubes, and ovaries are removed (unless following diagnosis of malignant or premalignant disease), the frequency of pelvic examination can be reduced to at least every 3 years. Breast examination and testing should continue to be performed as outlined in Chapter 15.

Not only gynecologic but also general medical assessments must be made by the physician providing gynecologic care. For many women, the gynecologist is the primary care physician and counselor. Complete historical information must be obtained at the initial visit and modified as necessary thereafter. A chronologic summary sheet listing diagnoses, surgical procedures, and medications with start and resolution dates is extremely helpful. Although the initial encounter will usually occur in a clinic or office setting, it may occur in a hospital room or emer-

gency room. For an established patient coming in for an annual physical examination and routine testing, only the interval history since the last encounter need be obtained. This information must be actively sought, however, as it may not be volunteered. For example, the patient may have developed an allergic reaction to a medication since her last visit, or a female relative may have developed breast cancer. The amount of information added to the chart may vary significantly at different visits, but the types of information sought should be essentially the same at each encounter.

History taking must be systematic so that omissions will be avoided. The history must be obtained in such a way that the patient does not feel rushed, and yet the process must be controlled for efficient use of time. A thorough history is especially important at the first encounter; it not only allows the practitioner to gain information necessary to make diagnoses and determine a management plan—it also enables the patient to evaluate and "get to know" the physician. Because the patient who does not trust her physician will not divulge information that may be vital to her care, trust must be established early. The initial scheduled appointment should be longer than follow-up visits to afford time for thorough evaluation.

The importance of interpersonal communication and development of that skill cannot be overemphasized. One may elect to obtain most historical information by questionnaire while the patient waits to be seen. For any problems identified in this way, there should be an explanation in the historical portion of the patient's medical record. Historical facts should be fully and accurately elicited, but recording does not necessarily require many pages. For example, a review of systems may take 15 minutes of interrogation but can be covered in writing by the simple comment, "noncontributory." One must, however, take whatever time is necessary to record important information, both positive and negative. *A complete and accurate medical record is the physician's best assistant.*

The experience of medical students and residents with history taking is deceptive because most or all of that training time is spent in a hospital setting. Most medicine, however, is practiced in an office. Therefore, one must de-

---

Terms Related to Vaginal Bleeding

Menarche: Age at first menstruation

Cycle length: The interval from the first day of one menstrual period to the first day of the next

Polymenorrhea (metrorrhagia): Bleeding between periods

Postcoital bleeding: Bleeding after intercourse

Hypermenorrhea (menorrhagia): Excessive menstrual flow

Menometrorrhagia (hyperpolymenorrhea): Prolonged bleeding at frequent and irregular intervals

Hypomenorrhea: Slight menstrual flow

Oligomenorrhea: Menstruation occurring less frequently than every 35 days

velop his or her own office record-keeping system rather than use one designed for hospital use.

Because it can be distracting for the patient to have the physician writing during the interview, information should if possible be retained for later entry into the chart. Brief jottings to help one remember what has been learned during the encounter are preferable to many pages of handwritten notes. Many physicians dictate results of encounters after the patient leaves the office.

Reason for Encounter (Chief Complaint)

The obvious starting point after introductory greetings—which are important and not to be dispensed with in the interest of time—is to learn why the patient is seeking medical care. She may have no specific complaint but may only want an annual physical examination. The main reason for the visit may not become obvious until after the examination or until both the history taking and physical examination have been completed. Often the true reason for the visit will not be ascertained until after the patient develops confidence in her doctor.

Present Illness

If an illness is present, it is important to determine its duration, the symptoms associated and what aggravates or relieves them, and the results of previous attempts at therapy of any kind. In the chapters that follow, symptoms associated with various diseases will be discussed. Deviations from what is normal *for the patient* must be identified and recorded. It must be remembered that what the patient considers to be normal may in fact be abnormal. Only thorough questioning will reveal such situations.

Menstrual History

It is important to establish the patient's age at first menstruation (**menarche**), the interval from the first day of one menstrual period to the first day of the next (**cycle length**), the duration of menstrual flow, the estimated amount of flow (number of pads), and whether there is bleeding between periods (**polymenorrhea, metrorrhagia**) or after intercourse (**postcoital bleeding**). One must establish the date of the first day of the last menstrual period (**LMP**) and determine whether the period was normal or abnormal, remembering that what is a normal period for one patient may not be normal for another. The number of tampons or sanitary napkins utilized per day is useful information only if one knows what prompts the changes. For example, some women may change when there is only a spot on a pad, and others may wait until the pad is saturated. Such factual information may help to explain cases in which two nulliparous women have similar menstrual histories and strikingly different hematocrits.

The mean length of "normal" menstrual flow is 5 days, with a range of 3–7 days. Bleeding that exceeds 7 days (**polymenorrhea, metrorrhagia**) is abnormal, and the cause should be determined just as when the menstrual flow is excessive (**hypermenorrhea, menorrhagia**). If prolonged bleeding occurs at frequent and irregular intervals, the term **menometrorrhagia** or **hyperpolymenorrhea** is used. Causes and diagnostic techniques are discussed in Chapter 21. The term describing slight ("light") menstrual flow, commonly observed in association with oral contraceptives, is **hypomenorrhea.** Menstruation occurring less frequently than every 35 days is called **oligomenorrhea.**

The practitioner must ascertain whether the patient is having **ovulatory menstrual cycles.** The normal cycle may vary between 21 and 35 days, but for most women it is around 28 days. A woman whose cycles are chronically anovulatory is at increased risk for anemia and endometrial carcinoma and suffers the potential embarrassment of unpredictable menses.

Ovulation usually can be verified by asking the patient if there are premonitory symptoms or signs (**molimina**) that enable her to anticipate menses. Common examples are bloating, increased appetite, specific food cravings (chocolate, potato chips, soft drinks), facial acne, breast tenderness (**mastodynia**) or enlargement, water retention, weight gain, irritability, depression, headache, cramps, backache, thigh ache, or, "I can just tell." Most women having ovulatory cycles will experience one or more of these premenstrual phenomena but are able to function normally. When these physiologic responses to ovulation are magnified and result in impairment of ability to function normally, they are referred to as **premenstrual syndrome (PMS),** which will be discussed in Chapter 10.

Another characteristic of ovulatory menses is occurrence at regular intervals. Women who ovulate usually have discomfort or cramps (**dysmenorrhea**) along with menstrual flow, and some have midcycle lower abdominal or pelvic pain (**mittelschmerz**) associated with ovulation. A woman who has a painless menstrual cycle every 3 months (oligomenorrhea) and no molimina is at increased risk for the development of endometrial cancer because she probably does not ovulate, and the endometrial cells are therefore exposed to estrogen only and never to progesterone.

Anovulatory menses are characterized by bleeding that is unpredictable as to onset, amount of flow, and duration of flow and is usually painless. On the other hand, if a woman has molimina prior to painful menstrual periods every 3 months, the physician need not be concerned about endometrial cancer but should be concerned about difficulty in achieving pregnancy if that is the patient's wish. Obviously, a woman who ovulates infrequently has fewer opportunities for conception.

Obstetric History

It is important to note the number of times a woman has been pregnant (**gravidity**) and the outcome of each pregnancy—living infant, stillborn infant, multiple pregnancy, miscarriage, etc. Abortion and miscarriage both connote early pregnancy loss without assigning guilt for the physician, but that is not always true for the patient. If the distinction between abortion and miscarriage is important to the patient, fetal loss can be recorded as "spontaneous" or "elective" without implying a judgment of any kind. Information regarding prior pregnancies may be withheld, but evidence of a previous pregnancy may be obvious upon examination of the cervix and uterus. Histologic or visual confirmation of the presence of pregnancy is important in cases where the patient says she has miscarried. For example, women with polycystic ovarian disease (Chapter 22) may say they have been pregnant four times and miscarried each time, whereas in fact they probably went through prolonged intervals without menses (**amenorrhea**) due to anovulation, and the anovulatory menses that then occurred were heavy. Dilation and curettage (D&C) or endometrial biopsy would confirm the presence or absence of pregnancy tissue. Accurate pregnancy tests now available have done much to eliminate this problem (see Pregnancy Tests, Chapter 8). This determination is important because if repeated miscarriages have occurred (**habitual abortion**), the management plan for that patient will be significantly different from that for a woman who is merely having anovulatory cycles (Chapter 9).

Gynecologic History

In addition to the menstrual history, a complete gynecologic history must include data about previous pelvic surgery, age at first intercourse, number of sexual partners, history of positive culture for *Neisseria gonorrhoeae* or other sexually transmitted bacteria or viruses or of treatment for suspected tubal or pelvic infection, and other sexually transmitted diseases. The patient should be questioned regarding her understanding about the transmission of potential pathogens, sequelae of infections, prevention of infections, symptoms or signs of infection in a sexual partner, and pregnancy prevention. Previous treatment for a Bartholin gland abscess or cyst should be recorded. The frequency and results of pelvic examinations and Papanicolaou testing should be noted as well as information regarding self breast examination and mammography.

Contraceptive History

Each method of contraception used, the duration and success of use, and any attendant problems should be documented. A history of unprotected intercourse not resulting in pregnancy is important information even if the patient was not actively seeking pregnancy during that time.

Past Medical History

Any significant medical or surgical illnesses should be recorded, as should previous transfusions, medications being taken, adverse reactions to medications, or other medical problems perceived by the patient even though treatment may not have been necessary.

Social History

Marital status data should include the current status and any previous marriages. The health of the spouse or partner and the quality of the relationship should be recorded. Discomfort during intercourse (**dyspareunia**) should be identified (Chapter 11). The health status of children should be recorded along with any of their problems, spe-

cial interests, or accomplishments. Personal habits such as sleep patterns, eating, smoking, drug use (prescribed or illicit), and alcohol use should be asked about. The patient may be unwilling at first to admit to abuse of alcohol or drugs, but when a trusting relationship is established that information may be forthcoming so that guidance can be offered.

System Review

Symptoms other than those related to the pelvis and reproductive organs should be elicited by organ system review. There may be overlap between the past medical history and the review of systems. The patient's general health should be assessed, including such things as weight stability or instability, appetite, and ability to function at home and at work.

Family History

The health status or the age at death and cause of death of grandparents, parents, and siblings must be recorded if known, since they may relate to management objectives. Such information may in some cases be used for the benefit of the individuals or the family unit as well as the patient.

PHYSICAL EXAMINATION

Anxiety about a possible illness or about the pelvic examination itself can increase discomfort and interfere with diagnosis. It is important that the patient be physically and mentally as relaxed as possible. This emphasizes the importance of establishing confidence during the process of taking the history. The practitioner must demonstrate not only courtesy and consideration but also patience, gentleness, and self-confidence. Throughout the examination, one must explain what will be done—and why—before it is done. This enables the patient to relax because she is concentrating on what is being said and trying to understand rather than on the discomforts associated with the examination. The examiner must be aware of the patient's responses and maintain a calm, confident, and sympathetic demeanor throughout the examination.

Because most examinations are for annual checkups and because most patients do not otherwise have complete physicals, it is important to perform a complete examination and not just a gynecologic examination. Performing a general physical examination prior to the pelvic examination also gives the patient time to develop confidence in the examiner.

Good lighting is mandatory. The examination room and the instruments used should be warm, and the examination table should be warm and comfortable. The patient should be asked to remove only enough clothing to allow access to areas that require examination, and a comfortable gown and other drapes should be provided. Ideally, a female assistant should be present when the examination is performed. If the examiner is a woman, that may be less important for the patient, but if the patient is emotionally disturbed, chaperoning is mandatory.

General Physical Examination

The patient's height, weight, and vital signs should be recorded. For certain conditions such as endocrinologic problems (see Chapter 20), other examinations and tests must be performed. Body habitus, stature, nutritional state, and the patient's general demeanor should be noted. The skin is inspected and palpated where there are abnormalities, and the findings are recorded.

Head & Neck

The hair, scalp, and skull should be inspected and examined, as should the eyes, ears, nose, mouth, oropharynx, tongue, and thyroid gland. Facial abnormalities should be noted—especially excessive facial hair.

Lymph Nodes

Anterior and posterior cervical, submental, supraclavicular, axillary, epitrochlear (cubital), and inguinal lymph nodes should be examined. There may be evidence of metastatic disease or infection in any of these locations before symptoms appear or the primary lesion becomes noticeable.

Back

The spine and the muscles of the back should be inspected and palpated. Costovertebral angle tenderness will be present with pyelonephritis and other renal diseases (see Chapter 16).

Heart & Lungs

Inspection, auscultation, percussion, and palpation of the anterior and posterior chest should be performed to evaluate function of the cardiorespiratory system. Abnormalities may indicate the need for antibacterial prophylaxis before certain surgical procedures, eg, in women with valvular heart disease, prosthetic valves, congenital heart disease (other than uncomplicated secundum septal defect), mitral valve prolapse with regurgitation, and idiopathic hypertrophic subaortic stenosis. Asthma and other pulmonary conditions require assessment prior to elective surgery as well.

Breasts

Inspection and palpation of the breasts are both important, but palpation much more so. All gynecologic patients should be encouraged to perform breast self-examination at home. Breast inspection is conducted with the patient's arms at the side, over the head, and pressed against her hips with elbows extended laterally. Alterations in contour with dimpling or flattening are sought.

For descriptive purposes, the breast is usually divided into four quadrants (Figure 2–1). Palpation is best performed with the patient supine, allowing breast tissue to distribute over the chest wall. A pillow under the shoulder on the side being examined facilitates nodule or mass detection (Chapter 14). The pads of three or four extended

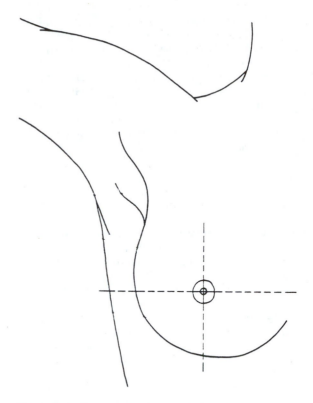

Figure 2–1. For purposes of description, the breast may be divided into four quadrants by horizontal and vertical lines crossing at the nipple. In addition, a tail of breast tissue frequently extends toward or into the axilla. An alternative method of localizing findings visualizes the breast as the face of a clock. A lesion may be located by the "time," eg, 4 o'clock, and by the distance in centimeters from the nipple. (Reproduced, with permission, from Bates B: *A Guide to Physical Examination,* Lippincott, 1974.)

fingers are utilized to gently compress the entire area of breast tissue against the chest wall.

Consistency, induration, masses, and tenderness are noted. It is common for breasts of ovulatory women to become more full and to harbor tender, nodular glandular tissue premenstrually. For that reason, the ideal time to perform the breast examination is about 5–7 days after onset of menses. If masses are present, they should be described by location, using quadrants or clockface systems and other landmarks, such as the nipple, the axilla, or the sternal border. The size of a mass should be recorded in centimeters, and the shape (contour), surface regularity, consistency, mobility with reference to overlying skin and underlying adjacent tissues, and tenderness should be noted, as well as alterations in the overlying skin. Edema or increased venous prominence may indicate underlying tumor.

The nipple and areola should be inspected and palpated—usually with the thumb and index finger, though both index fingers may be used. If nipple discharge is present or can be elicited, that should be noted. Discharge may be clear, white, red, green, black, gray, or yellow. The meanings of each type are discussed in Chapter 14.

The axillae may be examined with the patient supine or sitting. The pectoralis muscles should be relaxed and the arm abducted. The fingers should be bent slightly and inserted as high as is comfortably possible into the axillary apex. The fingers are brought down over the surface of the ribs by compression between the finger pads and chest wall. The anterior and posterior axillary folds should be palpated, as should the area overlying the humerus.

Abdomen

The patient's bladder should be empty. Abdominal examination is performed with the patient supine, arms at her sides, with a pillow under her head. It may be necessary to have the patient place her feet on the table, flexing her knees to further relax the abdominal wall. For descriptive purposes, the abdomen is usually divided into four quadrants (A) and three areas (B) as shown in Figure 2–2. The areas lateral to the umbilical region are called the flanks.

The abdomen should be inspected for masses and surgical scars. Abdominal contour, symmetry, venous pattern, pulsations, peristalsis, and distribution of sexual hair on the abdomen should be noted, as should the presence of stretch marks (**striae**).

Auscultation should be conducted in all quadrants and the epigastrium. The stethoscope should be warmed before use. The frequency and character of bowel sounds should be noted. Sounds may be gurgling, bubbling, or clicking in nature and normally occur at a rate of 5–34 per minute. Loud and prolonged sounds (**borborygmi**) may be normal "growling" or may indicate disease.

Percussion should be performed lightly in all areas to assess for dullness signifying masses (including normal organs) and tympany (gas) in the gastrointestinal tract. Areas of tympany and dullness may shift with body posi-

tion changes if the abdomen contains ascitic fluid. If abdominal discomfort is a complaint and if it can be localized, it is preferable to examine the remainder of the abdomen first, reserving the most tender areas for last. It is important when moving the abdominal wall during the examination to do so slowly and gently, with the pads of the fingertips. Some advocate placing the nonpalpating hand on top of the examining hand so that the passive examining hand can better palpate differences in resistance deep to the abdominal wall. However, with gentleness in examining the abdominal wall, one hand is usually sufficient. Light palpation is always performed initially, using approximated fingertip pads. *Warm* the hands if they are cold! Approach the abdomen slowly, with the examining hand and arm horizontal from the elbow, and tell the patient when the examination is about to commence. The fingers must be moved smoothly and without jabbing. The examiner is searching for areas of increased resistance or tenderness. Abnormalities sought by deep palpation include detection of masses or **organomegaly** (enlarged liver, spleen, kidneys, uterus, ovaries, bowel, or omentum), tenderness, or evidence of peritoneal irritation, whether caused by infection or chemical agents such as blood, bile, or a ruptured ovarian cyst. Gentleness is especially important when examining a patient with peritoneal irritation.

Rebound tenderness is a phenomenon that indicates the presence of abdominal peritonitis. It is elicited by gently depressing the abdominal wall and then suddenly removing pressure. As the abdominal wall bounces up and down, motion of the peritoneum causes excitation of the irritated dendrites, resulting in severe pain. The same information can be elicited by placing one's examining hand palm on the abdomen and gently shaking the abdomen laterally in both directions or superiorly and inferiorly. If peritoneal irritation is significant enough, the patient will reflexly maintain a rigid abdominal wall to prevent move-

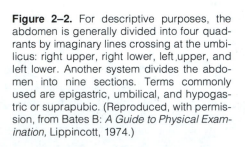

Figure 2–2. For descriptive purposes, the abdomen is generally divided into four quadrants by imaginary lines crossing at the umbilicus: right upper, right lower, left upper, and left lower. Another system divides the abdomen into nine sections. Terms commonly used are epigastric, umbilical, and hypogastric or suprapubic. (Reproduced, with permission, from Bates B: *A Guide to Physical Examination,* Lippincott, 1974.)

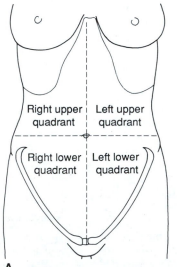

Right upper quadrant | Left upper quadrant
Right lower quadrant | Left lower quadrant

A

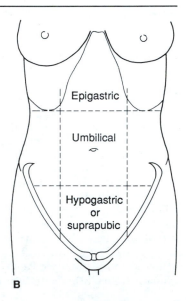

Epigastric

Umbilical

Hypogastric or suprapubic

B

ment of the peritoneum (**involuntary guarding**). Patients may guard voluntarily if they have been hurt during the examination (rebounding). Patients who have had an examination that elicited rebound will do everything in their power to prevent another examiner from reproducing the experience by guarding, or voluntarily holding the abdominal wall as rigid as possible.

Pelvic Examination

Examination of the external and internal genitalia may be difficult for the novice examiner because of its intimate and invasive nature. The experienced examiner should be able to convey a sense of "standard procedure" to the patient, but no patient ever really takes that attitude toward the pelvic examination. Gentle and considerate "good manners" in the preceding parts of the examination will help the patient to have confidence in the examiner and relax sufficiently for the pelvic examination. It is equally important, therefore, that the pelvic examination itself be performed gently, accompanied by explanations of what is being done and why.

The pelvis is examined with the patient in the lithotomy position, with her feet in stirrups and her arms by her sides. This flexes the thighs and allows abduction of the knees. Stirrups should be padded, or the patient may wear her shoes. Stirrups should extend far enough outward from the table so that the patient is not "sitting on her heels." The patient's head should be supported by a pillow, and the buttocks should extend slightly beyond the edge of the examining table. The patient should be appropriately draped. The examiner must have good lighting and warmed equipment.

Distribution of sexual hair should be noted, as should the appearance of the labia majora and minora, clitoris, and perineum. The labia must be moved in order to inspect and palpate these areas for altered pigmentation (red, white, brown, gray, black) or masses. The Bartholin gland areas should be inspected and palpated (Figure 2–3), as should the urethra. Skene's glands are normally situated in the distal inferior urethra. Bartholin glands, the urethra, and Skene's glands are frequently referred to as "**BUS.**"

The vagina and cervix are inspected utilizing metallic or plastic specula available in a variety of sizes and configurations (Figure 2–4). It may be necessary to utilize two specula—the second at right angles to the first—if there is significant vaginal wall relaxation. For speculum placement, the transverse perineal levator muscles must be relaxed. A comfortable way to facilitate relaxation is gentle introduction of a gloved index finger, exerting posterior pressure on the perineal body and levator muscles. It is more acceptable to the patient if the examiner's first touch is on the proximal inner thigh rather than the vulva. One can touch the inner thigh with the back of the examining hand and then roll the hand into contact with the vulva without startling the patient. The speculum, lubricated with warm water, should be introduced at approxi-

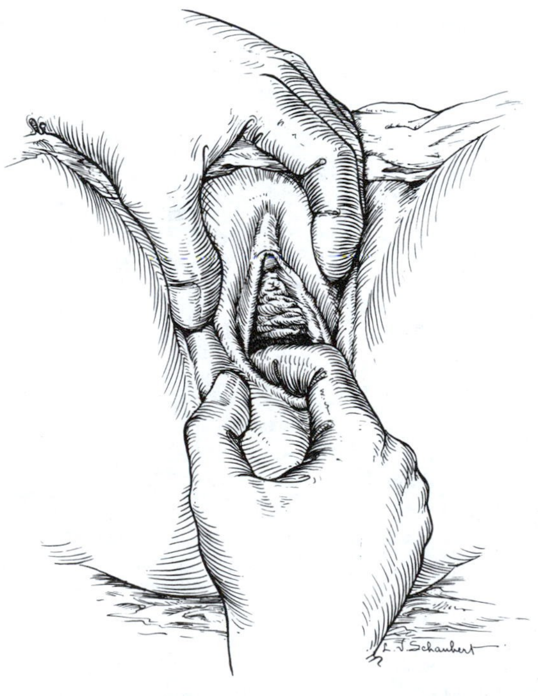

Figure 2–3. Palpation of major vestibular (Bartholin's) glands. (Reproduced, with permission, from Benson RC: *Handbook of Obstetrics & Gynecology,* 8th ed. Lange, 1983.)

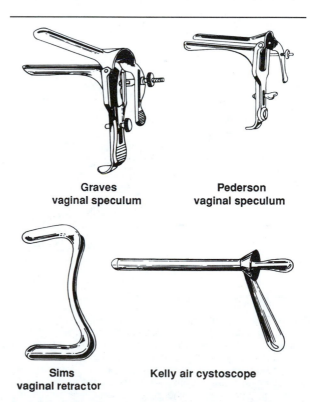

Graves vaginal speculum

Pederson vaginal speculum

Sims vaginal retractor

Kelly air cystoscope

Figure 2–4. Specula. (Reproduced, with permission, from Benson RC: *Handbook of Obstetrics & Gynecology,* 8th ed. Lange, 1987.)

mately a 45-degree angle to the introitus (Figure 2–5) until the leading portion of the speculum has traversed the vagina cephalad to the levator muscles. At this point, the axis of the speculum blades is rotated perpendicularly to the axis of the introitus. The speculum is then further introduced posteroinferiorly (Figure 2–6) and opened prior to complete insertion (Figure 2–7) so that the cervix can be inspected (Figure 2–8). Care must be taken to avoid upward pressure on the urethra.

The location of the cervix usually indicates where the corpus (body, or **fundus**) of the uterus is located except in cases of extreme flexion of the fundus or the cervix. If one sees principally the anterior lip of the cervix, the uterine fundus is probably anterior, and vice versa. If the anterior and posterior lips of the cervix are equally visible, the uterus is "midplane" and projects directly away from the upper end of the vagina.

Once the cervix is visualized, the distal speculum opening can be secured by setting the thumbscrew on the right of the metal speculum, freeing the hands of the examiner to perform maneuvers such as taking culture samples or material for Papanicolaou smears. The speculum should not be opened to its full excursion unless absolutely necessary, since doing so causes extreme discomfort. The proximal speculum opening can also be increased by loosening the thumbscrew in the handle of the instrument and pushing upward on the proximal (upper) blade.

Inspection of the cervix should include noting the color

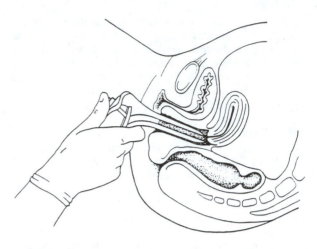

Figure 2–6. Speculum examination of the vagina. After the speculum has entered the vagina, fingers should be removed from the introitus and the blades of the speculum should be rotated into a horizontal position, maintaining the pressure posteriorly. (Reproduced, with permission, from Bates B: *A Guide to Physical Examination.* Lippincott, 1974.)

of the cervix and the characteristics of the opening (**cervical os**). The cervix is normally pink but may be purplish if the woman is pregnant or taking oral contraceptives. If a woman has never been pregnant or has not delivered vaginally, the os is small and round or oval (Figure 2–9). If the woman has delivered vaginally, the os is described as

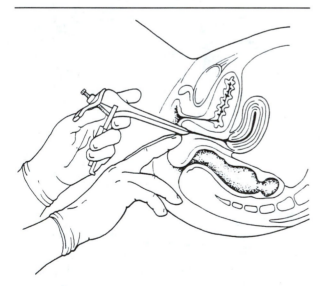

Figure 2–5. Speculum examination of the vagina. Place two fingers just inside or at the introitus and gently press down on the perineal body. With your other hand, introduce the closed speculum past your fingers at a 45-degree angle downward and a 45-degree angle off the horizontal. The blades should be held obliquely and pressure exerted toward the posterior vaginal wall in order to avoid the more sensitive anterior wall and urethra. Be careful not to pull on the pubic hair or to pinch the labia with the speculum. (Reproduced, with permission, from Bates B: *A Guide to Physical Examination. Lippincott,* 1974.)

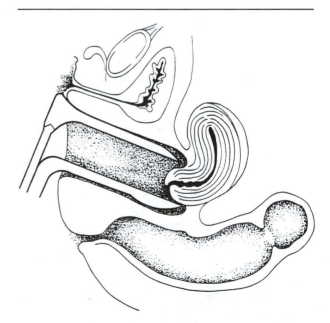

Figure 2–7. Speculum examination of the vagina. The blades should be opened after nearing full insertion and maneuvered so that the cervix comes into full view. (Reproduced, with permission, from Bates B: *A Guide to Physical Examination.* Lippincott, 1974.)

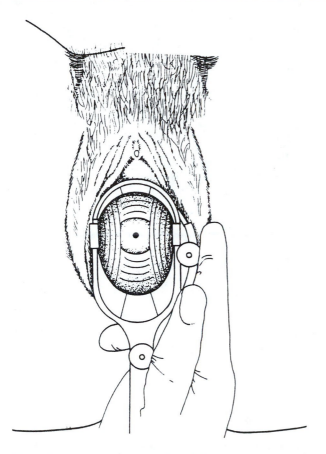

Figure 2–8. Speculum examination of the vagina. Inspect the cervix and its os. Note the color of the cervix and look for ulcerations, nodules, masses, bleeding, or discharge. (Reproduced, with permission, from Bates B: *A Guide to Physical Examination.* Lippincott, 1974.)

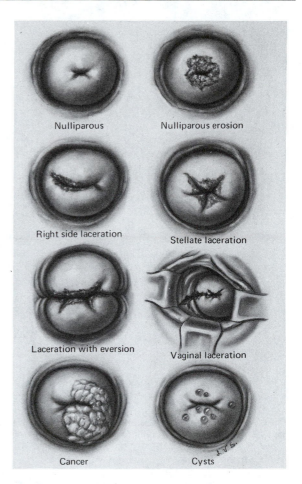

Nulliparous

Nulliparous erosion

Right side laceration

Stellate laceration

Laceration with eversion

Vaginal laceration

Cancer

Cysts

Figure 2–9. The uterine cervix: Normal and pathologic appearance. (Reproduced, with permission, from Bates B: *A Guide to Physical Examination.* Lippincott, 1974.)

parous and appears as a horizontal cleft, and delivery may result in cervical lacerations (Figure 2–9). Prior delivery, pregnancy, and oral contraceptives may result in lateral displacement of the squamocolumnar junction. The central more pink or reddish area is the endocervix, which is surrounded by smooth, light pink squamous epithelium. Any cervical discharge (mucus, pus, blood) should be noted, as should the presence of ulcers, nodules, cysts, or masses.

The tests most commonly started during this part of the examination are cervical cytologic examination, "a wet prep," and culture. Cells for cytologic evaluation should be obtained from the squamocolumnar junction, the endocervix, and the vaginal pool. Most premalignant cellular abnormalities (**dysplasia**) and carcinomas develop at the squamocolumnar junction. A wooden or plastic spatula cytobrush for endocervix is utilized to scrape this junction and then transfer the cells to a glass slide prelabeled with the patient's name and the date (Figure 2–10). The slide is immediately sprayed with fixative or dropped into a container of fixative. A cotton-tipped swab moistened

with saline or a cytobrush is gently inserted into the cervical os until resistance is met. The swab is then rotated first clockwise and then counterclockwise along the course of the endocervical canal. A cytobrush is rotated 90 degrees. The cells then are gently rolled onto another prelabeled glass slide and fixed with appropriate spray or placed in a jar of fixative. Either device may be utilized to obtain cells from the posterior vaginal pool; they are handled identically on a third slide. If no cervix is present, the distal vagina is sampled, as is any area that looks suspicious. In many instances, all cellular material is placed on one slide.

In some settings, endocervical culture to detect *Neisseria gonorrhoeae* is routinely performed in asymptomatic women. This should be done in all women complaining of vaginal discharge or those who may have upper reproductive tract infection. The culture material is obtained with a sterile, dry cotton-tipped applicator from the endocervical canal. The material is immediately inoculated into culture medium. A *Chlamydia trachomatis* specimen should also be obtained, preferably with a small brush, placed on a

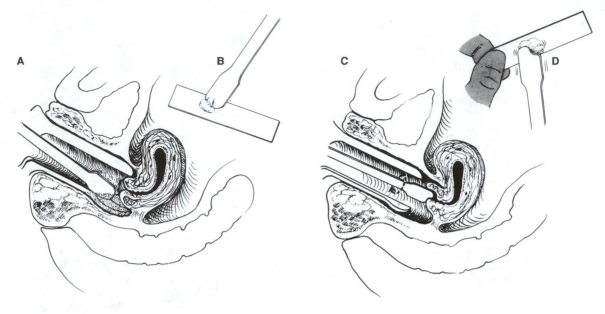

MATERIALS NEEDED

One cervical spatula, cut tongue depressor, or cotton swab.
One glass slide (one end frosted). Identify by writing the patient's name on the frosted end with a lead pencil.

One speculum (without lubricant).
One botttle of fixative (75% ethyl alcohol) or spray-on fixative, eg, Pro-fixx or Aqua-Net.

Figure 2–10. Cells being collected from the posterior fornix and cervix and applied to a glass slide. **A:** Vaginal pool material obtained. **B:** Adequate drop 2.5 cm from end of slide, smeared, fixed, and dried. **C:** Cervical scraping from complete squamocolumnar junction, taken by rotating spatula 360 degrees around external os, high up in the endocervical canal. **D:** The material is placed 1 inch from the end of the slide and then smeared, fixed, and dried. (Reproduced, with permission, from Benson RC: *Handbook of Obstetrics & Gynecology,* 8th ed. Lange, 1987.)

clean, dry slide, and submitted for testing by fluorescent antibody, monoclonal antibody, enzyme immunoassay, or culture if indicated. Women who complain of vaginal discharge should have a sample obtained for examination under a microscope (**wet prep**) to detect bacteria, protozoa, etc (Chapter 6). This sample is obtained with a saline-moistened cotton-tipped applicator from the vaginal pool or sidewall and placed on a slide to which a drop of saline and a coverslip are applied (Figure 2–10). Alternatively, the swab may be placed in a glass vial with 3 mL of saline solution for transport to the pathology laboratory. Another sample should be placed on a separate slide and 10% potassium hydroxide added before the coverslip for detection of yeast forms. Evidence of infection by herpes simplex virus (HSV) can be confirmed by culture or by monoclonal antibody or enzyme immunoassay testing; the sample is obtained with a sterile swab from the base of the suspicious vesicle.

After inspection and testing procedures have been completed, the speculum is gently removed and rotated as it is withdrawn to allow inspection of vaginal mucosa, noting color, inflammation, ulcers, discharge, or masses. It is important that the self-retainer of the speculum should be released prior to withdrawal. This is done by first increasing

the pressure on the opening device with a thumb and controlling the instrument so that vaginal or vulvar tissues are *not pinched* as the speculum blades come together (Figure 2–10).

Bimanual pelvic examination (Figure 2–11) will be very uncomfortable if the patient's bladder is full, so the patient should empty her bladder prior to the pelvic examination. Palpation of the internal genitalia is conducted from a standing position with one or two gloved and lubricated (sterile lubricant) fingers of one hand in the vagina and the other hand on the abdomen. The thumb adjacent to the fingers in the vagina should be abducted, and the ring and little (and perhaps middle) finger should be flexed into the palm. The urethra should be palpated along its entire length; this must be done as gently as if the patient had urethritis. The examiner is interested in knowing the caliber and consistency of the urethra as well as the point at which it disappears into the bladder neck. Support of this area (**the urethrovesical angle**) is very important. Positioning of the proximal urethra and bladder neck in the same pressure plane prevents loss of urine when intra-abdominal pressure is suddenly increased. With loss of pelvic support, this area will move caudad with increased intra-abdominal pressure, perhaps resulting in urine loss

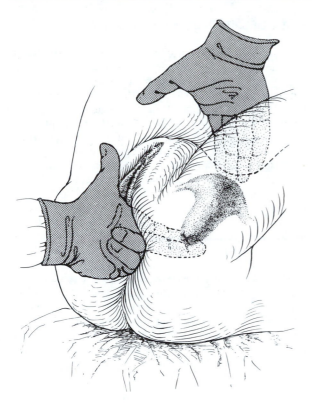

Figure 2–11. Bimanual pelvic examination. (Reproduced, with permission, from Bates B: *A Guide to Physical Examination.* Lippincott, 1974.)

(stress incontinence) due to pressure differences. It is important with each patient to correlate the position of the urethrovesical angle and its movement with increased intra-abdominal pressure (see Chapter 15).

The examiner's fingers are now in the anterior fornix of the vagina. The cervix should be completely palpated in either a clockwise or counterclockwise fashion, noting its consistency, shape, regularity, and the presence of masses, if any. Moving the cervix does not usually cause discomfort, though forceful cervical motion tenderness **(CMT)** can be elicited in any patient. The pelvic structures are then examined with the vaginal fingers in the anterior, both lateral, and posterior forniceal areas while pressure is exerted toward the pelvis, utilizing the abdominal hand as a paddle. Some advocate elevating the pelvic structures into the abdominal cavity and examining them through the abdominal wall. The rationale for this technique is dubious, and the examination is more painful when done in that way. Since the internal genitalia are pelvic organs, it seems reasonable to examine them in their normal location in the pelvis rather than after displacing them into the abdomen. The ovaries are difficult to palpate, and should be essentially impossible to palpate in prepubertal and postmenopausal women as well as in women taking birth control pills.

The position of the uterus should be noted as well as its size, consistency, contour, and mobility. Because three-dimensional assessment of uterine size is difficult to achieve, the size of the organ is often related to weeks of gestation—ie, as "a 6 weeks uterus," or 8 weeks, 10 weeks, or 12 weeks. Unfortunately, because what one examiner estimates as a 6-weeks uterus may be 8 weeks to another, it is better to use centimeter measurements. Each examiner should know the width and length of the index and middle fingers of the hand used for vaginal examinations. With experience, an accurate assessment of measurements in the pelvis can be made in this way.

Rectal examination. If the index and middle finger were inserted into the vagina, a new glove should be put on before examining the rectum to prevent spreading bacteria (*N. gonorrhoeae,* etc). Vaginal examination restricts one to the ability to examine only the anterior pelvis of a nonpregnant or early pregnant woman. The posterior pelvis can be examined through the rectum.

The anal sphincter is a voluntary muscle, but for practical purposes it becomes involuntarily contracted when touched. The examiner should place the lubricated pad of the gloved middle finger of the examining hand in the center of the sphincter and ask the patient to increase her intra-abdominal pressure **(Valsalva's maneuver),** which will do two things: (1) it will relax the anal sphincter, and (2) it will tighten the abdominal wall, making bimanual examination impossible. As the middle finger enters the anus, the index finger is inserted into the vagina. The examiner must now elevate the wrist, since the direction of continued insertion is posteroinferiorly. Once complete insertion has been achieved, the woman is asked to stop exerting pressure. This allows bimanual examination of the posterior pelvis, reexamination of the internal genitalia, and examination of the rectum (Figure 2–12). When palpated through the rectovaginal septum, the cervix has a firm, gritty texture. Thus, the vaginal index finger can identify the cervix; it also allows the examiner to measure pelvic structures.

The rectal examining finger must be withdrawn slowly

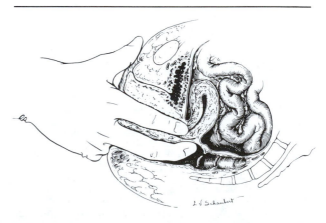

Figure 2–12. Rectovaginal examination. (Reproduced, with permission, from Bates B: *A Guide to Physical Examination.* Lippincott, 1974.)

to allow the patient to contract the sphincter so that fecal spilling does not occur. Reassurance is appropriate at this time.

Rectovaginal (RV) examination. The rectovaginal examination should be done as part of every pelvic examination until the examiner is comfortable with his or her ability to palpate pelvic structures. Thereafter, rectovaginal examination should be done in every woman with pelvic or lower abdominal complaints, in women who have had an abnormal vaginal bimanual examination, and in women 50 years of age or older. Some advocate its performance at every pelvic examination. It may well be more anxiety-producing than a pelvic examination for most women, so individualization is necessary. Testing for occult blood should be done when the examination is performed.

Extremities

Joint size and mobility should be noted. Subcutaneous growths, bony abnormalities, edema, and vascular abnormalities should be sought and recorded.

Neurologic Examination

The patient's gait should be observed at some point during the encounter. Facial nerves and deep tendon reflexes should be tested.

PLAN OF DIAGNOSIS & MANAGEMENT

The history and physical examination are performed so that the practitioner can identify problems or potential problems not only in symptomatic patients with presenting complaints but also in those who are asymptomatic. It may be necessary to await the results of laboratory tests before formulating a diagnosis and management plan. Diagnostic and treatment plans for the most frequent diseases or problems encountered by the gynecologist are presented in the chapters that follow. Each medical record should have in a prominent place a sheet listing in chronologic order the date of onset of any problem, the type of problem, and the date of resolution of each problem identified. Surgical procedures, medications, allergies, chronic medications, and Papanicolaou test results should also be included so that the practitioner can review that information at a glance.

The gynecologist must educate the patient regarding the frequency of pelvic examinations and Papanicolaou smears, when and how to do breast self-examinations, at what age routine annual mammography and estrogen replacement should be started, etc. If the patient has confidence in her physician, she will actively seek information about other health-related topics.

3

Benign Diseases of the Uterus

The uterus has an abdominal component, the corpus (fundus), and a vaginal component, the cervix. The uterus and the upper third of the vagina are derived from müllerian ducts. Benign diseases of the uterus are those most frequently diagnosed and treated by the gynecologist. Some diseases or abnormalities will be discussed elsewhere even though uterine tissue types are involved. Examples are adenomyosis and endometriosis (Chapter 23), endometritis (Chapter 8), and cervical cancer (Chapter 29).

LEIOMYOMA

Leiomyoma (myoma, fibroid, fibromyoma) is of smooth muscle origin and is the most common tumor of the female reproductive tract. The cause is not known. Heredity does not appear to play a role, though the tumors are up to ten times more common in black women. There is evidence that each tumor may be unicellular in origin.

The common terms "fibroid" and "fibromyoma" are not strictly accurate because the predominant element at histologic examination is a spindle-shaped smooth muscle cell with an elongated nucleus. Bundles of such cells are seen running in all directions, but there is a tendency to form a whorl-like pattern. The cells are uniform in size and shape if observed in the same plane. Mitoses are usually not found.

Grossly, leiomyomas are firm, rubbery white tumors with a characteristic whorled or trabeculated appearance on cross section. They have a pseudocapsule but not a true capsule, and this thin areolar tissue plane does permit surgical enucleation of the tumor from the uterine wall (myomectomy).

Autopsy studies show that about 20% of women over age 30 harbor uterine leiomyomas of varying sizes. Uterine leiomyomas are not usually detectable before puberty and grow only during the reproductive years, usually regressing in size after the menopause. They vary in size from microscopic growths (seedlings) to tumors weighing

more than 100 lb. Although leiomyomas can occur singly, they most often exist as multiple growths.

Under the hormonal stimulation of pregnancy, leiomyomas may enlarge and become softened and difficult to distinguish by palpation from surrounding normal uterine tissue. Tumor size usually diminishes after pregnancy.

Uterine leiomyomas may cause nausea and vomiting (due to intestinal obstruction), abdominal or pelvic heaviness, increased vaginal discharge, dysmenorrhea, abnormal uterine bleeding, urinary incontinence, frequent urination, inability to urinate, constipation, fatigue (due to anemia), dyspareunia, mucorrhea, mass, and pain.

Classification & Clinical Findings

Up to two-thirds of women with uterine leiomyomas have no symptoms. Some otherwise asymptomatic women may notice an abdominal mass, and some may believe they are pregnant—even without missing periods— if the mass is large enough.

Leiomyomas are classified according to their location in the uterine wall as subserous, intraligamentous, intramural, submucosal, or cervical (Figure 3–1).

A. Subserous Leiomyomas: Tumors arising from just under the peritoneal surface (serosa) of the uterus exist as small to large masses or knobby excrescences as they project from the uterine surface. They may develop distinct pedicles. Subserosal tumors may gain additional blood supply from omentum that has become adherent to the surface of the peritoneal uterus. When this occurs, the tumor gives a false appearance of arising primarily from omentum. These may become parasitic tumors, going where their blood supply leads them.

B. Intraligamentous Leiomyomas: Lateral growth may extend between the leaves of the broad ligament, or these tumors may actually arise in the broad ligament without uterine attachment.

C. Intramural Leiomyomas: Tumors within the wall of the uterus are referred to as intramural or interstitial tumors. If small, they may cause no change in uterine contour. As they enlarge, however, the uterus takes on a nodular, asymmetric shape. If these tumors become very

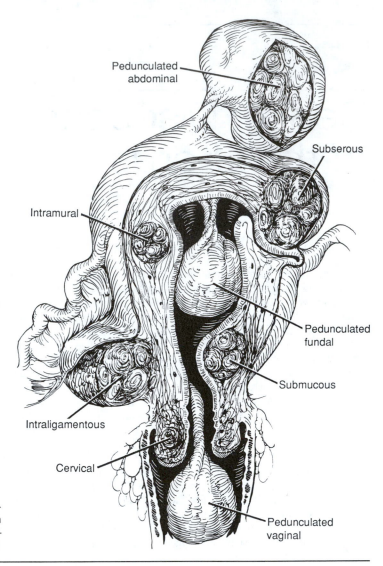

Figure 3–1. Locations of uterine leiomyomas. (Reproduced, with permission, from Pernoll ML, Benson RC (editors): *Current Obstetric & Gynecologic Diagnosis & Treatment,* 7th ed. Appleton & Lange, 1991.)

large, they will become—or will appear to be—both subserous and submucosal, ie, lying directly under the serosal peritoneum and the endometrium, respectively.

D. Submucosal Leiomyomas: Subserous or intramural uterine leiomyomas, even though they may attain significant size, may not cause symptoms. Submucosal leiomyoma is the least common type but the most important clinically because it most often causes symptoms. Excessive bleeding as a result of endometrial distortion associated with an enlarged uterus is one of the most frequent indications for hysterectomy in the United States. A submucosal tumor, however, even if small, is often associated with abnormal uterine bleeding, caused either by impingement on or compression of the blood vessels supplying the overlying endometrium or by contact with adjacent endometrium. Occasionally, submucosal tumors can develop a long stalk and can be delivered through the cervix. Associated symptomatology, though protracted over a long period of time, is that of labor, namely, uterine contrac-

tions causing lower abdominal or pelvic cramping, usually associated with hypermenorrhea. As these tumors project through the cervix, they not uncommonly become superficially ulcerated or infected, which also causes bleeding.

The overlying mucosa is thin and ulcerated, with histologic evidence of acute and chronic inflammatory responses. Upon inspection, the tumors may be confused with carcinoma of the cervix, and vice versa. If there is concern regarding possible cancer, biopsy should be performed prior to attempts at removal. Because these tumors prolapse from the endometrial cavity through the cervix, ascending infection in the uterus and upper tract may occur. In this case, pelvic infection is much more important than infection that may develop superficially in the leiomyoma or pseudocapsule. Parenteral antimicrobial therapy may be necessary if oral antibiotic therapy is not effective, and the tumor must be removed to prevent recurrences.

E. Cervical Leiomyomas: Cervical leiomyomas

occur most often in the posterior aspect and are usually asymptomatic. Anterior cervical leiomyomas frequently cause symptoms early because of bladder compression. The symptom most frequently reported is polyuria, and some women complain of stress incontinence. Urinary retention may result if tumors become very large.

Although the least common type of tumor, large cervical leiomyomas cause the greatest technical difficulties for the surgeon because of anatomic alterations and space restrictions. They may grow to such size that they become impacted in the pelvis, making it impossible to inspect or even palpate the cervix. This not only creates technical difficulties in removing the tumor but may also cause damage to adjacent organs such as the colon, ureters, or bladder.

When cervical tumors are lateral, ureteral displacement is the rule. The direction of displacement depends on the relationship of tumor origin to the uterine artery. The ureter passes under the uterine artery as the artery enters the uterus. When this occurs, not only uterine vessels but the ureters also can be displaced. It is extremely important that the ureters be identified at operation prior to removing any tissue, since a large lateral cervical myoma, for instance, can displace the ureter anterosuperiorly to as high as the level of the round ligaments.

Cervical leiomyomas may cause excessive mucus production and vaginal discharge (mucorrhea), dysmenorrhea due to obstruction of the normal diameter of the endocervical canal, dyspareunia because of the mass effect, and infertility.

F. Rare Types of Leiomyoma: There is a very rare condition associated with **intravenous extension** of benign leiomyoma into the pelvic veins. This intravenous leiomyomatosis is described as a benign but metastasizing lesion, since tumors are found in the lungs and other locations. Myomatous implants also can occur throughout the omentum and peritoneum to cause **leiomyomatosis peritonealis disseminata.** Patients with these very rare conditions have done well clinically when the uterus and its leiomyomas were removed along with the uterine tubes and ovaries. Hormone replacement is necessary.

Degenerative Changes

Under varying influences, leiomyomas can undergo five types of degenerative change: hyaline, cystic, calcareous, carneous, and myxomatous. Malignant change is rare, occurring in only 0.1–0.5% of cases (Chapter 30).

A. Hyaline Degeneration: The most frequently observed change is hyaline degeneration, which may occur as scattered patches or as interlacing fields that can be observed both grossly and microscopically throughout the large tumors. Hyaline degeneration can be identified grossly on cross section by loss of the whorl-like appearance as the tumor takes on a more homogeneous appearance. Such degeneration results in a tumor that is yellowish and softer than the normal myoma; on occasion, it may even become gelatinous.

B. Cystic Degeneration: The natural consequence of hyalinization and loss of vascular supply is liquefaction, which results in cystic degeneration. If this occurs in a large myoma that interferes with palpation of the normal uterus, the impression may be that of intrauterine pregnancy because of the softer consistency of the tumor.

C. Calcareous Degeneration: Calcification is observed most frequently in asymptomatic leiomyomas in the uteri of postmenopausal women. Either calcium carbonate or calcium phosphate may be deposited, and the calcified areas may be small and scattered or may form concentric rings. They are usually discovered in the course of radiographic studies of the abdomen and pelvis undertaken for unrelated reasons.

D. Carneous Degeneration: Necrosis may occur in all varieties of leiomyomas when the blood supply to the tumor has been compromised. Pedunculated subserous tumors may twist on their pedicle, resulting in necrosis and even sloughing from the uterus. Necrosis is more common centrally, but it can be observed at any location throughout a myoma. These areas are recognizable grossly when the normal white trabeculated whorl-like pattern is absent and has been replaced by a grayish-yellow, soft degenerated area. A predecessor to this—and a phenomenon seen frequently in pregnancy and associated with infarction, is carneous (red) degeneration; this striking appearance is caused by congestion and interstitial hemorrhage.

During pregnancy, carneous degeneration often is associated with a low-grade temperature elevation and mild leukocytosis. When this occurs acutely, the common complaint is pelvic pain, and the tumors usually are tender. This condition may be confused with placental abruption (Chapter 58), but pain in that case is usually more diffuse and commonly associated with vaginal bleeding. Chorioamnionitis is another possible diagnosis that might be suggested by fever and leukocytosis. Tenderness associated with this condition, however, is more diffuse, and fetal tachycardia is often present.

E. Myxomatous Degeneration: Myxomatous or fatty degeneration is a rare type undoubtedly related to late changes of hyaline degeneration or even necrosis, though metaplasia might be responsible.

Diagnosis & Differential Diagnosis

Only about 35% of leiomyomas cause symptoms, and most are undetected or are identified only at routine pelvic or abdominal examination because the uterus is enlarged. Since this condition affects women in their reproductive years, pregnancy should be ruled out even if the uterus is irregular in contour and firm. Tumors are occasionally diagnosed in women undergoing radiographic evaluation of the abdomen for unrelated reasons. Sonography or other specialized procedures such as CT scan or MRI may be useful in differentiating them from ovarian or colonic tumors. Small submucosal tumors may be diagnosed by hysterosalpingography (in the course of investigation of infertility) or by hysteroscopy (as part of the investigation of abnormal uterine bleeding). Hysterosalpingography is a radiologic study in which a radiopaque dye is injected through the cervix into the uterine cavity to outline the endometrial cavity, establish patency of the uterine tubes, and detect pelvic adhesions. Hysteroscopy is a surgical procedure in which a small scope is used to achieve direct visualization of the endometrial cavity (Chapter 17).

Complications

The incidence of spontaneous miscarriage is probably increased severalfold in women with detectable leiomyomas, and vaginal delivery may be prevented by large tumors because of uterine inertia, fetal malposition, or an obstructed birth canal. Placental abruption may occur as a result of large tumors, and postpartum hemorrhage may occur as a result of ineffective uterine contraction.

Large tumors may mask the presence of other significant disease in the ovaries or bowel and in pregnant women may cause discrepancies between uterine size and gestational age.

Treatment

The mere presence of one or more leiomyomas does not mandate therapy. With the advent of newer technology such as ultrasonography and computerized tomography (CT), and in an otherwise asymptomatic woman, an aggressive surgical approach may no longer be necessary. The presence of the leiomyoma does not necessarily affect endometrial histology. Because of diminution of blood supply to the endometrium, however, it is possible that the endometrium may be relatively atrophic and may have the histologic picture of chronic endometritis with lymphocytes and plasma cells. This likely is the consequence of a reduced blood supply (ischemia) rather than a primary infection. Decisions must be individualized depending upon the nature and severity of symptoms and the size and location of the leiomyomas, as well as age, parity, general health, and most importantly, desire for future pregnancy.

A. Surgical Treatment: If tumors cause uterine enlargement to above the level of the umbilicus (more than 20 weeks' gestational age), partial ureteral obstruction can occur, calling for treatment either by myomectomy or, preferably, hysterectomy. Small submucous tumors may be removed by hysteroscopy or dilatation and curettage (D&C). Tumors causing infertility—or large tumors in women who wish to preserve reproductive function—can sometimes be removed at laparotomy or laparoscopically without the need for entering the endometrial cavity. Any such uterine incision is at risk for dehiscence during subsequent pregnancy and labor.

If it is impossible to remove the tumors individually—and if they are causing significant symptoms—hysterectomy may be necessary.

B. Medical Treatment: Symptomatic women who are not good surgical candidates may be treated with gonadotropin-releasing hormone (GnRH) analogues or agonists. These drugs cause suppression of ovarian hormone secretion and regression of tumor size. Such treatment must be intermittent because prolonged therapy results in significant bone loss and may cause osteoporosis.

LYMPHANGIOMA & HEMANGIOMA

Lymphangiomas and hemangiomas are rare benign tumors not related to leiomyomas—usually incidental histologic findings reported by the pathologist. If symptomatic, they usually cause problems through mass effects.

MYOMETRIAL HYPERTROPHY

Myometrial hypertrophy is an ill-defined condition of unknown origin characterized by symmetric enlargement of the uterine walls without leiomyomas, hemangiomas, etc. Women with this condition frequently have hypermenorrhea, and a D&C or hysterectomy for leiomyomatosis may be performed for symptomatic treatment. The uterine weight is usually in the neighborhood of 120–200 g, and the uterus is at least twice normal size.

ENDOMETRIAL POLYPS

Benign endometrial abnormalities other than hyperplasia (Chapter 30) are much less common than those involving the myometrium—if one excludes endometritis. The next most common nonmalignant endometrial disease consists of a group of lesions described as polyps (Figure 3–2). The genesis of these structures is not known. In fact, a polyp is more of an architectural than a histologic diagnosis, because the growth is merely an extension or projection of tissue attached by a pedicle, or stem, to the organ

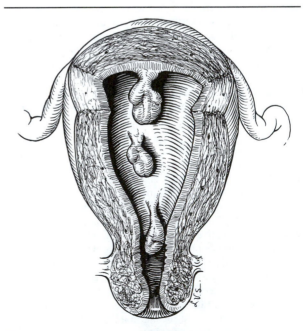

Figure 3–2. Endometrial polyps. (Reproduced, with permission, from Pernoll ML, Benson RC (editors): *Current Obstetric & Gynecologic Diagnosis & Treatment,* 7th ed. Appleton & Lange, 1991.)

of origin. Histologically, endometrial polyps have a central stromal element and blood supply with endometrium peripherally. The pedicle may be short and thick (sessile), or it may be thin and long enough so that the polyp protrudes through the cervical os (Figure 3–3), similar to a prolapsing pedunculated subserous leiomyoma. Polyps may be spheroidal or cylindric and single or multiple. Smaller polyps usually are unassociated with bleeding or other symptoms, whereas larger polyps cause abnormal bleeding by mass effect and pressure on adjacent endometrium or by outgrowing their blood supply, resulting in ulceration, degeneration, and bleeding (Figure 3–3). The tissue in these polyps may respond to hormonal stimulus, as does the normal endometrium. Furthermore, the endometrial component of some polyps may respond to estrogen only, with resultant hyperplasia—in contrast with surrounding normal endometrium. Polyps that do not respond normally to hormonal production are those frequently associated with bleeding at abnormal times during the menstrual cycle (intermenstrual bleeding), similar to anovulating menses. The symptoms and signs of ovulation are always present when ovulation occurs and do not disappear with the occurrence of polyps or leiomyomas. This bit of clinical history is important because in anovulatory women with abnormal uterine bleeding, organic disease must be considered as the cause of bleeding. Hormonal therapy is not indicated and will not correct the problem.

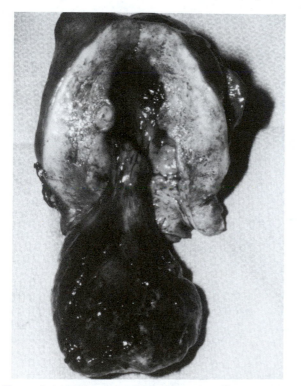

Figure 3–3. Large, partially infarcted endometrial polyp prolapsed through the cervical os. (Reproduced, with permission, from Pernoll ML, Benson RC (editors): *Current Obstetric & Gynecologic Diagnosis & Treatment,* 7th ed. Appleton & Lange, 1991.)

Surgical therapy is indicated and required to correct symptomatology.

CERVICAL ABNORMALITIES

The histologic condition most frequently encountered in the cervix is "chronic cervicitis." It is present in essentially every cervical biopsy and for that reason should probably be considered a normal finding. No treatment is required.

Cervical Erosion
Any process that results in destruction of the stratified squamous epithelium of the ectocervix is called cervical erosion, appearing as a usually painless, beefy-red, obviously inflammatory lesion. Bacteria have been cultured from the site. Mucopurulent vaginal discharge is often a presenting complaint, along with vaginal spotting or staining, especially after intercourse.

Antimicrobial therapy (Chapter 6) usually will reverse the symptoms. Biopsy should be performed to exclude carcinoma.

Cervical Ectropion
Endocervical tissue may appear to be swollen and congested and to "roll out" of the endocervical canal. Childbirth, pregnancy, and oral contraceptives all enhance this phenomenon, which requires no treatment.

Squamous Metaplasia & Nabothian Cyst Formation
A normal event occurring in all cervices is that of epidermization—a physiologic phenomenon in which stratified squamous epithelium replaces and "overgrows" the glandular columnar endocervical epithelium. Squamous metaplasia can be diagnosed with a special microscope called a colposcope; confirmation by biopsy is not necessary.

It is this process that covers the gland openings and results in retention (nabothian) cyst formation. One or many nabothian cysts are usually visible on the ectocervix of women during the reproductive years. They may vary in size from 1 mm to 6 cm and are filled with mucoid secretions of endocervical glands. Although the cysts may grossly appear to be clear, bluish, reddish, yellow, or white; when punctured, they usually yield a clear, viscous mucoid secretion. There is frequently increased vasculature over the cysts, sometimes raising a concern about cervical cancer. Treatment usually is not required.

Leukoplakia
As squamous metaplasia occurs, the redder endocervical tissue may appear to have white patches. Any white patch that is visible to the naked eye without application of any material such as acetic acid represents leukoplakia and may or may not be a sign of significant disease.

As will be elucidated in Chapter 29, any abnormal-appearing cervix deserves evaluation not only with a Papanicolaou smear but also with colposcopic examination and perhaps cervical biopsy. Any area of leukoplakia must be investigated by colposcopically directed cervical biopsy.

Leukoplakia must be differentiated from condylomata acuminata (venereal warts) and cervical intraepithelial neoplasia (CIN), a potentially premalignant disease discussed in Chapter 29.

Cervical Polyposis

Proliferation of endocervical tissue can result in polyp formation. The primary complaint associated with cervical polyps is intermenstrual and postcoital bleeding. Interestingly, this type of polyp formation is promoted by oral contraceptives and pregnancy. These lesions are generally small, though rarely they may reach a diameter of 1–2 cm. Pedicles are usually small, so that polyps can be easily removed in the clinic by snipping or twisting. The lesions should be examined histologically, as should any tissue removed from a patient. It is of paramount importance that the container with a biopsy specimen have a patient identifying sticker and source of specimen attached; it is also mandatory that the specimen be accompanied by an accurately completed request for histologic examination. The more historical and clinical information provided to the pathologist, the more likely the diagnosis is to be correct. Adding the patient's phone number to the slip and transposition of that number to the final typed pathology report will facilitate patient contact.

Other Cervical Disorders

Other rare conditions that may develop in the cervix include mesonephric cysts (Chapter 5), endometriosis (Chapter 23), pregnancy (Chapter 8), and metastatic gestational trophoblastic disease (Chapter 32). Infections are discussed separately in Chapter 6.

SUGGESTED READINGS

Horbst AL et al: *Comprehensive Gynecology.* Mosby, 1992.

Konrad P, Mellblom L: Intravenous leiomyomatosis. Acta Obstet Gynecol Scand 1989;68(4):371.

Kurman RJ: *Blaustein's Pathology of the Female Genital Tract,* 3rd ed. Springer, 1987.

McCarthy S: Gynecologic applications of MRI. Crit Rev Diagn Imaging 1990;31(2):263.

4

Benign Tumors of the Ovaries & Fallopian Tubes

Tumors of the ovaries are important gynecologic problems in all age groups. Careful follow-up is essential to rule out persistent mass which may be due to neoplastic disease. Fallopian tube tumors are rare and frequently asymptomatic.

BENIGN TUMORS OF THE OVARY

The ovary is the most likely site of a pelvic mass, and enlargement may be due to a physiologic cyst or ovarian neoplasm. Physiologic cysts tend to vary in size with the menstrual cycle and often are manifested by recognizable symptoms, such as alterations in menstrual patterns or by lower abdominal pain. Neoplasms produce few symptoms initially but persist or, more often, increase in size. Ovarian neoplasms may be benign or malignant and are either cystic or solid or a combination of both types. The diagnosis and management of malignant ovarian tumors are discussed in Chapter 31.

Management of an adnexal mass is a challenging task for the gynecologist. A functional cyst is best managed conservatively, whereas a benign ovarian tumor frequently requires operative treatment. The differential diagnosis of an adnexal mass varies with the patient's age. Table 4–1 lists the tumors most commonly seen in women of prepubertal, reproductive, and menopausal years.

Table 4–1. Ovarian tumor origin and incidence of malignancy grouped by reproductive age.

Prepubertal	Reproductive	Menopausal
Germ cell 80%	Functional 70%	Malignant 50%
Malignant 10%	Endometrioma 10% Neoplastic 20% Benign 85% Malignant 15%	

Nonneoplastic lesions of the ovary are briefly reviewed in the following sections.

FUNCTIONAL OVARIAN CYSTS

Follicular Cysts

Follicles become cystic in response to gonadotropic hormone stimulation. If ovulation does not occur, the follicle usually becomes atretic. In cases of persistent anovulation, there may be numerous cystic follicles. If ovarian follicular development occurs yet the follicle fails to rupture at ovulation, a follicular cyst forms.

These cysts are common and may vary in size. If the lesion is more than 2 cm in diameter, it is generally considered to be a follicular cyst; if less than 2 cm, it is considered to be a cystic follicle. Rarely are these cysts larger than 6–8 cm in size. One or more granulosa cell layers and a fairly prominent theca interna and externa are common histologic findings. The lesions are unilocular and can be hemorrhagic. Most resolve spontaneously and remain undetected. Hemorrhagic cyst's occasionally presents with hemoperitoneum and may require surgical exploration.

Corpus Luteum Cysts

Corpus luteum cysts usually arise if regression of a corpus luteum does not occur after the luteal phase. There may be central hemorrhage, which causes rupture of the cyst and occasional hemoperitoneum. Corpus luteum cysts are lined by a luteinized granulosa and theca layer. The typical gross appearance is of a corrugated bright yellow border, often with central hemorrhage or a cavity containing fibrin. A persistent corpus luteum cyst may be associated with a delay in menstruation followed by vaginal spotting and lower abdominal pain similar to the clinical findings of ectopic pregnancy. Lutein cysts are commonly larger than follicular cysts and may be firm to palpation and appear solid by ultrasound examination.

If pregnancy occurs and trophoblastic hCG (human chorionic gonadotropin) production ensues, the corpus luteum becomes a corpus luteum of pregnancy, and progesterone secretion is continued. If pregnancy does not occur, the corpus luteum normally regresses and forms the corpus albicans.

Functional cysts of corpus luteum or follicular origin typically undergo spontaneous regression. Cysts in a patient in her reproductive years should be followed closely for 2 months. Those that do not regress during the observation period should be evaluated by sonography and by laparoscopy or laparotomy. Because functional cysts are extremely rare in patients taking oral contraceptive pills, cysts in women using the pill or in prepubertal girls or postmenopausal women should be evaluated by sonography and usually by surgical exploration of the pelvis via laparoscopy or laparotomy.

Polycystic Ovaries

Polycystic ovaries are usually slightly enlarged, bilateral, and show a mixture of small follicular cysts and cystic follicles without evidence of ovulation. The surface may become thickened and take on a pearly-white appearance. In addition to the cystic follicles, both follicular and stromal hyperthecosis are present. Follicular hyperthecosis occurs when there is luteinization of the theca interna of the cystic follicles. Stromal hyperthecosis consists of isolated islands and nests of luteinized theca cells within the stroma of the ovary (Figure 4–1). The hyperthecotic areas secrete androstenedione and testosterone, and these patients frequently have hirsutism, anovulation, and oligomenorrhea (see Chapters 21 and 22).

Theca-Lutein Cyst, Hyperreactio Luteinalis, Luteoma

Theca lutein cysts, hyperreactio luteinalis, and luteoma are functional tumors of the ovary occurring in association with pregnancy and elevated levels of (or sensitivity to) hCG. Theca-lutein cysts may develop in patients with hydatidiform mole or choriocarcinoma (see Chapter 32) or in response to ovulation induction with menotropins (Pergonal) and hCG. Theca lutein cysts are dominated by the theca interna, with marked luteinization of the multiple follicles. Trophoblastic disease can cause massive bilateral theca-lutein cysts.

Hyperreactio luteinalis may occur in pregnancy, and the luteinized theca is the source of massive production of androstenedione. The presenting symptom in these patients may be the onset of virilization during pregnancy. Female fetuses, however, usually are protected from androgen excess by the aromatization of androgens to estrogens within the placenta. This condition regresses after pregnancy but may recur in subsequent pregnancies.

Pregnancy luteomas are usually solid and bilateral, with a typical dull tan appearance (Figure 4–2). There are multifocal and nodular coalescing masses of luteinized cells. The exact cause is unknown, but the lesions may represent exaggerated luteinization of preexisting stromal hyperthecosis. Stromal hyperthecosis has been demonstrated in some areas of the surrounding ovarian parenchyma. Some of these patients and their fetuses may be virilized as a result of production of certain androgens that are not substrates for placental aromatase.

These benign tumors regress after delivery.

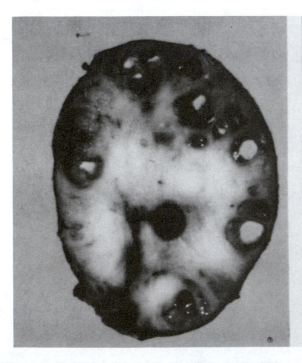 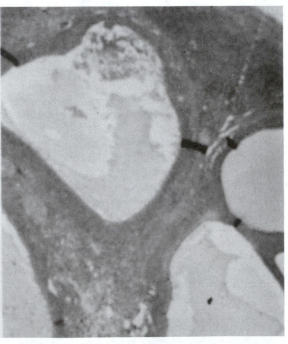

Figure 4–1. **A:** Gross specimen of polycystic ovary with thickened capsule and cystic follicles. **B:** Photomicrograph showing follicular and stromal hyperthecosis and cystic follicles. (Courtesy of J Sandstad.)

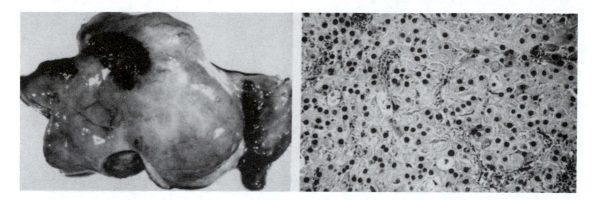

Figure 4–2. *A:* Ovary with large luteoma. *B:* Photomicrograph showing luteinized cell masses. (Courtesy of J Sandstad.)

NEOPLASTIC OVARIAN TUMORS

Ovarian neoplasms may arise from ovarian surface epithelium, from stromal components, or from germ cells. The single most common ovarian neoplasm is the dermoid tumor, arising from ovarian germ cells; but as a group, tumors arising from surface epithelium are even more common.

1. OVARIAN TUMORS OF SURFACE EPITHELIAL CELL ORIGIN

Epithelial tumors comprise about 80% of all ovarian neoplasms. They are presumed to arise from the surface epithelium of the ovary, which is derived from the same coelomic lining that gives rise to the müllerian ducts. Therefore, tumors that arise from the surface epithelium differentiate into cell types similar to those of müllerian origin, such as serous, mucinous, endometrioid, and Brenner tumors. Epithelial tumors should be classified according to the best-differentiated area and graded according to the least-differentiated area if more than 5% of the tumor is found to be of lesser differentiation.

Serous Tumors

Serous ovarian tumors are lined by ciliated epithelium resembling that of the uterine tube. Approximately 70% of serous tumors are benign, 10% are borderline malignant, and 20% are invasive carcinomas. Benign lesions are typically smooth and unilocular and contain a clear yellow liquid. Occasionally, internal or external papillary excrescences may be present, but these are usually minimal. One of the hallmarks of papillary serous tumors is the formation of psammoma bodies. Psammoma bodies are characteristically found in papillary serous tumors; however, they may also be found with borderline and malignant serous tumors. Benign serous tumors are bilateral in approximately 10% of patients. Borderline serous tumors are bilateral in approximately 25% of cases, and serous cystadenocarcinoma is bilateral in approximately two-thirds of cases.

Most serous tumors are asymptomatic and are found incidentally during routine pelvic examination. Occasional symptoms of "pelvic fullness" or abdominal distention occur in patients with very large tumors.

These tumors are best removed by a midline abdominal incision in order to allow for complete exploration of the pelvis and entire abdomen. Any solid or papillary areas identified in the cyst must be examined by frozen section technique to identify foci of malignancy.

Mucinous Tumors

Mucinous tumors are lined by columnar mucinous epithelium resembling that of the endocervix (Figure 4–3) and can grow to enormous size. The epithelial lining may resemble that of the intestine and may contain goblet cells. Mucinous neoplasms are usually multiloculated, and benign ones are bilateral in less than 5% of cases. Fortunately, over 85% of all mucinous tumors are benign. Rarely, a condition known as pseudomyxoma peritonei coexists with a mucinous tumor. In such cases, mucin spreads throughout the abdominal cavity. While this is not a malignant change, there are long-term complications with recurrence of abdominal mucin (mucinous ascites). Some authors suggest liquefying the mucin with 10% dextrose in water prior to evacuating the mucinous fluid from the abdomen.

Treatment is surgical. Conservative surgery is possible in young women with reproductive potential in whom benign lesions are found, but preferred therapy consists of total abdominal hysterectomy, bilateral salpingo-oophorectomy, and careful abdominal inspection (see Chapter 31).

Endometrioid Tumors

Endometrioid ovarian tumors have a high propensity for malignancy (endometrioid carcinoma). Benign endometrioid tumors of the ovary are most often endometriomas (Chapter 23) and are not surface epithelial tumors in the strictest sense. Endometriosis is not considered a premalignant forerunner of this ovarian tumor.

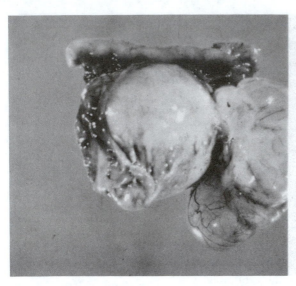 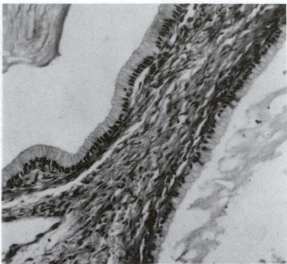

Figure 4–3. *A:* Fallopian tube and ovary containing mucinous cystadenoma. *B:* Columnar mucinous epithelium in mucinous cystadenoma. (Courtesy of J Sandstad.)

Brenner Tumors

Brenner tumors of the ovary consist of nests of transitional-like epithelium, usually with a central core of mucinous cells. These tumor cells have an appearance similar to that of transitional epithelium of the urinary bladder. Malignant Brenner tumors occur but very rarely. Most Brenner tumors are incidental findings and have the gross appearance of a white fibrous tumor similar to a fibroma. Ascites or Meigs' syndrome (ascites and right hydrothorax) may be associated with a Brenner tumor, and the patient may present with complaints of abdominal or pelvic fullness.

2. OVARIAN TUMORS OF STROMAL CELL ORIGIN (Gonadal Stromal Tumors)

Neoplasms arising from ovarian stroma may be endocrinologically active. Androstenedione, estrone, and estradiol all are produced by stromal cells; therefore, these tumors may be masculinizing or feminizing. Differentiation may be along ovarian cell lines (eg, granulosa-theca cell tumors) or along testicular lines (eg, Sertoli-Leydig cell tumors).

Granulosa Cell Tumors

These tumors often are feminizing and may cause precocious pseudopuberty (see Chapter 13) in children and postmenopausal bleeding with endometrial hyperplasia or carcinoma in postmenopausal patients. Cells have morphologic features of granulosa cells and form typical Call-Exner bodies, characterized by pseudorosettes around a central hyalinized area thought to be the residue of nuclear degeneration (Figure 4–4).

Ovarian stroma can contain luteinized theca cells that may lead to development of a granulosa-theca cell tumor. It is possible that many granulosa-theca cell tumors are granulosa cell tumors with a secondarily induced luteinized stroma. One of the characteristic histologic features is the coffee bean-type nuclear groove. Granulosa cell tumors are considered to be of low malignant potential and can persist or recur.

Treatment is by surgical removal. Since these tumors are bilateral in only 5% of cases, unilateral salpingo-oophorectomy is usual therapy in young patients. Total abdominal hysterectomy and bilateral salpingo-oophorectomy is done for bilateral disease or in older women.

Fibrothecoma

Fibrothecomas constitute another category of gonadal stromal tumors. At one end of the spectrum are pure fibromas not associated with abnormal steroid production. Pure fibromas are usually found in elderly patients. The tumors have a firm, smooth, white, whorled appearance, and they can become quite large and undergo central cystic degeneration. Fibroma has been described as occasionally causing ascites and Meigs' syndrome.

At the opposite end of the spectrum is the thecoma, which contains lipid-rich luteinized theca cells and is usually estrogenic in function. Most such tumors contain some component of both fibroma and thecoma; therefore, the term fibrothecoma is applied to the large number of tumors in this category. These tumors are almost invariably benign, with only rare reports of malignant cases.

Sertoli-Leydig Cell Tumors

These tumors differentiate toward a testicular cell line and often have virilizing effects such as hirsutism, bald-

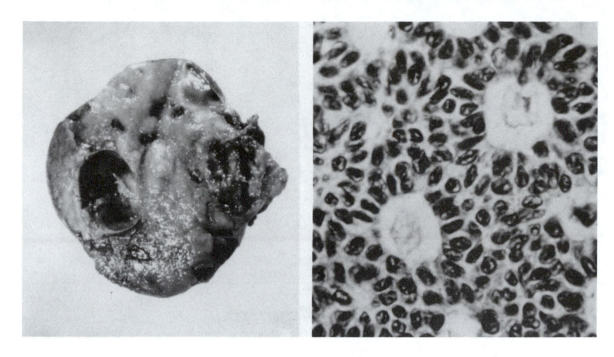

Figure 4–4. *A:* Cut surface of granulosa cell tumor. *B:* Typical Call-Exner bodies in granulosa cell tumor. (Courtesy of J Sandstad.)

ing, clitoromegaly, and muscle mass development. Most are combined Sertoli-Leydig cell tumors; however, pure Sertoli cell tumors do exist. The well-differentiated Sertoli cell tumor is composed of uniform tubules. These tumors can be estrogenic, yet most mixed Sertoli-Leydig cell tumors are androgenic and produce testosterone. The combined Sertoli-Leydig cell tumor can be well-differentiated, poorly differentiated, or may have intermediate morphologic features based upon the differentiation of the Sertoli cells. The Leydig cell component in all these tumors is fairly uniform, containing polygonal cells with abundant eosinophilic cytoplasm and occasional crystals of Reinke, which appear as elongated crystalline rectangles.

Hilus Cell Tumors

These lesions are similar to Leydig cell tumors and are differentiated by their anatomic location in the ovary. They contain a uniform population of Leydig cells with crystals of Reinke. If crystals of Reinke cannot be found, the tumor is placed in the more generic category of lipid cell tumor. Crystals of Reinke are reassuring signs of the benign nature of the tumor. In lipid cell tumors, the size of the tumor is prognostic. Tumors less than 9 cm in diameter have not been shown to exhibit aggressive behavior.

Gynandroblastoma

This is a rare tumor that differentiates along both ovarian and testicular cell lines.

OVARIAN TUMORS OF GERM CELL ORIGIN

All tumors of germ cell origin must be initially considered to be malignant with the possible exception of teratomas. This is fortunate, because in absolute numbers teratomas are the most frequently encountered of all ovarian tumors. Even so, there are malignant forms of teratoma, as explained below.

Although the remaining types of germ cell tumors are few in absolute numbers, when they do occur they are usually malignant. Specifically, gonadoblastoma is more often malignant than benign, and dysgerminomas and yolk sac or endodermal sinus tumors are always malignant. The latter two malignancies are mentioned only briefly below for completeness and are more extensively considered in Chapter 31.

Teratomas

Teratomas may be immature or mature. Mature teratomas of the ovary can be solid but are usually cystic. The mature teratoma (dermoid cyst) is the most common germ cell tumor and, as is true of most germ cell tumors, occurs in women under the age of 30. Abundant hair and keratinous debris may be present grossly. Bone and well-formed teeth can also be identified in the central area (Rokitansky's protuberance) (Figure 4–5), from which multiple pathologic specimens should be taken in order to identify immature components and any malignant transformation that may occur. Malignant transformation can occur in any of the components but most often the squamous cell component. Occasionally there may be prolifer-

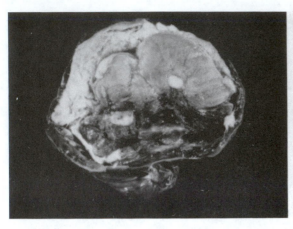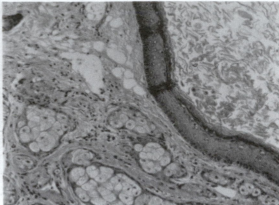

Figure 4–5. **A:** Mature cystic teratoma with areas of sebaceous material, bone, and striated muscle. **B:** Photomicrograph showing mature squamous epithelium and sebaceous glands. (Courtesy of J Sandstad.)

ation of active thyroid tissue within a teratoma (struma ovarii).

Mature teratomas usually can be removed as a simple ovarian cystectomy if future childbearing is desired. The incidence of bilaterality is 15%, so the opposite ovary should be carefully inspected and perhaps bivalved if it appears enlarged or suspicious.

Immature teratomas of the ovary are all considered to be malignant, with varying degrees of aggressiveness. These immature variants are characterized by the presence of immature fetal tissue, especially immature neural-epidermal tissue. Most immature teratomas are solid, but they may have cystic components. The size of the tumor, the clinical stage in which it is found, and its grade and the grade of its metastases are of value in estimating the prognosis (see Chapter 31).

Gonadoblastoma

This lesion is a combined germ cell and sex cord stromal tumor that contains cells resembling those of a dysgerminoma and either immature granulosa or Sertoli cells. These tumors tend to have marked calcifications. Most of them occur in patients with abnormal gonads, such as those with gonadal dysgenesis and an XY karyotype. Although the gonadoblastoma is benign in its early stages, there often is development of dysgerminoma or other malignant germ cell tumors.

Dysgerminoma

This tumor is the least well differentiated of all the germ cell tumors and most often occurs in patients under age 30 or in the streak gonads of patients with gonadal dysgenesis. The tumor is characterized by a uniform cell population of primitive germ cells with prominent nucleoli. Characteristic fibrosis and lymphocytic infiltration are present. Benign syncytiotrophoblastic differentiation can occasionally occur, which may result in the production of low levels of hCG. Grossly, the tumors are solid, with a

smooth surface, and they are usually unilateral. They are universally malignant and are discussed in greater detail in Chapter 31.

Yolk Sac or Endodermal Sinus Tumor

This tumor is considered to be a germ cell tumor that mimics the embryonic development of the yolk sac. Endodermal sinus tumors are rare but are the second most common malignant germ cell tumor in the ovary (see Chapter 31). They occur most commonly in children and adolescents and are rare over the age of 40 years. Patients usually present with a recent onset of abdominal pain and swelling. Grossly, the tumors are large, averaging around 15 cm. The external surface is predominantly smooth, but rupture sites are often present. The tumor is soft and friable, with areas of hemorrhage and necrosis. Cystic areas can be present, sometimes giving a honeycomb appearance to the cut surface. The tumors are usually unilateral, with bilateral involvement as a secondary process.

Schiller-Duval bodies have been described in over half of yolk sac tumors. Clinically, all yolk sac tumors should be considered malignant. Alpha-fetoprotein is a serum marker useful in following the treatment of these patients.

BENIGN TUMORS OF THE FALLOPIAN TUBES

Benign lesions of the fallopian tubes are frequently asymptomatic and found at the time of surgery for other causes. These include myomas, hemangiomas, and fibromas—all very uncommon lesions. Inflammatory lesions such as hydrosalpinx or pyosalpinx are frequently the cause of enlargement of the oviduct. The most common benign tumor of the fallopian tube is benign mesothelioma (adenomatoid tumor). This is a proliferation of the serosal mesothelial lining, giving rise to a firm nodule. The tumor is occasionally large enough to constrict the lumen. Similar lesions have been described in other mesothelium-lined surfaces. Epithelial papillomas and polyps occasionally occur.

Paratubal cysts may arise from either mesonephric (wolffian) duct remnants, paramesonephric (müllerian) duct remnants, or mesothelium. The hydatid cyst of Morgagni is the most common of these cysts and is a müllerian-derived structure lined by ciliated cells containing intracytoplasmic mucin.

SUGGESTED READINGS

Bloomfield TH: Benign cystic teratomas of the ovary: A review of seventy-two cases. Eur J Obstet Gynecol Reprod Biol 1987; 25(3):231.

Blustering A (editor): *Pathology of the Female Genital Tract.* Springer-Verlag, 1977.

Einhorn N et al: CA 125 assay used in conjunction with CA 15-3 and TAG-72 assays for discrimination between malignant and non-malignant diseases of the ovary. Acta Oncol 1989;28(5):655.

Meigs JV, Armstrong SH, Hamilton HH: A further contribution to the syndrome of fibroma of the ovary with fluid in the abdomen and chest, Meigs syndrome. Am J Obstet Gynecol 1943; 46:19.

Jones III HW, Wentz AC, Burnett LS (editors): *Novak's Textbook of Gynecology,* 11th ed. Williams & Wilkins, 1988.

Rome RM et al: Functioning ovarian tumors in postmenopausal women. Obstet Gynecol 1981;57:705.

Samah M, Woodruff JD: Paratubal cysts: Frequency, histogenesis and associated clinical features. Obstet Gynecol 1985;65: 691.

Shevchuk MM, Fenoglio CM, Richart RM: Histogenesis of Brenner tumors, I. Histology and structure. Cancer 1980;46: 2607.

Spanos WJ: Preoperative hormonal therapy of cystic adnexal masses. Am J Obstet Gynecol 1973;116:551.

Talerman A: Germ cell tumours. Ann Pathol 1985;5(3):145.

Young RH, Scully RE: Ovarian Sertoli-Leydig cell tumors: A clinicopathological analysis of 207 cases. Am J Surg Pathol 1985;9(8):543.

5

Embryology & Congenital Anomalies of the Female Reproductive Tract

Developmental anomalies of the female genital tract are not common, but even minor defects may result in an increased incidence of threatened abortion and abnormal fetal lie. More serious defects often result in significant fetal and maternal hazards. There is little familial tendency associated with spontaneous defects, which at most may be polygenic or multifactorial traits.

EMBRYOLOGY

Genitourinary anomalies result from some abnormality arising during the process of embryogenesis. Embryologic development begins when the metanephric ducts emerge and connect with the cloaca between the third and fifth gestational weeks. Between the fourth and fifth weeks, two ureteric buds develop distally from the mesonephric (wolffian) ducts and begin to grow upward (cephalad) toward the mesonephros. The paramesonephric (müllerian) ducts form bilaterally between the developing gonad and the mesonephros. The paramesonephric ducts extend downward and laterally to the mesonephric ducts and finally turn medially to meet and fuse together in the midline. The fused paramesonephric duct descends to the urogenital sinus to join Müller's tubercle. The close association between the paramesonephric and mesonephric ducts has clinical relevance, because damage to either duct system is usually associated with damage to both (uterine horn, kidney, and ureter).

The uterus is formed by union of the two paramesonephric ducts at about the tenth week of gestation. The fusion begins in the middle of what will become the uterus and then extends caudally and cephalad. The characteristic shape of the uterus is now formed, with cellular proliferation at the upper portion and simultaneous disso-

lution of cells at the lower pole, thus establishing the first uterine cavity. This cavity is at the lower pole, with a thick wedge of tissue above. The upper thick wedge of tissue (septum) is slowly dissolved, creating the ultimate uterine cavity. This process usually is completed by the 20th week. One might reasonably expect that any failure to fuse the two paramesonephric ducts or failure to reabsorb the tissue between them would result in separate uterine horns or some degree of persistence of the uterine septum.

The vagina is formed between the urogenital sinus and Müller's tubercle by dissolution of the cell mass (cord) between the two structures. It is believed that this dissolution starts at the hymen and moves upward toward the cervix, which is also being canalized. Failure of this process will be associated with persistence of the cell cord, and agenesis of the vagina or lesser abnormalities of this process will result in varying degrees of vaginal septum formation.

GENESIS & CLASSIFICATION OF PARAMESONEPHRIC DUCT ABNORMALITIES

Because fusion of the two paramesonephric ducts forms the vagina, cervix, and uterine body, the principal groups of deformities arising from three types of embryologic defects can be classified as follows:

(1) There may be defective canalization of the vagina, resulting in a transverse vaginal septum or, in the most extreme form, absence of the vagina.

(2) There may be unilateral maturation of one paramesonephric duct with incomplete or absent development of the opposite duct. The resulting defects often are associated with abnormalities of the upper urinary tract.

(3) The most common abnormality is absence or faulty midline fusion of the paramesonephric ducts. If there is complete lack of fusion, the result is two entirely separate uteri, cervices, and vaginas. With incomplete reabsorption of the tissue between the two fused paramesonephric ducts, a uterine septum results.

Various classifications of these anomalies have been proposed, none of them completely satisfactory. The terminology often is so complicated and erudite that their relative obstetric significance is obscured. The classification of paramesonephric duct abnormalities offered by Buttram and Gibbons is based upon failure of normal development and distributes diverse anomalies into groups with similar clinical characteristics, prognosis for pregnancy, and treatment (Table 5–1 and Figure 5–1). The classification also includes a category for abnormalities associated with in utero exposure to diethylstilbestrol (DES). These authors have emphasized that vaginal anomalies may exist alone or in association with other paramesonephric duct anomalies, but vaginal anomalies have not been classified because they are not associated with fetal loss. Vaginal anomalies using the scheme proposed by Buttram and Gibbons are most commonly associated with classes III and IV.

Types of Cervices

A. Single Cervix: The normal cervix.

B. Septate Cervix: A cervix consisting of a single muscular ring divided by a septum. The septum may be confined to the cervix or, more commonly, may be the downward continuation of a uterine septum or the upward extension of a vaginal septum.

C. Double Cervix: Two distinct cervices, each resulting from separate paramesonephric duct maturation. Both a septate and a true double cervix are frequently associ-

Table 5–1. Classification of müllerian anomalies.[1]

I. Segmental müllerian agenesis or hypoplasia.
A. Vaginal
B. Cervical
C. Fundal
D. Tubal
E. Combined anomalies
II. Unicornuate uterus
A. With rudimentary horn
1. With endometrial cavity
a. Communicating
b. Noncommunicating
2. Without endometrial cavity
B. Without rudimentary horn
III. Uterine didelphys
IV. Bicornuate uterus
A. Complete (division down to internal os)
B. Partial
C. Arcuate
V. Septate uterus
A. Complete (septum to internal os)
B. Partial
VI. Diethylstilbestrol-related

[1]Modified from Buttram VC, Gibbons WE: Müllerian anomalies: A proposed classification (and analysis of 144 cases). Fertil Steril 1979;32:40.

ated with a longitudinal vaginal septum, with the result that many septate cervices are erroneously classified as double. The diagnosis depends on visual and digital examination of the cervix and is of clinical importance.

D. Single Hemicervix: This anomaly arises from unilateral paramesonephric duct maturation.

Types of Vaginas

A. Single Vagina: The normal vagina.

B. Longitudinally Septate Vagina: One with a more or less complete longitudinal septum.

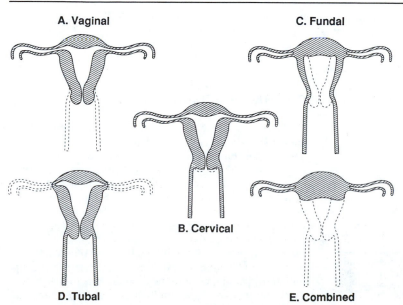

A. Vaginal

C. Fundal

B. Cervical

D. Tubal

E. Combined

Figure 5–1. Class I: Segmental müllerian agenesis or hypoplasia with subdivisions, I-A vaginal through I-E combined.

C. Double Vagina: It is often difficult to distinguish double vagina from the completely septate vagina. The true double vagina includes a double introitus and resembles a double-barreled shotgun, with each passage terminating in a distinct, separate cervix. In some cases, one of the two vaginas may end blindly.

D. Transversely Septate Vagina: Transverse vaginal septa are of different developmental origin, resulting from faulty canalization of the united paramesonephric duct anlage rather than faulty longitudinal fusion.

DIAGNOSIS OF ANOMALIES OF THE VAGINA & UTERUS

Physical Examination

Symptoms and signs are summarized in Table 5–2. Vaginal septa usually are discovered during routine examination by the physician or when the individual herself notices that vaginal tampons are not always effective in absorbing menses.

Uterine malformations are usually discovered by simple speculum inspection or during bimanual examination—or occasionally at cesarean section or during manual exploration of the uterine cavity after vaginal delivery. Fundal notching, palpated abdominally, most often is indicative of a malformed uterus, and the clinical impression can be confirmed by laparoscopy. Without radiologic examination, high-resolution sonography, or direct visualization of the uterine cavity—and often laparoscopic examination—it is difficult to distinguish septate from bicornuate uterus.

Table 5–2. Symptoms and Signs Associated with Female Genital Anomalies

Symptoms	
Primary amenorrhea	Leakage with tampon in place
Dyspareunia	Irregular vaginal bleeding
Dysmenorrhea	Habitual abortion
Cyclic pelvic pain	Spontaneous second trimester
Inability to achieve penile penetration	abortion
	Premature labor
Infertility	Postpartum hemorrhage

Signs	
Vaginal mass (hematocolpos, mucocolpos, Gartner's duct cyst)	Absent uterus/cervix
	Absent/short vagina
	Ambiguous genitalia
Abdominal mass (hematosalpinx, hematometra)	Absent pubic hair
	Fetal malpresentation
	Retained placenta

Reproduced, with permission, from Growdon WA: Embryology and congenital anomalies of the female genital system. In Hacker NF and Moore JG (eds): *Essentials of Obstetrics and Gynecology*, Philadelphia, PA, W. B. Saunders, 1986.

Hysteroscopy, Hysterography, Laparoscopy

Hysteroscopic examination and hysterography are of value in ascertaining the configuration of the uterine cavity. When these procedures are combined with laparoscopic confirmation of the absence or presence of an external division of the uterus and the presence or absence of a rudimentary uterine horn, virtually all uterine abnormalities can be accurately described and classified.

Sonography

Sonography may be used to identify abnormal uterine development, though it lacks the precision provided by hysteroscopy and hysterosalpingography. During actual or suspected pregnancy, however, sonographic examination can be quite informative.

Urologic Evaluation

When asymmetric development of the reproductive tract is found, urologic evaluation is indicated because of the frequent association of urinary tract anomalies. When there is uterine atresia on one side or when one side of a double vagina terminates blindly, an ipsilateral urologic anomaly is common.

SIGNIFICANCE OF SPONTANEOUS DEVELOPMENTAL ANOMALIES

PARAMESONEPHRIC DUCT HYPOPLASIA OR AGENESIS (Buttram & Gibbons Class I)

Vaginal hypoplasia or agenesis renders pregnancy virtually impossible, and even in those rare cases where a uterus is surgically attached to a neovagina, successful pregnancy is extremely rare. The various types of vaginal septa are easily dilated, displaced, or surgically divided. The septate cervix functions remarkably well, but during labor there is a danger of rupture and hemorrhage.

BUTTRAM & GIBBONS CLASSES II–V

The major obstetric difficulties arise from uterine anomalies. The uterus must dilate and hypertrophy sufficiently to accommodate a term-sized fetus in a longitudinal lie and, at the proper time, must contract efficiently to expel the fetus. Uterine defects that result from maturation of only one paramesonephric duct or from lack of fusion often give rise to a hemiuterus that fails to dilate and hypertrophy, resulting in a host of possible difficulties that include abortion, ectopic pregnancy, rudimentary horn pregnancy, preterm delivery, fetal growth retardation, abnormal fetal lie, uterine dysfunction, and even uterine rupture. Surprisingly, even in those conditions in which only a uterine septum is present, there is an appreciable increase in the incidence of abortion. Because of these obstetric problems, each uterine defect will be discussed within the classification suggested by Buttram and Gibbons (Table 5–1).

Reproductive Performance of Women With Unicornuate Uterus (Buttram and Gibbons Class II)

The incidence of unicornuate uterus in one series of 1160 uterine anomalies was 14%. In approximately 90% of cases of unicornuate uterus with rudimentary horns, there was no communication between the horns (Figure 5–2). This information has both gynecologic and obstetric significance.

As illustrated in Table 5–3, pregnancy outcome is poor. Reproductive failure is apt to be due to anatomic defects. For example, the increased incidence of abortion may be explained partially by the smaller uterine size and the possible implantation of the zygote in a communicating rudimentary horn. The smaller hemiuterine size almost certainly is an explanation for the increased rates of preterm delivery, fetal growth retardation, breech presentation, and abnormal uterine function in labor and for the increased incidence of cesarean section.

Tubal pregnancies and pregnancies in the rudimentary horn are special problems. In pregnancies with implantations in rudimentary horns, uterine rupture usually occurs prior to 20 weeks of gestation. Intraperitoneal hemorrhage may be massive and life-threatening.

Reproductive Performance in Women With Uterus Didelphys (Buttram and Gibbons, Class III)

Uterus didelphys (Figure 5–3) is distinguished from bicornuate uterus and septate uterus by the presence of complete reduplication of cervices and hemiuterine cavities. Although the problems associated with uterus didelphys are similar to those seen with unicornuate uterus (except for ectopic and rudimentary horn pregnancies), overall successful pregnancy outcome was 68%, with a 30% abortion rate and a perinatal mortality rate of only 4%.

Uterus didelphys may cause significant problems, however. In addition to the 30% abortion rate noted above, there was a preterm delivery rate of 21%, fetal growth retardation occurred in 11% and breech presentation in 43%, and the cesarean section rate was 82%.

It is unusual but not rare for twin pregnancies to occur in women with this anomaly. There is even one reported case of triplets with a delivery interval of 72 days.

Reproductive Performance in Women With Bicornuate & Septate Uteri (Buttram & Gibbons Classes IV and V)

In both of these categories, there is a marked increase in abortion rate except for the arcuate uterus, which is merely a slight deviation from normal. Pregnancy losses in the first 20 weeks were observed by Buttram and Gibbons to be 88% for septate and 70% for bicornuate uteri. The cause of this extraordinarily high pregnancy wastage is thought to be partial or complete implantation on the largely avascular septum and ultimate failure of the conceptus to acquire an adequate blood supply. Once pregnancy is well established, overall outcome is associated with an increased incidence of preterm delivery, abnormal fetal lie, and the need for cesarean section.

A hysterosalpingogram usually cannot be used alone to differentiate septate uterus and bicornuate uterus because of the difficulty of establishing the presence or absence of an external division of the uterus. Buttram and Gibbons

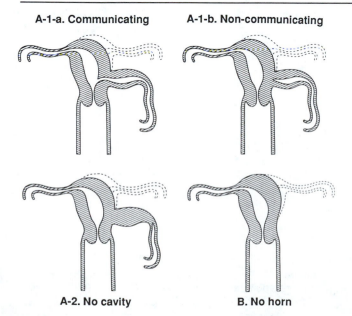

A-1-a. Communicating   **A-1-b. Non-communicating**

A-2. No cavity   **B. No horn**

Figure 5–2. Class II: Unicornuate uterus either with (II-A) or without rudimentary horn (II-B). Those with a rudimentary horn are divided into those with (II-A-1) or without an endometrial cavity (II-A-2). Those with an endometrial cavity either have (II-A-1-a) or do not have a communication with the opposite horn (II-A-1-b).

Table 5–3. Pregnancy outcome in women with a unicornuate uterus.[1]

	Semmens 1962	Beernink 1976	Andrews 1982	Heinonen 1982	Buttram[2] 1983	Fedele 1987
Patients	5	5	5	13	31	20
Conceiving	4	4	5	10	?	13
Pregnancies	11	8	13	15	60	29
Horn pregnancies	1	—	—	—	—	1
Abortion (%)	4 (36)	1 (12)	7 (54)	7 (47)	29 (48)	17 (59)
Premature labor (%)	?	3 (37)[3]	2 (15)	3 (20)	10 (17)	3 (10)
Term delivery	?	4	4	5	21	10
Live birth rate (%)	(63)	(75)	(45.1)	(40)	(40)	(38)

[1]Modified from Fedele L and associates: Reproductive performance of women with unicornuate uterus. Fertil Steril 1987;47:416.
[2]Partly personal data.
[3]One twin pregnancy.

have stressed the necessity for laparoscopy to establish the presence of an external uterine division.

OBSTETRIC & GYNECOLOGIC MANAGEMENT OF UTERINE ANOMALIES

Abnormal fetal presentations are common and in general are treated in the same way as when the uterus is normal. Attempts at external podalic version, however, are less apt to be successful and may prove dangerous. If uterine dysfunction develops, it is unwise to stimulate these defective uteri with oxytocin. Cesarean section is safer, but unfortunately the diagnosis often is not made in time.

Cerclage has been attempted in some cases in which cervical incompetence was suspected, and it may be indicated in unicornuate, didelphic, bicornuate, and septate uteri. The question of whether to place a suture in both cervices of a uterus didelphys is unresolved. There appears to be no reason for cerclage with arcuate uterus. If active labor supervenes, procrastination in severing a cerclage ligature must be avoided because of the increased risk of uterine rupture.

A woman with a uterine anomaly and a poor obstetric history—eg, repeated abortions not ascribable to some other cause—may benefit from metroplasty or plastic repair.

Women with septate or bicornuate anomalies and poor previous obstetric outcomes are likely to have good outcomes after repair. In bicornuate uteri (classes IV-A and IV-B, Figure 5–4), the method of repair is usually transabdominal metroplasty involving resection of the septum and recombination of the uterine fundus (Kessler et al, 1986).

With uterine septa (class V, Figure 5–5), the management of choice appears to be transcervical intrauterine resection of the septum, which is accomplished by scissors passed through a hysteroscope (Fayez, 1986).

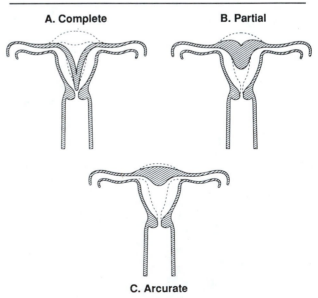

A. Complete   **B. Partial**

C. Arcurate

Figure 5–4. Class IV: Bicornuate uterus in which the septum is complete down to the internal os (IV-A), partial (IV-B), or arcuate (IV-C).

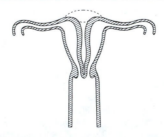

Figure 5–3. Class III: Uterine didelphys.

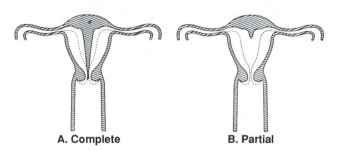

A. Complete

B. Partial

Figure 5–5. Class V: Septate uterus with complete septum to the internal or external os (V-A) or partial septum (V-B).

INDUCED DEVELOPMENTAL ABNORMALITIES OF THE REPRODUCTIVE TRACT; DIETHYLSTILBESTROL EXPOSURE IN UTERO

For nearly a quarter of a century from about 1950 until the early 1970s, diethylstilbestrol, a synthetic nonsteroidal estrogen, was prescribed for an estimated 3 million pregnant women in the United States. Enthusiastic endorsements published in early uncontrolled reports from prestigious medical centers soon established this drug as the obstetrician's "miracle drug" for prevention of most forms of pregnancy wastage, including those resulting from abortion, preeclampsia and other hypertensive disorders, diabetes, and preterm labor.

The first serious problem associated with the use of stilbestrol (other than that it did not live up to its early promise) was identification of clear cell adenocarcinoma of the vagina in some women who had been exposed in utero to stilbestrol (Herbst et al, 1971). It has been established subsequently that the risk of malignancy is slight but real (0.14–1.4 per 1000 exposed women followed through age 24 years).

More recently, impaired reproductive performances of women exposed in utero to stilbestrol have been recognized (Managan et al, 1982). A variety of reproductive tract deformities have been identified also (Figure 5–6).

The problems associated with administration of diethylstilbestrol to pregnant women will be of historical interest only as the affected generation ages.

A. Constriction bands

B. T-shaped

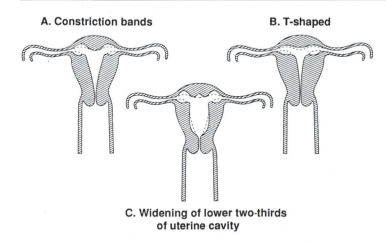

C. Widening of lower two-thirds of uterine cavity

Figure 5–6. Class VI: Diethylstilbestrol anomalies, including uterus with luminal changes, such as constriction bands in the uterine cavity (VI-A), T-shaped cavity (VI-B), and widening of the lower two-thirds of the uterine cavity (VI-C). (Modified from Buttram VC, Gibbons WE: Müllerian anomalies: A proposed classification. Fertil Steril 1979;32:40.)

SUGGESTED READINGS

Andrews MC, Jones HW Jr: Impaired reproductive performance of unicornuate uterus: Intrauterine growth retardation, infertility and recurrent abortion in five cases. Am J Obstet Gynecol 1982;144:173.

Beernink FJ, Beernink HE, Chinn A: Uterus unicornis with uterus solidaris. Obstet Gynecol 1976;47:651.

Buttram VC, Gibbons WE: Müllerian anomalies: A proposed classification (an analysis of 144 cases). Fertil Steril 1979;32:40.

Fayez JA: Comparison between abdominal and hysteroscopic metroplasty. Obstet Gynecol 1986;68:399.

Fedele L et al: Reproductive performance of women with unicornuate uterus. Fertil Steril 1987;47:416.

Fowler WC Jr et al: Risks of cervical intraepithelial neoplasia among DES exposed women. Obstet Gynecol 1981; 58:720.

Heinonen PK, Saarikoski S, Pystynen P: Reproductive performance of women with uterine anomalies: An evaluation of 182 cases. Acta Obstet Gynecol Scand 1982;61:157.

Herbst AL, Ulfelder H, Poskanzer DC: Adenocarcinoma of the vagina. N Engl J Med 1971;284:878.

Kessler I et al: Indications and results of metroplasty in uterine malformations. Int J Gynaecol Obstet 1986;24:137.

Mashiach S et al: Triplet pregnancy in uterus didelphys with delivery interval of 72 days. Obstet Gynecol 1981;58:519.

Semmens JP: Congenital anomalies of female genital tract: Functional classification based on review of 56 personal cases and 500 reported cases. Obstet Gynecol 1962;19:328.

Toaff R: A major malformation: Communicating uteri. Obstet Gynecol 1974;43:221.

Vessey MP: Epidemiological studies of the effects of diethylstilbestrol. IARC Sci Publ 1989;96:335.

6

Benign Diseases of the Vulva, Vagina, & Cervix

DISORDERS MANIFESTED BY VAGINAL DISCHARGE

Vaginal discharge is one of the three most common presenting complaints in gynecology (the others are abnormal vaginal bleeding and pelvic pain). The most common causes of inflammation of the lower genital tract (vulvitis-vaginitis-cervicitis) or similar complaints are discussed here. Herpes simplex infection, gonorrhea, and *Chlamydia trachomatis* infection cause vaginal discharge, but discussion of those disorders is deferred to the next chapter on sexually transmitted diseases.

Office Diagnosis

The office diagnosis is based upon an easily obtained history and physical examination and a carefully prepared saline wet mount. Each of the salient history and physical characteristics of these disorders is discussed under the appropriate etiologic heading, and the preparation of a wet mount is described below. The saline wet mount—a suspension of vaginal discharge in normal saline viewed at 400× magnification—is the first laboratory test performed and often the only one necessary to make a correct diagnosis of disorders causing vaginal discharge. Patients complaining of vaginal discharge or other symptoms consistent with vulvitis, vaginitis, or cervicitis should be advised not to douche for several days prior to examination, and appointments should be scheduled to avoid menses.

There are many ways to prepare the slide for examination. The following technique is commonly used.

(1) Place about ½ inch of normal saline in a 5-mL test tube, eg, a small red-topped tube for blood collection.
(2) After inspection of the vulva, vagina, and cervix, obtain a specimen of vaginal discharge on a cotton-tipped applicator. The specimen should be obtained from deep in the vagina at 3 and 9 o'clock next to the

cervix, as this area is relatively protected from cleansing by menstrual flow or douching.
(3) Place the cotton-tipped applicator in the collection tube with saline solution.
(4) Complete the pelvic examination.
(5) Stir the saline with the cotton-tipped applicator, and then use the applicator to place some of the suspension on a clean microscope slide. Cover with a cover glass and examine at 400× magnification.
(6) For suspected *Candida* infection, a second slide can be made with a drop of 10% potassium hydroxide added on the slide.

Clinical Diagnosis & Management

In Table 6–1 are summarized the major symptoms, findings, and therapy for the most frequent causes of vaginal discharge. Every effort should be made to arrive at a correct diagnosis and to provide specific therapy. "Shotgun" therapy should be avoided, since the antiseptics employed for that purpose are themselves potential chemical irritants of the vagina and often do more harm than good.

FUNGAL VULVOVAGINITIS

Candida albicans causes 67–95% of fungal infections of the vulva and vagina. Other candidal species and *Torulopsis glabrata* are responsible for the remainder of cases. *C albicans* is a dimorphic organism that ordinarily grows as a yeast form but is capable of taking on a stranded appearance under conditions of relative hypoxia. The yeast phase is thought to represent colonization; the stranded form is indicative of infection.

Factors predisposing to vaginal candidal infection include pregnancy, administration of broad-spectrum antibiotics, immunosuppression, and diabetes mellitus. Oral contraceptives were once thought to predispose to candidal infection, but the modern formulations do not appear to have this disadvantage. Candidal infection may be sexually transmitted, but most cases cannot be explained in this way.

Table 6–1. Diagnosis and management of vaginitis.

Cause	Major Symptom	Physical Findings	Diagnostic Tests and Procedures	Treatment
Candida albicans infection	Pruritus	Cheesy white exudate, pH 4.0–4.7	Wet prep or KOH prep	Clotrimazole, miconazole, Ketoconazole for refractory cases or immunocompromised patients.
Chlamydia trachomatis infection		Mucopurulent discharge, cervical erosion	Culture, immunofluorescent staining	Tetracycline, erythromycin, doxycyline.
Trichomonas vaginalis infection	Odor	Frothy greenish exudate, pH 5.0–7.0; strawberry cervix.	Wet prep, immunofluorescent staining	Metronidazole. All sex partners must be treated.
Gonorrhea		Cervical discharge	Cervical culture, Gram stain	Ceftriaxone, spectinomycin, ciprofloxacin or norfloxacin.
Genital herpes	Pain	Ulceration, vulval vesicles and ulcers	Tzank prep, virus culture	Oral acyclovir (intravenous if severe).
Bacterial vaginosis	"Fishy" odor	Thin gray discharge, pH 5.0–5.5	Wet prep, sniff test (gas chromatography)	Metronidazole, orally or topically. Topical clindamycin is an alternative drug.
Chemical exposure		Discharge, erythema; may be ulcerative	History and exclusion of other causes	Terminate contact.
Physiologic vaginitis		Discharge but no odor or erythema	Wet prep, history, exclusion of other causes	Reassurance

Clinical Findings

A. Symptoms and Signs: Most patients with *C albicans* infection complain of genital itching, which may be so intense that the vulva and vagina are not only erythematous but also edematous. Excoriations from scratching may be present. White or yellow adherent plaques may be visible in the vagina or on the vulva. The classic vaginal discharge associated with candidal infection is thick, white, and curdlike and is present in most but not all infected patients (Figure 6–1).

B. Laboratory Findings: The diagnosis is confirmed by demonstrating the stranded form of the organism in examination of a saline wet mount under a microscope. Recognition of the fungus may be aided by adding a drop of 10% potassium hydroxide to the specimen on the slide. Candidal cell walls are resistant to this concentration of alkali. Thus, all cells except those of the fungus will be destroyed.

The fungus may also be cultured on Sabouraud's or Nickerson's medium. Since both colonized and infected women will be culture-positive for *C albicans,* cultures are more helpful as a test of cure than as a diagnostic aid.

Treatment

The use of intravaginal antifungals should be delayed until the second or third trimester of pregnancy, but topical agents may be used on the skin of the vulva in early pregnancy to provide symptomatic relief. Treatment of sexual partners should be reserved for cases of recurrent or persistent infection. In such cases, sexual partners must be treated even if they are asymptomatic.

A. Topical Nystatin and Imidazoles: Topical miconazole, clotrimazole, terconazole, butoconazole, or tioconazole in ointment, cream, or suppository form applied once nightly for 3–7 days—or nystatin twice daily for 14 days—provides effective therapy for the vast majority of cases.

B. Topical Gentian Violet: Gentian violet is still useful for symptomatic relief in severe cases. A single application of 1% gentian violet solution to affected areas provides prompt relief. Repeated applications are necessary for cure. Staining is an aesthetic disadvantage.

C. Systemic Imidazole Therapy: Ketoconazole is an orally effective, relatively safe agent whose major disadvantage is its rare hepatocellular toxicity, which is usually reversible but may be fatal. Ketoconazole should not be used during pregnancy.

D. Management of Recurrences: A thorough medical history should be taken, with emphasis on the predisposing factors listed above. There should clear evidence of fungal infection or at least colonization before instituting therapy for recurrent fungal vulvovaginitis, since women may reexperience itching even months after cure without actually being reinfected. This itching usually will disappear without further therapy. Finally, therapy for recurrences must be provided for more than the surface of the vaginal mucosa, since *C albicans* may invade the deeper layers of the vaginal mucosa.

Recurrences may be treated by extended topical therapy for 14 or even 28 days. In addition, topical therapy may be prescribed for two subsequent menstrual cycles following a normal course of therapy, to be used only while bleeding continues. Prolonging therapy allows the deeper layers of the vaginal mucosa to move to the surface by the normal process of cell turnover and maturation and thus exposes these cells to the topical therapy. Systemic therapy with oral ketoconazole should be considered in resistant and protracted cases.

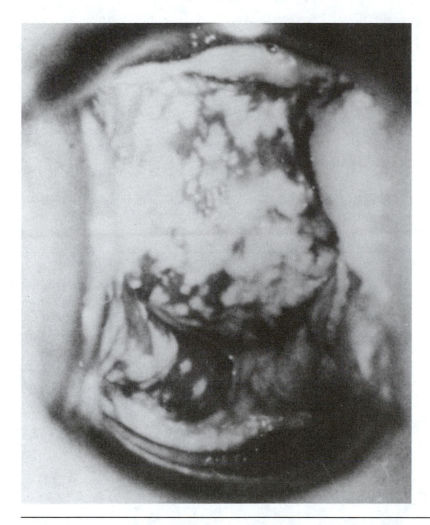

Figure 6–1. The curdlike discharge of candidal vaginitis. (Reproduced, with permission, from Lichtman R, Papera S: *Gynecology Well-Woman Care.* Appleton & Lange, 1990.)

TRICHOMONAL VAGINITIS

Trichomonas vaginalis is an anaerobic flagellate protozoan, oval in shape and slightly larger than a white blood cell, with four anterior flagella and an anterolateral undulating membrane. Humans are the only known host. Although the organism is not known to take the form of a cyst or other resistant form, the trophozoite itself is one of the most resistant to extremes of temperature and drying of all of the parasitic protozoa. It survives for 5 days or longer at 0 °C and prefers an environment in which the pH is 5.0 or slightly higher.

In women, the organism infects mainly the vagina and cervix, but the urethra and bladder may also be involved. It is estimated that 25% of women are infected with *T vaginalis,* but only 15–20% of infected women have symptoms.

Trichomonal vaginitis is sexually transmitted except in rare instances. Transmission via contaminated articles such as towels or douching equipment does occur. Most infected individuals of both sexes are asymptomatic. The rate of diagnosis in the sexual partners of infected women is low because of difficulties in securing adequate specimens.

Clinical Findings

A. Symptoms and Signs: The most common symptom is vaginal discharge with a foul odor. Most women will not volunteer information about the odor, which must therefore be solicited during the interview. Other symptoms consistent with *T vaginalis* infection include intermenstrual bleeding—particularly postcoital bleeding—vulvar or vaginal itching, and dyspareunia. Symptoms of urethritis such as dysuria and urinary frequency or urgency are uncommon, but trichomonal urethritis should be considered in patients with sterile urine cultures.

The discharge classically associated with trichomonal vaginitis has been described as watery, yellow-green, and foamy. Unfortunately, about 80% of symptomatic women do not have the classic picture.

The cervix may be involved in severe infections and may be dotted with subepithelial hemorrhages. The finding of colpitis macularis (strawberry cervix) is virtually pathognomonic of trichomonal infection (Figure 6–2).

B. Laboratory Findings: The diagnosis is confirmed by finding the motile flagellate protozoan on a saline wet mount. The sensitivity of the wet mount for this purpose has been reported to be as low as 50% and as high as 95%. *T vaginalis* can be cultured, but cultures are not commercially available. A direct immunofluorescent staining test is now available and may be useful for diagnosis in patients with suggestive symptoms but negative wet mounts.

Treatment

A. Curative Therapy: Curative treatment for symptomatic infection must include treatment of sexual part-ners as well as destruction or sterilization of all potentially contaminated clothing and other articles.

Metronidazole is the drug of choice. It is administered orally as a single dose of 2 g, or as two doses of 1 g taken 12 hours apart, or as 250 mg 3 times daily for 7 days. All methods are at least 95% effective. The single-dose regimen has the obvious advantage of ensuring patient compliance.

The side effects of metronidazole are numerous, uncomfortable, and dose-related. Treatment of resistant *T vaginalis* is with 1 g orally twice daily for 7 days. Intravenous metronidazole has been used successfully to treat resistant cases.

While there is no evidence that metronidazole adversely affects the fetus, the drug should be avoided during preg-

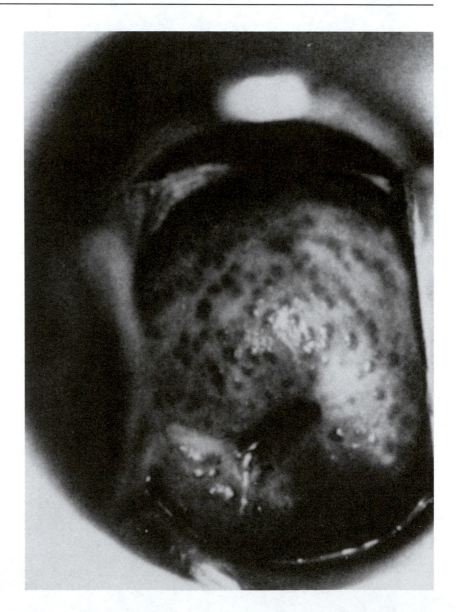

Figure 6–2. Colpitis macularis of trichomonal cervicitis. (Reproduced, with permission, from Lichtman R, Papera S: *Gynecology Well-Woman Care.* Appleton & Lange, 1990.)

nancy. If local therapy does not adequately relieve symptoms, metronidazole may be used after the first trimester.

B. Local Therapy: When treatment for cure is impossible or impractical, symptomatic relief may be provided by acidifying the vagina or asking the patient to douche with a mild antiseptic or detergent solution.

BACTERIAL VAGINOSIS

Bacterial vaginosis is not an infection in the ordinary sense but a malproportion of bacterial populations in which overrepresented and underrepresented species are normal residents of the human vagina. There are no known predisposing factors or etiologic agents. This entity is not thought to be sexually transmitted, since simultaneous treatment of sexual partners does not decrease the frequency of recurrences or lengthen the interval between recurrences. The overrepresented species in vaginal cultures of women with the disorder tend to be anaerobic bacteria, including *Gardnerella vaginalis*, *Mobiluncus* (a recently described small, curved, motile gram-negative rod), and some *Bacteroides* species.

Clinical Findings
A. Symptoms and Signs: The vast majority of patients complain only of a copious vaginal discharge that may or may not be accompanied by an offensive odor. When the offensive odor is present, it may be accentuated after coitus or after alkaline douching. The discharge is "nonspecific" in that it does not fit the classic description of the discharge caused by *C albicans, T vaginalis,* or *Neisseria gonorrhoeae*. It is usually thin, gray, and noncharacteristic of infection. This discharge will usually have a pH between 5.0 and 5.5.

B. Laboratory Findings: The diagnosis may be suggested by the appearance of a sample of discharge in saline wet mount. The discharge ordinarily contains many bacteria, and *Mobiluncus* may occasionally be observed. Stippled, granulated epithelial cells with obscure borders called "clue" cells may be seen. The clue cell represents a normal vaginal epithelial cell with many bacteria adherent to its surface. A paucity of white blood cells is characteristic.

The diagnosis is confirmed if 1 or 2 drops of 10% potassium hydroxide added to a suspension of discharge causes a fishy odor. This "whiff" or "sniff" test takes advantage of the fact that alkalinization of the discharge will volatilize the characteristic amines produced by certain anaerobic bacterial species.

Treatment
Metronidazole, 500 mg twice daily orally for 7 days, will achieve cure in about 90% of cases. Topical sulfonamides and antibiotic therapy with tetracycline or ampicillin are less successful alternatives. Topical metronidazole and topical clinclamycin are now available and may provide cure rates equal to oral metronidazole.

BACTERIAL VAGINITIS

Most true bacterial infections of the vagina occur in women with concurrent urinary tract infection and are probably secondary infections. In some cases, the urinary tract infection itself may be asymptomatic and the patient will present with a complaint of vaginal discharge and a foul odor. The discharge is usually nonspecific in appearance. The microscopic appearance is consistent with a diagnosis of bacterial vaginosis except that many white cells are present along with bacteria and clue cells. Symptoms of urinary tract infection can often be elicited, and suprapubic palpation frequently elicits tenderness. A positive urine culture confirms the diagnosis. Therapy should be aimed at the urinary tract infection. Separate or topical therapy for the vaginitis is unnecessary.

True bacterial vaginitis in the absence of urinary tract infection is uncommon and often difficult to treat. This entity is ordinarily caused by coliform bacteria and, in essence, represents fecal contamination of the vagina. The patient presents in the same way as the patient with secondary bacterial vaginitis, and the diagnosis is made by excluding urinary tract infection. The vaginitis should be treated with antibiotics chosen on the basis of bacterial cultures of the vaginal discharge followed by sensitivity tests. If no obvious cause for fecal contamination of the vagina can be found, occult rectovaginal fistula should be considered and attempts made to establish that diagnosis.

CHEMICAL VULVOVAGINITIS

Any chemical in contact with the vagina or vulva is a potential irritant. Examples include spermicides and their vehicles, douching agents, acetic acid, and the antimicrobials used to treat other forms of vaginitis and vulvitis. The patient usually complains of discharge with or without irritation. The discharge is ordinarily nonspecific in appearance and on microscopic examination characteristically consists chiefly of white blood cells. The diagnosis is made by excluding other causes of vaginitis and cervicitis, including gonorrhea and chlamydial infection. No therapy is necessary other than avoidance of the chemical irritant.

VAGINAL DISCHARGE DUE TO MIXED CAUSES

Patients with vaginal discharge of mixed origin present a diagnostic and therapeutic dilemma requiring expert clinical judgment that can only be acquired by experience. An obvious example is the patient with bacterial vaginosis and anything else that causes vaginal discharge. The discharge of bacterial vaginosis is characterized by a paucity of white blood cells, while the discharge associated with other causes, including chemical irritation, is characterized by the presence of white blood cells. In this example, the microscopic appearance of the discharge will be consistent with a diagnosis of bacterial vaginitis, perhaps secondary to urinary tract infection. Some guidelines for diagnosis and management can be offered as follows:

(1) Be wary of a diagnosis of bacterial vaginitis unless the patient also has a urinary tract infection. True bacterial vaginitis is uncommon. Vaginal discharge of mixed origin is more common.

(2) Be wary of a diagnosis based on the saline wet mount if the chief complaint is inconsistent with that diagnosis. Consider the possibility that the discharge is of mixed origin and that the saline wet mount results may be in error. Do not hesitate to make a second slide or even obtain a second specimen.

(3) Be wary of the diagnosis if the patient does not respond to therapy or gets worse during therapy.

(4) Treat asymptomatic gonorrhea and chlamydial infection whenever you find it.

(5) Treat whatever is causing the symptoms.

(6) Avoid simultaneous administration of medications that have the same or similar side effects.

HUMAN PAPILLOMAVIRUS INFECTION

Genital infection with human papillomaviruses is one of the leading causes of benign disease of the vulva, vagina, and cervix. The incidence is not known. Although it is sexually transmitted, genital papillomavirus infection is not a reportable sexually transmitted disease. Various indirect measurements are consistent with the view that the incidence increased fivefold during the decade of the 70s and continued to increase during the 80s.

The virus itself is a member of the papovavirus family. It has been difficult to characterize because it cannot be grown in cell cultures. Nevertheless, DNA hybridization techniques have allowed identification of over 50 different types of human papillomavirus which appear to be antigenically distinct.

The virus is capable of infecting squamous epithelium, where it ordinarily induces papillomatous proliferation. The skin tumors that result are known as condylomata acuminata, or genital warts. Papillomavirus types 6 and 11 are typically found in classic condylomata acuminata, but types 16, 18, 31, and 33 tend to occur in condylomas with accompanying atypias, dysplasia, carcinoma in situ, and invasive cancer.

The virus is capable of causing a second type of lesion in which the infected cells do not form a raised condyloma but rather a more nearly macular lesion known as a flat condyloma. Both types of lesions may be seen anywhere in the lower genital tract, but the virus has a propensity for causing condylomata acuminata on the vulva and flat condylomata on the cervix.

CONDYLOMATA ACUMINATA

Condylomata acuminata appear as exophytic, warty growths with a cauliflower-like appearance (Figure 6–3). Individual lesions are typically small, but they may coalesce to form bulky, warty excrescences. Any portion of the vulva may be affected. Perianal and anal involvement also may occur. In the vagina, the lesions tend to be small and multiple, some being clearly visible only with the aid of a colposcope. The introitus is commonly studded with small condylomata. Classic condylomata acuminata of the cervix are not common. Condylomata tend to increase in size during pregnancy and in association with immunodeficiency or poor hygiene, but the natural history is unpredictable. Left untreated, they may regress spontaneously or persist and spread. Occasionally, the differentiation between condylomata acuminata and the condyloma lata of secondary syphilis cannot be made clinically. In such cases, serologic testing should be done before therapy is started.

Therapy is aimed at elimination of the visible lesions. There is no specific antiviral therapy. Intralesional or parenteral interferon has been used with some success and may be tried in patients with severe or recurrent problems. More typically, however, the options for therapy vary from topical application of cauterizing agents such as podophyllum resin or trichloroacetic acid to local ablation by cryotherapy to laser vaporization to surgical excision. The choice of therapy is based on the number and location of lesions and whether they are primary or recurrent. The use of fluorouracil cream has proved to be beneficial in the treatment of multiple small condylomas of the vagina or cervix.

FLAT CONDYLOMA

Flat condylomata are typically the expression of papillomavirus infection of the cervix. Much less frequently, they may be found on the vaginal epithelium or on the vulva. The pathognomonic cytologic finding is that of koilocytosis, an empty or hollow-appearing cytoplasm surrounding an atypical nucleus. Koilocytosis tends to be prominent in the superficial and intermediate layers of the cervix and is therefore frequently seen by cytologists examining Papanicolaou smears. If the cytologist also observes nuclear atypia and cellular disorganization, the Pap smear will be read as consistent with dysplasia. In the absence of nuclear changes, the smear may be read as koilocytosis or koilocytotic atypia. While papillomavirus types 16, 18, 31, and 33 have been associated with the presence of dysplasia, the oncogenicity of the virus has been difficult to determine. Since 70–90% of cervical intraepithelial neoplasias and invasive cancers contain demonstrable papillomavirus structural antigens, the association is well established. Most investigators currently believe that the virus is probably an important cofactor in the etiology of squamous epithelial carcinogenesis but not necessarily a carcinogen. Flat condylomata are asymp-

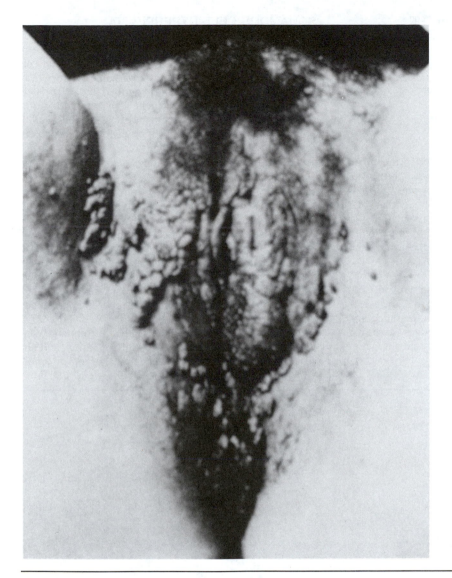

Figure 6–3. Vulvar condylomata acuminata. (Reproduced, with permission, from Lichtman R, Papera S: *Gynecology Well-Woman Care.* Appleton & Lange, 1990.)

tomatic, and unless the patient has coexistent condylomata acuminata of the vulva, the most likely presentation will be that of an abnormal Papanicolaou smear.

Some of these lesions may be visually detected as white patches on the cervix after application of 3% acetic acid. Most flat condylomata, however, will be subclinical. *Any patient with cytologic evidence of papillomavirus infection on a cervical smear or with evidence of vaginal or vulvar condyloma should undergo careful colposcopic evaluation of the cervix.* Biopsies must be performed to rule out coexistent intraepithelial neoplasia, particularly if the flat condyloma is near the squamocolumnar junction.

Therapy is aimed at eradicating the lesion by cryotherapy, laser vaporization, excisional biopsy, and fluorouracil cream. Evaluation and treatment of sexual partners is recommended in the event of recurrence.

VULVAR DYSTROPHY

Confusion has surrounded the nomenclature of several clinicopathologic vulvar skin conditions now grouped under the term vulvar dystrophy. By definition, the term "dystrophy" connotes abnormal nourishment of cells. The classification scheme recommended by the International Society for the Study of Vulvar Disease is shown in Table 6–2.

Vulvar dystrophy is a problem of postmenopausal women, though it may occasionally occur at a younger age. The cause is unknown, and the pathogenesis is poorly

Table 6–2. Classification of vulval dystrophies.[1]

I. Squamous cell hyperplasias (formerly hyperplastic dystrophy).
II. Lichen sclerosus.
III. Other dermatoses.

[1]International Society for the Study of Vulvar Disease.

understood. Controversy has existed as to the malignant potential of these lesions. Most vulvar dystrophies were considered premalignant in the older literature, whereas current knowledge is consistent with the view that their malignant potential is no more than 5%. This small malignant potential is realized only over a prolonged period of time, and in most verified cases the initial diagnostic biopsies have contained evidence of hyperplasia with or without atypia.

The most common complaint is vulvar pruritus, but patients may complain also of burning and dyspareunia. The lesions typically are white in appearance and may be extensive. Biopsy is required in every case, not only to establish the diagnosis, but also to rule out malignancy.

SQUAMOUS CELL HYPERPLASIA

Squamous cell hyperplasia is characterized by a thickened, keratinized white surface most frequently found on the labia, interlabial sulci, or posterior commissure. Occasionally it may appear as a poorly defined, red, excoriated lesion. Microscopic findings include hyperkeratosis and acantholysis, and cellular atypia may be present as well.

Treatment consists of application of topical corticosteroids, such as 1% hydrocortisone cream. In cases showing severe atypia, wide local excision is recommended.

LICHEN SCLEROSUS

Lichen sclerosus is the most common white lesion of the vulva. It usually affects both sides, presenting initially as white macules or coalescent plaques (Figure 6–4). At later stages, there is progressive atrophy of the epithelium, with destruction of the labial anatomy and development of fissures, synechiae, and introital stenosis which precludes intercourse in severe cases.

Microscopic features include epithelial thinning, with flattening of the rete pegs, edema, inflammation, and absence of elastic fibers. Treatment consists of topical appli-

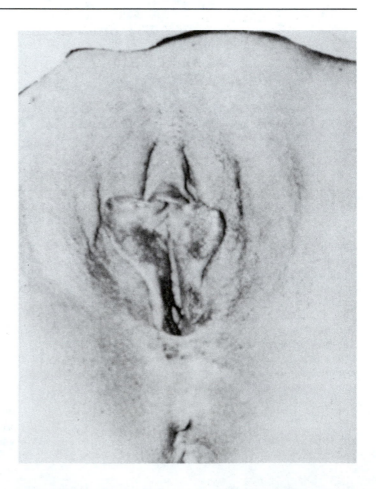

Figure 6–4. Lichen sclerosus. Whitish patches on labia minora and at fourchette. (Reproduced, with permission, from Lichtman R, Papera S: *Gynecology Well-Woman Care.* Appleton & Lange, 1990.)

cation of 2% testosterone propionate. Topical progesterone cream also has been advocated.

In some women, hyperplastic epithelium and lichen sclerosus coexist. This condition was formerly called mixed dystrophy and is associated with a higher incidence of atypical cellular changes seen at biopsy than is reported in either of the pure dystrophies. Treatment consists of a combination of corticosteroids and testosterone applications.

VULVAR CONDITIONS OF APOCRINE SWEAT GLAND ORIGIN

FOX-FORDYCE DISEASE

Fox-Fordyce disease consists of formation of multiple microcysts secondary to obstruction of apocrine gland ducts, with ensuing retention of sweat. The obstruction is due to hyperkeratinization of the follicular epithelium. The cause is not known. The lesions are most frequently seen over the mons, and the main symptom is pruritus. Topical estrogen creams, corticosteroids, and tretinoin (Retin-A) can be used for symptomatic treatment.

HIDRADENITIS SUPPURATIVA

Hidradenitis suppurativa is a chronic disorder caused by ductal obstruction and secondary infection of the apocrine glands (Figure 6–5). Initial symptoms usually are itching and burning. Later, the condition is characterized by multiple nodules, sinus tracts, abscesses, and scar tissue. Recurrent abscesses may appear and may drain spontaneously. Treatment is based on local hygiene, systemic antibiotics, and surgical drainage of infected areas. Significant scarring may occur in patients with recurrent hidradenitis.

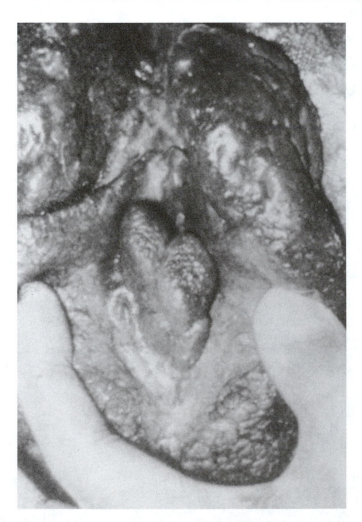

Figure 6–5. Hidradenitis suppurativa with distortion of the vulva. (Reproduced, with permission, from Lichtman R, Papera S: *Gynecology Well-Woman Care.* Appleton & Lange, 1990.)

BARTHOLIN GLAND CYST

Bartholin gland cyst is the most common benign vulvar tumor. The most important etiologic factor is obstruction of the opening of the main duct into the vestibule, with resulting enlargement. Small uncomplicated cysts are frequently asymptomatic. If they become large or infected (Bartholin abscess), symptoms such as pain and dyspareunia will rapidly develop. Most such cysts occur in the posterior part of the labia majora, and they may be clearly visible and easily palpable (Figure 6–6).

Therapy is not required for small asymptomatic cysts. Those that enlarge or form abscesses should be treated surgically. Marsupialization is the most successful surgical technique and is preferable to surgical excision of the gland, which may result in significant morbidity. Abscesses can also be drained via a Word catheter or pediatric Foley catheter.

CONDITIONS ASSOCIATED WITH IN UTERO EXPOSURE TO DIETHYLSTILBESTROL

Vaginal adenosis and malformations of the uterine cervix and corpus occur in about 20% of women who were exposed to diethylstilbestrol in utero. Both conditions are exceedingly rare except in association with diethylstilbestrol exposure (see also Chapter 5).

VAGINAL ADENOSIS

Vaginal adenosis consists of the presence of columnar epithelium and its secretory products within the vagina. It is often asymptomatic, though some patients complain of a profuse mucoid vaginal discharge. Careful evaluation of the entire vaginal canal is indicated and requires rotation of the speculum blades during the pelvic examination. Application of acetic acid allows easier identification of the lesions both visually and with the colposcope. Grossly, the lesions present as red patches on the vaginal mucosa, and at colposcopy there is a typical grapelike appearance. Biopsies should be obtained to confirm the diagnosis.

This lesion requires no treatment unless the vaginal discharge is incapacitating, but close follow-up is recommended because of the potential for malignant transformation to clear cell adenocarcinoma.

CERVICAL MALFORMATIONS

The most frequent macroscopic changes seen in the cervix of diethylstilbestrol-exposed women are the cocks comb (hood), collar (rim), and pseudopolyp. Biopsy usually reveals the presence of mucinous columnar cells with some degree of squamous metaplasia. Most women are asymptomatic, though an occasional patient may complain of mucous discharge.

Treatment is not required.

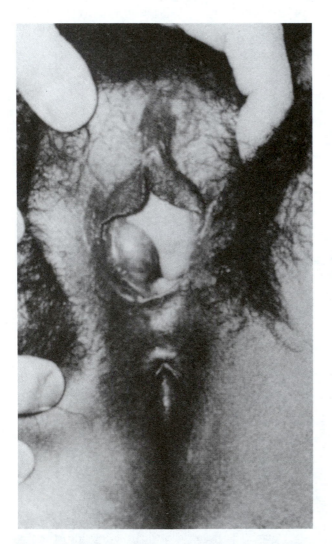

Figure 6–6. Bartholin gland cyst. (Reproduced, with permission, from Lichtman R, Papera S: *Gynecology Well-Woman Care.* Appleton & Lange, 1990.)

SELECTED READINGS

Friedrich DW Jr: Vulvar dystrophy. Clin Obstet Gynecol 1985;28:178.

Gardner HL, Kaufman RH: *Benign Diseases of the Vulva and Vagina.* GK Hall, 1981.

Kaufman RH, Faro S: Infectious diseases of the vulva and vagina. In: *Pathology of the Vulva and Vagina.* Wilkinson EJ (editor). Churchill Livingstone, 1987.

Kurman RJ (editor): *Blaustein's Pathology of the Female Genital Tract,* 3rd ed. Springer-Verlag, 1987.

Oriel JD: Genitoanal papillomavirus infection—a diagnostic and therapeutic dilemma. Semin Dermatol 1990;9(2):141.

Rodke G, Friedrich EG Jr, Wilkinson EJ: Malignant potential of mixed vulvar dystrophy. J Reprod Med 1988;33:454.

Welch WR et al: Pathology of colposcopic findings in 2635 diethylstilbestrol-exposed women. Gynecol Oncol 1985;21:277.

Woodruff JD: Noninfectious diseases of the vulva. In: *Ambulatory Gynecology.* Nichols DH, Evrard JR (editors). Harper & Row, 1985.

Woodruff JD: Noninfectious diseases of the vulva and vagina. In: *Obstetrics and Gynecology,* 5th ed. Danforth DN, Scott JR (editors). Lippincott, 1986.

zur Hausen H: Papillomaviruses in anogenital cancer as a model to understand the role of viruses in human cancers. Cancer Res 1989;49:4677.

7

Sexually Transmitted Diseases

A wide variety of diseases are attributable to bacterial and viral infections primarily acquired during sexual contact. These diseases are increasing in reported incidence at an alarming rate, undoubtedly because of increased sexual activity at younger ages, permissive sexual attitudes, the availability of effective contraception and abortion services, and increased physician awareness. Those at highest risk are young unmarried women with multiple sex partners. The most frequently encountered sexually transmitted diseases include bacterial infections caused by *Neisseria gonorrhoeae, Chlamydia trachomatis, Treponema pallidum, Haemophilus ducreyi,* and *Calymmatobacterium granulomatis* and viral infections caused by human papillomaviruses (Chapter 6), herpes simplex virus, and human immunodeficiency virus (AIDS). In most states, gonorrhea, syphilis, hepatitis, and AIDS are diseases that must be reported to appropriate health authorities. According to the Centers for Disease Control, the incidence of acute pelvic inflammatory disease is decreasing.

NEISSERIA GONORRHOEAE INFECTION

Neisseria gonorrhoeae is a gram-negative diplococcus specially adapted to thrive in moist columnar or transitional epithelium. It is a fragile organism, frequently not surviving sensitivity testing after isolation from culture material, so that a special culture medium (Thayer-Martin, Martin-Lester) is required. *N gonorrhoeae* is one of the few known pathogens that will infect the human uterine (fallopian) tube. When this organism is present, the bacterial agents of other sexually transmitted diseases such as *C trachomatis* and *Treponema pallidum* should be sought also. Up to 90% of women who are exposed to *N gonorrhoeae* will be colonized briefly; without therapy, only 10–20% will develop symptoms. Since gonococcal colonization (infection) is usually asymptomatic, cultures should be performed in all patients. Culture material for *N gonorrhoeae* is obtained with a sterile cotton swab from any area suspected of colonization. This material is transferred and applied to the special culture media mentioned above. Gonorrhea is a reportable disease. The endocervix

is the primary culture site. If there is no cervix, the distal urethra is the site to culture.

Clinical Findings

A. Symptoms and Signs: In many cases, colonization with *N gonorrhoeae* is asymptomatic, but symptomatic disease may follow after an incubation period of 2–7 days. Symptoms depend on the site involved, but usually there is pain and a purulent discharge. Affected organs include Bartholin's glands, Skene's glands, the urethra, the rectum, the endocervix, the endometrium and uterine tubes, the conjunctiva, and the oropharynx. Examination may show no abnormalities, or there may be swelling, erythema, tenderness, or purulent discharge. Abscesses may develop in Bartholin's or Skene's glands or in the oviducts. Prepubertal girls who develop gonococcal vulvovaginitis should be considered victims of sexual abuse until proven otherwise (see Chapter 13).

B. Laboratory Findings: The presumptive diagnosis of gonococcal infection is made by Gram stain, which shows intracellular gram-negative diplococci; by identifying oxidase-positive gram-negative diplococci from selective culture media; or by selective culture without specific carbohydrate fermentation testing. Definitive diagnosis is made by selective media culture with specific carbohydrate fermentation testing. In all cases, testing for β-lactamase enzyme production is desirable.

Complications

Systemic complications are uncommon but include the dermatitis-arthritis syndrome of tenosynovitis and dermatitis as well as purulent arthritis, endocarditis, and meningitis. A more common complication is salpingitis, which may progress to tubo-ovarian or pelvic abscess. Long-term sequelae of tubal infection include infertility, ectopic pregnancy, and chronic pelvic pain. Perihepatitis may occur as a result of gonococcal salpingitis; it may occur also in the absence of *N gonorrhoeae* or other sexually transmitted pathogens.

Treatment

Treatment for gonococcal infection depends on its location and severity. Current regimens recommended for the treatment of *N gonorrhoeae* infection, however, are not predictably curative for incubating syphilis. It is imperative to search for additional sexually transmitted diseases if one such disease is diagnosed. For example, adequate therapy for gonorrhea may result in partial treatment of syphilis. For that reason, it is very important to test for the presence of syphilis at the time of treatment for gonorrhea; 4–6 weeks later, the patient should be retested for evidence of infection with *T pallidum*. Beta-lactamase enzyme-producing strains of *N gonorrhoeae* are increasing, and their identification is important—especially if women are treated with penicillin, to which such strains are resistant. These strains of gonorrhea have been identified in southeast Asian immigrants and military personnel who have served in this area.

A. Uncomplicated Gonorrhea (Outpatient): Treatment regimens for uncomplicated gonorrhea are set out in Table 7–1. These regimens should be followed by doxycycline, 100 mg twice daily for 7 days, to cover *C trachomatis* infection. Tetracycline, 500 mg orally 4 times a day, may be substituted for doxycycline. Quinolones and tetracyclines should not be given to pregnant women; erythromycin or azithromycin is appropriate.

B. Complicated Gonorrhea (Hospitalization Recommended):

1. Disseminated—For disseminated disease, one of the third-generation cephalosporins is recommended as set forth in Table 7–1. Therapy may be switched to ampicillin or an equivalent if the species is sensitive and does not produce β-lactamase enzyme. Patients allergic to cephalosporins or who have a history of anaphylaxis to penicillin should be treated with spectinomycin, 2 g intramuscularly every 12 hours.

2. Endocarditis or meningitis—Give ceftriaxone as recommended in Table 7–1, with cardiologic or neurologic consultation.

3. Salpingitis—See Table 7–1 for drugs and dosages. Therapy should be continued for at least 48 hours after clinical improvement and then followed by doxycycline, 100 mg orally every 12 hours, for a total of 10–14 days of therapy.

C. Treatment of Sex Partners: Sex partners of women infected with *N gonorrhoeae* should be evaluated for gonococcal as well as other sexually transmitted diseases and treated empirically. If testing for *Chlamydia* is not performed, therapy should be given. Test-of-cure cultures are unnecessary after cephalosporin therapy. Experience is limited with quinolone therapy, and repeat culture 4–7 days after therapy is recommended, especially if there is pharyngeal disease.

CHLAMYDIA TRACHOMATIS INFECTION

The etiologic agent of **lymphogranuloma venereum** is *Chlamydia trachomatis*. Chlamydiae are bacteria with a cell wall similar to that of gram-negative bacteria. They are similar to viruses in that they can be grown only intracellularly and in tissue cultures. Except for L serotypes, chlamydiae invade only columnar epithelial cells. The population at risk for colonization and infection by chlamydiae is similar to that at risk for gonorrhea, ie, young single women with multiple sex partners (see Table 7–2).

Clinical Findings

A. Symptoms and Signs: Infected women may be asymptomatic or may have pain and discharge from affected sites. The organism may involve the urethra, Bartholin's glands, the rectum, the endocervix, the endometrium and uterine tubes, the conjunctiva, the oropharynx, the vulva, or the lung. Physical examination may disclose no abnormalities, or there may be a purulent discharge, erythema, and tenderness in affected areas. Children may develop vulvovaginitis.

B. Laboratory Findings: The diagnosis is usually made by fluorescent antibody testing of material taken by direct smear. This test is preferable to others because the results are available in only 20–40 minutes, sensitivity is usually over 90%, and specificity is 95% if the specimen has many columnar cells, few red blood cells, and little mucus, and if the patient is symptomatic. Although tissue culture has the highest sensitivity, it is also the most costly and time-consuming.

Complications

Complications of chlamydial salpingitis include infertility, ectopic pregnancy, and chronic pelvic pain. Peritoneal dissemination of salpingitis may cause perihepatitis, as is true for gonorrhea also. Infection in a pregnant woman may cause preterm labor, and the neonate may be infected in the birth canal, with resultant conjunctivitis or pneumonia.

Table 7–1. Treatment of gonorrhea.

Severity	Drug and Dosage
Uncomplicated (outpatient)	Ceftriaxone, 250 mg IM once (preferable) Ceftizoxime, 500 mg IM once Cefotaxime, 1 g IM once Ciprofloxacin, 500 mg PO once Norfloxacin, 800 mg PO once Cefuroxime axetil, 1 g PO once, with 1 g probenecid Spectinomycin, 2 g IM once
Complicated (inpatient) Disseminated	Ceftriaxone, 1 g IM or IV every 24 hours Ceftizoxime, 1 g IV every 8 hours Cefotaxime, 1 g IV every 8 hours
Endocarditis or meningitis	Ceftriaxone, 1–2 g IV every 12 hours for 2–4 weeks
Salpingitis	Cefoxitin, 2 g IV every 6 hours, *or* Cefotetan, 2 g IV every 12 hours, *plus* Doxycycline, 100 mg IV or PO every 12 hours, *or* Clindamycin, 900 mg IV every 8 hours, *plus* Gentamicin, 2 mg/kg IV as loading dose, then 1.5 mg/kg IV every 8 hours

Treatment

Because of its growth characteristics, chlamydial infections must be treated for at least 7 days. The drug of choice is doxycycline, 100 mg orally twice daily for 7 days, or tetracycline, 500 mg orally 4 times daily for 7 days. Alternative therapy for pregnant women or those allergic to tetracyclines is with erythromycin base, 500 mg orally 4 times daily for 7 days, or erythromycin ethylsuccinate, 800 mg orally 4 times daily for 7 days; or sulfisoxazole, 500 mg orally 4 times daily for 10 days, if erythromycin is not tolerated. Azithromycin is effective at a one time oral 1 g dose; it is expensive, but compliance can be guaranteed if furnished to the patient at the encounter.

Sexual partners (contact within 30 days) should be tested, and treated if positive. They should be treated if testing cannot be achieved. Test-of-cure cultures are unnecessary.

TREPONEMA PALLIDUM INFECTION

The incidence of syphilis is increasing. A 4-year period of decreasing incidence from 1982 to 1986 was followed by a 30% increase between 1986 and 1989. All persons at risk for sexually transmitted diseases should be tested for syphilis.

The etiologic agent of syphilis is *Treponema pallidum.* Between 10 and 90 days after treponemes gain access to the lymphatics and bloodstream through breaks in the skin or intact mucosal surfaces, evidence of primary infection appears as a chancre at the site of inoculation. If treatment is not given, signs of secondary syphilis appear as a generalized rash about 6 weeks later (2 weeks to 6 months). Even without treatment, this rash will disappear in 2–6 weeks. The infection may then become latent and remain so. Tertiary syphilis develops 4–20 or more years after untreated initial infection.

Sexual partners of patients with early syphilis should be evaluated clinically and serologically and treated presumptively if the exposure occurred within the preceding 90 days.

Clinical Findings

A. Symptoms and Signs: The manifestations of syphilis depend on the stage of infection. Primary syphilis is characterized by a painless indurated papule or ulcer with raised borders appearing anywhere on the mucous membranes or skin (Table 7–2). The characteristic dermatitis of secondary syphilis appears as a papulosquamous eruption that involves the soles and palms; the trunk may also be involved by a macular, maculopapular, or pustular rash. It is frequently accompanied by a viral-like syndrome of nonspecific symptoms and diffuse adenopathy. In latent syphilis, there may be recurrent episodes similar to those of secondary syphilis, though in most cases latent syphilis is asymptomatic.

B. Laboratory Findings: Only about 30% of those exposed become clinically infected. Definitive diagnosis is by darkfield examination or direct fluorescent antibody testing of material from an early lesion. Several presumptive serologic tests are in use, including the fluorescent treponemal antibody absorption (FTA-ABS) test, the microhemagglutination assay for antibody to *T pallidum* (MHATP), and nontreponemal tests in which the titer correlates with disease activity. Nontreponemal tests become positive 4–6 weeks after infection and include the Venereal Disease Research Laboratory (VDRL) and rapid plasma reagin (RPR) tests. It should be noted that false-positive VDRLs may occur in patients with connective tissue diseases and other patients with antiphospholipid antibodies in their plasma.

Complications

Most complications of syphilis result from failure to diagnose and treat. These complications involve not only the cardiovascular and central nervous systems but also the skeleton, skin, upper respiratory tract (nose, throat,

Table 7–2. Sexually transmitted diseases presenting as genital ulcers.

	Syphilis	Chancroid	Herpes Simplex	Lymphogranuloma Venereum	Granuloma Inguinale
Etiologic agent	*Treponema pallidum*	*Haemophilus ducreyi*	HSV-2	*Chlamydia trachomatis* L1–L3	*Calymmatobacterium granulomatis*
Primary lesion	Papule	Erythematous papule or pustule	Vesicle	Papule, pustule, or vesicle	Papule
Border	Sharp	Erythematous and undermined	Erythematous	Variable	Rolled and elevated
Depth	Superficial	Excavated	Superficial	Superficial	Elevated
Base	Red, smooth	Yellow, gray	Red, smooth	Variable	Red, rough
Secretion	Serous	Purulent, hemorrhagic	Serous	Variable	Scant
Induration	Firm	Soft	None	None	Firm
Number	Usually one	One to three	Multiple, may coalesce	One	One or more
Pain	Rare	Often	Common	Variable	Rare
Lymph nodes	Firm, nontender	Tender, may suppurate	Firm, tender	Tender, may suppurate	Enlarged

and larynx), oral mucous membranes, eye, liver, stomach, and lymph nodes.

Treatment

The treatment for syphilis depends on the stage and is characterized generally by protracted courses of penicillin in low doses.

A. Early Syphilis (Primary, Secondary, and Latent Less Than 1 Year):

1. Recommended–Benzathine penicillin G, 2.4 million units intramuscularly once.

2. Alternative for penicillin-allergic nonpregnant patients–Doxycycline, 100 mg orally twice daily for 14 days, or tetracycline, 500 mg orally 4 times daily for 14 days.

3. Alternative for pregnant (or any) patient– Erythromycin, 500 mg orally 4 times daily for 14 days, or ceftriaxone, 250 mg intramuscularly daily for 10 days.

B. Late Latent Syphilis (More Than 1 Year) or Cardiovascular Involvement:

1. Recommended–Benzathine penicillin G, 2.4 million units intramuscularly weekly for 3 weeks.

2. Alternative for penicillin-allergic nonpregnant patients–Same as for early syphilis.

C. Neurosyphilis:

1. Recommended–Aqueous crystalline penicillin G, 2–4 million units intravenously every 4 hours for 10–14 days.

2. Alternative (compliant patients)–Procaine penicillin, 2–4 million units intramuscularly daily for 10–14 days, plus probenecid, 500 mg orally 4 times daily for 10–14 days.

HAEMOPHILUS DUCREYI INFECTION

Genital *Haemophilus ducreyi* infections (chancroid) are increasing in prevalence. Outside the United States, chancroid is associated with increased rates of HIV infection. Other sexually transmitted diseases should be sought also. The incubation period is 2–5 days. Chancroid is a reportable disease.

Clinical Findings

A. Symptoms and Signs: Clinical findings include painful vulvar ulcers with a profuse contagious discharge; there is painful inguinal adenitis in over half of cases. Physical findings include a pustule that becomes a ragged ulcer surrounded by an erythematous wheal and associated regional lymphadenopathy.

B. Laboratory Findings: Definitive diagnosis is by culture using selective media; however, the organism is difficult to isolate. Clinical diagnosis is more practical.

Treatment

Treatment consists of inculcating habits of good personal hygiene plus antibiotic therapy with erythromycin base, 500 mg orally 4 times daily for 7 days, or ceftriaxone, 250 mg intramuscularly once. Alternative regimens include trimethoprim-sulfamethoxazole, 160/800 mg orally twice daily for 7 days; or amoxicillin-clavulanic acid, 500/125 mg orally 3 times daily for 7 days; or ciprofloxacin, 500 mg orally twice daily for 3 days.

Ulcers usually heal within 7 days, though it takes longer for adenopathy to regress. It may be necessary to drain the lymph nodes if they become fluctuant. This is best performed with needle aspiration through healthy adjacent skin rather than over the involved lymph node. Needle aspiration will greatly decrease the likelihood of fistula formation.

Sexual partners should be treated, as is true for all sexually transmitted diseases.

CALYMMATOBACTERIUM GRANULOMATIS INFECTION (GRANULOMA INGUINALE)

Infection with *Calymmatobacterium granulomatis* infection is rare in the United States. It is a chronic ulcerative granulomatous infection that affects the vulva, perineum, and inguinal regions. When the bacteria are encapsulated in mononuclear leukocytes, they are called Donovan bodies. The incubation period is 8–12 weeks.

Clinical Findings

A. Symptoms and Signs: Symptoms include painful ulcers on the vulva, perineum, or inguinal areas associated with a malodorous discharge. On physical examination, there are ulcers with a beefy-red base and clear, sharp edges. In late infection, inguinal lymph nodes may suppurate (buboes). Cervical lesions may mimic cervical carcinoma.

B. Laboratory Findings: Diagnosis is by identification of Donovan bodies with Wright's, Giemsa's, or silver stain.

Treatment

Treatment is with one of several bacteriostatic drugs for a minimum of 14 days: tetracycline, 500 mg orally 4 times daily for 14–21 days; doxycycline, 100 mg orally twice daily for 14–21 days; or erythromycin, 500 mg orally 4 times daily for 14–21 days.

HERPES SIMPLEX VIRUS INFECTION

Ninety percent of genital herpes simplex infection is due to herpes simplex virus type 2, with the remaining 10% due to type 1. It is endemic in the United States, and the incidence is highest in young, sexually active women. Susceptible individuals can acquire herpes from an asymptomatic carrier and may have severe infections. The incubation period is about 6 days and the attack rate about 70%.

Clinical Findings

A. Symptoms and Signs: The initial infection in the seronegative person is characterized by severe vulvar pain, burning, and pruritus, with urinary frequency and dysuria. There is usually fever, headache, and malaise. Clinical findings include single or multiple vesicles that rupture and form small, extremely tender ulcers, which may coalesce. Tender adenopathy may be present. The ulcers may take up to 1 month to heal completely. If the initial clinical infection occurs in a seropositive patient, these findings are attenuated. Thereafter, recurrent lesions show marked variation in the intensity, frequency, and duration of symptoms. For example, the average duration of a lesion is 7 days.

B. Laboratory Findings: A presumptive diagnosis is made clinically and by cytological techniques. Definitive diagnosis is made by isolation of virus in tissue culture.

Treatment

Supportive treatment is important and includes pain relief. Acyclovir therapy may attenuate these infections:

A. Primary Infection:

1. Outpatient–Acyclovir, 200 mg orally 5 times daily for 7–10 days.

2. Inpatient–Acyclovir, 5 mg/kg intravenously every 8 hours for 5–7 days or until resolution occurs.

B. Recurrent Episodes: If symptoms are severe, the following may be used: acyclovir, 200 mg orally 5 times daily for 5 days or 800 mg orally twice daily for 5 days. For individuals who have more than six episodes per year, daily suppressive doses of acyclovir (200 mg 2–5 times daily or 400 mg twice daily) may reduce the frequency of recurrences by at least 75%.

HUMAN IMMUNODEFICIENCY VIRUS INFECTION

By 1991, there were over 600,000 known cases of acquired immunodeficiency syndrome (AIDS) in the United States, the end result of infection caused by human immunodeficiency virus (HIV). Moreover, the Centers for Disease Control estimated that between 0.8 and 1.2 million persons in the United States had been infected by that time. This infection is most prevalent in homosexual or bisexual men, intravenous drug abusers, and hemophiliacs. Only about 10% of cases of AIDS in the United States have occurred in women, and most of these cases were clustered in the large metropolitan areas of New York City, New Jersey, and Miami. The majority were in women of reproductive age, which means that heterosexual and perinatal transmission are significant concerns. AIDS is a reportable disease.

As is true also for other types of sexually transmitted diseases, those at the highest risk are young, single women who may be intravenous drug abusers, contacts of men in high-risk groups, recipients of unscreened transfusions, and prostitutes.

The chance of acquiring HIV infection through sexual contact is unknown. Only about 5% of the cases reported to the Centers for Disease Control could have been acquired through heterosexual contact. There is a high concentration of the virus in semen, and coitus may cause breaks in introital mucosa. For these reasons, heterosexual infection is more often male-to-female than female-to-male. The presence of associated genital ulcer disease (Table 7–2) greatly increases the risk of infection because of the disrupted mucosa. The number of exposures to high-risk sexual partners and engaging in anal-receptive intercourse also increase the risk for infection. Heterosexual transmission and infection in women is the most rapidly expanding problem area.

Clinical Findings

A. Symptoms and Signs: The latent period between viral exposure and seroconversion is unknown but is estimated to be about 12 weeks. Between 45% and 90% of patients develop acute symptoms during the first few weeks after infection. Presentation is similar to that of mononucleosis, and symptoms may include an erythematous maculopapular rash, lymphadenopathy, pharyngitis, night sweats, fever, and weight loss. These manifestations resolve in several weeks without specific treatment. The interval between such an episode and development of the signs or symptoms of AIDS varies considerably, but about half of those infected become symptomatic within 10 years. The mortality rate of AIDS is presumed to be 100%, but this may be reduced somewhat by newly developed antiviral agents such as zidovudine (azidothymidine, AZT).

B. Laboratory Findings: Serologic testing for immunodeficiency virus should be conducted on persons at high risk or for those who request it. Pre- and post-test counseling about the interpretation of the tests is mandatory. Consent is obtained from the patient, and confidentiality must be maintained. Testing should be offered to the following groups: (1) women who consider themselves at risk for any reason, (2) women who received blood transfusions between 1978 and 1985, (3) women with infected sex partners or who are otherwise at risk for infection, (4) women undergoing medical evaluation or treatment for clinical signs or symptoms of HIV infection, (5) women who have lived in communities where prevalence of this infection was high, (6) women who have been correctional system inmates, (7) women who have sexually transmitted diseases, (8) women who have engaged in prostitution, and (9) women who have used intravenous drugs.

Antibody testing for immunodeficiency viral infection begins with a screening test, usually an enzyme-linked immunosorbent assay (ELISA). If the screening test is positive, it must be followed by a more specific confirmatory test. At present, the Western blot assay is commonly used.

Prevention

Prevention of HIV infection is currently the only realistic hope for control. Education of those potentially at risk and counseling for detection of the infection are difficult tasks that are the responsibility of all physicians. Behavior modification may be extremely difficult but should be attempted. Safety factors include reduction in the number of sexual partners, avoidance of partners who are in high-risk groups, use of condoms, and not sharing needles for intravenous drug abuse.

Nonoxynol-9 is a spermatocide that inactivates the virus in vitro. Whether it actually provides additional protection in actual use is speculative. It is used as a lubricant for many latex condoms.

Seropositive patients should be counseled about avoiding pregnancy, staying in a mutually monogamous sexual relationship, refraining from donation of blood, organs, or tissue, and using condoms lubricated with nonoxynol-9.

The treatment of established AIDS is beyond the scope of this book. Such patients do have a higher prevalence of pelvic inflammatory disease and *candidiasis* and should be screened more often for these diseases and when identified, aggressively treated. Clinics specializing in the counseling and treatment of patients who become seropositive and then develop clinical infection are expanding nationally.

SELECTED READINGS

Centers for Disease Control: 1989 sexually transmitted diseases treatment guidelines. MMWR 1989;38:S8.

Holmes KK et al: *Sexually Transmitted Diseases,* 2nd ed. McGraw-Hill, 1990.

8

Ectopic Pregnancy

The reproductive loss associated with failure of proper nidation has increased steadily for the past 15 years. Today, more than one in every 100 pregnancies in the United States is ectopic. The risk of death from an extrauterine pregnancy is 10 times greater than the risk associated with vaginal delivery and 50 times greater than that associated with induced abortion. Moreover, the prognosis for successful pregnancy is reduced significantly for women who have had one ectopic pregnancy—especially for primigravidas over age 30.

The key to effective management is early diagnosis, which is essential both for maternal survival and for conservation of reproductive capacity.

GENERAL CONSIDERATIONS

Definition

In a normal intrauterine pregnancy, the blastocyst implants in the endometrial lining of the uterine cavity. Implantation anywhere else constitutes ectopic pregnancy. Over 95% of ectopic pregnancies involve the uterine tubes.

Etiology

The following have been implicated as causes of ectopic pregnancy:

A. Mechanical Factors: Mechanical factors may prevent or retard the passage of the fertilized ovum into the uterine cavity.

1. Salpingitis–especially endosalpingitis, which causes agglutination of the arborescent folds of the tubal mucosa with narrowing of the lumen or formation of blind pockets.

2. Peritubal adhesions subsequent to postabortal or puerperal infection, appendicitis, or endometriosis, which cause kinking of the tube and narrowing of the lumen.

3. Developmental abnormalities of the tube, especially diverticula, accessory ostia, and hypoplasia.

4. Previous ectopic pregnancy–After one ectopic pregnancy, the incidence of another is 7–15%. The increased risk is probably due to previous salpingitis.

5. Previous operations on the tube, either to restore patency or, occasionally, the failure of sterilization.

6. Multiple previous induced abortions, increase the risk of ectopic pregnancy. The risk is unchanged after one induced abortion but doubled after two or more—probably as a result of small but significant increases in the incidence of salpingitis.

7. Tumors that distort the tube, such as uterine myomas and adnexal masses.

8. Tubal pregnancies are not increased by abnormal embryos.

9. Current use of intrauterine devices.

B. Functional Factors: Functional factors are those that delay passage of the fertilized ovum into the uterine cavity. Altered tubal motility may follow changes in serum levels of estrogens and progesterone—a change in the number and affinity of adrenergic receptors in uterine and tubal smooth muscle is probably responsible. An increased incidence of ectopic pregnancies has been reported after the use of progestin-only oral contraceptives in women who were exposed in utero to diethylstilbestrol.

External migration of the ovum is probably not an important factor except in cases of abnormal paramesonephric duct development resulting in hemiuterus with an attached noncommunicating rudimentary uterine horn (Chapter 5). Menstrual reflux has been suggested as a cause.

C. Tubal Mucosal Factors: Increase in receptivity of the tubal mucosa to the fertilized ovum favors tubal pregnancy. Ectopic endometrial elements may enhance tubal implantation.

Incidence

In the United States from 1970 through 1983, the rate of ectopic pregnancies tripled. The increase was greater for nonwhite than white women, and for both racial groups the incidence has increased with age. In 35- to 44-year-old white women, 1.3 of every 100 pregnancies were ectopic; however, this figure was 2.6 for nonwhite women. In patients under 25 years of age, the incidence of ectopic pregnancy almost doubled in the past decade.

Many cases are due to multiple causes, some of which

can be listed as follows: (1) increased prevalence of sexually transmitted tubal infection; (2) the popularity of contraception, which prevents intrauterine but not extrauterine pregnancies—especially intrauterine devices and perhaps low-dose progestational agents; (3) unsuccessful tubal sterilizations; (4) induced abortion followed by infection; (5) fertility induced by ovulatory agents; (6) previous pelvic surgery, including salpingotomy for tubal pregnancy and tuboplasty; (7) exposure to diethylstilbestrol in utero; and (8) better diagnostic techniques and earlier diagnosis.

Mortality Rate

Deaths from ectopic pregnancy in the United States decreased from 63 in 1970 to 46 in 1980 and 35 in 1983. Unfortunately, the percentage of all maternal deaths attributed to ectopic pregnancy increased from 8% in 1970 to 14% in 1980. *Ectopic pregnancy is now the second leading cause of maternal deaths in the United States.* The risk of death was greater in nonwhite than in white women; however, increasing age was not associated with an increased mortality rate.

In both racial groups, a dramatic fall which continued through 1983 has been documented in the death-to-case rate (Figure 8–1). Even so, it is estimated that the death rate from ectopic pregnancies might be reduced another 50% by even more prompt diagnosis and treatment—ie, another third of the deaths might be prevented if women were to seek earlier care.

ANATOMIC CONSIDERATIONS

The fertilized ovum may develop in any portion of the uterine tube. The ampulla is the most frequent site of implantation and the isthmus the next most common. Interstitial pregnancy is quite uncommon, occurring in only about 3% of all tubal gestations. From these primary types, certain secondary forms of tuboabdominal, tubo-ovarian, and broad ligament pregnancies occasionally develop.

Implantation of the Zygote

The fertilized ovum does not remain on the surface but promptly burrows through the epithelium. As the zygote penetrates the epithelium, it comes to lie in the muscular wall, since the tube lacks a submucosa. At the periphery of the zygote is a capsule of rapidly proliferating trophoblast, which invades and erodes the subjacent muscularis of the tube. The tube does not normally form an extensive decidua, though decidual cells can usually be recognized. The tubal wall in contact with the zygote offers slight resistance to invasion by the trophoblast, which soon burrows through it, opening maternal vessels.

Uterine Changes

In ectopic pregnancies, the uterus undergoes some of the changes associated with early normal pregnancy, including softening of the cervix and isthmus and increase in size. These changes in the uterus do not, therefore, rule out ectopic pregnancy.

In 1954, Arias-Stella described—as had others before him—changes in the endometrium associated with pregnancy. These endometrial changes have been collectively referred to as the **Arias-Stella reaction.** The cellular changes in the Arias-Stella reaction are not specific for ectopic pregnancy but may occur with either intrauterine or extrauterine gestations.

The external bleeding commonly seen in cases of tubal pregnancy is uterine in origin and associated with degeneration and sloughing of the uterine decidua. Soon after the death of the fetus, the decidua degenerates and is usually shed in small pieces, but occasionally it is cast off intact as a decidual cast of the uterine cavity. The absence of decidual tissue, however, does not rule out ectopic pregnancy.

NATURAL HISTORY OF TUBAL PREGNANCY

Tubal Abortion

A common termination of tubal pregnancy is separation of the products of conception from the implantation site and extrusion of the abortus through the fimbriated end of the oviduct. The frequency of tubal abortion depends in great part upon the site of implantation of the zygote. In ampullary tubal pregnancy, abortion is common, whereas rupture of the tube is the usual outcome in isthmic pregnancy. If separation is complete, the entire products may be extruded through the fimbriated end into the peritoneal cavity, and hemorrhage may cease and symptoms disappear.

Some bleeding usually persists as long as the products of conception remain in the oviduct, and the blood slowly trickles from the fimbriated end into the peritoneal cavity and typically pools in the rectouterine cul-de-sac. If the fimbriated extremity is occluded, the uterine tube may

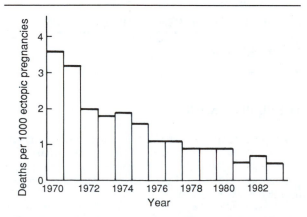

Figure 8–1. Mortality expressed as deaths per 1000 ectopic pregnancies for women with ectopic pregnancies in the United states, 1970–1983. (MMWR 1986;35:290.)

gradually become distended by blood, forming a hematosalpinx.

After incomplete tubal abortion, pieces of the placenta or membranes may remain attached to the tubal wall and, after being surrounded by fibrin, give rise to a placental polyp—as may occur in the uterus after incomplete uterine abortion.

Tubal Rupture

The invading, expanding products of conception may rupture the oviduct at any of several sites. As a rule, whenever tubal rupture occurs in the first few weeks, the pregnancy is situated in the isthmic portion of the tube a short distance from the cornu of the uterus. When the fertilized ovum is implanted well within the interstitial portion of the tube, rupture usually does not occur until later.

With intraperitoneal rupture, the entire products of conception may be extruded from the tube—or, if the rent is small, profuse hemorrhage may occur without extrusion. Commonly, the patient soon shows signs of collapse from hemorrhage and hypovolemia.

If an early conceptus is expelled essentially undamaged into the peritoneal cavity, it may reimplant almost anywhere, establish adequate circulation, and survive and grow, but this outcome is most unlikely because of damage during the transition. The products of conception, if small, may be reabsorbed; if larger, they may remain in the cul-de-sac for years as an encapsulated mass or even become calcified to form a lithopedion.

A. Abdominal Pregnancy: If only the fetus is extruded at the time of rupture, the effect upon the pregnancy will vary depending on the extent of injury sustained by the placenta. If the placenta is damaged appreciably, death of the fetus and termination of the pregnancy are inevitable; but if the greater portion of the placenta retains its attachment to the tube, further development is possible. The fetus may then survive for some time, giving rise to an abdominal pregnancy.

B. Broad Ligament Pregnancy: When the original implantation of the zygote is toward the mesosalpinx, rupture may occur at the portion of the tube not immediately covered by peritoneum, and the contents of the gestational sac may be extruded into a space formed between the folds of the broad ligament. This is called intraligamentous or broad ligament pregnancy.

Interstitial Pregnancy

When the fertilized ovum implants within the segment of the tube that penetrates the uterine wall, an especially grave form of tubal gestation results. Implantation at this site has also been referred to also as cornual pregnancy.

Interstitial tubal pregnancy accounts for about 3% of all tubal gestations. Because of the site of implantation, no adnexal mass is palpable, but rather there is variable asymmetry of the uterus that often is difficult to distinguish from an intrauterine pregnancy. Hence, early diagnosis is even more frequently overlooked than in other types of tubal implantation. Because of the greater distensibility of the myometrium covering the interstitial portion compared to the tubal wall (not surrounded by myometrium), rupture of an interstitial pregnancy is likely to occur somewhat later, at 9–16 gestational weeks. Because of the abundant blood supply from branches of both uterine and ovarian arteries immediately adjacent to the implantation site, the hemorrhage that attends the rupture may be rapidly fatal. In fact, tubal pregnancies in which the woman dies before she can be brought to the hospital are often of this type. Because of the large uterine defect, hysterectomy is commonly necessary. Very infrequently, an interstitial pregnancy may convert to a tubouterine pregnancy as described below.

Multifetal Ectopic Pregnancy

In rare instances, tubal pregnancy may be complicated by a coexisting intrauterine gestation, a condition designated as combined pregnancy. Gestational products are demonstrable ultrasonically within the uterine cavity in practically all instances of combined pregnancy.

Multifetal pregnancies at the same stage of development have been reported with embryos in the same tube as well as in different tubes.

Tubouterine, Tuboabdominal, & Tubo-ovarian Pregnancies

The so-called tubouterine pregnancy results from gradual extension into the uterine cavity of products of conception that originally implanted in the interstitial portion of the tube. Tuboabdominal pregnancy is a tubal pregnancy in which the zygote, originally implanted in the neighborhood of the fimbriated end of the tube, gradually extends into the peritoneal cavity.

Tubo-ovarian pregnancy occurs when the fetal sac is adherent partly to tubal and partly to ovarian tissue. Such cases arise from development of the zygote in a tubo-ovarian cyst or in a tube whose fimbriated extremity was adherent to the ovary at the time of fertilization or became so soon thereafter.

CLINICAL FEATURES & MANAGEMENT OF SPECIFIC TYPES OF ECTOPIC PREGNANCY

TUBAL PREGNANCY

Before tubal rupture or abortion, the manifestations of tubal pregnancy are diverse. Commonly, the individual believes she is normally pregnant or that she is aborting an intrauterine pregnancy. Less often, she does not even suspect that she is pregnant.

The Classic Presentation

In the so-called textbook case of ruptured tubal pregnancy, normal menstruation is replaced by variably delayed slight vaginal bleeding, usually referred to as "spotting." Suddenly, the woman is stricken with severe lower abdominal pain, frequently described as sharp, stabbing, or tearing in character. Vasomotor disturbances develop, ranging from vertigo to syncope.

Abdominal palpation discloses some tenderness, and vaginal examination—especially motion of the cervix—causes exquisite pain. The posterior fornix of the vagina may bulge because of blood in the cul-de-sac, or a tender, boggy mass may be felt to one side of the uterus.

Symptoms of diaphragmatic irritation, characterized by pain in the neck or shoulder especially on inspiration, develop in perhaps 50% of women who have significant intraperitoneal hemorrhage. This is caused by intraperitoneal blood irritating the cervical sensory nerves that supply the inferior surface of the diaphragm, especially on inspiration.

The woman with tubal rupture may or may not be hypotensive while lying supine. If she is not hypotensive when supine, she may become so when placed in a sitting position.

Clinical Findings & Diagnoses

In cases presenting as just described, diagnosis is not difficult. Even though the symptoms and signs of ectopic pregnancy often range from indefinite to bizarre before rupture or abortion, increasing numbers of women are seeking medical care before the classic clinical picture develops. The physician must make every effort to diagnose the condition before catastrophic events occur. The following symptoms, signs, and laboratory studies should be carefully evaluated.

A. Symptoms and Signs:

1. Pain–The most frequently experienced symptoms of ectopic pregnancy are pelvic and abdominal pain (100%) and amenorrhea with some degree of vaginal spotting or bleeding (60–80%). Gastrointestinal symptoms occur in 80% and dizziness or light-headedness in 58%.

Pain may be unilateral or bilateral, in the lower abdomen or generalized, or only in the upper abdomen. In the presence of hemoperitoneum, pain from diaphragmatic irritation may be experienced.

2. Amenorrhea–*The absence of a missed menstrual period in the history does not rule out tubal pregnancy.* One reason for this dictum is that the woman mistakes the uterine bleeding that frequently accompanies tubal pregnancy for menstrual bleeding and so gives an erroneous date for the onset of last menses.

3. Vaginal spotting or bleeding–As long as placental endocrine function persists, uterine bleeding is usually absent, but when endocrine support of the endometrium becomes inadequate, the uterine mucosa bleeds. Although profuse vaginal bleeding is suggestive of incomplete intrauterine abortion rather than an ectopic gestation, such bleeding can occur with tubal gestations.

4. Abdominal and pelvic pain–Exquisite tenderness on abdominal palpation and vaginal examination, especially on motion of the cervix, is demonstrable in over three-fourths of women with ruptured or rupturing tubal

pregnancies but occasionally may be absent prior to rupture.

5. Uterine changes–Because of the action of placental hormones, the uterus grows during the first 3 months of tubal gestation to nearly the same size as it would in an intrauterine pregnancy. Its consistency, too, is similar as long as the fetus is alive. The uterus may be pushed to one side by the ectopic mass.

6. Blood pressure and pulse–The early response to moderate hemorrhage is no change in pulse and blood pressure or occasionally a slight rise in blood pressure or a vasovagal response with bradycardia and hypotension. In the otherwise healthy young woman with an extrauterine pregnancy, only if bleeding continues and hypovolemia becomes intense, can the blood pressure be counted on to fall and the pulse rate to rise appreciably.

7. Hypovolemia–There are two simple means of detecting significant hypovolemia before development of hypovolemic shock: (1) The blood pressures and pulse rates in the sitting and supine positions are compared. A definite decrease in blood pressure and rise in pulse rate in the sitting position are usually indicative of a significant decrease in circulatory volume. (2) Urine flow is monitored carefully, since hypovolemia—in the absence of potent diuretic treatment—often causes oliguria before overt hypotension develops.

8. Temperature–After acute hemorrhage, the temperature may be normal or even low. Temperatures up to 38 °C may develop—perhaps related to hemoperitoneum—but higher temperatures are rare in the absence of infection. Fever is important, therefore, in distinguishing ruptured tubal pregnancy from acute salpingitis, in which the temperature is commonly above 38 °C.

9. Pelvic mass–A pelvic mass is palpable in only 20% of patients. Pain and tenderness often preclude identification of the mass by palpation.

B. Laboratory Findings: Measurement of hemoglobin, hematocrit, and leukocyte count and performance of pregnancy tests are useful if their limitations are understood.

1. Hemoglobin and hematocrit–After hemorrhage, the depleted blood volume is restored toward normal by hemodilution over the course of 1 or 2 days. Even after a substantive hemorrhage, therefore, the hemoglobin level or hematocrit reading may at first show only a slight reduction. For the first few hours after acute hemorrhage, a decrease in the hemoglobin or hematocrit level while the patient is under observation is a more valuable index of blood loss than is the initial reading.

2. Leukocyte count–The leukocyte count varies considerably in ruptured ectopic pregnancy. In about half of patients it is normal, but in the remainder varying degrees of leukocytosis up to 30 000/μL may be encountered.

3. Pregnancy tests–Ectopic pregnancy cannot be diagnosed by a positive pregnancy test alone. However, the key issue when confronted with the possibility of an ectopic pregnancy is whether the woman is in fact pregnant. In virtually all cases of ectopic gestation, chorionic gonadotropin will be detected in serum, but usually at a markedly reduced concentration compared to normal pregnancy. The problem is how to detect this marker of pregnancy in the most clinically efficacious manner.

Urinary pregnancy tests are most often latex agglutination inhibition slide tests with sensitivities for chorionic gonadotropin in the range of 500–800 mIU/mL. Their convenience is offset by their low sensitivity—ie, the chance of being positive in a woman with ectopic pregnancy is only 50–60%. Even when the tube-type tests are used (hemagglutination inhibition or latex agglutination inhibition), detection of the beta subunit of human chorionic gonadotropin is within the 150–250 mIU/mL range and is positive in only 80–85% of ectopic pregnancies.

Enzyme-linked immunosorbent assays (ELISA) are sensitive to 10–50 mIU/mL and are positive in 90–96% of women with ectopic pregnancies. This type of test also has the advantages of rapidity and ease of performance.

Serum radioimmunoassay for β-hCG is the most precise method, and virtually any pregnancy event can be detected in this way. In fact, because of the sensitivity of this assay, a pregnancy may be confirmed before there are pathologic changes in the uterine tube.

C. Other Diagnostic Aids: Because of the difficulties in diagnosis of ruptured tubal pregnancy, a variety of diagnostic aids other than tests for chorionic gonadotropin have been utilized. These include sonography, the combination of sonography and serum β-hCG determinations, culdocentesis, curettage, colpotomy, laparoscopy, and laparotomy.

1. Sonography–Identification of early products of conception in the uterine tube by this means is difficult, but if a gestational sac is clearly identified within the cavity of the uterus, it is most unlikely that an ectopic pregnancy coexists. Moreover, the absence of ultrasonic evidence of intrauterine pregnancy but a positive pregnancy test, fluid in the cul-de-sac, and an abnormal pelvic mass are practically diagnostic of ectopic pregnancy (Table 8–1). Unfortunately, sonographic findings at least suggestive of early intrauterine pregnancy may be present in some cases of ectopic pregnancy. What may appear on the sonogram as a small sac (very early pregnancy) or a collapsed sac (dead products of conception) may actually be a blood clot or decidual cast. Vaginal sonography reduces these errors. The presence of an intrauterine pregnancy usually is not recognized using real-time ultrasound until 5–6 menstrual weeks (see Chapter 35) or 28 days after timed ovulation. The identification with real-time sonography of fetal heart action clearly outside the uterine cavity provides firm evidence of ectopic pregnancy.

2. Quantitative β-hCG values and sonography–During the past decade, the clinical management of suspected ectopic pregnancy has changed remarkably. In essence, management is based upon the establishment or exclusion of pregnancy. If a sensitive urinary pregnancy test such as ELISA is positive, the diagnosis of pregnancy is established. A negative radioimmunoassay for serum β-hCG is required to exclude pregnancy.

When pregnancy is diagnosed in the hemodynamically stable woman with no abdominal ultrasonic evidence for ectopic pregnancy and a negative culdocentesis, subsequent management is based upon serial quantitative serum β-hCG values and abdominal sonograms. Kadar et al (1981a) described four clinical possibilities based upon quantitative β-hCG values:

(1) When the β-hCG value is above 6000 mIU/mL and an intrauterine gestational sac is seen using abdominal sonography, normal pregnancy is virtually certain.

(2) When the β-hCG value is above 6000 mIU/mL and there is an empty uterine cavity, a diagnosis of ectopic pregnancy is strongly suggested.

(3) When the β-hCG value is less than 6000 mIU/mL and a definite intrauterine ring of pregnancy is visualized, spontaneous abortion is likely to occur immediately or very soon. Ectopic pregnancy is still a possibility because of the degree of ultrasonic resolution available. A false diagnosis of a uterine gestational sac can be made when there are blood clots or decidual casts.

(4) When the β-hCG value is less than 6000 mIU/mL and there is an empty uterus, no definitive diagnosis can be made. Failure to visualize a gestational sac within the uterus is not unusual using abdominal sonography prior to 5 weeks' gestation. The methods of management in these circumstances are discussed below. If vaginal sonography is used, the critical β-hCG value is 2000 mIU/mL.

Some feel that with an empty uterus and any proof of

Table 8–1. Outcome in 94 women with possible ectopic pregnancy in whom ultrasonic findings are correlated with serum pregnancy test.[1]

	Serum LH/hCG Assay[2]			
	Positive		Negative	
Ultrasonic Findings	Ectopic	No Ectopic	Ectopic	No Ectopic
Empty uterus alone	10	6	0	16
Empty uterus + adnexal mass	13	2	0	11
Empty uterus + free fluid in cul-de-sac	9	0	1	5
Empty uterus + free fluid in cul-de-sac + adnexal mass	19	0	0	2
Total	51	8	1[3]	34

[1]Modified from Robinson HP et al: Aust NZ J Obstet Gynaecol 1985;25:49.
[2]Three different radioimmunoassays for β-hCG were used in this series. One assay cross-reacted with human luteinizing hormone (LH).
[3]Although a negative pregnancy test was noted, the ectopic pregnancy had been aborted from the uterine tube and was free in the hemoperitoneum.

pregnancy, laparoscopy or laparotomy is indicated. Another approach is to admit the patient to the hospital and perform serial hematocrits, monitor vital signs frequently, and order serial sonograms and β-hCG determinations. She will eventually continue with a normal pregnancy, abort, or develop clinical or ultrasonic evidence of ectopic pregnancy.

Kadar proposed another plan after observing that in women with normal pregnancies, the mean doubling time for β-hCG in serum was approximately 48 hours and the lowest normal value for this increase was 66%. They calculated this value by subtracting the initial value for β-hCG from the 48-hour value and dividing the result by the initial value, which is multiplied by 100 to obtain a percentage:

$$\frac{\text{β-hCG at 48 hours} - \text{Initial β-hCG}}{\text{Initial β-hCG}} \times 100$$

The authors cautioned that both β-hCG determinations must be performed simultaneously and that more reliable values could be obtained at 48-hour intervals. Failure to maintain this rate of increased β-hCG production, along with an empty uterus, was strong evidence for ectopic pregnancy. They further acknowledged that this plan would delay surgery at least 48 hours and that the test would still falsely identify 15% of normal women as likely to have an ectopic pregnancy and 13% of women with ectopic pregnancy as normal.

Finally, vaginal sonography plus quantitative serum β–hCG values have proven to be an even more sensitive method of establishing the presence or absence of an early intrauterine gestation.

3. Culdocentesis (Figure 8–2)–The simplest technique for identifying hemoperitoneum is culdocentesis, since it can be performed without hospitalization. As the cervix is pulled toward the symphysis with a tenaculum, a long 16- or 18-gauge needle is inserted through the posterior vaginal fornix into the cul-de-sac, whence fluid can be aspirated. Fluid containing fragments of old clots or bloody fluid that does not subsequently clot is compatible with the diagnosis of hemoperitoneum resulting from ectopic pregnancy.

Culdocentesis may be unsatisfactory in women with previous salpingitis and pelvic peritonitis, since the cul-de-sac may have been obliterated. Thus, failure to obtain blood from the cul-de-sac does not exclude the diagnosis of hemoperitoneum and certainly does not rule out ectopic pregnancy, either unruptured or ruptured.

4. Curettage–Differentiation between threatened or incomplete abortion of an intrauterine pregnancy and a tubal pregnancy may also be accomplished in many instances by curettage. If embryo, fetus, or placenta is identified, a simultaneous tubal pregnancy is very unlikely. When none of these structures are identified, tubal pregnancy is a probability. The identification of decidua alone in the uterine curettings strongly implies extrauterine pregnancy, but decidua alone may be present following a complete abortion.

5. Laparoscopy–Laparoscopy provides a means of diagnosing disease of the pelvic viscera, including ectopic pregnancy. Unfortunately, complete visualization of the pelvis may be impossible in the presence of pelvic inflammation or recent or remote bleeding. At times, identification of an early unruptured tubal pregnancy may be difficult using the laparoscope, even though the tube is fully visualized.

6. Laparotomy–If any doubt remains, laparotomy should be performed, since an unnecessary operation is far less tragic than death contributed to by indecision or delay. It is imperative that laparotomy not be delayed while laparoscopy is performed on the woman undergoing an obvious pelvic or abdominal catastrophe that requires immediate definitive treatment.

Differential Diagnosis

Prompt diagnosis of ruptured tubal pregnancy may be lifesaving, and the earlier an unruptured tubal pregnancy is diagnosed, the greater will be the likelihood of future reproductive success. There are few other disorders in obstetrics and gynecology that present so many diagnostic pitfalls.

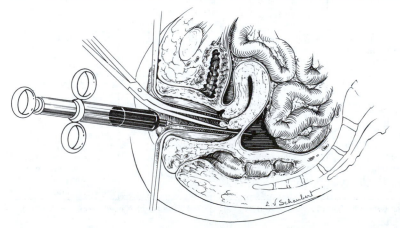

Figure 8–2. Culdocentesis. (Reproduced, with permission, from Pernoll ML (editor): *Current Obstetric & Gynecologic Diagnosis & Treatment,* 7th ed. Appleton & Lange, 1991.)

In the authors' experience, the following conditions are most frequently confused with tubal pregnancy: (1) acute or chronic salpingitis, (2) threatened or incomplete abortion of an intrauterine pregnancy, (3) rupture of a corpus luteum or follicular cyst with intraperitoneal bleeding, (4) torsion of an ovarian cyst, (5) appendicitis, (6) gastroenteritis, (7) discomfort from an intrauterine device, and (8) failure of tubal sterilization. (See Table 8–2.)

Treatment

Treatment of tubal pregnancy most often has been by salpingectomy with or without ipsilateral oophorectomy. The goal of such treatment was and should remain the preservation of the woman's life. Recently, treatment has changed from salpingectomy to procedures that favor tubal conservation. The traditionally more radical surgical approaches are presented first, followed by newer techniques designed to conserve uterine tube function. Some of these procedures can be done using a laparoscope.

A. Surgical Treatment:

1. Salpingectomy–In removing the oviduct, it is advisable to excise as a wedge certainly no more than the outer third of the interstitial portion of the tube (so-called cornual resection) in an effort to minimize the rare recurrence of pregnancy in the tubal stump without weakening the myometrium at that site of excision.

2. Ipsilateral oophorectomy–Most gynecologists leave the ovary when possible and, to minimize ovarian dysfunction and cyst formation, preserve the blood supply by clamping the vessels in the mesosalpinx close to the oviduct.

3. Sterilization–If the patient has reached her childbearing objectives and the ectopic pregnancy is the consequence of failed contraception, the decision may be for sterilization. Hysterectomy may be considered, or tubal sterilization can usually be performed quickly without increased risk. Conversely, all organs possible should be conserved in the woman of low parity with a strong desire for future pregnancies in spite of the increased risk of subsequent ectopic pregnancy.

4. Conservation of the uterine tube–In general, women under age 30 and those of higher parity have significantly higher fertility rates and more successful outcomes in subsequent pregnancies than older women of lower parity. A history of salpingitis and evidence of bilateral tubal disease are extremely bad prognostic signs. Finally, Sherman et al (1982) reported that *subsequent pregnancy and lower recurrent ectopic pregnancy rates were*

Table 8–2. Differential diagnosis of ectopic pregnancy.[1]

	Ectopic Pregnancy	Appendicitis	Salpingitis	Ruptured Corpus Luteum Cyst	Uterine Abortion
Pain	Unilateral cramps and tenderness before rupture.	Epigastric, periumbilical, then right lower quadrant pain; tenderness localizing at McBurney's point. Rebound tenderness.	Usually in both lower quadrants, with or without rebound. Dysuria sometimes present.	Unilateral, becoming general with progressive bleeding.	Midline cramps.
Nausea and vomiting	Occasionally before, frequently after rupture.	Usual. Precedes shift of pain to right lower quadrant.	Infrequent.	Rare. No symptoms or signs of pregnancy.	Almost never.
Menstruation	Some aberration; missed period, spotting.	Unrelated to menses.	Hypermenorrhea or metrorrhagia, or both.	Period delayed, then bleeding, often with pain.	Longer amenorrhea, then spotting, then brisk bleeding.
Temperature and pulse	37.2–37.8 °C (99–100 °F). Pulse variable; normal before, rapid after rupture.	37.2–37.8 °C (99–100 °F). Pulse rapid: 99–100.	37.2–40 °C (99–104 °F). Pulse elevated in proportion to fever.	Not over 37.2 °C (99 °F). Pulse normal unless blood loss marked, then rapid.	To 37.2 °C (99 °F) if spontaneous; to 40 °C (104 °F) if induced (infected).
Pelvic examination	Unilateral tenderness, especially on movement of cervix. Crepitant mass on one side or in cul-de-sac.	No masses. Rectal tenderness high on right side.	Bilateral tenderness on movement of cervix. Mass only when pyosalpinx or hydrosalpinx is present.	Tenderness over affected ovary. No masses. Uterus firm and not enlarged.	Cervix slightly patulous. Uterus slightly enlarged, irregularly softened. Tender only with infection.
Laboratory findings	White cell count of 15,000/μL. Red cell count strikingly low if blood loss large. Sedimentation rate slightly elevated.	Negative β-hCG. White cell count 10,000–18,000/μL (rarely normal). Red cell count normal. Sedimentation rate slightly elevated.	Negative β-hCG. White cell count 15,000–30,000/μL. Red cell count normal. Sedimentation rate markedly elevated.	Negative β-hCG. White cell count normal to 10,000/μL. Red cell count normal. Sedimentation rate normal.	White cell count 15,000/μL if spontaneous; to 30,000/μL if induced (infection). Red cell count normal. Sedimentation rate slightly to moderately elevated.

[1]Reproduced, with permission, from Pernoll ML (editor): *Current Obstetric & Gynecologic Diagnosis & Treatment,* 7th ed. Appleton & Lange, 1991.

observed in women in whom surgery was performed prior to rupture of the ectopic pregnancy.

If the woman has no history of infertility and no gross evidence of previous salpingitis, salpingotomy and salpingostomy result in equally favorable outcomes. Sherman reported intrauterine pregnancy rates for both groups to be more than 85%. If there is evidence for bilateral tubal disease, salpingostomy is clearly superior to salpingotomy.

Use of newer diagnostic techniques and surgical procedures to conserve damaged tubes will result in better subsequent pregnancy outcomes. Several of the surgical approaches for tubal reconstruction are discussed below.

5. Salpingostomy–This technique is used to remove a small pregnancy that is usually less than 2 cm in length and located in the distal third of the uterine tube (Figure 8–3). A linear incision, 2 cm in length or less, is made on the antimesenteric border immediately over the ectopic pregnancy. The conceptus usually will extrude from the incision and can be carefully removed. Small bleeding sites are controlled with needlepoint electrocautery or laser, and the incision is left unsutured to heal by second intention.

6. Salpingotomy–A longitudinal incision is made on the antimesenteric border of the uterine tube directly over the conceptus (Figure 8–4). The products of conception are removed with forceps or gentle suction, and the opened tube is irrigated with lactated Ringer's solution (not isotonic saline) so that bleeding sites can be identified and controlled.

When possible, the incision should not be extended through the end of the tube into the ampulla.

7. Segmental resection and anastomosis–This procedure is recommended for an unruptured ectopic pregnancy in the isthmic portion of the tube, since salpingotomy or salpingostomy would probably cause scarring

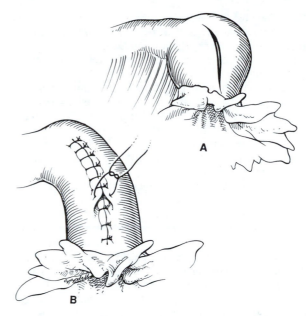

Figure 8–4. *A:* Linear salpingotomy for removal of an ectopic pregnancy larger than 2 cm in length from the distal third of the uterine tube. *B:* The incision is sutured, usually with a single layer of 7-0 interrupted sutures.

and subsequent narrowing of this small lumen (Figure 8–5).

8. Fimbrial evacuation–There is a temptation with distally implanted tubal pregnancies to evacuate the conceptual products by "milking" or "suctioning" the *ectopic*

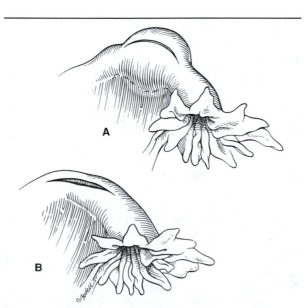

Figure 8–3. *A:* Linear salpingostomy for removal of a small tubal pregnancy in the distal third of the uterine tube. *B:* The incision is not sutured.

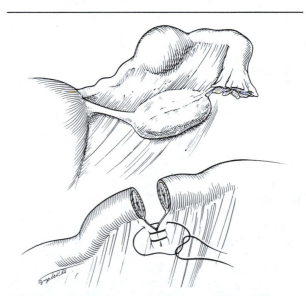

Figure 8–5. Segmental resection and anastomosis of the uterine tube for an unruptured ectopic pregnancy. Closure of the mesosalpinx results in reapproximation of the tubal segments. Anastomosis is accomplished with interrupted 7-0 vicryl sutures (see text).

from the tubal lumen. This is not recommended, since the practice is associated with an ectopic recurrence rate twice that of salpingotomy. There is also a high rate of surgical reexploration for recurrent bleeding from persistent trophoblastic tissue.

9. Other techniques–All of the above techniques can be done at a later time if the woman is in shock. The first rule must be that bleeding is rapidly arrested and cardiovascular resuscitation performed. If time and clinical circumstances permit, the above procedures can then be considered.If a tubal reconstructive procedure is done, all blood and debris should be irrigated from the abdomen and pelvis using lactated Ringer's solution. If a second procedure is planned for a later time, it is logical to obtain hemostasis with the least amount of tubal damage.

The risk of persistent tubal trophoblastic tissue following a tubal reconstructive procedure is real. For this reason, Bell et al (1987) recommend that another chorionic gonadotropin determination be performed 2 weeks later to compare with the original and to make certain that the value is falling. With persistent or increasing values, the choice of reexploration or chemotherapy with methotrexate (see below) must be made. Kamrava et al (1983) reported that values for chorionic gonadotropin usually are negative by 12 days following resection of tubal pregnancies, but occasionally they are elevated even 3 weeks after surgery.

B. Nonsurgical Management:

1. Methotrexate–Methotrexate is being used today as primary treatment in small unruptured tubal ectopic pregnancies (Stovall and Ling, 1992).

2. Anti-D immune globulin–If the woman is D-negative but not yet sensitized to D-antigen and the potential for reproduction persists, anti-D immune globulin should be administered to protect against isoimmunization. The D-negative patient should also receive anti-D immune globulin soon after platelet transfusion.

Prognosis

Spirtos et al (1987) reported that following resection of an ectopic pregnancy, approximately 14% of women ovulate by 19 days and 64% by 24 days. By the 30th postoperative day, almost three-fourths of women have ovulated. Thus, contraception should be started at the time of discharge from the hospital.

ABDOMINAL PREGNANCY

Typically, the growing placenta, after penetrating the wall of the oviduct, maintains to a degree its tubal attachment but gradually encroaches upon and implants in the neighboring serosa. Meanwhile, the fetus—usually but not always surrounded by amnion—continues to grow within the peritoneal cavity.

The condition of the fetus in abdominal pregnancy is exceedingly precarious, and the great majority have succumbed. About half of those that survive have an increased incidence of congenital malformations.

Clinical Findings

A. Symptoms and Signs: Since early rupture or abortion of a tubal pregnancy is the usual antecedent of an abdominal pregnancy, a history suggestive of the accident can usually be obtained in retrospect. By abdominal palpation, the abnormal position of the fetus—often a transverse or oblique lie—can frequently be confirmed. *Massage of the abdomen over the products of conception does not stimulate the mass to become more firm, as it most always does with advanced intrauterine pregnancy.* The cervix is usually displaced, depending in part on the position of the fetus, and it may dilate somewhat, but appreciable effacement is lacking.

B. Imaging Studies: Sonographic findings in abdominal pregnancy may not be clear enough to permit unequivocal diagnosis. However, if the fetal head is seen to lie immediately adjacent to the maternal bladder with no interposed uterine tissue, specific diagnosis of an abdominal pregnancy can be made.

MRI has been used to confirm abdominal pregnancy following a suspicious sonographic examination.

Treatment

The operation for abdominal pregnancy may precipitate massive hemorrhage. Without massive blood transfusion, the outlook for many such patients is hopeless. Hence, it is mandatory that at least 2000 mL of compatible blood be on hand in the operating room, with more blood readily available in the blood bank. Preoperatively, two intravenous infusion systems, each capable of delivering large volumes of fluid at a rapid rate, should be functioning. At the same time, techniques for monitoring the adequacy of the circulation should be employed. Whenever time allows, the bowel should be prepared using both mechanical cleansing and antimicrobial agents, since the bowel is often intimately adherent to the placenta and membranes.

Prognosis

Abdominal pregnancy is still one of the most formidable complications. Detection and eradication of ectopic pregnancies during the first trimester continue to be the most effective means of avoiding these terrible risks.

OVARIAN PREGNANCY

The criteria for diagnosis of ovarian pregnancy are that (1) the tube on the affected side must be intact, (2) the fetal sac must occupy the position of the ovary, (3) the ovary must be connected to the uterus by the ovarian ligament, and (4) unambiguously ovarian tissue must be found in the sac wall.

The symptoms and physical findings are likely to mimic those of tubal pregnancy or a bleeding corpus luteum. At the time of operation, early ovarian pregnancies are likely to be considered to be corpus luteum cysts or a bleeding corpus luteum.

Early ovarian pregnancies should be treated, when possible, by wedge resection or cystectomy; otherwise, oophorectomy is performed.

CERVICAL PREGNANCY

Cervical pregnancy is a rare form of ectopic gestation in which the ovum implants within the cervix below the internal os. The endocervix is eroded by the trophoblast, and the pregnancy proceeds to develop in the fibrous cervical wall.

Usually, painless bleeding appearing shortly after nidation is the first sign. As pregnancy progresses, a distended thin-walled cervix with the external os partially dilated may be evident. Bleeding without pain is the common clinical characteristic. Above the cervical mass, a slightly enlarged uterine fundus may be palpated.

Cervical pregnancy rarely goes beyond the 20th week of gestation and is usually terminated surgically because of bleeding. Since attempts at removal of the placenta vaginally may result in profuse hemorrhage and even death of the patient, methotrexate is the preferred method of treatment (Yankowitz et al, 1990).

SELECTED READINGS

Abbott J, Emmans LS, Lowenstein SR: Ectopic pregnancy: Ten common pitfalls in diagnosis. Am J Emerg Med 1990; 8(6):515.

Arias-Stella J: Atypical endometrial changes associated with the presence of chorionic tissue. Arch Pathol 1954;58:112.

Bell OR, Awadalla SG, Mattox JH: Persistent ectopic syndrome: A case report and literature review. Obstet Gynecol 1987;69: 521.

Bohm-Velez M, Mendelson EB, Freimanis MG: Transvaginal sonography in evaluating ectopic pregnancy. Semin Ultrasound CT MR (Feb) 1990;11(1):44.

Cunningham FG et al: Ectopic Pregnancy. In: Cunningham FG, MacDonald PC, Gant NF, Leveno KJ, Gilstraph LG (editors): *Williams Obstetrics,* 19th ed. Appleton & Lange, 1993.

DeCherney AH, Jones EE: Ectopic pregnancy. Clin Obstet Gynecol 1985;28:365.

Dorfman SF: Deaths from ectopic pregnancy, United States 1979 to 1980. Obstet Gynecol 1983;62:344.

Dorfman SF et al: Ectopic pregnancy mortality, United States, 1979 to 1980: Clinical aspects. Obstet Gynecol 1984; 64:386.

Kadar N, Caldwell BR, Romero R: A method of screening for ectopic pregnancy and its indications. Obstet Gynecol 1981b; 58:162.

Kadar N, DeVore G, Romero R: The discriminatory hCG zone: Its use in the sonographic evaluation for ectopic pregnancy. Obstet Gynecol 1981a;58:156.

Kamrava MM et al: Disappearance of human chorionic gonadotropin following removal of ectopic pregnancy. Obstet Gynecol 1983;62:486.

Leach RE, Ory SJ: Modern management of ectopic pregnancy [see comments]. J Reprod Med (May) 1989;34(5):324.

MacKay HT, Hughes JM, Hogue CR: Ectopic pregnancy in the United States, 1979–1980. MMWR 1984;33:1SS.

Robinson HP et al: Ectopic pregnancy: Potentials for diagnosis using ultrasound and urine and serum pregnancy tests. Aust NZ J Obstet Gynaecol 1985;25:49.

Sherman D et al: Improved fertility following ectopic pregnancy. Fertil Steril 1982;37:497.

Stock RJ: Ectopic pregnancy: A look at changing concepts and problems. Clin Obstet Gynecol 1990;33(3):448.

Stovall TG, Ling FW: Some new approaches to ectopic pregnancy. Contemp Obstet Gynecol 1992;37:35.

Strafford JC, Kagan WD: Abdominal pregnancy: Review of current management. Obstet Gynecol 1977;50:548.

Yankowitz J et al: Cervical ectopic pregnancy: Review of the literature and report of a case treated by single-dose methotrexate therapy. Obstet Gynecol Surv 1990;45:405.

Abortion

Abortion is defined as termination of pregnancy by any means before the fetus is sufficiently developed to survive. When abortion occurs spontaneously, the lay term "miscarriage" is often used. In the United States, the term "abortion" denotes termination of pregnancy before the 20th completed week of gestation, or 139 days, counting from the first day of the last normal menses. Another commonly used criterion for "abortion" is delivery of a fetus or neonate weighing less than 500 g.

Abortion may be spontaneous or induced, and both are discussed in turn below.

SPONTANEOUS ABORTION

Incidence

The incidence of spontaneous abortion is commonly stated as 10% of all pregnancies. However, the incidence is difficult to determine precisely, since as many as 30% of abortions may go unrecognized. Unrecognized losses occur early, and clinically recognized losses are likely to include a number of abortions in which the fetus died several weeks before the products were expelled.

Pathology

Hemorrhage into the decidua basalis and necrotic changes in the tissues adjacent to the bleeding usually accompany abortion. The ovum becomes detached entirely or in part and, presumably acting as a foreign body in the uterus, stimulates uterine contractions that result in expulsion. There may be no visible fetus in the sac, the so-called **blighted ovum.**

The **blood mole (carneous mole)** is an ovum that is surrounded by a capsule of clotted blood. The capsule is of varying thickness, with degenerated chorionic villi scattered through it. **Tuberous mole** and **tuberous subchorial hematoma of the decidua** are other names for the same lesion.

In abortions occurring after 12 weeks of gestational age, several outcomes are possible: (1) The retained fetus may undergo maceration. In such circumstances, the bones of the skull collapse, the abdomen becomes distended with blood-stained fluid, and the entire fetus takes on a dull reddish color. At the same time, the skin softens and peels off in utero or at the slightest touch, leaving behind the corium. The internal organs degenerate and undergo necrosis. (2) The amnionic fluid may be absorbed when the fetus becomes compressed upon itself and desiccated to form a **fetus compressus.** (3) Occasionally, the fetus eventually becomes so dry and compressed that it resembles parchment, the so-called **fetus papyraceus.** This latter outcome is relatively frequent in twin pregnancy if one fetus has died early and the other has gone on to full development.

Resumption of Ovulation

Ovulation may occur as early as 2 weeks after an abortion. A surge of luteinizing hormone (LH) has been detected in women as early as 16–22 days after abortion in 15 of 18 women studied. Moreover, the plasma progesterone level, which had plummeted after the abortion, increased soon after the LH surge. Therefore, it is important that effective contraception be initiated soon after abortion. The use of various contraceptive techniques following abortion is discussed in Chapter 26.

Etiology

More than 80% of abortions occur in the first 12 weeks of pregnancy, and the rate decreases rapidly thereafter. *Chromosomal anomalies cause at least half of these early abortions.* The risk of spontaneous abortion appears to increase with parity as well as with maternal and paternal age. The frequency of clinically recognized abortion increases from 12% in women under 20 years of age to 26% in those over age 40. Finally, the incidence of abortion is increased if a woman conceives within 3 months of a live birth.

A. Abnormal Development of the Zygote: The most common morphologic finding in early spontaneous abortion is abnormal development of the zygote, the embryo, the early fetus, or, at times, the placenta. Disorganized fetal growth has been identified in 40% of abortuses (both embryos and fetuses) that were expelled spontaneously before 20 weeks. Among embryos (< 30 mm crown-rump length), the frequency of abnormal morphologic development was 70%. Of the embryos on which tissue culture and chromosomal analyses were performed, 60% were demonstrated to have a chromosomal abnormality. For fetuses (30–180 mm crown-rump length), the frequency was 25%.

Abnormal fetal development, especially in the first trimester, may be classified as that associated with an abnormal number of chromosomes (aneuploidy) or with a normal number (euploidy).

1. Aneuploid abortion–Fifty to 60 percent of early spontaneous abortions are associated with a chromosomal anomaly of the conceptus (Table 9–1).

2. Euploid abortion–Chromosomally normal abortuses usually are lost later in gestation. Three-fourths of aneuploid abortions occur at or before 8 weeks, while euploid abortions peak at about 13 weeks. The incidence of euploid abortions increases dramatically after a maternal age of 35 years. The reasons for both observations are unknown. In fact, the reasons for euploid abortions generally are unknown, but there appear to be at least two possibilities: (1) a genetic abnormality, such as an isolated mutation or polygenic factors; and (2) a variety of maternal factors that will be discussed subsequently.

A **genetic mechanism** has been proposed by Simpson (1980), who observed that only about 0.5% of liveborn infants have chromosomal abnormalities whereas at least 2% of liveborn infants have diseases associated with a single-gene mutation or a polygenic mechanism of inheritance. He reasoned that these more common defects could produce abortions by altering various fetal functions or by altering differentiation.

Table 9–1. Chromosomal findings in human abortuses.[1]

	Percent	
Chromosomal Studies	Kajii et al (1980)	Simpson (1986)
Normal (euploid) 46 XY and 46XY	46	54
Abnormal (aneuploid) Autosomal trisomy	31	22
Monosomy X (45,X)	10	9
Triploidy	7	8
Tetraploidy	2	3
Structural anomaly	3	2
Double trisomy	2	0.7
Triple trisomy	0.4	NL
Others: XXY, monosomy 21	0.8	NL
Autosomal monosomy G	NL	0.1
Mosaic trisomy	NL	1.3
Sex chromosome polysomy	NL	0.2
Abnormality not specified	NL	0.9

[1]From Kajii T et al: Anatomic and chromosomal anomalies in 639 spontaneous abortuses. Human Genet 1980;55:87, and Simpson JL: CREOG Basic Science Monographs in Obstetrics and Gynecology. ACOG, 1986.
NL = not listed.

B. Maternal Factors: Maternal diseases usually are associated with euploid abortion. These losses peak at 13 weeks, and because of the later time, a correctable cause can sometimes be identified. Thus, a midtrimester abortion should be investigated in an effort to find the cause. A variety of diseases and developmental abnormalities have been implicated in euploid abortion, though the evidence is not convincing in all instances.

1. Chronic infections–*Listeria monocytogenes* and *Toxoplasma gondii* can cause abortion, though this happens less often in the United States than in other parts of the world. The isolation of *Mycoplasma hominis* and *Ureaplasma urealyticum* from the genital tract of some women who have aborted has led to the hypothesis that such infections might be abortifacients. Of the two organisms, *U urealyticum* appears to be the major offender. The evidence that genital herpes might cause abortion is weak.

2. Endocrine effects–An increased incidence of abortion has been attributed to hyperthyroidism, diabetes mellitus, and progesterone deficiency. Inadequate glucose control in diabetes may increase the incidence of abortion. Progesterone deficiency due to insufficient secretion of the corpus luteum or the placenta has been associated with an increased incidence of abortion.

It has been suggested that abnormal levels of one or more hormones might help to predict abortion or even serve as therapeutic guides. Unfortunately, reduced levels of these hormones usually are the consequence rather than the cause of irreversible damage to the fetoplacental unit. There are now well-documented cases of luteal phase defects, but they appear to be uncommon. The issue of how to make the diagnosis either by serum progesterone measurements or endometrial biopsy as well as the best therapy with clomiphene citrate or progesterone has been recently reviewed by Lee (1987) and by Check et al (1987a and 1987b), who reported that progesterone alone is effective as long as there is ultrasonic evidence of normal follicular maturation and normal estrogen production. As yet, there is no convincing evidence in well-controlled, randomized studies that progesterone therapy is efficacious. Progesterone therapy is not associated with an increased incidence of fetal malformations.

3. Recreational drugs and environmental toxins–A variety of agents have been reported to be associated with an increased incidence of abortion. As more information accumulates, not all such reports have been confirmed.

Tobacco has been linked with an increased incidence of euploid abortion. **Alcohol,** even in moderation, has been implicated as increasing the incidence of euploid abortion. Increased euploid abortion is strong evidence that both tobacco and alcohol are embryotoxins.

Radiation in sufficient doses is a recognized abortifacient. The abortifacient dose in humans is not precisely known, but a minimum lethal fetal dose is believed to be about 5 cGy.

Contraceptives were at one time linked with an increased incidence of abortion, but there now appears to be no such association. This is true both for oral contraceptives and for spermatocidal agents used in contraceptive creams and jellies. Intrauterine devices, however, are associated with an increased incidence of septic abortion after contraceptive failure.

Environmental toxins such as arsenic, lead, formaldehyde, benzene, and ethylene oxide may increase the abortion rate, but anesthetic gases do not have a similar effect.

4. Immunologic factors–There are two major mechanisms whereby immunologic abnormalities may cause abortion: autoimmune and alloimmune. **Autoimmune mechanisms** are those by which a cellular or humoral response is directed against a specific site within the host. Autoimmune disorders such as lupus erythematosus have been reported to be associated with an increased rate of abortion and fetal death. The antiphospholipid antibodies, including lupus anticoagulant and other anticardiolipin antibodies, are other examples. Both of these antiphospholipid antibodies are directed against platelets and vascular endothelium, which results in vascular destruction, thrombosis, abortion, and placental destruction.

Allogeneity denotes genetic dissimilarities in different animals of the same species. The human fetus is an allogeneic transplant that is tolerated by the mother for reasons that are incompletely understood, though several immunologic mechanisms are reported to prevent fetal rejection. These mechanisms include histocompatibility factors, circulating blocking factors, local suppressor factors, maternal or antipaternal antileukocytotoxic antibodies, and probably others. Therefore, some possible causes of recurrent abortion may be related to an abnormal maternal immune response that is turned against antigens on placental or fetal tissues. There is strong evidence that maternal-fetal histoincompatibility is essential to successful human pregnancy and that if mother and fetus are "too compatible," reproduction failure develops. In some cases of recurrent abortion, there is an increased sharing of maternal and paternal human lymphocyte antigens (HLA). The strongest association with fetal loss is with the HLA-DR locus.

5. Aging gametes–The age of both sperm and egg may influence the spontaneous abortion rate. Aging of gametes within the female genital tract before fertilization increases the chance of abortion.

6. Laparotomy–The trauma of laparotomy may occasionally provoke abortion. In general, the nearer the site of surgery to the pelvic organs, the greater the risk.

7. Uterine defects–Abnormalities of the uterus can be separated into those that are acquired and those that are developmental, resulting from spontaneous abnormalities (müllerian anomalies) or induced abnormalities from diethylstilbestrol (DES) exposure. These defects and their consequences are discussed in Chapter 5.

Intrauterine adhesions (synechiae; Asherman's syndrome) are usually due to curettage for an infected or missed abortion or for postpartum complications. Destruction of large areas of endometrium results in amenorrhea and recurrent abortions, believed to be due to insufficient endometrium to support implantation of the conceptus. Treatment is discussed in Chapter 24.

8. Physical and emotional trauma–There is no ev-idence to support the common belief that either intercourse or physical or emotional trauma causes or contributes to the risk of abortion.

C. Paternal Factors: Little is known about the role of paternal factors in the genesis of spontaneous abortion. Chromosomal translocations in sperm can of course lead to a zygote with too little or too much chromosomal material, resulting in abortion.

SPECIFIC TYPES OF SPONTANEOUS ABORTION

It is convenient to consider the clinical aspects of spontaneous abortion under five subgroups: threatened, inevitable, incomplete, missed, and recurrent abortion (Figure 9–1).

Threatened Abortion

Threatened abortion is vaginal bleeding or any bloody vaginal discharge during the first half of pregnancy. About 20–25% of women have this symptom, and half of those do in fact abort. The bleeding is frequently slight, but it may persist for days or weeks. There is an increased risk of suboptimal pregnancy outcome—preterm delivery, low birth weight, and perinatal death—but the risk of birth defect does not appear to be increased significantly.

Most cases of threatened abortion probably progress to the next stage no matter what is done. Therefore, the patient should be instructed to notify her physician immediately whenever vaginal bleeding occurs during pregnancy. If the bleeding is slight and no cause is ascertained after careful inspection of the vagina and cervix, she should be so informed. If an intrauterine device is still present and the "string" is visible, the device should be removed.

The pain of threatened abortion may be anterior and clearly rhythmic, simulating mild labor; a persistent low backache, associated with a feeling of pelvic pressure; or a dull, midline, suprasymphyseal discomfort accompanied by tenderness over the uterus. Whichever form the pain takes, the prognosis for continuation of the pregnancy in the presence of bleeding and pain is poor.

Careful examination is required to determine if the cervix is already dilated (abortion inevitable) or if there is a serious complication such as extrauterine pregnancy or torsion of an unsuspected ovarian cyst. The patient may be kept at home in bed with analgesics for pain, but if symptoms are severe she should be hospitalized. If blood loss is sufficient to cause anemia, evacuation of the products of conception is generally indicated. If bleeding is severe enough to cause hypovolemia, termination of the pregnancy is mandatory.

Slight hemorrhage may persist for weeks, raising a question about the status of the fetus. (The continued presence of chorionic gonadotropin in blood or urine does not indicate whether the fetus is alive or dead.) If the uterus—accurately measured over a period of time—does not increase in size or if it becomes smaller, one can conclude that the fetus is dead. An increase in uterine size indicates

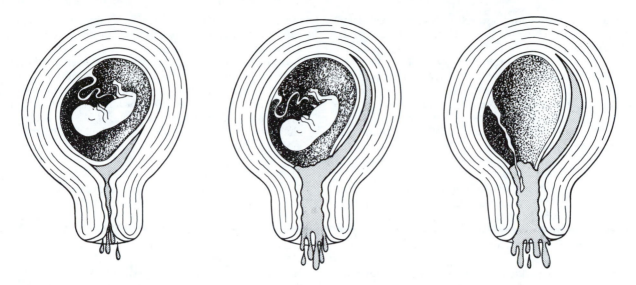

Figure 9–1. Types of abortions. **A:** Threatened. **B:** Inevitable. **C:** Incomplete.

that the fetus is still alive or that a hydatidiform mole is present.

The demonstration by sonography of a distinct, well-formed gestational ring with central echoes from the embryo implies that the products of conception are reasonably healthy. A gestational sac with no central echoes from an embryo or fetus implies probable death of the conceptus.

When abortion is inevitable, the mean diameter of the gestational sac is frequently smaller than appropriate for gestational age. Moreover, at 6 weeks' gestation and thereafter, fetal heart action should be discernible using real-time ultrasound. Most often, however, a single examination is insufficient to determine the likelihood of abortion. Serial sonographic observations to document lack of fetal growth are useful. After death of the conceptus, the uterus usually should be emptied.

Inevitable Abortion

Inevitability of abortion is signaled by gross rupture of the membranes along with cervical dilatation. Under these conditions, imminent abortion is almost certain.

If in early pregnancy the sudden discharge of fluid, suggesting rupture of the membranes, occurs before any pain or bleeding, the patient may be put to bed and observed for further leakage of fluid, bleeding, cramping, or fever. If after 48 hours there has been no further escape of amnionic fluid, no bleeding or pain, and no fever, she may get up and, except for any form of vaginal penetration, continue her usual activities. If, however, the gush of fluid is accompanied or followed by bleeding and pain—or if fever ensues—abortion should be considered inevitable and the uterus emptied.

Incomplete Abortion

The fetus and placenta are likely to be expelled together

in abortions occurring before the tenth week but separately thereafter. With abortions of pregnancies that are more advanced, bleeding is often profuse and may occasionally be massive, to the point of producing profound hypovolemia. If the placenta is partly attached and partly separated, the splintlike action of the attached portion of the placenta interferes with myometrial contraction in the immediate vicinity, and hemorrhage ensues. The vessels in the denuded segment of the placental site, deprived of the constriction provided by contraction and retraction of the myometrium, bleed profusely.

In instances of incomplete abortion, it is often unnecessary to dilate the cervix before curettage. In many cases, the retained placental tissue simply lies loose in the cervical canal and can be lifted from an exposed external os with ovum or ring forceps. Hemorrhage from incomplete abortion is occasionally severe but rarely fatal. Fever is not a contraindication to curettage once appropriate antibiotic treatment has been started.

Missed Abortion

Missed abortion has been arbitrarily defined as retention in utero of dead products of conception for 4–8 weeks or more. The rationale for this rigid time limitation is not clear and serves no purpose—retention for any prolonged period is sufficient to constitute missed abortion. Upon death of the ovum, there may or may not be vaginal bleeding or other symptoms signifying threatened abortion. For a time, the uterus then seems to remain stationary in size, but the mammary changes usually regress. The patient is likely to lose a few pounds in weight. Thereafter, careful palpation and measurement of the uterus shows that it has not only ceased to enlarge but has become smaller as a result of absorption of amnionic fluid and maceration of the fetus. If missed abortion terminates spontaneously, as most of them do, the process of expulsion is the same as in

any abortion. If retained several weeks after fetal death, the product is a shriveled sac containing a greatly macerated embryo.

Occasionally, after prolonged retention of the dead products of conception, serious coagulation defects develop, especially when gestation had reached the second trimester before the fetus died. The pathogenesis and treatment of coagulation defects and any attendant hemorrhage in instances of prolonged retention of a dead fetus are considered in Chapter 58.

Recurrent Spontaneous Abortion

Recurrent spontaneous abortion has been defined by various criteria of number and sequence, but probably the most generally accepted definition today requires three or more consecutive spontaneous abortions. Recurrent spontaneous abortions are chance phenomena in most cases.

It is important to differentiate spontaneous abortions that result from problems within the zygote from those much less common abortions that are due to maternal factors. In early abortions, a nonrecurring aneuploid abnormality of the conceptus is probably responsible. In late abortions, fetal development is more likely to have been euploid, with a maternal abnormality causing the abortion.

Several investigators now recommend karyotyping the parents after they have experienced two or three spontaneous abortions. When karyotyping is performed, chromosomal banding techniques should be used.

With the exception of the antiphospholipid antibodies and an incompetent cervix, the apparent cure rate after as many as three spontaneous abortions will range between 70% and 85% no matter what treatment is used. In other words, the loss rate will be higher—but not a great deal higher—than that anticipated for pregnancies in general. In fact, the likelihood of recurrent abortion is 25–30% regardless of the number of previous abortions. Poland et al (1977) noted that if a woman previously had delivered a liveborn infant, the risks for each recurrent abortion were approximately 30%, but if the woman had no liveborn infants and had experienced at least one fetal loss (spontaneous abortion, fetal or neonatal death), the risk of abortion was 46%. Following successful delivery, the likelihood of an abnormal child is not increased; however, the risk for preterm and small-for-dates infants is increased significantly.

INCOMPETENT CERVIX

Incompetent cervix is a discrete obstetric entity characterized by painless dilatation of the cervix in the second trimester or early in the third trimester, with prolapse of membranes through the cervix and ballooning of the membranes into the vagina, followed by rupture of the membranes and subsequent expulsion of a fetus that is so immature it is likely to succumb. Unless effective treatment is provided, this same sequence of events tends to be repeated with each pregnancy. Thus, the diagnosis remains difficult and is a clinical one based upon a carefully observed and recorded sequence of events that includes painless cervical dilatation and spontaneous rupture of the membranes.

Although the cause of cervical incompetence is obscure, previous trauma to the cervix—especially in the course of dilatation and curettage, conization, cauterization, or amputation—appears to be a factor in many cases. In other instances, abnormal cervical development, including that following exposure to diethylstilbestrol in utero, plays a role.

Treatment

Cervical incompetence calls for surgical reinforcement by some kind of purse-string suture (cerclage). It is best performed after the first trimester but before cervical dilatation of 4 cm is reached. Bleeding, uterine contractions, and ruptured membranes are contraindications to surgery.

A. Preoperative Evaluation: Cerclage should be delayed until after 14 weeks of gestation so that early abortions due to other factors will be completed. Sonography is mandatory to exclude major fetal anomalies and confirm the presence of a living fetus. Cervical cytologic tests should be negative. Obvious cervical infection should be treated, and cultures for gonorrhea, chlamydial infection, and group B streptococci are recommended by some. If culture results are positive, both sexual partners should be treated as described in Chapter 7. Sexual intercourse should be avoided for at least a week before and after surgery.

B. Cerclage Procedures: Two main types of operation are in current use during pregnancy. One very simple procedure recommended by McDonald consists of placement of a purse-string suture around the outside of the cervix. The Shirodkar operation is more complicated, and for that reason the McDonald procedure is associated with less trauma and blood loss. Success rates approaching 85–90% are achieved with both techniques.

There is no good evidence that prophylactic antibiotics to prevent infection or progestational agents or beta-mimetic drugs to prevent uterine contractions are of any value. If the operation fails and signs of imminent abortion or delivery develop, the suture must be released at once, since failure to do so may result in rupture of the uterus or cervix.

Transabdominal cerclage placed at the level of the uterine isthmus has been recommended in some instances. The procedure requires one laparotomy for placement of the suture and another for its removal or for delivery of the pregnancy products.

INDUCED ABORTION

THERAPEUTIC ABORTION

Therapeutic abortion is termination of pregnancy before the time of fetal viability for the purpose of safeguarding the life or health of the mother.

Until the United States Supreme Court *Roe v Wade* decision of 1973, only therapeutic abortions could be legally performed in most states. The most common legal definition of therapeutic abortion until then was termination of pregnancy before the period of fetal viability for the purpose of saving the life of the mother.

Indications

Some of the indications for therapeutic abortion are discussed in other chapters along with the diseases that commonly lead to the operation. Well-documented indications are persistent heart disease in the wake of previous cardiac decompensation, advanced hypertensive vascular disease, and invasive carcinoma of the cervix. Although it is impossible to predict what the acceptable indications for therapeutic abortion will be in the future, the therapeutic abortion policy formerly established by the American College of Obstetricians and Gynecologists seems most rational. According to that policy, therapeutic abortion may be performed for the following medical indications:

(1) When continuation of the pregnancy may threaten the life of the mother or seriously impair her health. In determining whether or not there is such a risk to health, account may be taken of the patient's total environment, actual or reasonably foreseeable.

(2) When pregnancy has resulted from rape or incest. In such cases, the same medical criteria should be employed in evaluation of the patient.

(3) When continuation of the pregnancy is likely to result in the birth of a child with severe physical deformities or mental retardation.

ELECTIVE (VOLUNTARY) ABORTION

Elective abortion is interruption of pregnancy before fetal viability at the request of the patient but not for reasons of maternal risk or fetal disease. At present in the United States, approximately one elective abortion is performed for every three live births.

Fetal Viability

The term "viable" is widely used to signify a reasonable chance of survival if the fetus were to be removed from the uterus. Termination of pregnancy before 38 weeks of gestation but after the fetus has achieved some potential for survival is referred to as preterm delivery. In many states, a birth certificate is prepared for any infant delivered at 20 weeks' gestational age or more or for any infant that weighs 500 g or more.

The United States Supreme Court, in its ruling on the legality of abortion, used the term "viability" but did not define it. Moreover, the Court stated,

. . . We need not resolve the difficult question of when life begins. When those trained in the respective disciplines of medicine, philosophy, and theology are unable to arrive at any consensus, the judiciary, at this point in the development of man's knowledge, is not in a position to speculate as to the answer.[1]

Counseling Before Elective Abortion

Especially in the circumstances usually surrounding the decision for or against abortion, knowledgeable and compassionate counselors are invaluable. There are, however, only three choices available to the woman considering an abortion: continued pregnancy, with its risks and responsibilities; continued pregnancy, with its risks but with adoption anticipated; or abortion with its risks. In some instances, the pregnant woman considering abortion may prefer to avoid abortion and allow the pregnancy to continue if social and economic problems can be resolved.

TECHNIQUES FOR ABORTION

The various techniques for performing elective abortion currently in use are outlined in Table 9–2 and discussed below. Requiring a positive pregnancy test before abortion induction will avoid a needless procedure on a nonpregnant woman whose period has been delayed for other reasons.

Surgical Techniques

The products of conception may be removed surgically through an appropriately dilated cervix or transabdominally by either hysterotomy or hysterectomy. These techniques were recently reviewed by the American College of Obstetricians and Gynecologists (Technical Bulletin No. 109, 1987). The techniques of cervical dilation, uterine evacuation, and associated complications are discussed in Chapter 17.

A. Transcervical Evacuation: Surgical abortion through the cervix is performed by first dilating the cervix and then evacuating the products of conception by mechanically scraping out the contents (sharp curettage) or by vacuum aspiration (suction curettage), or both. The likelihood of complications—uterine perforation, cervical laceration, hemorrhage, incomplete removal of the fetus and placenta, infection—increases after the first trimester and especially after about 16 weeks. For this reason, D&C or vacuum aspiration is best performed before 16 weeks.

1. Laminaria tents–Mechanical dilatation of the "undilated and uneffaced" cervix at the time of abortion is a

---

[1] Row v Wade (1973), 410 US 113.

Table 9–2. Techniques for accomplishing abortion.

I. Surgical
  A. Cervical dilatation followed by evacuation of uterine contents
    1. Curettage
    2. Vacuum aspiration (suction curettage)
    3. Dilatation and evacuation
  B. Laparotomy
    1. Hysterotomy
    2. Hysterectomy
II. Medical
  A. Oxytocin intravenously
  B. Intra-amnionic hyperosmotic fluid
    1. 20% saline
    2. 30% urea
  C. Prostaglandins E_2, F_{2a}, and prostaglandin analogues
    1. Intra-amnionic injection
    2. Extraovular injection
    3. Vaginal insertion
    4. Parenteral injection
    5. Oral ingestion
  D. Various combinations of the above
  E. Antiprogesterone RU 486

potentially traumatic procedure. The risk of trauma can be minimized by inserting into the cervical canal an agent that will slowly swell and dilate the cervix. Laminaria tents are used commonly to help dilate the cervix for abortion. The stems are packaged according to size (small, 3–5 mm in diameter; medium, 6–8 mm; and large, 8–10 mm). The strongly hygroscopic laminaria are thought to act by drawing water from proteoglycan complexes, causing them to dissociate and thereby allowing the cervix to soften and dilate.

2. Menstrual aspiration–Aspiration of the endometrial cavity using a flexible 5- or 6-mm Karman cannula and syringe within 1–3 weeks after failure to menstruate has been variously referred to as menstrual aspiration, menstrual extraction, menstrual induction, instant period, atraumatic abortion, and miniabortion. Problems include the absence of pregnancy, missing the implanted zygote with the curette, failure to recognize an ectopic pregnancy, and, rarely, uterine perforation.

3. Anti-D immunoglobulin–Treatment of D-negative women after abortion with Rh_o immune globulin (RhoGAM) is recommended, since about 5% of D-negative women undergoing abortion become immunized.

B. Hysterotomy or Hysterectomy: In a few circumstances, abortion by abdominal hysterotomy or hysterectomy is preferable to either D&C or medical induction (see below). If significant uterine disease is present, hysterectomy may be the ideal treatment. If sterilization is to be performed, either hysterotomy with interruption of tubal continuity or hysterectomy may on occasion be more advisable than curettage or medical induction followed by partial resection of the oviducts.

Medical Induction of Abortion

Very few safe and effective safe abortifacient drugs have been discovered, though throughout history many naturally occurring substances have been tried by women desperate not to be pregnant. Serious systemic illness or even death—but not abortion—has been the common result.

A. Oxytocin: Induction of second-trimester abortion is possible with high doses of oxytocin administered in small volumes of intravenous fluids. One regimen is as follows:

1. To 1000 mL of lactated Ringers' injection, add ten 1-mL ampules of oxytocin (10 IU/mL). The resulting solution contains 100 mU of oxytocin per milliliter.

2. Start an intravenous infusion at a rate of 0.5 mL/min (50 mU/min) and increase at 20- to 30-minute intervals up to a maximum rate of 2 mL/min (200 mU/min). If effective contractions are not established at this rate, the oxytocin concentration must be increased.

3. Discard all but 500 mL of the remaining solution, which contains a concentration of oxytocin of 100 mU/mL. To this 500 mL, add five 1-mL ampules of oxytocin, so that the resulting solution contains 200 mU/mL.

4. Reduce the rate of infusion to 1 mL/min (200 mU/min), and increase at 20- to 30-minutes intervals up to a rate of 2 mL/min (400 mU/min).

5. Continue at this rate for an additional 4–5 hours or until the fetus is expelled.

After each increase in infusion rate, careful attention must be directed to the frequency and intensity of uterine contractions, since each increase in infusion rate markedly increases the amount of oxytocin infused.

There are complications from the use of oxytocin. If appreciable volumes of electrolyte-free solution are administered along with oxytocin, water intoxication may develop (see Chapter 44).

B. Intra-amnionic Hyperosmotic Solutions: In order to achieve abortion during the second trimester, 20–25% saline or 30–40% urea has been injected into the amnionic sac to stimulate uterine contractions and cervical dilatation. These techniques are now being used less often than before. The mechanism of action is not clear.

C. Prostaglandins: Prostaglandins are now being widely used to terminate pregnancy, especially in the second trimester. Compounds commonly used are prostaglandin E_2 (dinoprostone), prostaglandin $F_{2\alpha}$ (dinoprost tromethamine), and certain analogues, especially carboprost methyl (15-methylprostaglandin $F_{2\alpha}$ methyl ester). The probable mode of action of the prostaglandins on the uterus and cervix is discussed in Chapter 37.

Prostaglandins can act effectively on the cervix and uterus (1) when placed in the vagina in the form of a suppository immediately adjacent to the cervix, (2) when administered as a gel through a catheter into the cervical canal and lowermost uterus extraovularly, or (3) when injected into the amnionic sac by amniocentesis. These three approaches reduce appreciably—but do not eliminate—the unpleasant systemic effects, especially gastrointestinal upset, that accompany oral or parenteral administration. At the same time, administration of prostaglandins by the three routes does cause cervical softening, uterine contractions, cervical dilatation, and expulsion of the products of conception in the great majority of cases, though repeated doses may be required.

D. Mifepristone (RU 486): A recently developed oral antiprogesterone called mifepristone (RU 486) has been used clinically to effect abortion in early human gestation, either alone or in combination with oral prostaglandins. Mifepristone soon will be available in the United States for use as an abortifacient.

CONSEQUENCES & COMPLICATIONS OF ELECTIVE ABORTION

Maternal Morbidity & Fatalities

Serious morbidity and even deaths have followed some elective abortions. Nonetheless, legally induced abortion is a relatively safe surgical procedure, especially when performed during the first 2 months. The risk of death from abortion performed during the first 2 months is about 0.6 per 100,000 procedures. *The relative risk of dying as the consequence of abortion is approximately doubled for each 2 weeks of delay after 8 weeks of gestation.*

Impact on Future Pregnancies

In a scholarly review of the impact of elective abortion upon subsequent pregnancy outcome, Hogue (1986) concluded as follows:

(1) Fertility is not affected by elective abortion.

(2) Vacuum aspiration for a first pregnancy results in no increased incidence of midtrimester spontaneous abortions, preterm deliveries, or low-birth-weight deliveries in subsequent pregnancies when compared to primigravida controls. However, dilatation and curettage in primigravidas results in an increased risk for subsequent ectopic pregnancy, midtrimester spontaneous abortion, and low-birth-weight infants.

(3) Subsequent ectopic pregnancies are not increased if the first termination is done by vacuum aspiration.

(4) Multiple elective abortions may increase various risks in subsequent pregnancies, but insufficient information is available to assess the risks accurately.

(5) Placenta previa probably is not increased by elective abortion.

(6) Induced midtrimester abortions apparently carry little risk to subsequent pregnancies if injection techniques are used. Unfortunately, there are not enough procedure-specific data available to form valid conclusions regarding the risks to future pregnancies following midtrimester abortion.

There is overwhelming proof that forceful dilatation of the cervix by any procedure, whether in a first- or second-trimester abortion, predisposes a subsequent pregnancy to increased risks.

Septic Abortion

Serious complications of abortion have been most often associated with criminal abortion (ie, one performed by an unlicensed practitioner). Severe hemorrhage, sepsis, bacterial shock, and acute renal failure all have developed in association with legal abortion, but at a much lower frequency.

Sepsis from abortion is most often caused by pathogenic organisms of the bowel and vaginal flora. Infection most commonly is confined to the uterus in the form of metritis, but parametritis, peritonitis (localized and general), and septicemia are by no means rare.

Treatment of the infection includes prompt evacuation of the products of conception. Although mild infections can be treated successfully with broad-spectrum antibiotics in the usual dosages, any serious infection should be attacked with great vigor from the very start. An example is clindamycin given along with gentamicin; however, several other regimens are equally effective.

Septic Shock

Endotoxemia and exotoxemia are likely to cause severe and even fatal shock. Septic shock, which fortunately now is rare, was previously seen most often in women of reproductive age in connection with induced abortion, though it can occur as a result of infection in the genital or urinary tract at any time during pregnancy or the puerperium. This complication is discussed in detail in Chapter 50 and the hematologic consequences of disseminated intravascular coagulation in Chapter 58.

Acute Renal Failure

Persistent renal failure in abortion usually stems from multiple effects of infection and of hypovolemia. Less commonly, it has been induced by toxic compounds employed to produce abortion, such as soap, hexachlorophene, or Lysol. Whereas very severe forms of bacterial shock are frequently associated with intense renal damage, the milder forms rarely lead to overt renal failure. Early recognition of this very serious complication is most important.

Renal failure is likely to be most severe when the cause of the sepsis includes *Clostridium perfringens,* which produces a potent hemolytic exotoxin. Whenever marked hemoglobinemia complicates clostridial infection, renal failure is the rule. At the outset, plans should be made to start effective dialysis early, before metabolic deterioration becomes severe.

SUGGESTED READINGS

American College of Obstetricians and Gynecologists: Methods of midtrimester abortion. Tech Bull No. 109, October 1987.

Atrash HK, Hogue CJ: The effect of pregnancy termination on future reproduction. Baillieres Clin Obstet Gynaecol (Jun) 1990;4(2):391.

Centers for Disease Control: Abortion surveillance: Preliminary analysis—United States, 1982–1983. MMWR 1986;35:7SS.

Check JH, Adelson HG: The efficacy of progesterone in achieving successful pregnancy: II. In women with pure luteal phase defects. Int J Fertil 1987a;32:139.

Check JH et al: The efficacy of progesterone in achieving successful pregnancy: I. Prophylactic use during luteal phase in anovulatory women. Int J Fertil 1987b;32:135.

Grimes DA et al: Early abortion with a single dose of the antiprogestin RU-486. Am J Obstet Gynecol 1988;158:1307.

Harlap S, Shiono PH, Ramcharan S: A life table of spontaneous abortions and the effects of age, parity and other variables. Page 145 in: *Human Embryonic and Fetal Death*. Porter JH, Hook EB (editors). Academic, 1980.

Herbst AL et al: Reproductive and gynecologic surgical experience in diethylstilbestrol-exposed daughters. Am J Obstet Gynecol 1981;141:1019.

Hogue CJR: Impact of abortion on subsequent fecundity. Clin Obstet Gynaecol 1986;13:95.

Kajii T et al: Avirachan S: Anatomic and chromosomal anomalies in 639 spontaneous abortions. Hum Genet 1980;55:87.

Kline J et al: Environmental influences on early reproductive loss in a current New York City study. Page 225b in: *Human Embryonic and Fetal Death*. Porter IH, Hook EB (editors). Academic, 1980.

Lähteenmäki P, Luukkainen T: Return of ovarian function after abortion. Clin Endocr 1978;8:123.

Lee CS: Luteal phase defects. Obstet Gynecol Surv 1987;42:267.

Poland BJ et al: Reproductive counseling in patients who have had a spontaneous abortion. Am J Obstet Gynecol 1977;127:685.

Scott JR, Rote NS, Branch DW: Immunologic aspects of recurrent abortion and fetal death. Obstet Gynecol 1987;70:645.

Shirodkar VN: A new method of operative treatment for habitual abortions in the second trimester of pregnancy. Antiseptic 1955;52:299.

Simpson JL: Genes, chromosomes, and reproductive failure. Fertil Steril 1980;33:107.

Stein Z et al: Maternal age and spontaneous abortion. Page 129 in: *Human Embryonic and Fetal Death*. Porter IH, Hook EB (editors). Academic, 1980.

Supreme Court of the United States Syllabus, Roe et al v Wade, District Attorney of Dallas County, Texas, January 22, 1973.

Warburton D et al: Chromosome abnormalities in spontaneous abortion: Data from the New York City study. Page 261 in *Human Embryonic and Fetal Death*. Porter IH, Hook EB (editors). Academic, 1980.

10

Chronic Pelvic Pain, Dysmenorrhea, & Premenstrual Syndrome

One of the most challenging problems for the gynecologist is the management of chronic pelvic pain. Unfortunately, the diagnosis is often obscure and relief difficult to achieve for many types of pain of apparent gynecologic origin.

CHRONIC PELVIC PAIN

Etiology

Many causes of chronic abdominal and pelvic pain are listed in Table 10–1.

The presence of adhesions cannot be correlated with pain; many patients with extensive adhesions may have no symptoms, and, contrariwise those with minimal adhesions may have severe symptoms. Unless the adhesions obstruct bowel or cause other significant anatomic alterations, it is unlikely that they are a cause of pelvic pain in a significant number of cases.

History

A thorough history is the physician's main resource in the investigation of chronic pelvic pain (see Chapter 2). Women with chronic pelvic pain often have two or more complaints, which should be listed at the first interview. The longer the list, the greater the likelihood that the origin of the pain might be unrelated to any identifiable organic cause.

Specific variables to be asked about are the location and timing of pain, its quality and severity, what brings it on, and what relieves it.

A. Location and Timing: The more accurately the patient can pinpoint the site of the pain, the more likely it is that a definitive diagnosis can be made. The onset of pain may be unrelated to any particular daily activity or time of the month, or there may be clear relationships to meals, sleeping, exercising, intercourse, prolonged standing, and phases of the menstrual cycle.

B. Quality and Severity: Pain should be character-ized as steady or intermittent; as mild, moderate, or severe; and as sharp and piercing or dull aching. If pain is intermittent, one should ask whether it remains steady or gradually increases in intensity.

C. Palliation: Pain may be relieved by eating, lying down, cessation of menses, etc.

Physical Examination

If abdominal or pelvic examination discloses a mass, hernia, bleeding, or pus, the diagnosis may be obvious. Tenderness alone may not be of much help.

Laboratory Investigation & Imaging Studies

Testing should be directed toward areas indicated by the history and physical examination. Obviously, the patient should have a Papanicolaou smear, and occult blood should be tested for in the rectum. Pregnancy and pregnancy-related entities should be excluded. A complete blood count, sonography, CT scan, and barium studies of the small and large bowel may be necessary.

Laparoscopy

At some point, if no cause has been determined, consideration should be given to laparoscopy. In one study of 1194 patients evaluated for chronic pain, Cunanan et al (1983) reported that 355 (30%) had normal pelvic and abdominal organs on laparoscopy and therefore an undiscovered reason for pain (and an unnecessary surgical procedure in retrospect).

Physiology of Pain Perception

The patient's perception of pain is modified by its chronicity. Transmission of "signals of discomfort" by peripheral nerve fibers can be stimulated by heat, pressure, or chemical mediators of inflammation. Bidirectional signals from the periphery to the brain and from the brain to the spinal cord may be modified by both affective states and motivational states. Modulation is accomplished through descending impulses that release neuromodulators in the

Table 10–1. Causes of chronic pelvic pain.

I. **Nongynecologic causes:**
  A. Abdominal wall:
    1. Lipoma
    2. Muscle strain or hematoma
    3. Hernia
  B. Peritoneum:
    1. Adhesions
    2. Endometriosis
  C. Gastrointestinal:
    1. Inflammatory:
      a. Ulcerative colitis
      b. Crohn's disease
      c. Diverticular disease
      d. Gastroenteritis
      e. Cholecystitis
      f. Pancreatitis
      g. Hepatitis
    2. Tumor:
      a. Cyst
      b. Polyp
      c. Carcinoma
    3. Obstruction, constipation
    4. Metabolic, malabsorption syndromes
    5. Adhesions
    6. Ulcer
  D. Urinary:
    1. Renal:
      a. Stone
      b. Infection
      c. Tumor
    2. Ureteral:
      a. Stone
      b. Obstruction, external
    3. Bladder:
      a. Infection:
        (1) Cystitis
        (2) Interstitial cystitis
      b. Tumor
      c. Stone
  E. Pneumonia
  F. Porphyria
II. **Gynecologic causes:**
  A. Uterine tube:
    1. Infection:
      a. Acute PID
      b. Chronic PID
      c. Actinomycosis
      d. Tuberculosis
    2. Pregnancy (chronic ectopic)
    3. Torsion (hydatid)
    4. Tumor
    5. Endometriosis
    6. Adhesions
  B. Ovary:
    1. Cyst, variable
    2. Tumor
    3. Torsion (with uterine tube)
    4. Endometriosis
  C. Uterus:
    1. Leiomyoma
    2. Infection
    3. Endometriosis
    4. Pregnancy
    5. Cancer
  D. Other:
    1. Pelvic congestion
    2. Adhesions
    3. Retrograde menstruation
    4. Pelvic relaxation
    5. Normal pelvis (no identifiable abnormalities)

spinal cord, the release mechanism thus acting as a "gate" that regulates transmission of peripheral signals to the brain via spinothalamic pathways. These modulators include serotonin and endorphins, both of which are linked to mood and pain perception. Any patient with chronic pain over a prolonged period develops depression, which may not be recognized. Depression may increase pain by opening the "gate" and allowing more signals of discomfort to enter.

Psychologic Aspects

Patients with chronic pain understandably develop psychologic responses and need understanding and sympathetic care. The physician must be on guard against attributing the pain to these responses.

Psychologic factors responsible for pain perception may have their origin in early life experiences. For example, several reports have linked chronic pelvic pain with childhood sexual abuse. For that reason, it is important to take a developmental, past medical, family, and social history as well as a review of systems.

Treatment

The best solution for a patient with chronic pelvic pain is a specific diagnosis followed by successful specific treatment. In all cases in which no specific cause can be identified, supportive management is required. Important aspects of treatment include spending more time with the patient, a willingness to listen, and a readiness to repeat the evaluation or undertake further studies when indicated. A multidisciplinary approach gives the best results. Psychologic evaluation is beneficial in many cases. Biofeedback training, transcutaneous nerve stimulation, and acupuncture may benefit some patients. Group and couple therapy is often helpful.

The patient should be told that her doctor knows she is experiencing pain even if no "physical cause" can be identified initially. Reassurance should be given that her natural concerns about cancer or other serious disease are groundless, since the history and physical examination would have led to their diagnosis.

Some discussion should be offered as to the teleological function of pain perception in calling attention to disease. It can be explained that when patients have chronic pain for which no cause can be found, the signals being sent are "false" ones and that the aim of medical treatment then is to find some means of interrupting or stopping the transmission of false messages.

Prostaglandin synthetase inhibitors should be used as necessary. Several are listed in Table 10–2. Sedatives should not be used because they may worsen the depression and psychomotor retardation associated with chronic pain. Anxiolytic drugs such as diazepam are not beneficial for chronic pain. Low-dose tricyclic antidepressants may be of benefit but should be given under the supervision of a physician knowledgeable about their effects. Narcotics are not indicated.

Table 10–2. Dosages of prostaglandin synthetase inhibitors.

Drug	Dosage[1]
Aspirin	600–1200 mg every 4–6 hours
Fenoprofen (Nalfon)	300–600 mg every 6 hours
Ibuprofen (Advil, Motrin, Nuprin, Rufen)	400–600 mg every 6 hours
Indomethacin (Indocin)	25–50 mg every 8 hours
Mefenamic acid (Ponstel)	500 mg initially, then 250 mg every 6 hours
Naproxen (Anaprox)	550 mg initially, then 275 mg every 8 hours
(Naprosyn)	500 mg initially, then 250 mg every 8 hours

[1]Use the smallest dose that produces relief.

PHYSIOLOGIC PAIN OF UTERINE ORIGIN (Primary Dysmenorrhea)

Prior to the early 1970s, many physicians believed that severe menstrual pain not associated with some obvious cause such as adenomyosis, endometriosis, uterine leiomyomatosis, or intrauterine contraceptive devices was of psychologic origin. Gynecologists now understand that menstrual cramps which begin with menarche or shortly thereafter and do not significantly worsen but remain essentially the same in intensity and duration from cycle to cycle are physiologic in origin. This form of dysmenorrhea is thought to be caused by uterine contractions induced by the prostaglandin $F_{2\alpha}$ that is normally formed as a consequence of estrogen-progesterone withdrawal at the end of a normal ovulatory cycle. The pain may precede menstrual flow by as much as 24 hours but most commonly occurs concomitantly with onset of bleeding.

Treatment

Most women with physiologic menstrual pain obtain significant or complete relief from suppression of ovulation with a low-dose combination oral contraceptive. The prostaglandin synthetase inhibitors listed in Table 10–2 provide relief for women who desire pregnancy or in whom oral contraceptives are contraindicated. Anticipatory treatment with these drugs offers no benefit with the exception of aspirin, which should be started 3–4 days before the expected menses.

Laparoscopy is indicated for women unresponsive to medical therapy. Some gynecologists perform laparoscopic uterine nerve ablation (LUNA) at the time of diagnostic laparoscopy if no disease or only stage I endometriosis is demonstrated. This relatively new procedure is reported to relieve pain in about 60% of women with dysmenorrhea unresponsive to medical management.

PREMENSTRUAL SYNDROME

Premenstrual syndrome consists of diverse symptoms that occur cyclically 1–14 days prior to the onset of menstrual bleeding, are relieved by the onset of bleeding, and are followed by a symptom-free interval of at least 7 days. Symptoms that have been reported include headache, breast swelling or tenderness, abdominal bloating, nausea, constipation, edema, backache, pelvic pain, increased thirst or appetite, cravings for sweet or salty foods, palpitations, hives, seizures, poor coordination, fatigue, depression, irritability, anxiety, lack of concentration, insomnia, aggressiveness, moodiness, indecision, forgetfulness, confusion, and feelings of loneliness. The syndrome affects between 20% and 60% of women of reproductive age and seems to increase in incidence and severity with age. The peak incidence occurs in the fourth decade.

The diagnosis is based on the history. If confirmation is required, a carefully maintained menstrual calendar that documents the occurrence of symptoms is useful. Some gynecologists ask for weekly calendars mailed to the office, feeling that more accurate histories can be compiled in that way. Documented relief of symptoms coinciding with menstrual bleeding followed by a symptom-free interval is critical to the diagnosis.

The syndrome is of unknown cause. Considering the diversity of reported symptoms, it seems likely that there is no single cause for all of the symptoms. The great majority of gynecologists agree that premenstrual syndrome, while it may include a number of physiologic symptoms, is not of psychologic origin.

Treatment

Clinical trials of various modes of therapy have been hampered by problems of patient selection and experimental design and by a 40–50% positive response to placebo. In general, the placebo affect provides only temporary relief.

Bromocriptine, pyridoxine, and prostaglandin synthetase inhibitors have been tried with questionable benefit. Progesterone administration has not been consistently helpful in controlled studies. Mild diuretics appear to relieve symptoms, perhaps resulting from salt and water retention late in an ovulatory cycle.

Psychologic depression is not commonly the chief manifestation, but when it does occur it is the most difficult symptom to treat. A recent report that naltrexone—a narcotic antagonist with dose-related hepatotoxicity—may be useful in the treatment of cyclic depression is therefore encouraging.

Psychologic support and reassurance from the physician and family members appear to be as effective as currently available pharmacologic therapy.

SUGGESTED READINGS

Cunanan RG Jr, Corey NG, Lippes J: Laparoscopic findings in patients with pelvic pain. Am J Obstet Gynecol 1983;146:587.

Gise LH (editor): *The Premenstrual Syndromes.* Churchill Livingstone, 1988.

Harrop-Griffiths J et al: The association between chronic pelvic pain, psychiatric diagnosis, and childhood sexual abuse. Obstet Gynecol 1988;71:589.

Lurie S, Borenstein R: The premenstrual syndrome. Obstet Gynecol Surv (Apr) 1990;45(4):220.

Magos A: Advances in the treatment of the premenstrual syndrome. Br J Obstet Gynaecol (Jan) 1990;97(1):7.

Rapkin AJ: Adhesions and pelvic pain: A retrospective study. Obstet Gynecol 1986;68:13.

Reading AE: A critical analysis of psychological factors in the management and treatment of chronic pelvic pain. Int J Psychiatry Med 1982-83;12:129.

Reiter RC: A profile of women with chronic pelvic pain. Clin Obstet Gynecol (Mar) 1990;33(1):130.

Reiter RC: Occult somatic pathology in women with chronic pelvic pain. Clin Obstet Gynecol (Mar) 1990;33(1):154.

11

Sexuality: The Gynecologist as Counselor

Awareness of the wide variations of normal in sexual behavior and of the common occurrence of psychosexual problems is vital for effective patient management in gynecologic practice. The gynecologist deals regularly with matters related to sexuality and is often the first physician to elicit complaints of sexual dysfunction. It is important for the physician to be well informed about sexuality, comfortable and nonjudgmental in dealing with patients' sexual concerns, and aware of suitable referral sources within the community when problems of sexual dysfunction seem to be beyond the scope of his or her training.

THE ROLE OF THE GYNECOLOGIST AS A COUNSELOR

In dealing with such sensitive issues as contraception, fertility, dyspareunia, and vaginal or pelvic pain, the gynecologist's role is to be a caretaker of each patient's reproductive system and an expert adviser about specific female sexual functions and dysfunctions. If the physician is judgmental or is clearly uncomfortable in dealing with matters of sexuality, the patient will easily sense this and will likely withhold comments or questions pertaining to sexual matters. Important information may in that way go unrecorded, with adverse implications for diagnosis and therapy.

According to large surveys of married couples, approximately 50% experience some form of sexual dysfunction. Disorders of desire or arousal are common complaints, as well as orgasmic dysfunction, dyspareunia, impotence, and premature ejaculation. The physician who is aware of the high incidence of sexual dysfunction and deals objectively and sensitively with these matters may be in a position to offer much-needed help to his or her patients.

Eliciting Complaints of Sexual Dysfunction

Because of social mores and cultural taboos, some problems of sexual function may be repressed, and the patient may present instead with complaints of anxiety or depression, chronic pelvic pain, fatigue, or headache. The physician should be aware that these common complaints may be the result of sexual problems or abuse and should attempt to elicit further data from the sexual history that may suggest a cause. Direct questions in a structured "yes or no" interview may not allow the inhibited patient to express her concerns. The physician must be alert to nonverbal clues that may signal the presence of underlying difficulties. A thorough sexual history should be aimed at identifying sexual dysfunction or the patient's misconceptions about sexuality. The history can be obtained in written or oral format, but the latter permits more interaction with the physician and contributes to greater understanding of important issues. The history should include specific questions and encourage comments and questions from the patient.

Typical questions in the sexual history are listed in Table 11–1.

Interpretation of Complaints

While complaints of anxiety, depression, and pelvic pain may have underlying causes related to sexual dysfunction, some forms of sexual dysfunction may be due to incompatibility of the sexual partners and deep discord in

---

Table 11–1. Common questions asked in a sexual history.

1. From whom did you receive early information on sex?
2. Age at menarche?
3. Age at first sexual experience?
4. Do you desire and enjoy sexual activities?
5. Do you have orgasms?
6. What percentage of the time are you orgasmic?
7. Have you ever been sexually abused or raped?
8. Do you masturbate?
9. How often do you have intercourse?
10. What percentage of the time are you orgasmic with intercourse?
11. Does your partner function satisfactorily?
12. Does your partner experience impotence, premature ejaculation, or lack of sexual desire?
13. Do you experience vaginal dryness or pain with intercourse?
14. Do you communicate well with your partner during sexual activities?
15. Do you have questions regarding sexual practices or problems you may experience?

the relationship. These difficulties are best handled by a marriage counselor.

When complaints relating specifically to sexual function are elicited, it is important to obtain a clear understanding of exactly what the symptoms are, the frequency of their occurrence, and any precipitating factors the patient can identify. It is sometimes useful for the physician to "sum up" the complaints for the patient to make certain the interpretation is correct. Both parties should participate in the discussion. The goal of treatment or its expected outcome should be expressly stated and agreed on as a guide to therapy.

Basics of Counseling

History taking is an individualized skill and may vary with the time allotted for the interview, the patient's style of communication, and the physician's background. A combination of directive and nondirective interview techniques allows the patient to discuss issues freely and gives the physician an opportunity to clarify and investigate certain issues more deeply. Even if the patient is hesitant about exploring some areas on the first visit, she may feel more free to discuss them at a later appointment.

Listening to the patient is a vital feature of the interview, permitting her to articulate her problems and obtain some relief from just talking about them. In some cases, the patient needs to be told that sexual practices such as masturbation and oral sex are acceptable types of sexual activity. Some of course are not, such as rape, child sexual abuse, and infliction of sexual trauma, and in appropriate cases the patient should be referred for psychiatric therapy and the circumstances reported to the responsible authorities or agencies. Some patients merely require straightforward information about sexual anatomy and physiology.

Counseling for the Physician

Most gynecologists do not choose to undertake intensive counseling with their patients unless they have had special training and a continuing desire to devote a great deal of time to that type of practice. However, many complaints of sexual dysfunction may be dealt with by the gynecologist. Most communities have access to psychiatrists or psychologists with special expertise in sexual problems for the patient who requires more intensive therapy.

HUMAN SEXUAL RESPONSES

The human sexual response is basically similar in both sexes. Sexual stimulation leads to vascular engorgement, muscular tension, and their physiologic consequences. The four phases of the sexual response, as described by Masters and Johnson, are **excitement, plateau, orgasm, and resolution.** The excitement phase is the longest. It may be induced by somatic or psychogenic stimuli and delayed or interrupted voluntarily. The neural functions of these responses are outlined in Table 11–2.

Whereas the female may have multiple orgasms in rapid succession, the male undergoes a refractory period of 5–30 minutes during which orgasm cannot be achieved by any means. Ordinarily, orgasm in the male is reached faster and more directly than in the female, for whom physical contact appears to be a less significant erotogenic factor. The intensity of the female reaction may depend upon the amount and type of foreplay. Direct contact with the clitoris is not usually achieved during intercourse in the "missionary position" (man over woman), since the clitoris normally retracts under the symphysis. Effective stimulation of the clitoris is better achieved by digital manipulation.

Because there is relatively little difference in size among most erect penises, the issue of penile size and level of enjoyment for the female is debatable unless the erect penis is very small or very large. Circumcision does not seem to decrease sensation for the male or delay ejaculation. The physician should recognize that sexual incompatibilities are usually psychogenic rather than physical and should attempt to identify serious psychosexual disorders and obtain psychiatric consultation as needed.

The details of the human sexual response have been described in the writings of Masters and Johnson. In general,

Table 11–2. Neuroanatomy of Excitement and Orgasm[1]

Reflex	Mediation	Afferent (Sensory) Connections	Spinal Cord Centers	Efferent (Motor) Connections
Excitement	Parasympathetic	From clitoris via the dorsal nerve of clitoris to the pudendal nerve.	S2–S4	Preganglionic fibers travel via the pelvic nerve (nervus erigentes) to the vesical and uterovaginal plexuses.
		From anterior labia via ilioinguinal nerve and the perineal branch of the posterior femoral cutaneous nerve.	T11–L2	Postganglionic fibers travel to the erectile tissue.
Orgasm	Sympathetic	Same	T11–L2	Preganglionic fibers travel via the splanchnic nerve to the inferior mesenteric ganglion and ganglia in the hypogastric, vesical, and pelvic plexuses. Postganglionic fibers pass to genital smooth muscle.
			S3–S4	Pudendal nerve to striated muscle (ischiocavernosus and bulbocavernosus).

[1]Reproduced, with permission, from *Essentials of Obstetrics and Gynecology.* Hacher, NF, Moore, JG (editors), WB Saunders, 1986.

there is great similarity in the genital and extragenital responses in both men and women during the four phases.

Female Sexual Responses

A. Genital Responses: During the **excitement phase** in women, there is tumescence of the glans of the clitoris, vasocongestion, and an increase in diameter and length of its shaft. The vagina provides lubrication within 10–30 seconds after stimulation, and the vaginal tube expands and assumes a darker purplish hue. The uterus is partially elevated, and the corpus becomes irritable. The labia majora in the nullipara undergo flattening, separation, and elevation away from the vaginal outlet. The labia minora undergo slight thickening and expansion.

In the **plateau phase,** the clitoris retracts under the symphysis. The vagina forms an orgasmic platform at its outer third and undergoes further increases in width and depth. The corpus and cervix are fully elevated, and there is further increase in irritability of the corpus. The labia majora become engorged. The labia minora undergo a striking change in color from bright red to dark red, indicating impending orgasm. At this stage, Bartholin's glands secrete one or more drops of mucoid material.

At **orgasm,** contractions of the orgasmic platform in the vagina are noted at intervals of 0.8 second, recurring 6–12 times. The uterus undergoes contractions to an extent that parallels the intensity of the orgasm.

During the phase of **resolution,** the clitoris returns to its normal position. Five to 10 seconds after orgasm, the platform ceases to contract and undergoes rapid detumescence. The vaginal walls relax, and their normal color returns within 10–15 minutes. The uterus returns to its normal position, but the external os continues to gape for about 20–30 minutes. In the nullipara, the labia majora return to their normal thickness and midline position; in the multipara, labial vasocongestion subsides. The labia minora change in color from bright red to light pink within 15 seconds, and their size decreases.

B. Extragenital Responses: Numerous extragenital reactions occur during the various phases of the female sexual response.

During **excitement,** several changes occur in the breasts. The nipples become erect and increase in size, with concomitant tumescence of the areolae. A maculopapular rash (sexual flush) develops late in the phase of excitement, beginning over the epigastrium and spreading over the breasts. Myotonia increases, both voluntary and involuntary. Tachycardia parallels the degree of sexual tension.

During the **plateau** phase, the nipples become turgid. The breasts increase further in size, and the areolae undergo further erection. The sexual flush is better developed and myotonia increases, accompanied by spastic contractions. Tachycardia increases to as high as 175/min, accompanied by increases in systolic and diastolic blood pressures of 20–60 and 10–20 mm Hg, respectively.

At the time of **orgasm,** the sexual flush parallels the intensity of the reaction. Myotonia is maximal, with loss of voluntary control, accompanied by involuntary contractions of the rectal sphincter. The respiratory rate increases to as high as 40/min and tachycardia to between 110 and 180/min. Blood pressure rises by about 30–50 mm Hg systolic and 20–40 mm Hg diastolic.

During **resolution,** rapid detumescence of the nipples and areolae occurs. The decrease in volume of the breasts is slower. The sexual flush disappears rapidly. Myotonia rarely continues for more than 5 minutes after orgasm. Hyperventilation and tachycardia return rapidly to normal. A film of perspiration appears on the body, unrelated to the extent of physical activity.

Male Sexual Responses

A. Genital Responses: In the male, the genital and extragenital reactions are similar to those just described in the female.

During **excitement,** the most obvious change is rapid erection of the penis. Erection may be lost and regained or inhibited by numerous stimuli during this phase. There is tensing and thickening of the scrotal skin and elevation of the sac. The testes are elevated as a result of shortening of the spermatic cords.

During the **plateau** phase, the penis undergoes an increase in circumference at the coronal ridge and in some cases a change in color of the corona. The testes may undergo enlargement of 50% over their nonstimulated state. Full elevation of the testes indicates impending ejaculation. Cowper's glands provide preejaculatory emission of a few drops of fluid containing numerous active spermatozoa.

At **orgasm,** the penis undergoes contraction along the entire length of the penile urethra. The contractions start at intervals of 0.8 second. After the first three or four contractions, the expulsive force is reduced.

During **resolution,** the penis undergoes detumescence in two stages: rapid and slow. The scrotum rapidly loses its congestion, and its normal folds reappear. The testes return to normal size and position.

B. Extragenital Responses: The male also undergoes certain extragenital reactions.

In **excitement,** there is occasional erection of the nipples, myotonia (including voluntary and involuntary components), and tachycardia and hypertension in proportion to the degree of sexual tension.

During the **plateau** phase, an inconsistent further increase in erection of the nipples occurs. A maculopapular rash develops late in this phase. The rash originates over the epigastrium and spreads to the chest wall, neck, forehead, and other locations. Myotonia is characterized by a further increase in voluntary and involuntary components. Hyperventilation occurs late in this phase, and tachycardia may range between 100 and 175/min, with an increase in blood pressure by about 20–80 mm Hg systolic and 10–40 mm Hg diastolic.

At **orgasm,** a well-developed sexual flush is seen in about 25% of men. Myotonia is characterized by loss of voluntary control and by involuntary contractions and spasm. The rectal sphincter undergoes contractions occurring at intervals of 0.8 second, and the respiratory rate may rise to as high as 40/min. Tachycardia ranges from 110 to 180/min, and a rise in blood pressure by about 40–100 mm Hg systolic and 20–50 mm Hg diastolic occurs.

During **resolution,** there is involution of erection of the nipples and rapid disappearance of the sexual flush. Myotonia disappears within 5 minutes after the end of orgasm. The increased blood pressure, heart rate, and respiratory rate return to normal. Perspiration in the male is inconsistent and usually confined to the palms and soles.

SEXUAL FUNCTION IN MARRIAGE & SIMILAR INTIMATE RELATIONSHIPS

Free sexual expression of desires and individual sexual needs is one of the most highly valued aspects of loving relationships. Many factors can cause sexual dysfunction, leading to disorders of desire, problems with lubrication, or difficulties in achieving orgasm or ejaculation.

Sexual Problems in Women

A. Anorgasmia: Lack of orgasm is a common complaint of women who present with sexual problems. It may be the result of not knowing "how" to be orgasmic, of not receiving adequate stimulation from a partner, or of having lost a previously established ability to have orgasms.

Many women experience orgasm only with oral or manual clitoral stimulation and have difficulties in achieving orgasm with penile thrusting alone. Some women may be orgasmic in some situations and not in others. These are normal variations, yet the patient may desire a change in her sexual response and should be offered help and advice about how to do this.

A woman with primary anorgasmia usually has had insufficient stimulation from her partner or from self-manipulation. It is useful to encourage these patients to achieve orgasm through masturbation as a way of finding out how much and what type of self-stimulation is necessary to achieve orgasm. She can then teach her partner techniques that have proved to be successful. These techniques may also be helpful for women with situational anorgasmia. When direct clitoral stimulation is included in foreplay and interspersed throughout penile thrusting, the intensity of response is increased. The "female above" position may be recommended for some couples, since it may allow for greater stimulation of the clitoris by the penis or symphysis and gives the woman better control of clitoral stimulation.

It is important for the anorgasmic woman to explore—alone and with a partner—factors that may affect whether or not she is orgasmic. Increased communication with the sexual partner may contribute greatly to orgasmic success.

B. Loss of Desire: This is a frequent complaint in women who may be under psychologic stress resulting from fatigue, boredom, anger, or loss of trust in a relationship. Effective treatment must include direct counseling about the goals and motivations of the partners. If partners are unwilling to engage in useful dialogue regarding their relationship, there is little chance for success.

C. Vaginismus: Vaginismus is involuntary and occasionally painful spasm of the pubococcygeal muscles. It is common in young girls during the first pelvic examination or in women with local vaginal infection or introital trauma. Affected women may be unable to allow penile penetration or digital examination of the vagina. Vaginismus may also occur in women following a traumatic sexual experience such as rape or incest.

In psychogenic vaginismus, the examination reveals no organic disease but the external paravaginal muscles are tight, and vaginal penetration by speculum or examining finger is painful and difficult or impossible. Forcible entry should be avoided. Therapy is aimed at deconditioning or desensitization of the vaginal spasm. This requires motivation and understanding of the woman and her partner. It is important to emphasize that vaginismus is beyond conscious control. Slow, gentle dilatation of the vagina with a series of graduated, lubricated vaginal dilators along with reassurance and sexual education are the mainstays of therapy. Psychotherapy may be necessary if these measures are unsuccessful.

D. Dyspareunia: Painful intercourse is frequently due to some primary physical disorder such as vaginal irritation associated with infection or decreased lubrication or to pelvic or perineal disease. Episodes of pain may seriously detract from the enjoyment of sexual activity, leading to loss of desire for intercourse.

The examination is aimed at searching for local causes of vaginal irritation such as involutional changes associated with the menopause or signs of infection. Pelvic disease such as endometriosis, salpingitis, or adherence of ovarian tissue to the vaginal cuff after hysterectomy may also be causes of dyspareunia.

Sexual Problems in Men

Impotence and premature ejaculation are the most frequent causes of sexual dysfunction in men.

A. Impotence: Impotence may be due to organic disease such as diabetes, cancer, or vascular insufficiency. Use of alcohol, tranquilizers, and many antihypertensive drugs may be associated with impotence. Most cases of impotence, however, have an underlying psychologic origin, often demonstrated by the fact that patients have penile erections upon awakening or during masturbation but are incapable of obtaining erectile capacity necessary for intercourse with a partner. If the relationship is stable, with no overt problems, therapy is frequently successful. Changes in medications or decreased use of alcohol or other depressants may be warranted. In psychogenic impotence, a well-motivated couple may practice noncoital stimulation. As the male reaches full erection and is able to sustain it, vaginal penetration with thrusting is encouraged. When vaginal containment is successful, the man should perform gentle thrusting movements followed by resting periods and eventually coitus.

B. Premature Ejaculation: Premature ejaculation is a too-rapid ejaculatory response—ie, within seconds to minutes after insertion into the vagina and before female orgasm occurs. The cause is almost always psychogenic, yet complete urologic evaluation is warranted to search for a medical or anatomic cause.

Ejaculatory control to the point of pacing in sexual arousal is the goal of therapy. Use of the "start-stop" technique has been helpful in these patients. The woman is encouraged to stimulate the patient's penis almost to the point of orgasm and then stop, employing the "squeeze" technique if necessary. The penis is then stroked to the point of excitement again and the procedure repeated. In the squeeze technique, stimulation is allowed just short of ejaculation. The penis is then grasped firmly between the thumb and forefinger and squeezed. These methods are repeated on a regular basis until the male can achieve vaginal penetration and coitus.

SUGGESTED READINGS

Baucom DH, Aiken PA: Sex role identity, marital satisfaction, and response to behavioral marital therapy. J Consult Clin Psychol 1984;52:438.

Cole M: Sex therapy: A critical appraisal. Br J Psychiat 1985; 147:337.

Goldstein MK, Teng NN: Gynecologic factors in sexual dysfunction of the older woman. Clin Geriatr Med (Feb) 1991;7(1):41.

Goldstein S, Preston J: Marital therapy for the elderly. Can Med Assoc J 1984;15:1551.

Hahlwes K, Revenstorf D, Schindler L: Effects of behavioral marital therapy on couples' communication and problem-solving skills. J Consult Clin Psychol 1984;52:553.

Jacobson NS: A component analysis of behavioral marital therapy: The relative effectiveness of behavior exchange and communication/problem-solving training. J Consult Clin Psychol 1984;52:295.

Masters WH, Johnson VE: *Human Sexual Response.* Little, Brown, 1966.

Tuohey MK: Working women, working lovers: The effect of our multiple roles on intimacy. J Am Med Wom Assoc 1985;40:92.

12

Sexual Assault

Sexual assault is a violent crime, as attested to by the number of cases of rape in women associated with significant physical trauma. Since sexual assault may result in protracted and significant psychologic as well as physical trauma, it is of paramount importance to have an understanding of the nature and impact of this crime directed primarily (although not entirely) against women.

RAPE

INCIDENCE & EPIDEMIOLOGY

The actual incidence of sexual assault in the United States is unknown. However, according to the American College of Obstetricians and Gynecologists, rape accounts for 10–20% of all reported crime. Moreover, this is an underreported crime.

The age of sexual assault victims varies from the very young to the very old. In a 2-year (1986–1987) survey of rape examinations at Parkland Hospital in Dallas, 1989 rape examinations were performed, and the ages of the victims ranged from 2 years to 83 years. Astonishingly, 70 (4%) of the patients examined were 6 years of age or younger! Almost one-fifth (18.6%) of the cases involved girls aged 15 years or younger. Considering that approximately 10% of rape cases are reported in Dallas, it is estimated that almost 20,000 rapes occurred in Dallas County over the 2-year period. Approximately 2% of the rapes reported occurred in pregnant women.

DEFINITIONS

There are many definitions of rape, often varying from state to state. All definitions share a common denominator, however: absence of consent of the victim. The most common form of rape is forcible vaginal penetration by a penis. Ejaculation does not have to occur as a requirement for defining rape, and in many cases it does not occur.

As recently pointed out by the American College of Obstetricians and Gynecologists, the definition of rape has evolved to include penetration by any object or body part into the vagina, oral cavity, or anus. In short, rape or sexual assault is a forcible sexual act, often violent, inflicted upon the victim without her consent.

Males of any age may also be victims of rape. Intercourse with a female below the statutory age of consent—usually 18 years—has classically been defined as statutory rape.

THE ASSAILANT

There is no one stereotype that fits all rapists. Individuals who commit this crime come from a wide variety of ethnic, racial, and socioeconomic backgrounds, and the ages of assailants may range from young teenagers to old men. Often the assailant may be an acquaintance, friend, or even a relative. Another form of rape usually involving a nonstranger is the date rape. From recent surveys of college students, it appears that this form of rape is increasing in frequency. Many such assaults go unreported. Thus, probably in only 50% of cases or less is the assailant actually a stranger.

Almost all cases of rape involve aggressive behavior, including murder of the victim. At Parkland Memorial Hospital, some form of nongenital trauma occurs in 40% of victims. Common areas involved were the head, neck, and extremities. Three percent of victims had stab or gunshot wounds. Only 7% had evidence of genital tract trauma.

Many assailants experience some form of sexual dysfunction, as evidenced by the absence of ejaculation in many cases of rape. At Parkland Hospital, sperm are found in 50% or less of the specimens obtained from victims.

THE RAPE SURVIVOR

Just as there is no single stereotype for all rapists, there is none that fits all rape survivors. Age varies greatly, and rape victims may be married or single women from all racial and socioeconomic groupings.

MANAGEMENT OF RAPE SURVIVORS

The rape survivor is often emotionally distraught, beset by feelings of anger, shame, and helplessness. By the time she is ready to be seen by a gynecologist, she probably has been subjected to several hours of questioning by the local authorities. As a result, she often is both emotionally and physically fatigued. Thus, the examiner must start with empathy and understanding of what the patient has endured both in the actual assault and in its aftermath.

History

The key features of the rape examination are summarized in Table 12–1. Consent for the examination should be obtained by explaining its purpose. The exam should include a brief but pertinent history and physical examination, collecting specimens for evidence, treatment of significant trauma, and prophylactic treatment for prevention of certain sexually transmitted diseases. A summary of the history portion of the rape protocol utilized at Parkland Hospital is shown in Table 12–2.

Physical Examination

Consent should be obtained prior to the examination, and a chaperone should be present during the examination. The physical exam (Table 12–3) should include a complete survey of the body for bruises, scratches, and lacerations. A thorough pelvic examination should be done for evidence of trauma. All areas of trauma should be noted on a diagram of the body and genital tract (Figure 12–1). A thorough written description of all areas of trauma also should be included. The absence of any signs

Table 12–1. Summary of rape examinations performed at Parkland Memorial Hospital during 1986–1987.[1]

	1986	1987	Total
Total Examinations	1031	958	1989 (100%)
Ages (years)[2]			
>15	843	776	1619 (81.4%)
<15	188	182	370 (18.6%)
<12	79	83	162 (8.1%)
< 6	38	32	70 (3.5%)
Pregnant victims	23	22	45 (2.3%)
Trauma[3]			
Nongenital			40%
Genital			7%

[1]From Wendel and Stone (personal communication, 1989).
[2]Age range 2 years to 83 years.
[3]Estimated from a smaller subset of the sample.

Table 12–2. Key features of the history portion of the rape protocol at Parkland Memorial Hospital.

General information
  Date and time of assault
  Age, race, and parity
  Date and character of last menses

Sexual history
  Recent coitus prior to assault
  Contraceptive
  Douching practice

Alleged assault
  Penetration of mouth, vulva, vagina, and rectum
  Use of condom

Other sexual acts

Trauma

of trauma per se does not rule out the possibility of sexual assault.

Laboratory & Specimen Collection

One of the most important segments of the rape examination is the collection of potential evidence. As outlined in Table 12–4, collection of evidence includes diagrams or photographs of significant trauma. X-rays should be taken when indicated. Slides should be made for examination for motile sperm from all areas of penile penetration. Sufficient material should also be taken for later examinations by a forensic science laboratory for either sperm or acid phosphatase. With the recent advances in molecular genetic techniques, it also may be possible to analyze sperm or semen in an attempt to match the DNA with that of an accused assailant by the method of DNA fingerprinting. Fingernails should be examined for the presence of blood, skin, or other tissue and specimens sent to the forensic laboratory. Pubic hair combings may provide useful evidence if pubic hairs from the assailant are recovered. Clothing worn by the victim should be sent to the forensic laboratory if not already collected by other legal authorities. Blood for toxicology screening should be sent when indicated. All specimens should be meticulously labeled. A strict "chain of evidence" protocol must be followed with regard to the handling of all specimens. At Parkland Memorial Hospital, such specimens are placed in a sexual

Table 12–3. Physical examination of the rape survivor.

General
  Vital signs
  Emotional status

Body Surface[1]
  Bruises, lacerations, scratches

Genital Tract[1]
  External genitalia
  Hymen or hymenal ring
  Vagina
  Cervix, uterus, and adnexa
  Anus and rectum

[1]A sketch of all positive findings should be made.

____
Patient's Name or Stamp

PHYSICAL EXAMINATION

A) Patient's B.P.: ____________ Pulse: ____________ Temp: ____________

B) Patient's general appearance: ________________________

C) Patient's emotional status: ________________________

D) Clothing stains: ________________________

Bruises?	Yes ❑	No ❑
Scratches?	Yes ❑	No ❑
Lacerations?	Yes ❑	No ❑
Bite marks?	Yes ❑	No ❑

If yes, note and describe on anatomical drawings below

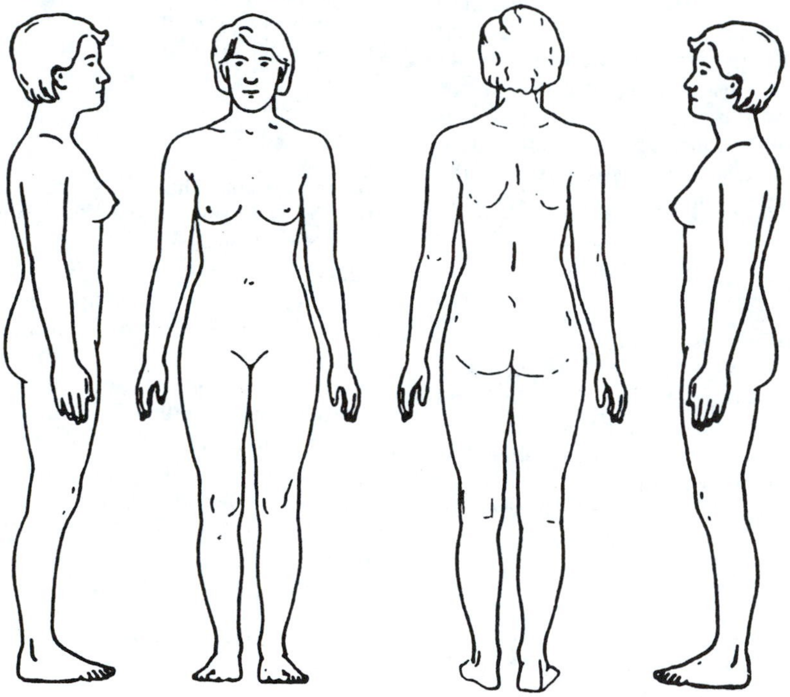

__________________ Date

__________________ M.D. Physician's Signature

Page 3 of 5 Pages

Figure 12–1. Physical examination for alleged sexual assault victims. (Used with permission of Irving Stone, PhD, Chief, Physical Evidence Section, Southwestern Institute of Forensic Sciences, Dallas, Texas.)

_____

Patients Name or Stamp

PELVIC EXAMINATION (use a non-lubricated speculum)

Vulva: Normal ❑
Abnormal ❑ Describe: _____

Perineal: Normal ❑
Abnormal ❑ Describe: _____

Hymen: Normal ❑
Abnormal ❑ Describe: _____

Vagina: Normal ❑
Abnormal ❑ Describe: _____

Cervix: Normal ❑
Abnormal ❑ Describe: _____

Uterus: Normal: ❑
Abnormal ❑ Describe: _____

Adnexa: Normal ❑
Abnormal ❑ Describe: _____

Recto-vaginal: Normal ❑
Abnormal ❑ Describe: _____
Not Done ❑

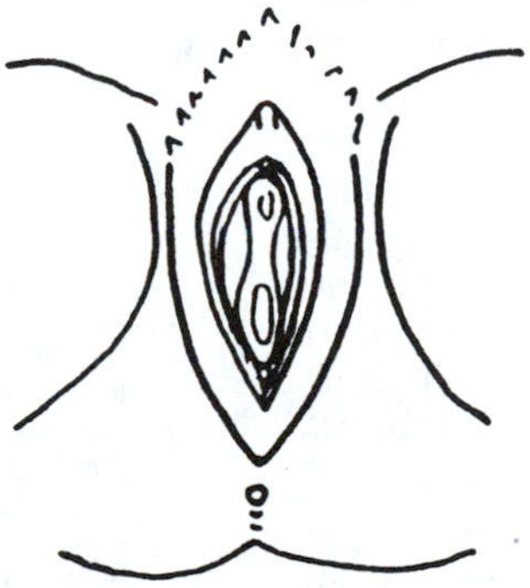

A) Were spermatozoa observed in the vaginal vault?   YES ❑ NO ❑
B) Were these motile?   YES ❑   NO ❑
C) Where intercourse is reported more than 24 hours prior to examination,
   were spermatozoa observed in cervical mucous?   YES ❑ NO ❑

NOTE: DISCARD PIPET AND SLIDES AFTER EXAMINATION FOR SPERMATOZOA.

_____   _____ M.D.
        Date   Physician's Signature

Page 4 of 5 Pages

Figure 12–1. continued

Table 12–4. Collection of evidence and laboratory evaluation.

Sketches, diagrams, and description of all trauma
Photographs when indicated
X-rays when indicated
Toxicology screening for alcohol or drugs when indicated
Wet preps for identification of motile sperm from all cases involving penile penetration
Specimens for forensic laboratory for detection of sperm, semen, acid phosphatase, from all areas of penile penetration
Collection of clothing for forensic examination
Nail clippings and pubic hair combings, as indicated

assault kit, and the box is labeled and sealed. The history and physical examination forms, along with all sketches and photographs, are also placed in the kit prior to sealing. The kit is then placed in a locked box in the emergency room by the examining physician. Any pertinent clothing, such as underwear, is also collected, labeled, and sealed in a bag and placed in the locked box. The specimens are then picked up by forensic science personnel who have approved access to the locked box.

Treatment

All trauma should be treated appropriately, and prophylaxis should be given for common sexually transmitted diseases (Table 12–5). One regimen recommended by the Centers for Disease Control is ceftriaxone, 250 mg intramuscularly, followed by tetracycline, 500 mg orally 4 times a day for 7 days, or oral doxycycline, 100 mg twice a day for 7 days. This regimen will provide satisfactory prophylaxis for the majority of cases of incubating syphilis, gonorrhea, and chlamydia. All areas of penetration should be cultured for *Neisseria gonorrhoeae,* and blood should be taken for serologic testing for syphilis. The rape survivor may also be a candidate to receive 0.5 mL of tetanus toxoid intramuscularly if needed to maintain current immunization status.

Prevention of pregnancy as a result of rape is of crucial importance. It is common practice in many centers, including Parkland Hospital, to provide prophylactic estrogen therapy in an attempt to prevent pregnancy in in-

Table 12–5. Recommended treatment for the rape survivor.

Attention to lacerations and other trauma
Culture for *Neisseria gonorrhoeae* and serologic tests for syphilis
Antibiotic prophylaxis:[1]
   Ceftriaxone, 250 mg IM, followed by tetracycline, 500 mg PO qid for 7 days, or–
   Doxycycline, 100 mg PO bid for 7 days
Tetanus toxoid, 0.5 mL IM as indicated
Consideration for estrogen therapy:
   Ethinyl estradiol, 1.5 mg PO tid for 5 days, or–
   Diethylstilbestrol, 25 mg PO bid for 5 days
Emotional support and counseling
   Rape crisis center
   Other
Follow-up

[1]Adapted from CDC: 1989 Sexually Transmitted Disease Treatment Guidelines. MMWR 1989;38 (No. 5–8):41.

dividuals who are at risk and who desire such therapy. However, patients should be counseled regarding the potential risk after receiving these estrogens of fetal abnormalities should they already be pregnant. Serum β-hCG determination will help avoid this problem. The specific estrogens and doses recommended are outlined in Table 12–5.

Most rape survivors need some form of emotional support and may benefit from the services offered by a rape crisis center. It is important to ensure that the patient has the availability of follow-up for both emotional support and evaluation of possible sexually transmitted diseases.

A growing and significant concern by victims of rape is the risk of HIV exposure during sexual assault—especially if anal penetration has occurred. The actual risk is unknown but appears to be very low, and the patient can generally be reassured. If the patient is to be tested, it is best to obtain an initial screening for HIV at 6 weeks to 3 months following the assault. At present, there are no recommendations for use of prophylactic zidovudine (Retrovir)—formerly called azidothymidine (AZT).

The true incidence of serious psychologic sequelae or post-traumatic stress syndrome that occurs as a consequence of rape is not known. If, however, such complications develop, it is imperative that the astute physician promptly recognize the problem and intervene in a timely fashion. The diagnostic criteria for post-traumatic stress disorders are listed in Table 12–6.

Table 12–6. Diagnostic criteria for post-traumatic stress disorder.

A. Existence of a recognizable stressor that would evoke symptoms of distress in almost everyone
B. Reexperiencing the trauma, as evidenced by at least one of the following:
   1. Recurrent and intrusive recollections of the event
   2. Recurrent dreams of the event
   3. Suddenly acting or feeling as if the traumatic event were recurring because of an association with an environmental or ideational stimulus
C. Numbing of responsiveness to or reduced involvement with the external world, beginning some time after the trauma, as shown by at least one of the following:
   1. Markedly diminished interest in one or more significant activities
   2. Feeling of detachment or estrangement from others
   3. Constricted affect
D. At least two of the following symptoms that were not present before the trauma:
   1. Hyperalertness or exaggerated startle response
   2. Sleep disturbance
   3. Guilt about surviving when others have not or about behavior required for survival
   4. Memory impairment or trouble concentrating
   5. Avoidance of activities that arouse recollection of the traumatic event
   6. Intensification of symptoms by exposure to events that symbolize or resemble the traumatic event

Reprinted with permission from the American Psychiatric Association Committee on Nomenclature and Statistics, Diagnostic and Statistical Manual of Mental Disorders. 3rd ed. Washington, DC, American Psychiatric Association, 1980.

THE BATTERED WOMAN

The subject of the battered woman has received significant media attention, and domestic violence appears to be more widespread than previously thought. This is especially true regarding wife abuse.

DEFINITION & INCIDENCE

Spouse abuse (most often the wife) may vary from simple verbal abuse to the infliction of physical trauma. A battered woman, obviously, is one who has actually undergone physical trauma. According to a recent publication on the subject by the American College of Obstetricians and Gynecologists, a battered woman is "any woman over the age of 16 with evidence of physical abuse on at least one occasion at the hands of an intimate male partner." In the case of spouse abuse, such physical abuse is almost always repetitive.

Although the exact incidence of spouse abuse is difficult to ascertain, some have estimated that it may occur in up to 50% or more of families in the United States.

DIAGNOSIS

In one study of battered women conducted by Yale University (1977–78), almost one-fifth of the battered women had head injuries and approximately 80% of the women required some medical treatment because of the injuries.

The key to diagnosis, in the absence of signs of overt trauma, is a high degree of suspicion. Some of the signs and symptoms of abused women are summarized in Table 12–7. One should be suspicious if a given patient is noted to have bruising on several visits.

THERAPY

Most battered women are reluctant to either report abuse to the authorities or to leave their family situation. These women should be offered support and counseling.

Most cities have some form of shelter and social services for them and their children. Equally important is to provide counseling for the children in these families. It may be necessary to place these children in temporary foster homes for their own safety. Many states have laws requiring the reporting of suspected or known child abuse.

Finally, it is important to provide counseling for the male partner who is responsible for the abuse. This is often very difficult since many of these offenders are reluctant to admit that they indeed abuse their spouses or children—thus the frequent need for legal assistance.

INCEST & SEXUAL ABUSE

INCIDENCE

According to a recent technical bulletin published by the American College of Obstetricians and Gynecologists (1990), almost 40% of girls less than 18 years of age have been sexually abused—either via intrafamilial or extrafamilial abuse.

DEFINITION

Sexual abuse can be defined as sexual activity, often sexual intercourse, of a nonvoluntary nature in a young girl and may include incest or sexual molestation of young females outside the family. Incest can be defined as intrafamilial sexual intercourse, or intercourse between close family members such as father and daughter or brother and sister.

DIAGNOSIS

Unfortunately, many cases of sexual abuse, especially of an incestuous nature, do not come to light until after a girl reaches adulthood and after much emotional and psychologic trauma has occurred. As pointed out by the American College of Obstetricians and Gynecologists,

Table 12–7. Common signs and symptoms in abused women.

- Headaches, chest, back, or pelvic pain
- Insomnia
- Choking sensation
- Hyperventilation
- Gastrointestinal symptoms
- Emotional instability
- Shyness, fright, or embarrassment
- Alcohol or substance abuse
- Trauma

Adapted from American College of Obstetricians and Gynecologist, Technical Bulletin, No. 124, January. 1989.

Table 12–8. Possible signs of sexual abuse or incest in young girls.

- Recurrent sexually transmitted diseases
- Alcohol or substance abuse
- Poor school performance and truancy
- Runaways
- Recurrent urinary tract infections
- Perineal warts
- Recurrent pregnancies or abortions
- Psychosomatic disorders

Adapted from American College of Obstetricians and Gynecologists. Technical Bulletin No. 145, September 1990.

certain signs should alert the clinician to the possibility of incest or sexual abuse (Table 12–8).

TREATMENT

Therapy should consist primarily of removal of the individual from the environment of sexual abuse. This often requires legal assistance, and most states have laws and guidelines for reporting such abuse. Young girls will also often require protracted counseling from qualified individuals. Finally, these young girls need medical care to rule out the presence of sexually transmitted diseases and possibly even obstetrics care and support in the case of pregnancy.

SUGGESTED READINGS

American College of Obstetricians and Gynecologists: The adolescent obstetric-gynecologic patient. ACOG Technical Bulletin. No. 145, (Sept) 1990.

American College of Obstetricians and Gynecologists: The battered woman. ACOG Technical Bulletin. No. 124, (Jan) 1989.

American College of Obstetricians and Gynecologists: Sexual Assault: ACOG Technical Bulletin No. 172, (Sept) 1992.

Centers for Disease Control: 1989 sexually transmitted disease treatment guidelines. MMWR 1989;38:41.

Felitti VJ: Long-term medical consequences of incest, rape, and molestation. South Med J 1991;84:328.

Goldberg WG, Tomlanovich MC: Domestic violence, victims and emergency departments: New findings. JAMA 1984; 251:3259.

Hicks DJ: Rape: Sexual assault. Am J Obstet Gynecol 1980; 137:931.

Rounsaville B, Weissman MM: Battered woman: A medical problem requiring detection. Int J Psychiatr Med 1977–78;8:191.

Russell DEH: The incidence and prevalence of intrafamilial and extrafamilial sexual abuse of female children. Child Abuse Negl 1983;7:133.

Shepard M: How to manage the victim of rape. Contemp Ob/Gyn 1983;22:253.

Woodling BA, Evans JR, Bradbury MD: Sexual assault: Rape and molestation. Clin Obstet Gynecol 1977;20:509.

13

Pediatric & Adolescent Gynecology; Normal & Abnormal Puberty

The reproductive tract in children and adolescents is somewhat different in structure, hormonal support, and function from that of adult females, yet many of the same gynecologic disorders occur in both groups.

Gynecologic examination in the child requires patience, gentleness, and the use of special instruments and techniques. Knowledge of developmental stages and the endocrine physiology of these age groups is necessary for proper evaluation. When careful examination is impossible because of the patient's inability to cooperate, examination under anesthesia may be necessary.

DEVELOPMENTAL ENDOCRINE & PHYSIOLOGIC CHANGES

Infancy

Neonatal follicle-stimulating hormone (FSH) and luteinizing hormone (LH) levels rise with the withdrawal of maternal estrogens that occurs as a result of separation from the placenta at delivery. Some estrogen effect due to stimulation from maternal placental estrogen sources occurs—along with production of endogenous estrogen in modest amounts—for up to 6–8 weeks. The newborn female, therefore, may exhibit estrogenic effect with cervical mucus production, maturation of vaginal epithelial cells, and occasional breast budding and rare estrogen withdrawal bleeding and follicular cyst development. The labia minora and majora are larger and thicker than in a prepubertal child, and the clitoris appears disproportionately large. The hymen may appear thickened and enlarged in this age group as a consequence of estrogen exposure. The uterus and cervix are about 4 cm long, with the uterine cervix being three times the length of the body of the uterus. The uterus is palpable on rectal examination of a newborn. Lactobacilli populate the vaginal mucosa, leading to an acidic pH. Vaginal discharge or uterine bleeding may occur in the first 2 weeks, again as a result of recent exposure to and withdrawal from placental estrogens. By 6–8 weeks, estrogen levels have dropped, and atrophic and involutional changes of the vagina and uterus occur.

Early Childhood

In early childhood (under age 1 year to 7 years), there are changes in the hypothalamic-pituitary-gonadal axis with the development of an extremely sensitive negative feedback system as well as central inhibition of gonadotropin-releasing hormone (GnRH) release. Sex steroid levels fall, and the female reproductive tract is not exposed to endogenous hormones at this time. Pubic and axillary hair and breast budding have not yet appeared. The labia are thin and do not completely protect the introital opening. The pH of the vagina is alkaline, the vagina is reddened and thinned, and vaginal irritation is common. The clitoris is small, and the uterine corpus to cervix ratio is 2:1.

Late Childhood & Adolescence

In late childhood, there is gradual reawakening of the hypothalamic-pituitary-ovarian axis, with early nighttime peaks of LH. Adrenarche, thelarche, and finally menarche and ovulation occur. The average age at menarche is about 12½ years. The vaginal mucosa becomes thicker, the labia minora and majora plumper and thicker. The ratio of uterine corpus to cervix is 1:1.

In young adolescence, the development of secondary sexual features continues, and the external genitalia take on their adult appearance. Physiologic leukorrhea may occur.

GYNECOLOGIC EXAMINATION OF CHILDREN

Examination of Infants

All newborn infants require careful inspection of the external genitalia at the time of birth as well as in the event of abnormal vaginal bleeding or discharge. A general examination should be conducted to look for other anomalies such as cardiac and gastrointestinal (including anal) malformations. With the infant's thighs and legs spread, the examiner depresses the perineum, exposing the vaginal introitus. The clitoris is inspected to rule out enlargement associated with androgen excess in utero (Chapter 20). Posterior labial fusion is also associated with excess androgen exposure or simple labial agglutination. The vaginal opening is inspected to rule out imperforate hymen or vaginal agenesis. Some vaginal and cervical mucus is normal in the newborn. The inguinal and labial areas should be palpated to rule out the presence of a mass, which may be an undescended testis in a male pseudohermaphrodite. Rectoabdominal examination is performed to palpate for a uterus. Ovaries are not generally palpable at this time unless pathologically enlarged.

Examination of Prepubertal Children

Prepubertal children may be very sensitive to genital examination, and it is important to gain their confidence and support before proceeding. It may be helpful to examine small children in a parent's lap to lessen apprehension. Common complaints in this age group include infections and foreign bodies within the vagina, labial adhesions, precocious pubertal development, anorectal or urinary tract disorders. Inspection of the external genitalia is usually possible, as is collection of vaginal discharge for culture by insertion of a saline-moistened cotton swab. Vaginoscopy is essential for visualization of the vagina and cervix in patients with vaginal bleeding or purulent discharge or if there is a suspicion of foreign body or tumor within the vagina. Cultures for gonorrhea or chlamydial infection should be performed if there is a purulent discharge.

Examination of the small child can be accomplished either in the frogleg or the knee-chest position. The vagina and cervix may be visualized with the use of a nasal speculum or otoscope. Cervical inspection is not always warranted, and in some case only visualization of the vagina and genitalia is necessary.

Examination of Adolescent Girls

A pelvic examination in an adolescent girl is similar to an adult examination. It is useful to ask the patient if she would like to have her mother in the room or not. Small, narrow speculums are necessary and less painful than adult sizes. First pelvic examinations are usually much easier if explanations of procedures are given.

COMMON GYNECOLOGIC DISORDERS IN CHILDREN & ADOLESCENTS

Vulvovaginitis

The most common gynecologic complaint in this age group is vulvovaginitis. Poor perineal hygiene is a common cause, as is the use of irritating soaps or clothing. Proper cleansing of the vaginal and anal areas should be taught and encouraged. The etiologic classification for childhood vulvovaginitis is listed in Table 13–1.

Sitz baths are effective in relieving irritation that has progressed to labial agglutination. The addition of an estrogenic cream nightly for about 2 weeks will allow for normal separation of agglutinated labia. Digital or forced opening of agglutinated labia is contraindicated as worse scarring and agglutination usually develops. The majority of cases resolve spontaneously at puberty.

Sexually transmitted organisms such as *Neisseria gonorrheoae* and *Chlamydia trachomatis* can be grown in cultures using appropriate Thayer-Martin plates or test kits. Gonorrheal vulvovaginitis is treated with penicillin G, 100,000 units/kg intramuscularly, along with probenecid, 25 mg/kg. Penicillin-allergic patients or patients with chlamydial infections can be treated with tetracycline, 40 mg/kg orally for 7 days.

Nonspecific vulvovaginitis may be treated with appropriate antibiotics. Pinworm *(Enterobius vermicularis)* infection may also present as vulvovaginitis and is diagnosed by direct observation of pinworms and stool cultures. Treatment is with pyrantel pamoate, 11 mg/kg orally as a single dose. Therapy with mebendazole is also effective.

Vaginal Bleeding

Vaginal bleeding in a prepubertal age girl may be due to many different problems. It is important to elicit a history of possible vulvar trauma, discharge, exposure to estrogen-containing compounds, or foreign body insertion. Examination should include observation for signs of precocious pubertal development, which may indicate the presence of premature reawakening of the hypothalamic-pituitary axis, a hormonally active tumor, central nervous system disorder, or exogenous hormone exposure in the form of medication (oral contraceptive pills or conjugated estrogens). The presence of purulent bloody discharge may signify an inflammatory vulvovaginitis with bleeding from irritated sites. Evidence should be sought of sexual trauma with tearing of the hymen or posterior fourchette abrasion. Foreign bodies in the vagina such as game pieces or wads of toilet paper are common causes of bleeding, and examination under anesthesia may be necessary to reveal and remove them.

Cervical visualization may be important to rule out pol-

Table 13–1. Classification of vulvovaginitis according to cause.

Nonspecific vulvovaginitis
  Polymicrobial infection associated with disturbed homeostasis; secondary to poor perineal hygiene or a foreign body
Vulvovaginitis due to secondary inoculation
  Infection resulting from inoculation of the vagina with pathogens affecting other areas of the body by contact or blood-borne transmission: secondary to upper respiratory tract infection or urinary tract infection
Specific vulvovaginitis
  Specific primary infection, most commonly sexually transmitted: *Neisseria gonorrhoeae, Gardnerella vaginalis, herpesvirus, Treponema pallidum,* others

yps or sarcoma botryoides. Urinary tract infections may be disguised as vaginal bleeding. A clean-catch midstream urine specimen may reveal the presence of hemorrhagic cystitis. Prolapse of the distal urethra may also present as lower genital tract bleeding. It is more common in young black females. Urethral prolapse appears as a red, irritated, fluffy ring over the urethral opening. Treatment is with sitz baths, estrogen cream application, and distal urethral resection in persistent cases.

Dysfunctional Uterine Bleeding

Another problem reported in the adolescent group is irregular, sometimes heavy, menstruation. Young adolescents are prone to anovulation and hence irregular menses, but other causes of abnormal bleeding are common. The early maturing hypothalamic-pituitary axis may be prone to defects in positive feedback and the establishment of ovulatory cycles. Anovulatory cycles may be common for one to two years after menarche. Observation and reassurance are in order unless bleeding is bothersome. Low dose oral contraceptives will establish regular menstruation without inhibiting growth and skeletal maturation.

In sexually active adolescents all common disorders of pregnancy can occur with threatened abortion, ectopic pregnancy, molar pregnancy, or others. A sensitive pregnancy test is essential in establishing an early pregnancy event. PID with salpingitis or endometritis may be associated with dysfunctional uterine bleeding (DUB). Cultures for Chlamydia and GC are important in evaluating sexually active teens.

Blood dyscrasias are found in up to 19% of adolescents presenting with menorrhagia. These patients usually have other associated physical findings such as petechiae, ecchymoses, or epistaxis, but the first presentation may be menorrhagia or prolonged menstrual bleeding. Laboratory evaluation including a bleeding time, PT, PTT, CBC with platelet count, and factor VII levels are necessary. Thrombocytopenia, clotting disorders, von Willebrand's disease, and other disorders of platelet function may present with prolonged or profuse menstruation.

Anatomic abnormalities of the reproductive tract may also be associated with DUB. Vaginal carcinoma or adenosis due to DES exposure, cervical carcinoma, or hemangioma are rare causes. Uterine myoma, carcinoma, IUD devices, polyps, or breakthrough bleeding due to surreptitious oral contraceptive use may occur. Functional ovarian cysts or tumors may also occur in this age group. Cystic lesions will resolve in approximately 70% of patients whereas solid tumors are more likely to be pathologic. Foreign bodies such as retained tampons, condoms, etc, may be associated with DUB. Congenital anomalies like partially obstructed outflow tract may present with cyclic menstruation followed by chronic bloody discharge or cyclic abdominal pain, amenorrhea, and a vaginal pelvic mass due to hematocolpos. Diagnosis may be made by careful examination, sonography and hysterosalpingography. A surgical procedure is indicated for opening an imperforate hymen or transverse vaginal septum, or obstructed hemi-vagina in uterine didelphys.

NORMAL PUBERTAL DEVELOPMENT

Puberty is the period of transition between childhood and adulthood, a time of accelerated growth, sexual maturation, and profound psychologic change. The hormonal changes that signal the onset of puberty are complex and only partially understood. On average, the pubertal sequence of accelerated growth, pubarche, and the development of secondary sexual characteristics requires about 4½ years to complete. The range of development is 1½–6 years.

Secondary Sexual Characteristics (Figures 13–1 to 13–3)

Objective criteria are available for classifying individuals as to pubertal development. These descriptive norms were published by Marshall and Tanner in 1969–1970.

The earliest sign of pubertal development in females is the onset of breast development. Ovarian estrogen is the

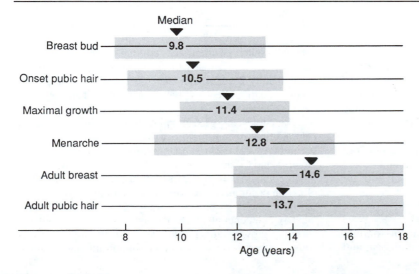

Figure 13–1. Chronologic relationship of pubertal events. (Reproduced, with permission from Speroff L, Glass RH, Kase NG: *Clinical Gynecologic Endocrinology and Fertility,* 3rd ed. Williams & Wilkins, 1983.)

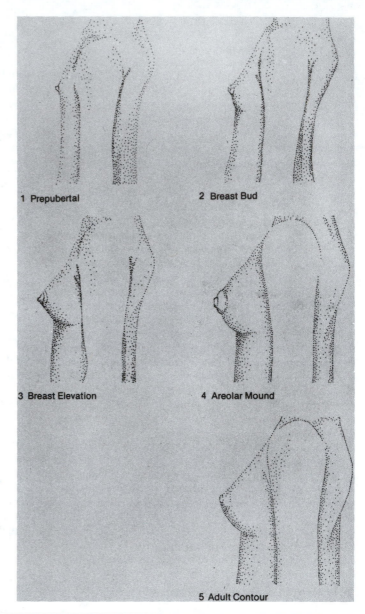

1 Prepubertal   2 Breast Bud

3 Breast Elevation   4 Areolar Mound

5 Adult Contour

Figure 13–2. Stages of breast development: **A, Stage 1:** Prepubertal breast. **B, Stage 2:** Breast bud stage. **C, Stage 3:** Further breast and areolar enlargement. **D, Stage 4:** Areola and papilla form a secondary mound. **E, Stage 5:** Mature stage. Only papilla projects, areola recessed to general contour of breast. (Reproduced, with permission, from Styne DM, Grumbach MM: Puberty in the male and female: Its physiology and disorders. In: *Reproductive Endocrinology.* Yen SCC, Jaffe RB (editors). Saunders, 1978.)

hormonal source of breast growth stimulation. Figure 13–1 shows the timing and sequence of events at puberty in girls. Pubic and axillary hair growth is under adrenal androgen and ovarian control. Menarche (the first menstrual period) is a later event in the pubertal process. Cycles may not be ovulatory in the first few months after menarche, leading to episodes of irregular menses.

Physical changes of puberty occur 6–12 months later in boys than in girls. Growth of the penis and scrotum occurs at about the same time as pubic hair development; both are under androgenic control.

Growth Spurt

Hormonal control of the adolescent growth spurt in girls is via the action of estradiol, growth hormone, and perhaps other ovarian and adrenal androgens. (Males begin growth and reach the peak of growth velocity approximately 2 years later than girls. In boys, the growth spurt is stimulated by the action of testosterone and growth hormone.)

The adolescent growth spurt proceeds in three stages: (1) the time of minimal growth velocity at the beginning of puberty, (2) the time of rapid growth (peak height velocity), and (3) decreased velocity and cessation of growth with epiphyseal fusion. Since epiphyseal fusion and ossification occur as the bony skeleton matures, measurement of bone age is an objective indicator of overall maturity that is independent of chronologic age, body habitus or size, or growth rate. In children with delayed or precocious puberty, bone age is an important measurement

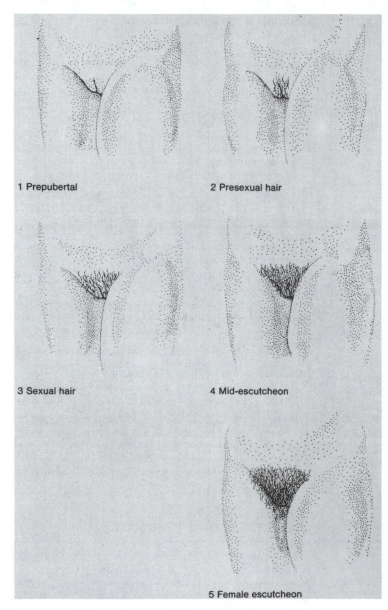

1 Prepubertal

2 Presexual hair

3 Sexual hair

4 Mid-escutcheon

5 Female escutcheon

Figure 13–3. Stages of pubic hair development. **A, Stage 1:** No pubic hair. **B, Stage 2:** Sparse hair on labia majora. Darker, coarser hair extending to mons pubis. **D, Stage 4:** Adult hair without spread to medial thighs. **E, Stage 5:** adult hair with spread to medial thighs. (Reproduced, with permission, from Styne DM, Grumbach MM: Puberty in the male and female: Its physiology and disorders. In: *Reproductive Endocrinology.* Yen SCC, Jaffe RB (editors). Saunders, 1978.)

of the amount and duration of pubertal hormonal elaboration.

Hormonal Changes of Puberty

An initial surge in gonadotropin levels follows birth as a result of loss of negative feedback as placental estrogens are withdrawn. Throughout childhood, there is increasing sensitivity of the "gonadostat" or hypothalamic-pituitary axis, and levels of FSH, LH, and steroid hormones fall. There is also evidence for the existence of a central nonsteroidal suppressor of endogenous GnRH and gonadotropin synthesis. Gonadotropin levels reach a nadir and remain suppressed throughout childhood.

At puberty, there appears to be a gradual release of inhibition of the hypothalamic-pituitary axis with the appearance of increasing amplitude and frequency of GnRH pulses, first at night and then throughout the day and night. Gonadotrope cells become more sensitive to GnRH, and FSH and LH secretion occurs. As gonadotropin levels rise, gonad-derived sex steroid levels increase, and positive and negative feedback of steroid levels to the pituitary and hypothalamus becomes operational.

ABNORMAL PUBERTY

Abnormalities of puberty can occur as a result of problems at any level of the hypothalamic-pituitary axis. Aberrations can result in the early onset of puberty (precocious puberty) or a delay in pubertal maturation (delayed puberty).

PRECOCIOUS PUBERTY

A child in whom pubertal changes occur more than 2.5 SD below the mean is said to be undergoing precocious puberty. In the United States, onset of pubertal events prior to age 8 in girls and age 9 in boys is considered precocious. Several forms of precocious puberty exist, and categorization is important to aid in diagnosis.

Isosexual precocity is a disorder in which the precocious characteristics are appropriate for the child's genetic and gonadal sex. True isosexual precocity results from premature activation of the hypothalamic-pituitary-gonadal axis, and the rise in gonadotropin levels following a bolus injection of GnRH is indistinguishable from normal pubertal response.

Heterosexual precocity occurs when sexual characteristics are inappropriate for the genetic sex, ie, feminizing syndromes in boys or virilizing syndromes in girls.

1. ISOSEXUAL PRECOCITY

The three categories of isosexual precocity are (1) true precocious puberty, or complete isosexual precocity; (2) isosexual precocious pseudopuberty, or incomplete isosexual precocity; and (3) isolated forms of pubertal development.

True Precocious Puberty

True precocious puberty is characterized as an early but otherwise normal sequence of female pubertal development. Maturation of the hypothalamic-pituitary-ovarian axis occurs, leading to the onset of regular cyclic menstruation and ovulation. Bone age is advanced, growth spurt and pubarche occur. No cause for premature activation of the axis can be found in 90% of cases, and these are referred to as constitutional or idiopathic. The remaining 10% have some form of organic brain disease such as tumor (hamartoma, germinoma, neurofibroma) or other central nervous system disorders such as meningitis, encephalitis, or head injury. Many of these patients will have other neurologic signs or symptoms or a history of central nervous system disorder. Evaluation of these patients includes careful neurologic examination, electroencephalography, and imaging of the head by MRI or CT scan.

Incomplete Isosexual Precocity

Incomplete isosexual precocity occurs in girls exposed endogenously or exogenously to a source of estrogen. Feminization will occur, but the progression to adult patterns of LH and FSH secretion and ovulatory cycles will not. A prepubertal response to a GnRH bolus will exist. Ovarian cysts or tumors that secrete estrogen (granulosa or thecal cell tumors) are the most frequent cause. These tumors can often be palpated during pelvic or abdominal examination and confirmed by pelvic ultrasound or CT scan. Adrenal adenomas or carcinomas can also produce hormones leading to isosexual precocity. McCune-Albright syndrome is the triad of café au lait spots, polyostotic fibrous dysplasia, and precocious puberty. The cause is unknown, but there is increased estrogen secretion from autonomous functioning ovarian cysts. Hypothyroidism may occasionally present with precocious puberty, ovarian cysts, and galactorrhea. Elevated thyroid-stimulating hormone (TSH), estrogen, prolactin, and gonadotropins are found. Certain estrogen-containing medications such as oral contraceptives, estrogens for menopausal replacement, and even estrogen-contaminated meat or other food products may lead to precocious pseudopuberty.

Isolated Forms of Sexual Precocity

Isolated pubertal signs such as early breast budding (premature thelarche) or premature development of axillary or pubic hair (premature adrenarche) may also occur. These rare events are usually due to some transient increase in estrogen or adrenal androgen secretion or end organ sensitivity. They are usually self-limited and resolve spontaneously. Most patients then experience pubertal events at an appropriate time.

2. HETEROSEXUAL PRECOCITY

Masculinization or virilization of a prepubertal female is usually due to congenital adrenal hyperplasia or to excess androgens secreted by an adrenal or ovarian tumor. Measurements of serum 17 hydroxy-progesterone dehydroepiandrosterone sulfate (DHEAS), and testosterone, may aid in the diagnosis. Imaging of the ovaries or adrenal by ultrasound, CT scan, or MRI may also reveal an endocrine tumor in those organs.

The clinical findings of the above disorders are contrasted in Table 13–2.

EVALUATION & TREATMENT OF SEXUAL PRECOCITY

The history and physical examination, including pelvic examination or rectoabdominal examination, may often suggest the diagnosis. Imaging of the head by CT scan or MRI is required to rule out a central nervous system tumor. Ultrasound or CT scan of the pelvis or adrenals, bone age determinations, and measurement of TSH, LH,

Table 13–2. Clinical findings in premature thelarche, premature adrenarche, and pseudoprecocious puberty.

Findings	Premature Thelarche	Premature Adrenarche	Pseudoprecocious Puberty				
			Isosexual			Heterosexual	
			Ovarian Tumor	Adrenal Tumor	Exogenous Estrogens	Ovarian Tumor	Adrenal Tumor
Breast enlargement	Yes	No	Yes	Yes	Yes	Yes	Yes
Pubic hair	No	Yes	Yes	Yes	Yes	Yes	Yes
Vaginal bleeding	No	No	Yes	Yes	Yes	Yes	Yes
Virilizing signs	No	No	No	Yes	No	Yes	Yes
Bone age	Normal	Normal to Minimally Advanced	Advanced	Advanced	Advanced	Advanced	Advanced
Neurologic deficit	No	No	No	No	No	No	No
Abdominopelvic mass	No	No	Usually	No	No	Occasional	No

Modified with permission from Ross GT, Vande Wiele RL: The ovaries. In Williams RH (ed): Textbook of Endocrinology. 6th ed. Philadelphia, WB Saunders Co, 1981, p 379.

FSH, and steroid hormones are other essential tests. A GnRH stimulation test is done to evaluate the degree of maturation of the hypothalamic-pituitary axis. A bolus of 100 µg of GnRH (Factrel) is given intravenously and serum measurements of FSH and LH are done at 0, 15, 30, and 60 minutes.

Treatment of ovarian or adrenal tumors is surgical. Operative removal or radiation treatment of central nervous system tumors may be indicated. Current treatment of constitutional or idiopathic precocious puberty is with a GnRH analogue (eg, leuprolide) for suppression of LH and FSH. Regression of breast development and cessation of vaginal bleeding occurs promptly with this therapy. Therapy is continued until age 10. The patient will then go through puberty at an appropriate time. Ketoconazole and testolactone (an aromatase inhibitor) have been shown to cause regression of pubertal events in patients with McCune-Albright syndrome.

DELAYED PUBERTY

Delay of pubertal events beyond age 13 in girls and age 14 in boys is considered abnormal, and evaluation is warranted in such cases. Constitutional delay occurs in 0.6% of teenagers. There is often a family history of delayed puberty, and these adolescents are usually short for their chronologic age and have been smaller than their peers for years. Bone age is usually retarded, but as bone age reaches 11–13 years in girls (12–14 in boys), pubertal events will spontaneously occur.

Certain hypothalamic tumors may result in pituitary hormone deficiencies by interfering with pulsatile secretion of gonadotropin-releasing hormone (GnRH). Gonadotropin deficiency may also arise from lesions or defects that involve the pituitary directly. Isolated gonadotropin deficiency occurs in Kallman's syndrome, which is associated with olfactory aplasia, anosmia, and absence of GnRH neurons. Kallman's syndrome patients are treated with low-dose estrogens to effect breast development and pubertal maturation. A typical regimen is oral conjugated estrogens 0.3 mg daily for 6 months, 0.625 mg daily for 6 months, then 1.25 mg daily. Oral progestins are added when breakthrough bleeding occurs or after about 6 to 9 months of therapy. Once pubertal development is complete, oral contraceptives may be used as an easy and reliable form of hormone replacement.

Primary gonadal failure and the impaired secretion of gonadal steroids lead to decreased negative feedback and elevated LH and FSH levels consistent with hypergonadotropic hypogonadism. In the female, the most common form of hypogonadism is the syndrome of gonadal dysgenesis (Turner's syndrome). Hormone therapy is similar to Kallman's syndrome.

SUGGESTED READINGS

Dewhurst CJ: *Practical Pediatric and Adolescent Gynecology.* Marcel Dekker, 1980.

Emans SJH, Goldstein DP: *Pediatric and Adolescent Gynecology,* 3rd ed. Little, Brown, 1990.

Kingsbury A: The clinical importance of vaginal discharge in childhood. Aust NZ J Obstet Gynaecol 1984;24:135.

Larvey JP, Sanfilippo JS: *Pediatric and Adolescent Obstetrics and Gynecology.* Springer-Verlag, 1985.

Paradise JE et al: Vulvovaginitis in premenarcheal girls: Clinical features and diagnostic evaluation. Pediatrics 1982; 70:193.

Rimsza ME: An illustrated guide to adolescent gynecology. Pediatr Clin North Am (Jun) 1989;36(3):639.

Speroff L, Glass RH, Kase NG: *Clinical Gynecologic Endocrinology and Fertility,* 4th ed. Williams & Wilkins, 1989.

Styne DM, Grumbach MM: Puberty in the male and female: Its physiology and disorders. In: *Reproductive Endocrinology.* Yen SCC, Jaffe RB (editors). Saunders, 1991.

14

Breast Disease

As the primary health care provider for a large proportion of American women, gynecologists have accepted the responsibility for the detection and, in some cases, treatment of disorders not occurring within the female genital tract. Hypertension, hypercholesterolemia, and thyroid disorders are examples.

The breast is hardly foreign territory to the gynecologist. As physicians who see the vast majority of their patients annually or even more frequently, gynecologists are ideally situated to provide effective screening for breast cancer and ongoing therapy for most benign breast disorders. Until recently, this responsibility could not be approached with enthusiasm since clinically detectable breast cancer traditionally doomed a patient to a disfiguring, defeminizing surgical procedure with statistically disappointing success. The recent validation of safe and effective screening techniques for breast cancer, the development of office procedures for the evaluation of breast masses, clarification of the relationship between benign breast disorders and breast cancer, and the availability of medications effective in the treatment or prevention of benign breast disorders have provided the gynecologist with effective means to serve their patients.

BREAST CANCER

Incidence & Epidemiology

It is estimated that one out of 10 American women will develop breast cancer during her lifetime. The estimated incidence in the United States in 1979 was 75 cases per 100,000 women of all ages. The incidence rises up to age 45 and then plateaus or falls slightly for approximately 5–10 years, only to increase rapidly again thereafter.

The major epidemiologic factors that increase or decrease the risk for development of carcinoma of the breast are listed in Table 14–1. Breast cancer appears to be a disease of Western civilization. Oriental women have a lower incidence of breast cancer than Caucasian Americans; however, among Japanese moving to Hawaii, a definite increase in breast cancer incidence has been demonstrated over successive generations. An increased risk of breast cancer among women receiving high doses of irradiation to the breast has been demonstrated among survivors of atomic bomb explosions and among women who have received multiple fluoroscopies during treatment for tuberculosis. Early menarche (age < 12 years) and late menopause (age ≥ 55 years) increase the risk for breast cancer slightly. Surgical menopause prior to age 50 and especially prior to age 35 appears to be protective. Nulliparous women have been thought to be at increased risk for breast cancer suggesting that pregnancy itself may be protective. The actual relationship between pregnancy and breast cancer risk is more complex. Women who give birth to their first child prior to the age of 30 seem to be at lower risk for breast cancer than nulliparous women, whereas women who bear their first child after the age of 30 are at increased risk. It should be noted that the relationship between breast cancer risk and first birth has been studied only in relation to full-term births; the effects of spontaneous abortion and premature birth on the risk of breast cancer are unknown. Lactation and breast feeding do not appear to influence breast cancer risk. Hormonal therapy with estrogen and progestin, either in the form of oral contraceptives or as agents used in the management of postmenopausal symptoms, may increase the risk of breast cancer slightly. (See Chapters 15 and 26.) Alcohol consumption in excess of 5 grains per day (approximately three drinks per week) increases the risk for breast cancer. Caffeine and cigarette smoking do not appear to influence the risk. The influence of the amount and type of fat in the diet on the risk of breast cancer is controversial.

The most important epidemiologic factor influencing the risk of breast cancer is the family history. A positive family history increases the risk of developing breast cancer prior to age 60 and particularly prior to the onset of menopause. The risk is greater if the afflicted family member is a first-degree relative (mother, sister, daughter) but is still increased if the member is a second-degree relative (aunt, grandmother). The risk is further increased if the afflicted member developed cancer prior to the age of menopause or if two first-degree relatives have a history of breast cancer. A family history in which one first-degree relative and one second-degree relative have breast

Table 14–1. Epidemiologic factors for breast cancer.

Increase Risk	Uncertain or No Effect	Decrease Risk
Western hemisphere	Lactation	Oriental country
Caucasian	Estrogen therapy	Oriental or Native American
Irradiation	Oral contraceptive use	Surgical menopause
Menarche < 12 years	Caffeine consumption	Age at first obstetric delivery < 25
Menopause > 55 years	Cigarette smoking	years
Age at first obstetric delivery > 30 years	Dietary fat intake	
Alcohol consumption		
Positive family history		

cancer confers no greater risk than that of a single first-degree relative with breast cancer. The influence of a family history of other malignant neoplasms on the risk of breast cancer is unknown.

Although the cause of breast cancer is unknown, it seems likely that hormones play at least a permissive role in its development. Men develop breast cancer very rarely; surgical menopause appears to be protective; exogenous estrogen or progestin may influence breast cancer risk; and estrogen or progesterone receptor protein is detectable in some breast cancers. The epidemiologic evidence is consistent with the view that breast cancer is due to a complex combination of environmental and genetic influences.

Some women continuously secrete and resorb fluid within the alveolar ductal system of the nonlactating breast. Interestingly, a higher proportion of Caucasians are secretors than Orientals or Native Americans, and the incidence of breast cancer is also higher in Caucasian women than in Oriental or Native American women. It is theoretically possible that any dietary or environmental chemical making its way into the blood will be secreted into this breast fluid and perhaps concentrated within the breast. Malignant transformation of epithelium appropriately proliferating in response to hormonal influences could then occur.

Breast Cancer Screening

A. Examination by the Physician and Self-Examination: Careful physical examination of the breasts by the physician should be performed on each patient at least annually, and more frequent examinations may be appropriate for patients at high risk. It is now apparent, however, that this examination is not sufficient to screen for breast cancer, since up to half of palpable breast cancers already have nodal metastasis at the time of discovery. This probably reflects the physician's inability to detect lesions smaller than 1–2 cm in diameter and the relative infrequency of examination (every 6–12 months).

All women over the age of 20 should practice breast self-examination. There is reason to believe that a woman who carefully examines her breasts 12–13 times a year will be able to detect lesions earlier than if she depends on the physician's examination performed only once a year.

A woman should examine her own breasts at a specified time in her cycle, such as a few days following cessation of menstrual flow or, if she is acyclic, on a specified day of the month. Women should be instructed to continue breast self-examination on a monthly basis after menopause, since the incidence of breast cancer increases dramatically after menopause.

All students of gynecology should be able to instruct a patient in breast self-examination. The following set of instructions and illustrations are reprinted here with the permission of The American College of Obstetricians and Gynecologists:

1. Self-examination should always be performed in good light. Stand or sit in front of a mirror, arms at your sides.
2. Look for dimpling or puckering of the breast skin, retraction (or pushing in) of the nipples, and changes in breast size or shape. Look for the same signs with your hands pressed tightly on your hips and then with your arms raised high.

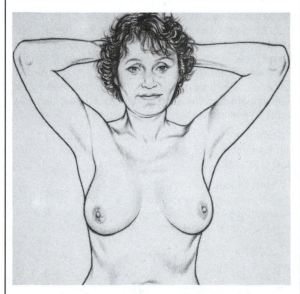

3. Lie flat on your back. Place a folded towel or a pillow under your left shoulder and place your left hand under your head.
4. With your right hand, keeping the fingers flat and together, gently feel your left breast without exerting too much pressure. Use small circular motions with your fingers.

continued on next page

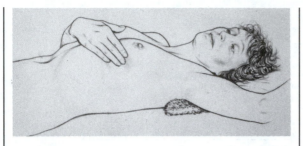

5. Picture your breast as the face of a clock. Begin your small circles at 12 o'clock at the very top of your breast. Repeat the circular motion at 1 o'clock, 2 o'clock, and so on. When your hand returns to 12 o'clock, move it closer to the nipple and repeat the process. Do this in smaller and smaller circles until you have examined all the breast tissue.

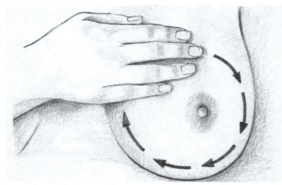

6. Examine the nipple area in the same way and check for any discharge.

7. Be sure to examine the area below the armpit, which also contains breast tissue and should not be missed.

8. Lower your right arm to your side and reverse the procedure: Place the folded towel or pillow under your right shoulder, right hand under your head, and use your left hand to feel your right breast.

Steps 4–8 can also be done when showering or bathing. Examination of the breasts is easier when they are smooth and wet with soap and water.

What to look for:

Many women have lumps in their breasts. The important thing for you to keep in mind is that you are looking for something new or unusual:

___ New lumps
___ Puckering
___ Dimpling
___ Thickening or hardening under the skin
___ Retraction of the nipple
___ Bleeding or discharge from the nipple
___ Any other unusual appearance of the skin or nipple

If you find any of these signs, alert your doctor as soon as possible.

Breast self-examination has the obvious advantage that frequent examinations are more likely to detect masses as soon as they become clinically palpable. Women with dense, very large, or irregular breasts encounter the same difficulties with breast self-examination as the clinician performing the annual examination for the reason that small, subtle changes are not readily detectable.

B. Mammography: A number of imaging techniques have been recommended for breast cancer screening, but the only technique of proved utility is mammography. Figure 14–1 depicts the theoretic growth of a breast cancer based on the assumption of 100 days' doubling time. Mammography is capable of detecting breast cancer approximately 3 years before it reaches clinically detectable size. The survival rate at 5 and 8 years for women with breast cancer that was less than 1 cm in diameter at the time of starting therapy is virtually identical with that of women with carcinoma in situ and approaches 100%. Mammography is a screening technique that now offers truly early detection and increased chances for survival.

Timing and scheduling of screening mammography. Opinion differs, but it seems reasonable to obtain an initial mammogram in an asymptomatic patient between the ages of 35 and 40—closer to age 35 in women at increased risk and closer to age 40 in women with no risk factors. Beginning at age 40, mammography should be performed annually in women at increased risk and every other year in women with no increased risk. Beginning at age 50, mammography should be performed annually in all women.

Mammography at its best is still an imperfect tool. Although the American College of Radiology now certifies diagnostic radiology centers and specifies the number of views, radiation dose, and type of equipment for mammography according to standards agreed upon by the American College of Radiology and the American Cancer Society, one must accept the human factors of variations in technique and expertise in interpreting the mammogram. In addition, it is estimated that 5–10% of palpable breast carcinomas are not visualized on mammography. As useful and potentially beneficial as the technique is, it is not a replacement for breast self-examination and physical examination by a physician.

C. Other Imaging Techniques:

1. Thermography, measuring temperatures in the breast, and diaphanography, transillumination of the breast with visible or infrared light, are imaging techniques capable of demonstrating larger (1–5 cm in diameter) tumors but are unreliable in detecting small tumors. They are therefore not useful as screening procedures. Ultrasound is useful in differentiating between a solid and a fluid filled mass. Ultrasound may also be used as a guide for needle aspiration. Computerized tomography (CT) of the breast involves higher doses of radiation, takes longer to perform, and is more costly than standard mammography. The one advantage of CT, the ability to image the extreme lateral and medial portions of the breast, may prove useful in carefully selected patients.

2. Magnetic resonance imaging (MRI) has great promise as a breast imaging technique. MRI involves no

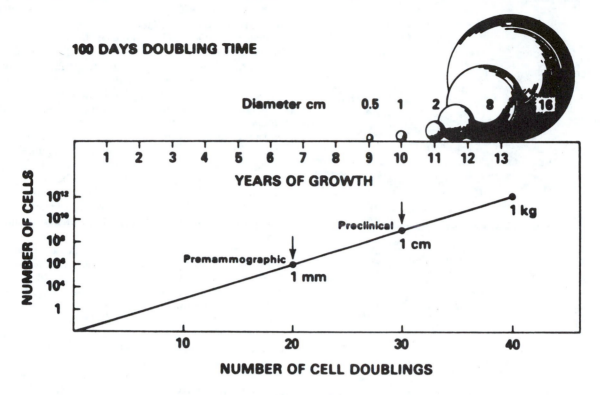

Figure 14–1. Theoretic growth of a breast cancer based on the assumption of 100 days' doubling time.

ionizing radiation, may be capable of differentiating between benign and malignant tissue saving some women the expense and trauma of biopsy while providing other women with preoperative staging of breast cancer, and may be capable of performing some chemical analysis of tissue. High cost and lack of scientific demonstration of efficacy cause MRI to be considered an experimental breast imaging technique for the present.

Diagnosis

The definitive diagnosis of breast cancer can only be made histologically. The tissue sample for histologic examination may be obtained by open biopsy, traditional needle biopsy, or the newer technique of fine-needle aspiration. Fine-needle aspiration cytology (FNA) is a technique of obtaining cellular material from a breast mass with a needle of less than 1.0 mm external diameter. This is a relatively simple office procedure. A 22 or 23 gauge needle is most often employed and local anesthesia is optional. FNA will probably become a necessary skill for all gynecologists within 10 years. False positives are rare. The false negative rate is currently considered to be about 5%, but this is likely to rise as more inexperienced physicians take up the technique.

Treatment & Prognosis

The treatment of breast cancer lies outside the province of the practicing gynecologist. Nevertheless, it is important for the gynecologist to understand the principles of surgical decision making. Patients with breast cancer require extensive counseling, and many women faced with the finding of a breast mass or an abnormal mammogram want that counseling to begin in the gynecologist's office.

A. Prognostic Indicators: In general, the prognosis for breast cancer is determined by the apparent extent of disease at the time of initial diagnosis and by the tendency for any particular patient's tumor to behave aggressively. In turn, the prognostic indicators are used as a guide to therapy.

The apparent extent of disease is codified in a staging system that takes into account the size and other clinical characteristics of the primary tumor (T), the presence and clinical characteristics of palpable axillary or supraclavicular nodes (N), and the presence of distant metastases (M).

Breast tumors spread by direct infiltration, through the lymphatic drainage of the breast, and by hematogenous metastasis. Clinical evidence of direct infiltration includes fixation of the tumor to underlying fascia, muscles, or chest wall and changes in the skin overlying the tumor such as edema, ulceration, or the presence of satellite skin nodules. The lymphatic drainage of the breasts is illustrated in Figure 14–2. Palpation of the axillary nodes is an important aspect of clinical staging. A portion of the drainage from the axillary nodes is to the supraclavicular nodes. Involvement of the supraclavicular nodes implies excessive involvement of the axillary nodes and a poor prognosis. The parasternal node chain cannot be ignored.

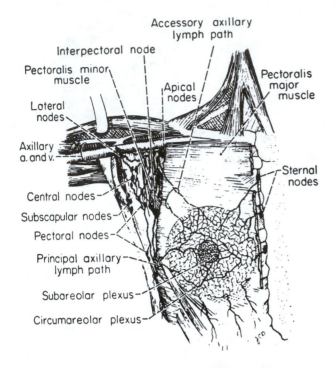

Figure 14–2. The axillary lymph node system and the parasternal lymph node chain constitute the major routes of lymph drainage from the breast. (From Woodburn, RT: *Essentials of Human Anatomy,* New York, Oxford University Press, 1983.)

Forty to fifty percent of breast cancer patients with axillary lymph node metastases also have parasternal node metastases and about 4% of breast cancer patients have parasternal node metastases only. The most common sites of distant metastasis are bone (particularly vertebrae), pelvis, lung, liver, and brain.

The details of this "TNM" classification of breast cancer are presented in Table 14–2, which also includes a description (in TNM notation) of the four stages of disease. Staging is done clinically and is used to provide a first estimate of prognosis and as a guide to individualization of therapy. The correlation between prognosis and clinical stage is set forth in Table 14–3. While tumor size and the presence or absence of distant metastases are obvious prognostic indicators, refinements in prognosis can be made only after operation. For example, the status of axillary lymph nodes is a significant prognostic indicator (Table 14–4). Forty percent of patients judged clinically to be free of axillary node involvement will have positive axillary nodes noted by the pathologist. Conversely, 25% of patients judged clinically to have node involvement will have no histologic evidence of tumor in resected axillary nodes.

By collating the prognostic features of histologic type and histologic grade, the presence or absence of hormone receptors, and the presence or absence of vascular invasion, one can estimate the aggressiveness of the tumor.

Breast cancer arises from the epithelium of large or intermediate sized ducts and is called "ductal," or from the epithelium of the terminal ducts of the lobules and is called "lobular." Other histologic types are variants of ductal carcinoma with histologically distinctive features. Infiltrating ductal carcinoma is by far the most common histologic type of breast cancer and does not carry a favorable prognosis. A summary of the proportion of breast cancers of various histologic types is presented in Table 14–5 along with a note indicating which types carry a favorable prognosis. Table 14–5 shows that those histologic types which carry a favorable prognosis tend to be the less common tumors. Low histologic grade of tumor is also associated with a favorable prognosis, but most breast cancers are neither highly undifferentiated nor highly differentiated but rather of intermediate grade. It is apparent that some tumors of intermediate histologic grade behave quite aggressively whereas others do not. Evidence of vascular invasion—particularly invasion of dermal lymphatics (inflammatory carcinoma)—implies a poor prognosis.

Hormone receptors. Attempts have been made recently to measure molecular markers in the hope that these measurements would be more reflective of the functional differentiation of the tumor cells and thus provide more prognostic information than histologic study alone. Measurement of hormone receptors—receptors for both estrogen and progesterone—in breast cancers has provided a first approximation of functional differentiation. The logic is straightforward: tumors that contain estrogen receptors (ER+) should be better differentiated biologically than tumors which do not (ER–). Furthermore, tumors capable of responding to estrogen by the production of progesterone receptors (PR+) should be better differentiated than tumors which do not contain progesterone receptor sites (PR–). Well-differentiated tumors should carry a better prognosis.

While the presence of progesterone receptor in breast cancers correlates moderately well with a favorable prognosis, the measurement of estrogen and progesterone receptors has proved to be most useful as a predictor of which tumors will respond favorably to endocrine therapy.

Prognostic indicators that may have clinical application in the near future include measurements of cell ploidy or chromosomal content and measurements of the extent of expression of certain oncogenes.

B. Surgical Options: For most of this century, the standard therapy for carcinoma of the breast was radical mastectomy as originally described by Halsted: en bloc removal of the breast, pectoral muscles, and axillary lymph nodes. Although the disfiguring Halsted operation was associated with significant postoperative problems, it probably provided rational therapy for the vast majority of patients presenting with advanced disease, as was so often the case in the first half of the century. The addition of modern radiotherapy techniques, hormonal therapy, and cytotoxic chemotherapy as potential choices in breast cancer therapy, along with the tendency of the modern woman to present with less advanced disease, has made it

Table 14–2. TNM (tumor-node-metastasis) classification of breast cancer.[1]

T Primary tumors

TIS	Paget's disease of the nipple with no demonstrable tumor
T1	Tumor <2 cm T1a, T2a, T3a with *no* fixation
T2	Tumor 2–5 cm T1b, T2b, T3b with *fixation* to underlying pectoral fascia or muscle
T3	Tumor >5 cm
T4	Tumor of any size with direct extension to chest wall or skin
T4a	With fixation to chest wall (including ribs, intercostal muscles, and serratus anterior muscle *but not* pectoral muscle)
T4b	With edema (including peau d'orange), ulceration of skin of breast, or satellite skin nodules on same breast
T4c	Both T4a and T4b
T4d	Inflammatory cancer

Dimpling of the skin, nipple retraction, or any other skin changes except those in T4b may occur in T1, T2, or T3 without changing the classification

N Reginal lymph nodes

N0	No palpable ipsilateral axillary nodes
N1	Movable ipsilateral axillary nodes
	N1a Nodes *not* considered to contain growth
	N1b Nodes considered to contain growth
N2	Ipsilateral nodes considered to contain growth and fixed to one another or to other structures
N3	Ipsilateral supraclavicular or infraclavicular nodes considered to contain growth, or edema of the arm

M Distant metastases

M0	No known distant metastases
M1	Distant metastases *present*

Definitions of Clinical Stages I–IV Using TNM Classification			
Stage I	T1a	N0 or N1a	M0
	T1b	N0 or N1a	M0
Stage II	T0	N1b	M0
	T1a	N1b	M0
	T1b	N1b	M0
	T2a	N0, N1a, or N1b	M0
	T2b	N0, N1a, or N1b	M0
Stage III	T3	Any N	M0
	Any T	N2	M0
Stage IV	T4	Any N	Any M
	Any T	N3	Any M
	Any T	Any N	M1

[1]Staging system of the International Union Against Cancer and the American Joint Committee for Cancer Staging and End Results Reporting.

possible to achieve results that are at least as good as those of the Halsted mastectomy by employing simpler, less disfiguring surgical approaches. These less extensive procedures include lumpectomy (wide local excision of primary tumor), partial mastectomy (excision of the segment or quadrant of the breast containing the primary tumor), and simple mastectomy (excision of the entire breast containing the primary tumor). Axillary node dissection is usually

performed with any of the less extensive procedures not to control the tumor but to provide prognostic indicators and guide adjuvant chemotherapy or radiotherapy. The combination of simple mastectomy with axillary node dissection is often called "modified radical mastectomy."

There is controversy about the extent of surgery indicated for various stages of the disease. The patient herself should participate in the decision. It is generally agreed that for patients with early disease, one of the less exten-

Table 14–3. Breast cancer: Survival correlated with clinical staging.[1]

Clinical Staging	Five-Year Survival (%)
Stage I	85
Stage II	66
Stage III	41
Stage IV	10

[1]Modified from Giuliano AE: Breast. Chapter 12 in: *Current Medical Diagnosis & Treatment 1991*. Schroeder SA et al (editors). Appleton & Lange, 1991.

Table 14–4. Histologic staging of breast carcinoma.[1]

	Crude Survival (%)	
Axillary Lymph Node Status	**Five Years**	**Ten Years**
Negative	78	65
One to 3 positive	62	38
Four or more positive	32	13

[1]Modified from Giuliano AE: Breast. Chapter 12 in: *Current Medical Diagnosis & Treatment* 1991. Schroeder SA et al (editors). Appleton & Lange, 1991.

Table 14–5. Classification of breast cancers by histologic type. (FP = favorable prognosis.)

Histologic Type	Percent of All Breast Cancers
Infiltrating ductal (not otherwise specified)	70–80
Medullary (FP)	5–8
Mucinous (FP)	2–4
Tubular (FP)	1–2
Papillary	1–2
Invasive lobular	6–8
Other	< 1
Secretory (FP)	
Adenoid cystic (FP)	
Epidermoid	
Sudiferous	

sive surgical procedures can be recommended; and that for all patients with advanced disease, the addition of radiation therapy, chemotherapy, or hormonal therapy can be recommended.

C. Hormonal Therapy: In general, the objective of hormonal therapy is to remove hormonal stimulation from those tumors that seem to be hormone-responsive. This has traditionally been accomplished by performing bilateral oophorectomy. The orally effective antiestrogen tamoxifen has been used in some patients instead of bilateral oophorectomy with equal success.

The potential response to hormonal therapy may be predicted by the presence and concentration of estrogen and progesterone receptors in the primary tumor. About 40% of primary tumors may be expected to be PR-positive, and 70–80% of patients harboring such a tumor will respond to hormonal therapy. Slightly over one-fourth of primary tumors contain neither estrogen nor progesterone receptors, and patients harboring such tumors do not usually respond to hormonal therapy. The remaining tumors contain estrogen receptor but not progesterone receptor. In these cases, the amount of estrogen receptor is predictive of response to hormonal therapy, with those tumors containing the highest concentrations of estrogen receptor per milligram of protein responding most favorably.

D. Cytotoxic Chemotherapy: Combination therapy can be used as adjuvant therapy in the treatment of breast cancer. Combinations of adriamycin/vincristine, 5 fluorouracil/adriamycin/cyclophosphamide, and adriamycin/cyclophosphamide have been reported to improve survival in cases of advanced disease. While combinations that do not include adriamycin have been studied, such combinations seem to be less effective.

While the timing and duration of hormonal therapy or cytotoxic chemotherapy remains a matter of debate, a consensus of which tumors would best be treated with one or the other form of adjuvant therapy is presented in Table 14–6.

E. Very Early Disease: While the concept remains controversial, a number of experts have suggested that stage 0 or minimal breast cancer should include invasive cancers less than 0.5 cm in diameter and carcinoma in situ of the breast. Long-term survival in patients with this so-called stage 0 breast cancer approaches 100% at 15 years,

but to date these results have been achieved only with treatment by mastectomy. Whether equally good results can be obtained with more conservative approaches has yet to be demonstrated.

FIBROCYSTIC DISEASE OF THE BREAST

The broad term "fibrocystic disease" is a misnomer. Biopsies performed on patients with so-called fibrocystic disease may be read by the pathologist as adenosis, apocrine metaplasia, cysts, fibrosis, mastitis, periductal mastitis, squamous metaplasia, ductal ectasia, fibroadenoma, hyperplasia, papilloma, or atypical hyperplasia. As more women undergo routine mammography for breast cancer screening, radiologists become more convinced that radiographic evidence of so-called fibrocystic disease is detectable in over 90% of women aged 40 or older.

Many women present with complaints of breast pain with or without nodularity that may or may not be cyclic in nature. A patient with a palpable, distinct, dominant mass requires immediate evaluation. Aspiration of a cystic mass may be both diagnostic and therapeutic. The aspirated fluid may be submitted for cytologic examination, and a cystic mass that completely disappears with aspiration and does not recur within 3–6 months may be followed without further evaluation. Solid masses require histologic study. The specimen may be obtained by fine-needle aspiration or by open biopsy. The patient in whom no distinct dominant mass is palpable should receive a benign diagnosis such as physiologic nodularity or cyclic mastalgia. Mammography may be indicated if the patient is over 35 or is at high risk for the development of breast cancer.

Table 14–6. Summary of NIH Consensus Conference and Clinical Alert on Adjuvant Chemotherapy.

Premenopausal Women[1]		
Nodal Involvement	Estrogen Receptors	Adjuvant Systemic Therapy
Yes	Positive	Combination chemotherapy
Yes	Negative	Combination chemotherapy
No	Positive	Probably tamoxifen
No	Negative	Probably combination chemotherapy

Postmenopausal Women		
Nodal Involvement	Estrogen Receptors	Adjuvant Systemic Therapy
Yes	Positive	Tamoxifen
Yes	Negative	Probably combination chemotherapy
No	Positive	Probably tamoxifen
No	Negative	Probably combination chemotherapy

[1]Modified from Giuliano, AE: The Breast. Chapter 60 in *Current Obstetric & Gynecologic Diagnosis & Treatment.* 7th ed, Pernoll ML, Appleton & Lange, 1991.

There has been confusion about whether biopsy-proved fibrocystic changes are associated with an increased risk for breast cancer. It is now clear that all nonproliferative and some proliferative lesions do not increase the risk. Lesions that do not increase cancer risk include sclerosing adenosis, apocrine metaplasia, ductal ectasia, fibroadenoma, fibrosis, mild hyperplasia, periductal mastitis, and squamous metaplasia. Therefore, patients with symptomatic nodularity or with mastalgia are best treated medically.

Treatment

Oral contraceptives, danazol, tamoxifen, and bromocriptine have been used. Considering the cost and side effects, low-dose oral contraceptives seem to be a good first choice.

Danazol therapy provides rapid and almost universal symptomatic relief. Unfortunately, the drug is expensive and causes a number of unpleasant side effects. Moreover, over half of patients treated with danazol will develop symptoms again within 12 months after discontinuing therapy.

The response to tamoxifen is similar, but there may be a lesser tendency to recurrence.

The use of bromocriptine appears to be limited only by its propensity to cause nausea and vomiting.

Investigators have been unable to substantiate the initial observation that reducing methylxanthine consumption is effective therapy for mastalgia or physiologic nodularity. Nonetheless, there may be some effect, pharmacologic or placebo, and since there is little or no expense to the patient, it may be worth trying.

BENIGN NEOPLASMS OF THE BREAST

Fibroadenoma

Fibroadenoma is the most common benign neoplasm of the breast. This tumor tends to occur in younger women, the peak age being between 21–25 years. The patient usually complains of a breast mass, which may be found at breast examination. The mass tends to be smooth, well-circumscribed, firm, mobile, and rubbery in consistency. Since very large, tense cysts may have a similar feel, sonography may be used to differentiate between a cystic and solid mass. Fine-needle aspiration will establish the diagnosis.

Some fibroadenomas respond to medical therapy with danazol or tamoxifen, but definitive therapy usually consists of simple excision of the tumor.

Intraductal Papillomas

Intraductal papillomas are the most common cause of unilateral and uniductal discharge and of bloody nipple discharge. Nipple discharge that is not milk (see Chapter 21) should be considered a symptom or sign of malignancy until proved otherwise. This is particularly true if the discharge is thinner than toothpaste and is associated with a breast mass. Intraductal papilloma is a benign lesion of the lactiferous duct. It is usually solitary, but patients with multiple papillomas or papillomatosis have been reported.

Therapy consists of excision at the time of diagnosis. Papillomas with fibrovascular cores increase the risk for development of carcinoma.

MAMMARY DUCT ECTASIA

Ductal ectasia is a disorder of perimenopausal patients, who usually present with a mass and a red, tender breast that is diffusely hard. This is accompanied by a nipple discharge that may appear to be gray or green to black in color and has the consistency of toothpaste. Ductal ectasia is probably the most common cause of nipple discharge in women over age 55. Because ductal inflammation is associated with the disorder, local lymph nodes may be swollen. The combination of dominant mass and local lymph node involvement usually indicates the need for surgery because of concern for the possibility of carcinoma. Ductal ectasia may resolve spontaneously if the discharge is expressed. Observation, at least for a brief time, is justified if this diagnosis is likely.

HYPERPLASIA & ATYPIA

Significant hyperplasia of ductal epithelium with or without accompanying atypia increases the risk for development of carcinoma of the breast. Because these lesions are diagnosed histologically following excisional biopsy, it is impossible at present to classify them as premalignant. Nevertheless, a conservative approach would be to consider benign breast lesions accompanied by significant hyperplasia or by atypical hyperplasia to be premalignant. These lesions would include intraductal papillomas with fibrovascular cores, moderate or severe ductal hyperplasia, and atypical hyperplasia, either ductal or lobular. Women who have had one of these proliferative mastopathies must have annual mammograms and must practice breast self-examination. The use of oral estrogen or progestin in such women is a subject for debate.

SUGGESTED READINGS

Giuliano AE: Breast. Chapter 12 in: *Current Medical Diagnosis & Treatment 1991.* Schroeder SA et al (editors). Appleton & Lange, 1991.

Hindle W: *Breast Disease for Gynecologists.* Appleton & Lange, 1989.

15

Pelvic Relaxation & Urinary Incontinence

PELVIC RELAXATION

"Pelvic relaxation" is a nonspecific term that may denote one or more of the following conditions: (1) cystocele, (2) stress urinary incontinence, (3) rectocele, (4) enterocele, and (5) uterine or vaginal prolapse. These conditions occur chiefly as a result of weakness or defect in the supporting tissues, including the muscles of the pelvic diaphragm, ligaments, and fascia. They may be related to inherent weaknesses in the supporting structures but more commonly are associated with the trauma of childbirth. Thus, they are most often seen in older, multiparous women. They may also occur following pelvic surgery (especially vaginal prolapse).

VAGINAL PROLAPSE

Relaxation of the tissues supporting the pelvic organs may cause downward displacement of one or more of these organs into the vagina, which may result in their protrusion through the vaginal introitus.

CYSTOCELE

The main support of both the urethra and the bladder is the pubo-vesical-cervical fascia, and a cystocele is primarily a hernia in the anterior vaginal wall secondary to weakness or defect in this fascia (Figure 15–1). The incidence of symptomatic cystoceles is unknown, but most parous women probably have some degree of defect in the anterior vaginal fascia.

Clinical Findings

Most cystoceles are asymptomatic and are diagnosed at the time of routine vaginal examination. When symptoms do occur, they consist mainly of feelings of vaginal or pelvic pressure accompanied by a bulge or mass in the vagina. Unless very large in size, cystoceles rarely are associated with urinary retention or difficulty in voiding.

Traditionally, cystoceles were classified as grades I, II, or III according to their relationship to the vaginal introitus (a grade III cystocele was one that prolapsed through the introitus). This classification has little clinical utility and often is confusing. It is best to describe what one sees in the simplest of terms—ie, a cystocele that prolapses to within so many centimeters of the introitus or to the introitus, or through the introitus.

Treatment

A useful guide to therapy of any kind is that it is difficult to make a patient better than "asymptomatic." Thus, it is generally neither necessary nor desirable to repair a small asymptomatic cystocele.

For most patients who have large cystoceles prolapsing to or through the vaginal introitus and significant symptoms, surgical repair is the treatment of choice. Repair is accomplished vaginally in most patients, especially if the cystocele is very large. The primary vaginal procedure is anterior colporrhaphy, or "anterior repair," which consists simply of surgical plication of the anterior vaginal fascia supporting the bladder (Figure 15–2). If the uterus is still present, this procedure usually is performed in conjunction with vaginal hysterectomy.

Small cystoceles can also be repaired abdominally by removal of a small V-shaped wedge from the anterior vaginal wall. "Overcorrection" of a cystocele, however, may so reduce the urethrovesical angle as to lead to urinary incontinence. For this reason, most clinicians include plication of the urethrovesical angle at the time of cystocele repair.

Patients unable to tolerate surgery may be treated with a vaginal pessary, though not often with success (Figure 15–3). For older patients who are no longer sexually ac-

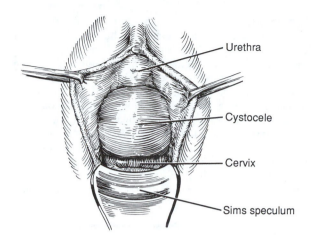

Figure 15–1. Sims speculum used to inspect the anterior vaginal wall. The anterior blade of a bivalved speculum does not allow adequate visualization and may support the vaginal wall, leading to errors in judgment of the degree of relaxation. (Reproduced, with permission, from Pernoll ML (editor): *Current Obstetric & Gynecologic Diagnosis & Treatment,* 7th ed. Appleton & Lange, 1991.)

tive, either partial (LeFort) or complete obliteration of the vagina ("colpocleisis") may be accomplished.

RECTOCELE

A rectocele is chiefly a hernia in the posterior vaginal wall secondary to weakness or defect in the rectovaginal septum (fascia) and portions of the levator ani muscle. This defect probably results from damage or stress secondary to childbirth (Figure 15–4).

Clinical Findings

Most rectoceles are asymptomatic and are detected incidentally at routine vaginal examination. Patients with large rectoceles may complain of difficulty in evacuation of stool, a vaginal mass, and a sensation of fullness. Rectoceles are relatively easy to detect on pelvic examination. Rectovaginal examination with one finger in the vagina and one finger in the rectum shows the hernia projecting into the vagina and often out through the introitus.

Treatment

It is not necessary to repair small rectoceles, especially if the patient is asymptomatic. For patients with rectoceles prolapsing through the introitus or those who have significant symptoms, the principal mode of therapy is surgery—usually posterior colporrhaphy, which consists chiefly of opening the posterior vaginal wall over the hernia site and plication of the rectovaginal fascia. The levator ani muscles are also approximated in the midline (Figure 15–5). Excessive or redundant vaginal mucosa is excised.

Patients who refuse or cannot tolerate surgery may receive temporary relief from medical management, consisting of laxatives and stool softeners. Vaginal pessaries are generally not helpful in patients with significant rectoceles.

ENTEROCELE

An enterocele is a hernia of the rectouterine pouch (cul-de-sac, pouch of Douglas) into the rectovaginal septum (Figure 15–6). Rarely, a similar hernia may also occur anteriorly. Although the cause of enterocele is not known in every case, these lesions are probably related to vaginal trauma during childbirth.

Clinical Findings

Patients with enteroceles may be asymptomatic. The most common symptoms are fullness and vaginal pressure. The patient also may palpate a mass in her vagina.

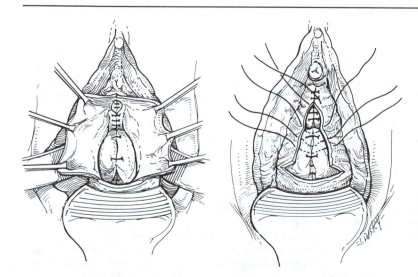

Figure 15–2. Repair of cystocele and plication of urethra for correction of stress incontinence of urine. (Modified and reproduced, with permission, from Pernoll ML (editor): *Current Obstetric & Gynecologic Diagnosis & Treatment,* 7th ed. Appleton & Lange, 1991.)

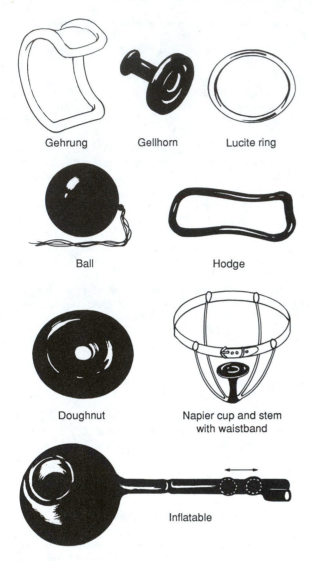

Gehrung   Gellhorn   Lucite ring

Ball   Hodge

Doughnut   Napier cup and stem with waistband

Inflatable

Figure 15–3. Types of pessaries. (Reproduced, with permission, from Pernoll ML (editor): *Current Obstetric & Gynecologic Diagnosis & Treatment,* 7th ed. Appleton & Lange, 1991.)

On physical examination, an enterocele may be confused with a rectocele. The former is usually a bulging from the upper posterior vaginal wall and the latter a bulging from the lower posterior vaginal wall. Enterocele can usually be confirmed on rectovaginal examination by palpating a mass between the two fingers when one finger is in the rectum and one in the vagina. Rarely, bowel peristalsis may be seen or palpated in the mass.

Patients with large posterior enteroceles often have associated uterine prolapse, cystoceles, and rectoceles. Rarely, an anterior enterocele may be confused with a cystocele. Palpation of the mass with a Foley catheter in place can help delineate these two conditions.

Treatment

As with cystoceles and rectoceles, the primary mode of therapy is surgery. The repair can be accomplished either transabdominally or vaginally. If the patient does not have an associated rectocele or cystocele, the abdominal approach is generally best. This consists of ligation of the hernia sac along with obliteration of the rectouterine pouch with one or more purse-string sutures. If the patient has an associated rectocele or cystocele, the vaginal approach is best and consists primarily of "high ligation" of the hernia sac and approximation of the uterosacral ligaments. If a uterus is still present, hysterectomy is generally performed, along with repair of other vaginal hernias such as a cystocele or rectocele.

UTERINE PROLAPSE

The uterus is supported principally by the endopelvic fascia and the cardinal and uterosacral ligaments. Prolapse of the uterus usually occurs as a consequence of weakness in these support structures. As with all genital tract hernias, this is usually associated with trauma secondary to childbirth. Any condition associated with increased abdominal pressure such as neoplasms or ascites may also cause uterine prolapse.

Clinical Findings

Most parous women have some degree of uterine prolapse or descensus, and the majority of such affected women are asymptomatic. In symptomatic cases, the uterus may prolapse down to or through the introitus and present as a "mass." The patient may complain of significant pressure and the feeling of a bulge in her vagina. Patients often complain of feeling a firm mass in the vagina. Rarely, the uterus may prolapse completely outside the vagina. Women with uterine prolapse frequently also have one of the hernias mentioned above.

The diagnosis of uterine prolapse is relatively easy to make on pelvic examination. Uncommonly, an extremely elongated cervix with little or no descent in the uterine fundus may be confused with uterine prolapse. Uterine fibroids, polyps, or tumors also may be confused with uterine prolapse.

Treatment

In asymptomatic patients with minimal uterine descensus, no therapy is required. Patients who are postmenopausal and not receiving estrogens may benefit from estrogen therapy. This is especially true if the patient has an atrophic vagina. Estrogen therapy will also improve the tone of the tissue such that the tissue planes will be much more easy to dissect if surgery is required.

For asymptomatic patients with significant uterine descensus, surgery is the primary mode of therapy. Oper-

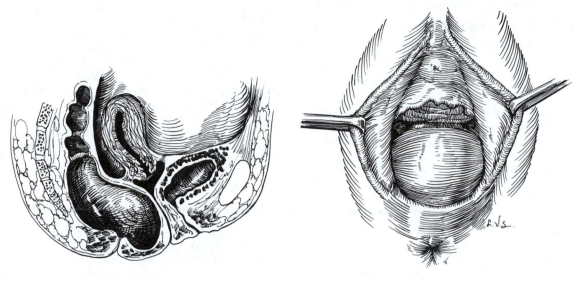

Figure 15–4. Rectocele. (Reproduced, with permission, from Pernoll ML (editor): *Current Obstetric & Gynecologic Diagnosis & Treatment,* 7th ed. Appleton & Lange, 1991.)

ation consists of hysterectomy performed either abdominally or vaginally depending upon the degree of prolapse and other associated hernias, such as rectoceles, cystoceles, or enteroceles. The surgical approach is also somewhat dependent on the status of the viscera—whether or not there are significant adhesions from previous surgery, previous pelvic inflammatory disease, etc. The abdominal approach is generally preferred in the presence of these complications.

Patients with uterine descensus also commonly have

loss of support of the vaginal apex and require either vaginal or abdominal suspension of the vaginal cuff following hysterectomy.

For patients who are unable to tolerate surgery, a vaginal pessary may be useful. Such patients should also receive estrogen therapy unless contraindicated.

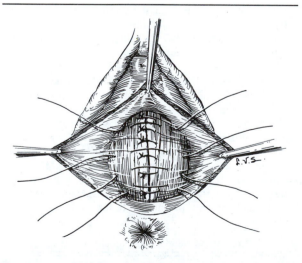

Figure 15–5. Approximation of levator ani muscles for repair of rectocele. (Reproduced, with permission, from Pernoll ML (editor): *Current Obstetric & Gynecologic Diagnosis & Treatment,* 7th ed. Appleton & Lange, 1991.)

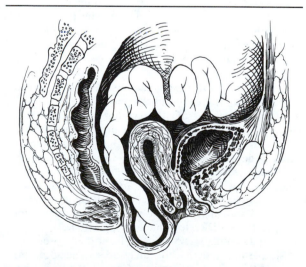

Figure 15–6. Enterocele. (Reproduced, with permission, from Pernoll ML (editor): *Current Obstetric & Gynecologic Diagnosis & Treatment,* 7th ed. Appleton & Lange, 1991.)

URINARY INCONTINENCE

Urinary incontinence may be classified as genuine stress incontinence, urge incontinence, or overflow incontinence. Leaking of urine or incontinence can also result from an abnormal opening or fistula between the urinary and genital tracts. Total incontinence is most often due to a fistula between the bladder or urethra and the vagina. Because of the rarity of this condition today, it is mentioned here only for completeness of coverage.

GENUINE (TRUE) STRESS INCONTINENCE

True stress incontinence occurs chiefly in women who are ordinarily continent at rest or with minimal activity. In the presence of stress, as with exercise, coughing, sneezing, or heavy lifting, they become incontinent of urine. This type of incontinence results from an increased pressure gradient between the bladder and the proximal urethra. Normally, the functional portion of the urethra is "intra-abdominal" (ie, above the urogenital diaphragm) such that increased abdominal pressure acts equally on the bladder and the proximal urethra. When the urethrovesical junction descends so that the functional urethra is no longer an intra-abdominal organ, increased intra-abdominal pressure may result in incontinence.

Clinical Findings

A. Symptoms and Signs: The diagnosis of genuine stress incontinence is based principally on the history of loss of urine with stress or activity and the absence of urgency, frequency, and dysuria. Physical examination may reveal some loss of anterior support, and the patient may also have a cystocele. It is not uncommon for these patients to have other defects also, such as rectoceles, enteroceles, or uterine prolapse. The patient may demonstrate loss of urine with coughing or sneezing during the examination.

A simple neurologic examination should be performed in the perineal area to detect both sensory and motor deficits. The sensory test can be accomplished via pinprick and the motor test by stroking each side of the anal orifice, which will generally elicit contraction of the sphincter muscle—the so called "anal wink"—in a normal patient.

B. Laboratory Findings: Laboratory evaluation should begin with urinalysis and urine culture, especially if the patient has urgency, frequency, or dysuria. If the patient has abnormal sensory and motor tests, a glucose tolerance test and VDRL test should also be done.

C. Cystometry: The most useful test is cystometry. The simplest form of this test can be done as an office procedure with a Foley catheter and a large (50 mL) syringe. After the patient voids, a Foley catheter is inserted to measure residual urine, which should be less than 50 mL.

Next, the syringe (minus the plunger) is attached to the Foley catheter, and 50-mL increments of sterile saline solution are instilled into the bladder. The first urge to void should normally be recorded after instillation of 150–200 mL of saline. The column of fluid in the syringe should be observed for unusual movements or waves suggestive of uninhibited bladder contractions or **detrusor dyssynergia.** The maximum capacity of the bladder is reached when the patient feels she can no longer hold her urine (approximately 450–500 mL) (Table 15–1). Next, approximately 250 mL of fluid is removed along with the Foley catheter, and the patient is asked to cough. A sudden loss of urine is consistent with genuine stress incontinence. A delay in loss of urine is suggestive of detrusor dyssynergia and is an indication for urologic consultation. If the patient is continent while lying down, she should be asked to cough while standing, as many patients will be continent in the recumbent position.

If the patient loses urine in either the recumbent or standing position, a Bonney test should be performed. This test involves gently supporting the bladder neck either with a finger on each side of the urethra or with a Kelly clamp (with care taken not to compress the urethra) and asking the patient to cough again. If the patient is continent, surgical repair likely will be successful.

Cystoscopy and more elaborate types of cystometry are generally not indicated unless the patient has a large residual capacity, a very small capacity, or urge incontinence suggestive of either detrusor dyssynergia, infection, or inflammation (Table 15–2).

Treatment

Once the diagnosis of genuine stress incontinence is made, therapy consists primarily of some type of surgical repair. Estrogen therapy in the postmenopausal patient may provide some measure of relief or improvement. Surgical repair may be accomplished either vaginally or abdominally. If a uterus is present, hysterectomy is also generally performed at the same time.

The vaginal approach is generally utilized in patients who have other associated conditions such as cystoceles, rectoceles, enteroceles, or uterine prolapse. The technique of vaginal repair is illustrated in Figure 15–2 and consists primarily of plication of the anterior vesicovaginal fascia, especially in the area of the urethrovesical junction.

There are numerous abdominal operations for genuine stress incontinence. All result primarily in elevation and support of the vesical neck. The simplest and probably most common abdominal procedure is the Marshall-Marchetti-Krantz procedure. This consists primarily of placing sutures in the paravaginal tissues next to the bladder neck and securing the sutures to the back of the sym-

Table 15–1. Normal values for cystometry.

Residual volume	< 50 mL
First urge to void	150–200 mL
Maximum capacity	450–500 mL
Uninhibited contractions	None

Table 15–2. Criteria for diagnosis of genuine stress incontinence.

Normal urinalysis, negative urine culture
Normal neurologic examination
Poor anatomic support (cotton-tipped applicator test, x-ray, or ure-throscopy)
Demonstrable leakage with stress (stress test or pad test)
Normal cystometrogram or urethrocystometry (normal residual urine volumes, bladder capacity, and sensation; no involuntary detrusor contractions)

physis pubis (Figure 15–7). A variation on this technique is called the Burch procedure, which involves suturing the paravaginal fascia next to the bladder neck to the ileopectineal ligaments instead of the symphysis pubis. There also are various sling procedures. All of these techniques utilize either a portion of fascia or synthetic material to elevate and support the bladder neck.

Although opinion differs about which of these procedures are best, it is generally accepted that abdominal procedures will result in a higher cure rate than those done via the vaginal approach. Reported cure rates range from 65% to 95% depending on the specific procedure.

URGE INCONTINENCE

Urge incontinence is loss of urine associated with an almost uncontrollable urge to void. The urge to void usually occurs suddenly and catches the patient off guard. Urge incontinence can be secondary to either uninhibited detrusor contractions (so-called "unstable bladder") or can occur as a result of chronic irritation. This latter category may be secondary to chronic infection, irritation, or to tumors such as fibroids or cancer.

Clinical Findings

The diagnosis of urge incontinence is based primarily upon the history. It should be noted that patients with urge incontinence may also have a form of stress incontinence. Patients who have detrusor dyssynergia or an unstable bladder demonstrate uninhibited contractions on cystometry (Figure 15–8). Patients who have urge incontinence secondary to an irritable bladder generally will not demonstrate uninhibited detrusor contractions but will often demonstrate a smaller bladder capacity at the time of cystometry. Infection, inflammation, or a neoplasm can also be demonstrated with cystoscopy.

Treatment

The primary treatment for urge incontinence is medical unless stress urinary incontinence is also present. Medications for unstable bladder secondary to uninhibited detrusor contractions are most often anticholinergic agents (Table 15–3).

Patients with urge incontinence secondary to an irritable bladder may respond to antibiotics as suppressive therapy. An acceptable regimen is with nitrofurantoin macrocrystals (Macrodantin), 100 mg at bedtime. For patients with significant inflammation, instillation of anti-inflammatory agents into the bladder may be helpful. Patients with tumors or neoplasms may require surgery.

OVERFLOW INCONTINENCE

Overflow incontinence results primarily from a neurogenic bladder, which in turn may be due to a variety of causes including multiple sclerosis, trauma, and diabetes. A neurogenic (neuropathic) bladder is one in which the normal innervation to the bladder is either absent or damaged secondary to a neurologic disorder or disease, resulting in loss of the usual vesical reflexes and sensation associated with normal bladder emptying. Patients who have undergone radical hysterectomy may also have neurogenic bladder. Psychologic factors may occasionally con-

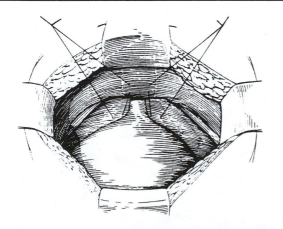

Figure 15–7. Marshall-Marchetti-Krantz procedure. (Reproduced, with permission, from Creighton SM, Stanton SL: Suprapubic surgery for stress incontinence. *Contemp Ob/Gyn* 1989;33:74–85.)

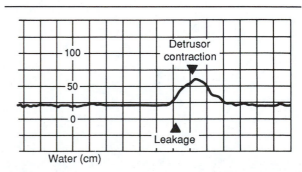

Figure 15–8. Unstable bladder. The cystometrogram reveals a detrusor contraction and associated leakage, both involuntary. (Reproduced, with permission, from Pernoll ML (editor): *Current Obstetric & Gynecologic Diagnosis & Treatment,* 7th ed. Appleton & Lange, 1991.)

Table 15–3. Anticholingergic agents for the treatment of the unstable bladder (detrusor instability).

Propantheline bromide (Pro-Banthine), 15–30 mg every 4–6 hours
Oxybutynin chloride (Ditropan), 5–10 mg 3–4 times daily
Flavoxate hydrochloride (Urispas), 100–200 mg 3–4 times daily
Hyoscyamine sulfate (Cystospax, others), 0.125–0.25 mg 3–4 times daily

tribute to an overdistended bladder with overflow incontinence.

Clinical Findings

Besides loss of urine, patients with an overdistended bladder leading to overflow incontinence may also complain of a full sensation and increased pressure. The diagnosis of overflow incontinence usually is confirmed by cystometry, which reveals a very large bladder capacity. Patients may tolerate the instillation of more than 1000 mL of saline solution without discomfort. There also is absence of uninhibited bladder contractions.

Treatment

The treatment of overflow incontinence is primarily medical. Cholinergic agents that increase bladder tone and contractility may prove effective. An example is bethanechol (Urecholine), 10–15 mg orally 3–4 times daily (Table 15–3).

SUGGESTED READINGS

American College of Obstetricians and Gynecologists: *Urinary Incontinence*. ACOG Technical Bulletin No. 100, 1987

Creighton SM, Stanton SL: Suprapubic surgery for stress incontinence. Contemp Ob/Gyn 1989;33:74.

Robertson JR, Hebert DB: Gynecologic urology. Chapter 41 in: *Current Obstetric & Gynecologic Diagnosis & Treatment,* 7th ed. Pernoll ML (editor). Appleton & Lange, 1991.

Stenchever MA: Diagnosis and management of urinary incontinence. Compr Therapy 1986;12:58.

Symmonds RE: Relaxation of pelvic supports. Chapter 40 in: *Current Obstetric & Gynecologic Diagnosis & Treatment,* 7th ed. Pernoll ML (editor). Appleton & Lange, 1991.

16

Urinary Tract Infections

The urinary tract is a frequent site of infection in women. Both the upper and lower tracts may be involved, and infection may be symptomatic or asymptomatic (Table 16–1).

The acquisition of bacteriuria in females occurs early in life—in contrast to males, in whom the frequency approaches that of the female only in later life. It has been estimated that as many as 5% of school-aged girls will have bacteriuria, and as many as 15–20% of adult women will experience a urinary tract infection during their lifetime.

ETIOLOGY

Most uropathogens are acquired from the gastrointestinal tract. The Enterobacteriaceae (Table 16–2) account for approximately 85–95% of infections, with *Escherichia coli* being the single most commonly isolated organism, especially in infections that are community-acquired.

The major reason urinary tract infections are more common in women than men is anatomic. The female urethra is relatively short, averaging 3–4 cm in length, and thus forms less of a barrier to invading pathogens. Moreover, it is in relatively close proximity to both the vagina and the rectum and therefore may be more readily colonized by enteric organisms. Urinary tract infections have been reported to be more common in young, sexually active women, probably as a consequence of urethral trauma during intercourse.

Certain bacteria have a unique ability to attach themselves to the uroepithelium of the lower urinary tract, which probably accounts for their increased virulence. An example is found in the P-fimbriated strains of *E coli,* which attach to specific receptors in the uroepithelium. This may explain why some women have a higher frequency of persistent or recurrent urinary tract infections and why some are more susceptible to upper tract infections such as acute pyelonephritis.

ASYMPTOMATIC INFECTIONS

Asymptomatic infection of the lower urinary tract ("asymptomatic bacteriuria") is the presence of significant bacteria (by definition, $\geq 100,000$ of a single uropathogen per milliliter of urine collected via clean-voided midstream sampling) without associated symptoms such as dysuria or suprapubic discomfort. Counts of less than 100,000/mL or specimens yielding two or more organisms probably represent contamination and not infection. An exception is a urine specimen containing less than 100,000 organisms/mL of a single uropathogen that was obtained by suprapubic aspiration or bladder catheterization. The accuracy of a diagnosis based on a specimen obtained via the clean-voided technique, if confirmed by culture of a second clean-voided specimen, approaches that obtained by culture of a specimen obtained by catheterization.

The most common organisms isolated in patients with asymptomatic bacteriuria are listed in Table 16–2.

Treatment

Most women with asymptomatic bacteriuria go undetected, probably suffer no long-term ill effects, and require no treatment. An exception is the woman who becomes pregnant. Approximately 5–6% of all pregnant women have detectable bacteriuria at the first prenatal visit, and without treatment about 25% of these women will develop symptomatic infections such as acute pyelonephritis, with significant risks to mother and fetus (see Chapter 60). Treatment in such cases consists of a short course of one of several antibiotics such as nitrofurantoin, sulfisoxazole, ampicillin, or a cephalosporin.

Nonpregnant women with asymptomatic bacteriuria who have a history of frequent urinary tract infections require treatment also as outlined above, and the results are comparable.

Table 16–1. Urinary tract infections in women.

Lower tract
 Asymptomatic bacteriuria (positive urine culture)
 Symptomatic (urgency, frequency, suprapubic discomfort, dys-
  uria)
  Acute urethral syndrome (negative urine culture)
  Acute cystitis (positive urine culture)
Upper tract
 Symptomatic (fever, chills, nausea, vomiting, flank pain, positive
  urine culture)
  Acute pyelonephritis

SYMPTOMATIC INFECTIONS

LOWER TRACT INFECTIONS (Acute Cystitis)

Symptomatic infection of the lower urinary tract is manifested by dysuria, frequency, urgency, and suprapubic pressure in addition to a positive urine culture. In the absence of upper tract involvement, these patients do not have systemic symptoms such as flank pain or fever.

Cystitis is the most common type of urinary tract infection encountered by the gynecologist. The diagnosis is based chiefly on clinical symptoms and a positive urine culture. If acute dysuria is present, bacteria counts of less than 100,000 organisms/mL of urine may be significant. Urinalysis will generally reveal numerous bacteria and leukocytes. Occasionally, patients will have microscopic and, rarely, gross hematuria ("hemorrhagic cystitis"). The most common bacterial isolates are listed in Table 16–2.

Treatment

Management of acute cystitis consists primarily of documentation of infection by urine culture and by ruling out other causes of symptoms and other infections such as vaginitis or sexually transmitted disease (Table 16–3). Patients who have significant dysuria but a negative urine culture and no bacteriuria or pyuria are generally classified as having **acute urethral syndrome.** In such cases, culture of urine for chlamydial organisms is required.

Antimicrobial agents effective against uropathogens are listed in Table 16–4. Since most infections are due to *E coli,* therapy should be directed toward this organism until the results of urine culture are reported. In the past, stan-

Table 16–2. Commonly isolated pathogens in women with urinary tract infections.

Escherichia coli [1]
Klebsiella-Enterobacter [1]
Streptococcus
Staphylococcus
Proteus
Pseudomonas

[1]Account for approximately 95% of all community-acquired urinary tract infections.

Table 16–3. Management of symptomatic lower urinary tract infections (ie, cystitis).

Documentation of infection
 Urinalysis
 Urine culture
Rule out other infections
 Vaginitis
 Sexually transmitted disease
Appropriate antimicrobial therapy
Reassurance

dard therapy consisted of antibiotics given 3 or 4 times a day for a 7–10 days; however, shorter courses of therapy have recently been shown to be efficacious in women with uncomplicated infections. In fact, several "single-dose" regimens have been shown to be very effective in eradicating bacteria and providing relief. Commonly used single-dose oral regimens for uncomplicated lower urinary tract infections include amoxicillin (3 g), trimethoprim-sulfamethoxazole (two double-strength or four single-strength tablets), or sulfisoxazole (2 g) (Table 16–5). Nitrofurantoin as a single 200-mg oral dose may also be effective.

Complicated cases (persistent infections, frequent recurrent infections, or infections associated with obstruction) should be treated with conventional 7- to 10-day regimens. Protracted therapy with ampicillin or a cephalosporin may significantly alter the gastrointestinal and genital tract flora and predispose to yeast vaginitis. The newer fluorinated quinolones (eg, norfloxacin) may be useful in chronic or recurrent urinary tract infections in nonpregnant women. The usual dose is 400 mg orally twice daily for 7–10 days.

Common characteristics repeatedly observed in women with urinary tract infections are listed in Table 16–6. The newly married or recently sexually active woman commonly develops acute infections that may be especially worrisome if she suspects she has a "venereal disease." Such infections may in their turn result in sexual dysfunction. Therapy in such cases consists of reassurance as well as antimicrobial therapy. For women who have recurrent symptoms after intercourse, a single dose of an antibiotic such as nitrofurantoin given soon after intercourse is usually effective. Voiding before and after intercourse should also be encouraged.

Frequent recurrent or chronic urinary tract infection is a debilitating disorder that may have significant psychologic effects. Patients may have been treated by other physicians with only temporary success. They are often re-

Table 16–4. Antimicrobial therapy for symptomatic lower urinary tract infections in women.

Sulfisoxazole
Trimethoprim-sulfamethoxazole
Ampicillin or amoxicillin
Cephalosporin
Nitrofurantoin
Norfloxacin

Table 16–5. Single-dose oral regimens for treatment of urinary tract infections in women.

Amoxicillin, 3 g
Trimethoprim-sulfamethoxazole, two double-strength tablets or four single-strength tablets
Sulfisoxazole, 2 g
Nitrofurantoin, 200 mg

Table 16–7. Management of recurrent or chronic urinary tract infections.[1]

Understanding
Reassurance
Increase fluid intake
Avoid delays in urination
Suppressive therapy
Self therapy

[1]Modified from Schaeffer AJ: Postgrad Med 1987;81:51.

ferred to the gynecologist to rule out anatomic causes such as cystocele and uterine fibroids. They require special attention as outlined in Table 16–7. As is true of many conditions encountered in gynecology—examples are chronic vaginitis and chronic pelvic pain—the first step in management is convincing the patient that her physician understands she has a problem but that reassurance is appropriate. Urinary infections almost never result in end-stage renal disease and can often be treated successfully with low-dose suppressive therapy (after an initial standard course of therapy for 7–10 days) for 6–12 months. A single dose of an antimicrobial agent such as nitrofurantoin, trimethoprim-sulfamethoxazole, or one of the new fluorinated quinolones such as norfloxacin—given once a day, usually at bedtime—is generally effective. Such therapy will have little effect on the gastrointestinal or vaginal flora.

Most women so treated will be asymptomatic during therapy and for many months thereafter. Unfortunately, recurrent infections are relatively common. Patients with frequent recurrences may also initiate self-therapy when they first experience symptoms of infection. Antibiotics such as nitrofurantoin or norfloxacin are useful for self-start therapy.

ACUTE URETHRAL SYNDROME

The acute urethral syndrome is characterized by frequency and dysuria. The diagnosis is based primarily on the absence of the usual uropathogens such as *E coli* on culture. The urethra should be cultured for *Chlamydia* as well as *Neisseria gonorrheae*.

Treatment

Specific therapy for women with acute urethral syndrome depends on the organism isolated. Since chlamydiae may be found, empiric therapy with tetracycline is usually effective for nonpregnant patients. Tetracyclines are contraindicated in pregnant women because of the risk of discoloration of fetal deciduous teeth.

Table 16–6. Common associated features in women with urinary tract infections encountered by the gynecologist.

Newly married
Recently sexually active
Recurrent infections associated with intercourse
Chronic urinary tract infections
Psychologic effects (anxiety, depression)

UPPER TRACT INFECTIONS (Acute Pyelonephritis)

Common symptoms of acute pyelonephritis include fever, chills, and back pain. Patients may also have nausea and vomiting. On physical examination, the patient generally will have fever and costovertebral angle tenderness. Pyuria and white cell casts are often found on urinalysis.

Treatment

In the nonpregnant patient, therapy may be either oral or parenteral depending on the severity of symptoms.

A. Oral Therapy: Women who are not dehydrated and who are able to tolerate oral intake may be treated as outpatients, with ampicillin or a cephalosporin. Therapy generally is continued for 7–10 days. Since many strains of *E coli* are resistant to ampicillin, the β-lactamase inhibitor clavulanic acid plus amoxicillin may prove useful.

B. Parenteral Therapy: Women with nausea and vomiting, those who are dehydrated, or those who are pregnant should be hospitalized, parenteral therapy should be started. Although therapy ultimately should be based on the results of sensitivity tests, ampicillin or a cephalosporin can be started empirically. An aminoglycoside should be added for patients with proven sepsis or shock or those who have had a recurrence of infection. Single-agent therapy with some of the newer broad-spectrum penicillins or cephalosporins may also be effective in these latter patients. Parenteral therapy should be continued until the patient has been afebrile for 24–48 hours, after which she can be started on oral antibiotics to complete a 10- to 14-day course of therapy. Patients with persistent or recurrent episodes of acute pyelonephritis should have further urologic evaluation to rule out obstruction.

NOSOCOMIAL INFECTIONS

Hospital-acquired urinary tract infections are relatively common and may be a source of significant morbidity and extended hospitalization. Such infections are more common in older and debilitated women. Organisms such as *Proteus, Enterobacter, Pseudomonas, Streptococcus faecalis (enterococcus; group D streptococcus),* and *Staphylococcus* are more likely to be isolated from the urine of patients with nosocomial infections than community-acquired infections, though *E coli* also is commonly isolated. Most of these infections are associated with the use of an indwelling Foley catheter. Since many hospital strains of *E coli* as well as other uropathogens are resistant to ampicillin, therapy should consist of one of the newer broad-spectrum penicillins (especially in combination with a β-lactamase inhibitor) or with a cephalosporin. The newer fluorinated quinolones, such as norfloxacin, may also be effective.

The mainstay in the treatment of nosocomial infections is prevention. Indwelling catheters should be used only when necessary and removed as soon as possible. Only catheters with a closed, sterile drainage system should be used. Prophylactic antibiotics for indwelling Foley catheters may induce bacterial resistance, especially if used for more than a few days. If prophylactic antibiotics are used, an antibiotic such as nitrofurantoin, 100 mg orally daily, should be considered.

UROLOGIC REFERRAL

Urologic evaluation may be indicated for women with incumbent or persistent urinary tract infections as well as those with hematuria or suspected obstruction. Such evaluation usually includes cystoscopy, intravenous pyelography, and ultrasonography.

SUGGESTED READINGS

Givens CD, Wenzel RP: Catheter-associated urinary tract infection in surgical patients: A controlled study on the excess morbidity and costs. J Urol 1980;124:646.

Parsons CL: Criteria for selecting an antibiotic. Contemp Obstet Gynecol 1988;32:103.

Schaeffer AJ: How bacterial adherence promotes recurrent urinary infection. Contemp Obstet Gynecol 1988;32:94.

Schaeffer AJ: Recurrent urinary tract infections in women: Pathogenesis and management. Postgrad Med 1987;81:51.

Stamm WE: Dysuria: Establishing a diagnostic protocol. Contemp Obstet Gynecol 1988;32:81.

Stamm WE: Prevention of urinary tract infections. Am J Med 1984;76:148.

Stamm WE et al: Causes of the acute urethral syndrome in women. N Engl J Med 1980;303:409.

Stamm WE et al: Diagnosis of coliform infection in acutely dysuric women. N Engl J Med 1982;307:463.

Tuomala R: Confronting issues that sidetrack optimal care. Contemp Obstet Gynecol 1988;32:109.

17

Gynecologic Surgery

Four of the most frequently performed elective surgical procedures are pelvic operations performed by the obstetrician and gynecologist. This chapter outlines the indications and contraindications of these and other surgical procedures, with guidelines and comments about technique and postoperative management. Complications of the procedures are discussed in Chapter 18.

MINOR SURGICAL PROCEDURES

Minor pelvic surgical procedures are usually performed in day surgery (ambulatory surgery, same-day surgery) units, because hospitalization is not required before or after. It is a principle of surgical practice that patients should not be removed from their normal routines sooner than necessary and that they should be returned to normal activity status as quickly as possible—for both physical and psychologic reasons. The advent of day surgery has provided greater opportunities to act on that principle and has significantly reduced the cost of health care. Same-day admissions for major surgical procedures are also becoming the standard of care for much the same reasons.

DILATION & CURETTAGE (D&C)

Indications & Contraindications

The indications and contraindications for D&C are listed in Table 17–1. Abortion is discussed in Chapter 9,

and the causes of abnormal uterine bleeding are discussed in Chapter 21. Before undertaking D&C for abnormal uterine bleeding, one must be certain that the bleeding is not pregnancy-related.

Endometrial biopsy has replaced D&C as a diagnostic test in many instances, and hormonal therapy will correct many functional causes of abnormal bleeding. Endometrial biopsy may be impossible because of cervical stenosis, however—as frequently happens in postmenopausal women.

D&C is performed therapeutically for endometrial polyps or small, pedunculated submucous leiomyomas; endometrial hyperplasia is more completely removed hormonally than mechanically. Suction curettage removes more tissue than sharp curettage and should be used routinely for diagnostic as well as therapeutic procedures.

Technique
(See accompanying box.)

D&C is performed with the patient in the dorsal lithotomy position. The patient should have voided recently. It may be necessary to drain the bladder with a catheter if it fills again before the procedure is started.

Pain management can range from simple analgesia with nonsteroidal anti-inflammatory agents to general anesthesia. If general anesthesia is unnecessary or contraindicated, pain control can be achieved by paracervical block or epidural or regional spinal analgesia. In nonpregnant patients, the latter is usually preferred because of the discomfort associated with retraction and cervical dilation.

If general anesthesia is required, the extremities should be padded to prevent undue pressure by stirrups. The occiput, scapulae, and arms should be protected also.

A thorough pelvic examination should be performed

Surgery Checklist: Dilation & Curettage

Anesthesia	Sounding the uterus
Examination	Cervical dilation
Dorsal lithotomy position—pad pressure points	Polypectomy
Vaginal and vulval surgical scrub	Endometrial curettage
Drape	Pathology specimens and report
Endocervical curettage	Operative note, both dictated and handwritten

Table 17–1. Minor gynecologic procedures: Indications and contraindications.

	Indications	Contraindications
Dilation and curettage (D&C)	**Diagnosis and treatment** of abnormal uterine bleeding: heavy or prolonged periods, postmenopausal bleeding. Abortion management. Removal of "lost" intrauterine device.	Anticoagulation with warfarin; any condition in which regional or general anesthesia is contraindicated.
Conization of the cervix	**Diagnosis:** Extent of CIN-dysplasia or - (1) Neoplasia on biopsy with unsatisfactory colposcopy (2) Neoplasia on endocervical curettage (3) Significant discrepancy in degree of neoplasia between Papanicolaou smear and colposcopically directed cervical biopsy (more than one step difference, with more disease indicated on Papanicolaou smear than on biopsy—eg, CIN III on smear and CIN I on biopsy). (4) Microinvasive squamous cell cancer on biopsy **Treatment:** CIN III (> 2 quadrants), large acetowhite lesion (> 2 quadrants) with neoplasia on biopsy.	Antiicoagulation with warfarin; any condition in which regional or general anesthesia is contraindicated.

before preparation of the patient to determine uterine and adnexal size, position, and abnormalities. The vulva and vagina should be prepared with povidone-iodine or an equivalent antiseptic. Most gynecologists use drapes for this procedure, though the infection rate with or without drapes is virtually nil.

A handle-weighted, single-blade speculum is inserted into the vagina and self-retracts posteriorly. Another retractor is gently inserted into the anterior fornix, allowing maximal visualization of the cervix, which is then grasped on the portio at 12 o'clock with a single-toothed tenaculum for stabilization. This also allows for complete visualization of the vaginal fornices because it affords controlled movement of the cervix (Chapter 9).

When D&C is performed for diagnosis of abnormal bleeding or potential neoplasia, samples should be segregated to ensure accurate localization of disease. The first specimen is from the endocervix, before cervical dilation. Special curettes (Kevorkian, Gusberg) are designed for this purpose, and the specimen should be collected on Telfa (coated cellulose sponge) for submission to the surgical pathology laboratory as a separate specimen. Collection is achieved by inserting the curette to the internal os, withdrawing it completely, and depositing the specimen on to the Telfa. This process is then repeated so that most of the endocervix is sampled. Uterine depth is then measured by gently inserting a uterine sound or graduated, soft metal probe. The depth recorded should agree roughly with the physical assessment of uterine size. The angle of insertion is determined by the position of the uterus. Insertion is safest if the operator places the last three fingers of the hand used to insert the instrument on the patient's vulva and uses the thumb and index finger to gently advance the sound into the uterine cavity while stabilizing the cervix with the tenaculum, which is held in the other hand.

Dilators are blunt, slightly curved, numbered metal instruments that are gently inserted through the cervix as described above until the opening allows insertion of a metal or suction curette. Hanks dilators are gradually tapered, have a cervical stop ring, and are measured in French (F) sizes. Hegar dilators are blunt, and calibrated in millimeters of diameter (20F = 9 mm).

The uterine cavity is then explored with forceps designed for polyp removal. Forceps insertion is performed as with the sound, in the plane of least resistance, and to the fundus. The forceps is then slightly opened, rotated 90 degrees, closed, and removed. This technique is repeated until the cavity has been thoroughly explored. Specimens are segregated for separate submission to the pathology laboratory.

The endometrial cavity is then sequentially covered with a suction curette. When the endometrial cavity is explored with the curette, contour aberrations are noted. Many gynecologists segregate the endometrial specimen obtained from the lower half of the uterus from that obtained from the fundal area by placing each on a separate piece of Telfa and submitting them to the pathologist in separate jars. The uterus should again be "sounded" after the procedure to detect perforation.

Each specimen bottle should have a label bearing the patient's name, the date, the time, the doctor's name, and other hospital stamp information. The origin of each specimen (type of tissue) must also be on the label. The request slip should convey sufficient information to enable the pathologist to provide a comprehensive interpretation of the specimens.

Finally, the operative report must be dictated immediately after the procedure and not postponed for any reason. A concise and complete handwritten operative note should also be made part of the patient's record, since dictations may be lost, machines may malfunction, etc.

CONIZATION OF THE CERVIX

Indications & Contraindications

The indications and contraindications for cervical conization are listed in Table 17–1.

Colposcopy, or examination of the cervix with a variable magnification microscope, has significantly reduced the number of operations (conization) undertaken because of an abnormal Papanicolaou smear. Cervical intraepithelial neoplasia (dysplasia) is discussed in Chapter 29.

Conization may be used not only diagnostically but therapeutically as well, especially if the patient desires future childbearing and the specimen includes the entire lesion. The best evidence that therapy has been adequate is a surgical margin without dysplasia. If there is dysplasia at an ectocervical margin, the patient must be followed with Papanicolaou smear, colposcopy, and biopsy as indicated. If the endocervical margin is positive, the patient must be followed by endocervical curettage in addition to the Papanicolaou smear. If both margins are positive, the above tests are combined.

Hysterectomy may be required for patients with extensive and advanced dysplasia.

Technique
(See accompanying box.)

Conization begins in the same way as D&C. Preparation of the vagina must not be so vigorous that cervical tissue is removed, since neoplastic tissue is fragile. The lesion must be completely removed with a margin of several millimeters of presumably normal tissue. This determination can be made with a colposcope and acetic acid for cervical dehydration—or with a concentrated iodine solution. Normal squamous epithelium of the cervix and vagina contains glycogen; these cells stain dark brown when iodine is applied. Neoplastic tissue does not contain glycogen and therefore will not "stain" with iodine. The internal margin of the surgical specimen is usually the internal os, which is identified with the uterine sound.

The descending (cervical) branches of the uterine artery are located laterally at about 3 and 9 o'clock. To ensure hemostasis, these vessels are usually ligated with absorbable suture before the procedure begins. Epinephrine or oxytocin can be mixed with saline and injected circumferentially into the cervix to induce vasospasm and achieve hemostasis. The sample is then removed sharply with a knife or scissors—or with a CO_2 laser and then scissors for the base. Any remaining canal is curetted to ensure complete removal of the lesion and to detect residual neoplasia.

The cone specimen may be long and narrow or short and wide. One should always leave as much normal cervical stroma and endocervical glandular tissue as possible, especially in women who desire future fertility.

Hemostasis may be adequate after removal of the specimen or can be achieved with running or interrupted absorbable sutures, cauterization, or Monsel's stiptic solution (ferric subsulfate).

The endocervical curettage and cone specimens are sent to the pathologist separately. The cone specimen must be oriented for the pathologist either by opening at 12 o'clock or by placing a suture at 12 o'clock. The pathologist may prefer that the specimen be sent fresh or in formalin opened and pinned to a tongue blade.

The operator should label the specimen containers, complete the surgical pathology sheet (including marker identification), and dictate the operative note immediately.

MAJOR SURGICAL PROCEDURES

HYSTERECTOMY
(Figures 17–1 to 17–6)

Hysterectomy is the major surgical procedure most frequently performed on women of reproductive age. It can be performed abdominally or vaginally, depending on specific indications. Vaginal hysterectomy is preferred because there is no abdominal incision, the hospital stay is shorter, and recuperation is quicker. In the past, a 10- to 14-day hospital stay was not uncommon following hysterectomy. Today, a 3- to 4-day stay is common after abdominal hysterectomy and a 2- to 3-day stay after vaginal hysterectomy.

Many insurance companies will not pay for the night preceding surgery as a hospital night unless there is a medical reason for the patient to be in hospital. Laboratory testing and consultation should therefore be performed on an outpatient basis prior to hospital admission whenever possible and appropriate.

If the principal reason for hysterectomy is stress urinary

Surgery Checklist: Conization of the Cervix

Anesthesia
Examination
Dorsal lithotomy position—pad pressure points
Gentle vaginal and vulval surgical scrub
Drape
Identify outer margins of lesion
  Colposcope with acetic acid
  Concentrated iodine solution (Lugol's)
Identify inner margin (often the internal os)
Hemostasis
  Sutures at 3 and 9 o'clock
  Saline with epinephrine or saline with oxytocin injection

Specimen removal
Curettage above proximal margin
Hemostasis
  Sutures
  Cautery
  Ferric subsulfate (Monsel's solution)
Pathology specimens and report
Operative note, both dictated and handwritten

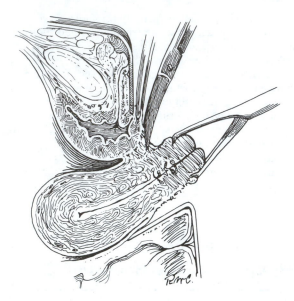

Figure 17–1. Lateral view of dissection of the base of the bladder from the cervix and lower uterine segment. Note that scissors are directed toward the uterus. (Reproduced, with permission, from: Mattingly RF, Thompson JD [editors]: *TeLinde's Operative Gynecology,* 6th ed. Lippincott, 1985.)

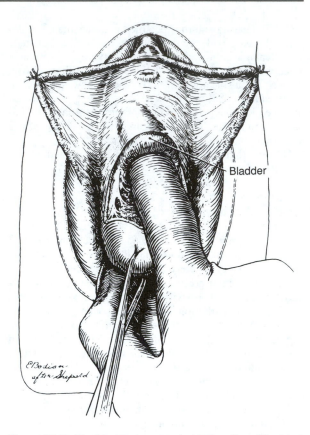

Bladder

Figure 17–2. The bladder is separated to the plica of the bladder peritoneum by blunt finger dissection. (Reproduced, with permission, from: Mattingly RF, Thompson JD [editors]: *TeLinde's Operative Gynecology,* 6th ed. Lippincott, 1985.)

incontinence, the choice of route—abdominal or vaginal—will depend on which type will achieve the best result. Although it is not mandatory that hysterectomy be performed as part of surgical correction for incontinence, the benefits of surgery without hysterectomy may be lost if pregnancy followed by vaginal delivery should occur.

The patient must be informed about the nature of her problem, alternative methods of treatment, and the complications that might result from any of the treatments or from no treatment. This should be done in the office before admission to the hospital and again in the hospital, and her partner, if applicable, should be present on one or both occasions. Documentation in a format other than the signed informed surgical consent form is important, and the office record is the logical place to preserve the signed form.

Only benign diseases will be discussed in this chapter.

1. ABDOMINAL HYSTERECTOMY
(See accompanying box.)

The uterus is usually completely removed—ie, total hysterectomy is usually performed. In rare circumstances, hysterectomy may be partial, with the cervix left in situ (subtotal hysterectomy, supracervical hysterectomy). To the lay public, "partial hysterectomy" means removal of the uterus and "complete hysterectomy" means removal of the tubes and ovaries as well, or salpingo-oophorectomy. However, the term "hysterectomy" properly refers only to uterine removal. Unilateral or bilateral salpingo-

oophorectomy is performed frequently at abdominal hysterectomy, depending on what lesions are present or the age of the patient. There is controversy about the appropriate age for "prophylactic" removal of otherwise normal ovaries. Older women with adnexal disease requiring surgical removal will usually also undergo hysterectomy.

In most instances, the abdominal approach is utilized when the uterus is too large to be removed vaginally or when disease involves the adnexa. The most frequent indication is uterine leiomyomatosis. Hysterectomy is almost always elective and is not performed until medical alternatives have been exhausted.

Antibiotic prophylaxis (one dose) may be beneficial.

Preoperative counseling should emphasize the importance of early ambulation, deep breathing, and calf exercises. Early ambulation has greatly reduced the incidence of pulmonary embolism while hastening the return of normal gastrointestinal function. If it is anticipated that ambulation will not be possible soon after operation, the prophylactic administration of heparin by subcutaneous injection is believed to be beneficial. Some surgeons administer heparin to all women undergoing abdominal hysterectomy. In certain cases, laparoscopy will enable the

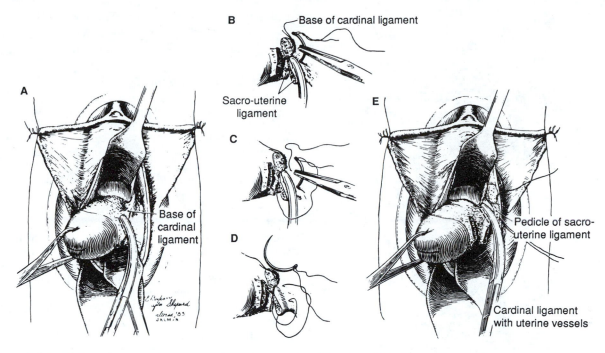

Figure 17–3. **(A)** The left cardinal ligament is clamped to be cut at dotted line. **(B, C, D)** Transfixion of the uterosacral ligament. **(E)** The base of the broad ligament with the uterine vessel is clamped to be cut at dotted line. (Reproduced, with permission, from: Mattingly RF, Thompson JD [editors]: *TeLinde's Operative Gynecology,* 6th ed. Lippincott, 1985.)

Surgery Checklist: Abdominal Hysterectomy

Anesthesia

Examination

Supine position—pad pressure points

Abdominal, vaginal, and vulval surgical scrub

Insertion of indwelling urethral catheter

Drape

Abdominal incision
  Vertical
  Horizontal

Exploration of upper abdomen, including lymph nodes

Self-retaining retractor

"Pack" small and large bowel out of pelvis

Restore normal anatomic relationships

Ureteral identification

Successive clamping, incising, and individual delayed absorbable suture ligatures of the following: round ligaments, infundibulopelvic ligaments (if salpingo-oophorectomy), uterine tubes and utero-ovarian ligaments (if ovaries retained), broad ligaments, uterine arteries and veins, cardinal ligaments, uterosacral ligaments

Incising vagina circumferentially (excises uterus)

Delayed absorbable suture ligature of vaginal margin (cuff): interrupted, running

Ureteral examination

Ensure hemostasis

Approximate pelvic parietal peritoneum (optional), running, delayed absorbable suture

Approximate abdominal wall peritoneum (optional), running, delayed absorbable suture

Approximate abdominal wall fascia, delayed absorbable suture: running, interrupted

Approximate abdominal wall skin: suture, clips, staples

Sterile dressing

Pathology specimens and report

Operative note, both dictated and handwritten

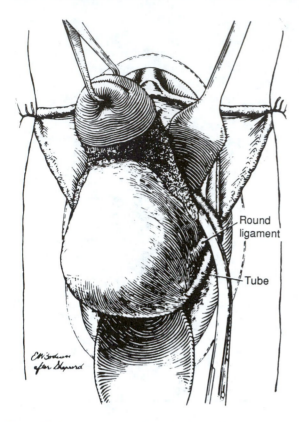

Figure 17–4. The upper portion of the broad ligament, including the tube, the ovarian ligament, and the round ligament, is clamped. (Reproduced, with permission, from: Mattingly RF, Thompson JD [editors]: *TeLinde's Operative Gynecology,* 6th ed. Lippincott, 1985.)

patient to undergo vaginal hysterectomy because contraindications can be removed with laparoscopic surgery.

2. VAGINAL HYSTERECTOMY

Vaginal hysterectomy requires a shorter hospital stay and is associated with less pain and morbidity—other than infection—than abdominal hysterectomy. With a single preoperative intravenous dose of antibiotic, the morbidity rate from infection can be reduced to 5% or less. The infection rate is higher after this procedure than after abdominal hysterectomy because contamination begins with the first incision and continues throughout the procedure. In abdominal hysterectomy, contamination occurs only at the end of the procedure, when the vaginal canal is entered.

Since there is no abdominal incision with vaginal hysterectomy, there are fewer respiratory problems, less pain, and earlier ambulation.

Contraindications to vaginal hysterectomy are chiefly anatomic—related to uterine size or the presence of adnexal disease. The pubic arch should be 100 degrees or more. Multiple prior pelvic surgical procedures—but not cesarean section—are a contraindication in the minds of most surgeons. Undiagnosed disease may be encountered, so it should be clearly understood by the patient—and documented—that the procedure may require completion transabdominally. Some vaginal surgeons may routinely remove uteri of up to 16 weeks' gestational size; training and experience are the deciding factors. Day surgery vaginal hysterectomy has been reported.

Technique
(See accompanying box.)

The technique for vaginal hysterectomy is basically the reverse of that for abdominal hysterectomy, with the important exceptions that upper abdominal exploration is impossible and ureteral identification is more difficult. Adnexa can be removed, if necessary. Bladder drainage can be done before the procedure, but many wait until after anterior colpotomy is performed because with the

Figure 17–5. Adnexal removal. When removal of adnexa is indicated *(A)*, the pedicle to the tip of the broad ligament is pulled into the operative field and two Heaney clamps are placed on the infundibulopelvic ligament. The ligament is excised, and the tube and ovary are removed. *(B)* The ligament is ligated with a free-tie of No. 0 delayed-absorbable suture, which is placed behind the inner clamp, *(C)* transfixed to the tip of the clamp, *(D)* tied firmly before removal of the outer clamp. (Reproduced, with permission, from: Mattingly RF, Thompson JD [editors]: *TeLinde's Operative Gynecology,* 6th ed. Lippincott, 1985.)

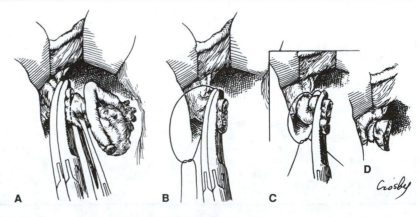

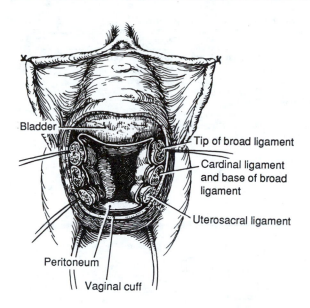

Figure 17–6. Cut surface of the tip of the broad ligament, the cardinal ligament, and the uterosacral ligament. (Reproduced, with permission, from: Mattingly RF, Thompson JD [editors]: *TeLinde's Operative Gynecology,* 6th ed. Lippincott, 1985.)

bladder distended it is easier to notice when cystotomy occurs.

Anterior colpotomy is a crucial part of the procedure. Some surgeons perform anterior colpotomy immediately after posterior colpotomy but others wait until after the uterosacral and cardinal ligaments are "clamped, cut, and tied" because uterine descent occurs with the latter, and identification of the anterior peritoneal reflection is thus more easily made. Some surgeons inject a dilute solution of epinephrine (eg, 1:100,000) or saline-oxytocin solution at the junction of the vagina and cervix for hemostasis.

LAPAROSCOPY

This transperitoneal endoscopic technique is assuming an increasingly important role in gynecologic surgery. With the use of improved laparoscopic techniques, many conditions can be diagnosed and treated as outpatient (ambulatory) same-day surgery procedures because laparotomy can be avoided.

Instruments are of various diameters and provide visualization of a 180-degree viewing angle. It is necessary to create a pneumoperitoneum with CO_2 in order to allow complete visualization of the pelvic organs. This is accomplished with a special needle and a pneumatic insufflator that will allow careful monitoring of the pressure, flow rate, and volume of gas used for inflation. A fiberoptic light source and cord are also necessary. Different laparoscopes are used for diagnosis and therapy, and some are of single-puncture and some of double-puncture design. Instruments available for the operative laparoscope include those for biopsy, coagulation, manipulation, incision, aspiration, clip or Silastic ring application, and even knot tying. Attachments for laser therapy and videotaping enhance the wide variety of applications of this procedure.

Indications
(Table 17–2)

The indications for this surgical procedure are expanding yearly. With the aid of colpotomy, adnexectomies are now being performed. General surgeons are evaluating the effectiveness and safety of laparoscopic laser cholecystectomies. The technique is being used to evaluate response to therapy for acute salpingitis, for appraisal of bowel viability after surgery, and for other diagnostic and therapeutic purposes not requiring hospital admission or laparotomy.

Technique
(See accompanying box and Figure 17–7.)

Laparoscopy is a "blind procedure," since the operator

Surgery Checklist: Vaginal Hysterectomy

Anesthesia
Examination
Dorsal lithotomy position—pad pressure points
Vaginal and vulval surgical scrub
Drape
Circumferentially incise vagina
Posterior colpotomy
Advance bladder (Figs 17–1 and 17–2)
Anterior colpotomy

Successive clamping, incising, and individual delayed
  absorbably suture ligatures of:
  Uterosacral ligaments (Fig 17–3)
  Cardinal ligaments (Fig 17–3)
  Uterine arteries, veins (Fig 17–3)
  Broad ligaments (Fig 17–3)
  Uterine tubes, utero-ovarian ligaments (ovaries retained)
    (Fig 17–4)
    Infundibulopelvic ligaments (ovaries excised)
    (Fig 17–5)
Ensure hemostasis, inspect pedicles (Fig 17–6)
Approximation of pelvic parietal peritoneum (optional):
  running
Approximation of vagina (vaginal cuff), delayed absorb-
  able suture: interrupted, running

Table 17–2. Major gynecologic surgical procedures: Indications and contraindications.

	Indications	Contraindications
Abdominal hysterectomy	Symptomatic uterine leiomyomas (pain, pressure, bleeding) Asymptomatic leiomyomas (12–14 weeks' gestational size, rapid growth) Symptomatic endometriosis refractory to medical management Chronic pelvic pain refractory to medical management Symptomatic dysfunctional uterine bleeding refractory to medical management Uncontrollable bleeding after obstetric delivery (uterine atony, placenta accreta or percreta, uterine rupture) Infection unresponsive to medical management Stress urinary incontinence	**Contraindications to elective procedure:** Undiagnosed abnormal uterine bleeding Unknown results of Pap smear Active infection Pregnancy Warfarin anticoagulation Any condition in which regional or general anesthesia is contraindicated
Vaginal hysterectomy	Pelvic relaxation Stress urinary incontinence Cervical intraepithelia neoplasia, high-grade Dysfunctional uterine bleeding unresponsive to medical management Symptomatic uterine leiomyomas of 10–12 weeks' gestational size or less	Uterus larger than 10–12 weeks' gestational size Adnexal disease Warfarin anticoagulation Any condition in which general or regional anesthesia is contraindicated Operator dependent
Laparoscopy	**Diagnosis:** Cause of chronic pelvic pain (endometriosis, infection) Genital anomalies Cause of acute pelvic pain (ectopic pregnancy, ruptured ovarian cyst, adnexal torsion, appendicitis, salpingitis, leiomyoma) **Photodocumentation** (for teaching, patient understanding) **Therapy:** Sterilization Salpingostomy for ectopic pregnancy Endometriosis (fulguration, laser vaporization) Lysis of adhesions Salpingitis–aspiration of purulent material for culture Salpingostomy for tubo-ovarian abscess, pyosalpinx Removal of extruded IUD Myomectomy Ovum collection for in vitro fertilization Gamete intrafallopian transfer (GIFT) Wedge resection of ovaries	**Absolute:** Intestinal obstruction Generalized peritonitis Large pelvic or abdominal mass Large-volume hemoperitoneum (cardiovascular instability) Warfarin anticoagulation Any condition in which regional or general anesthesia is contraindicated **Relative:** Severe cardiac or pulmonary diseases Multiple previous surgical procedures Obesity
Tubal sterilization	Desire for sterility	Uncertainty about motivation Pelvic infection Legal guardianship Young age[1] Warfarin anticoagulation Any condition in which regional or general anesthesia is contraindicated

[1]There may be statutory bars to sterilization of minor females.

does not know the condition of the abdominal cavity or the location of its contents. If the patient has had prior abdominal surgical procedures, adhesion formation and organ fixation increase the risk of operative injury. The advent of "open" laparoscopy allows its performance in many patients listed in the relative contraindication category.

The periumbilical area can be blocked with 15 mL of 1% lidocaine. The oviduct is pain-sensitive and may be locally anesthetized with 2% lidocaine. Many patients prefer general anesthesia, however, because steep Trendelenburg positioning makes it difficult to breathe.

A uterine manipulator is usually inserted so that all areas of the pelvis can be visualized. A small trocar inserted through a transverse incision in the midline about 8 inches below the laparoscope facilitates further manipulation and is necessary for more extensive surgery.

TUBAL STERILIZATION
(See accompanying box and Figures 17–8 to 17–11.)

Over a million women a year elect tubal sterilization, and most such procedures are performed laparoscopically. This operation is for practical purposes irreversible—

Surgery Checklist: Laparoscopy

Anesthesia

Examination

Procedure begins in modified dorsal lithotomy
   position;
   pad pressure points

Surgical scrub:
   Abdomen
   Pelvis

Drape

Insertion of Veress needle through 1 cm
   subumbilical incision through fascia

Pneumoperitoneum, 2–3 L of gas

Needle removal

Laparoscopic trocar or cannula placement
   through same hole

Trocar removal

Laparoscopic placement:
   Patient placed in Trendelenburg position
      (Fig 17–7)
   Diagnosis
   Therapy

Evacuation of insufflated gas

Closure of skin incisions, subcuticular with
   absorbable suture

---

there is 1:400 failure rate—and should not be done if the patient is not certain she will never regret the decision. Most decisions for sterilization are based on the assumption that family size will not change, but fatal diseases, accidental deaths, and divorce may make a difference in the patient's life. Many tubal sterilizations are performed immediately after delivery, and when this is so the decision must be firm irrespective of the newborn's health. If the patient conditions her consent upon the birth of a healthy baby, it is better to postpone the procedure.

The importance of counseling before tubal sterilization cannot be overstated. All types of sterilization for both sexes should be described, along with their advantages and risks. In 1979, the United States Department of Health and Human Services published regulations about providing specific information about surgical contraception, a standardized consent form, and a mandatory 30-day waiting period for women whose care is federally funded. There is no requisite parity level, and the United States Supreme Court has ruled that the husband's consent is not required—though his involvement would be beneficial if he is supportive and not coercive.

POSTOPERATIVE CARE
(See accompanying box.)

The first 48–72 hours after operation are the most critical. Monitoring of cardiovascular, pulmonary, and renal system reserves and their responses to surgery allows accurate assessment of the patient's condition. Postoperative care actually begins before the procedure is performed; for example, patients with chronic obstructive lung disease should undergo intensive pulmonary therapy prior to surgery in order to minimize postoperative pulmonary complications.

CARDIOVASCULAR SYSTEM

Careful monitoring of blood pressure and pulse is usually all that is necessary. In rare cases, it may be necessary—utilizing central lines or Swan-Ganz catheters—to monitor central venous pressure or the pulmonary artery and pulmonary capillary wedge pressures.

Lability of the autonomic nervous system immediately after surgery can cause wide swings in blood pressure. There is usually some shift in plasma volume, and hidden hemorrhage may occur. Vasoconstriction and tachycardia ascribed to pain or excitement may mask this loss temporarily, coupled with intravenous fluids administered during the procedure. It is mandatory to monitor and record

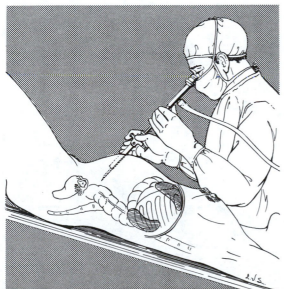

Figure 17–7. Pelvic laparoscopy with the patient in the Trendelenburg position. (Reproduced, with permission, from Pernoll ML, Benson RC (editors): *Current Obstetric & Gynecologic Diagnosis & Treatment,* 6th ed. Appleton & Lange, 1987.)

Procedures for Tubal Sterilization

Laparoscopy:
    Electrocauterization: unipolar, bipolar
    Silastic band (Falope ring) application
    Clip (Hulka) application
Laparotomy, mini-laparotomy:
    Pomeroy (Fig 17–8)
    Irving (Fig 17–9)
    Uchida (Fig 17–10)
    Fimbriectomy (Fig 17–11)

Vaginal:
    Pomeroy
    Silastic band
    Hulka clip
    Fimbriectomy

---

fluid administration and urinary output over short intervals initially; the intervals can then be extended.

Tachycardia must be carefully evaluated. A loss of 25–30% of intravascular volume is required for hypotension to develop. Peripheral vasoconstriction with cold, clammy, pale extremities is further evidence of hypovolemia. Concealed bleeding may occur into intraperitoneal or retroperitoneal spaces. Severe pain, either in the recovery room or on the nursing floor, is a signal that such bleeding may be occurring. Frequent hematocrits should confirm blood loss, and sonography may identify the site of bleeding. Reoperation is usually necessary to achieve hemostasis in these rare instances.

Patients with known cardiovascular disease are usually under the care of a cardiologist or internist, who should be consulted preoperatively and who may be needed postoperatively. Medications being given for cardiovascular disease prior to surgery usually can be continued without interruption. Patients with valvular heart disease require antimicrobial prophylaxis to prevent infective endocarditis. A preoperative electrocardiogram should be obtained from women over 40 years of age and from those with known cardiovascular disease.

PULMONARY SYSTEM

Hypoventilation is the most common postoperative pulmonary problem. Pain that limits respiratory excursion is one reason, and the other is the fact that patients usually sleep "deeply" because of the anesthesia and the parenteral pain medication.

Alveolar ventilation must be assured. Preoperative discussion with the patient should stress the importance of

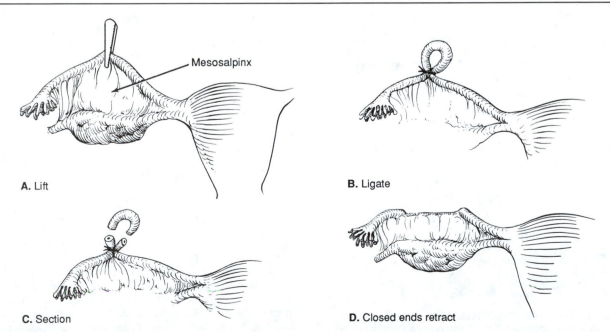

A. Lift   Mesosalpinx

B. Ligate

C. Section

D. Closed ends retract

Figure 17–8. Pomeroy method of sterilization. (Reproduced, with permission, from Benson RC: *Handbook of Obstetrics & Gynecology*, 8th ed. Lange, 1983.)

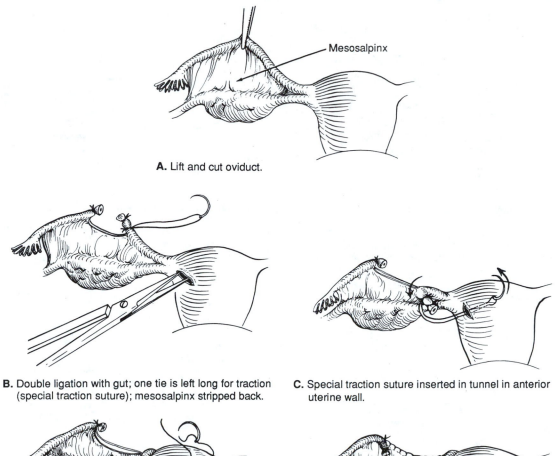

A. Lift and cut oviduct.

B. Double ligation with gut; one tie is left long for traction (special traction suture); mesosalpinx stripped back.

C. Special traction suture inserted in tunnel in anterior uterine wall.

Figure-8 fixation suture

D. Traction suture tied and proximal tube sutured in tunnel.

E. Implantation of the proximal tubal limb into a tunnel in the anterior uterine wall.

Figure 17–9. Irving method of sterilization. (Reproduced, with permission, from Benson RC: *Handbook of Obstetrics & Gynecology,* 8th ed. Lange, 1983.)

deep breathing, which should be practiced beforehand. Patients with any degree of restrictive or obstructive lung disease should avoid elective procedures unless conditions are optimal, which in occasional cases may require early admission and intensive pulmonary toiletry. The physician managing the pulmonary disease must be consulted preoperatively and as needed postoperatively.

A preoperative chest x-ray should be ordered for women over 40 and those with known pulmonary disease. Women with respiratory disease should have, in addition, preoperative pulmonary function tests.

URINARY SYSTEM

Monitoring urinary output is a means of monitoring the cardiovascular and renal systems provided one knows what fluid has been administered and what the combined fluid losses have been. Preoperative laboratory testing routinely includes measurement of serum electrolytes and creatinine. Patients with impaired kidney function require different fluid therapy intraoperatively and postoperatively. Preoperative consultation should be obtained for patients with abnormal renal function.

For patients undergoing hysterectomy, an indwelling

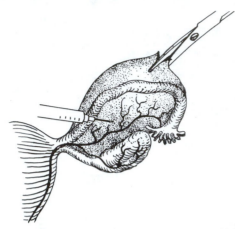

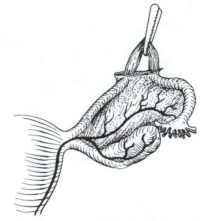

A. Saline with epinephrine injected below serosa, which becomes inflated locally. Muscular tube, and even blood vessels, can be separated from serosa, which is then cut open.

B. Muscular tube emerges through opening or is pulled out to form a U shape.

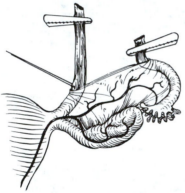

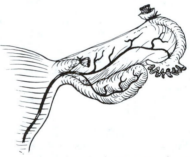

C. Fimbriated end is untouched, while the end leading to the uterus is stripped of serosa. This can usually be done without damaging blood vessels.

D. About 5 cm of muscular tube is cut away; the end is buried automatically in serosa. Fimbriated end and serosa opening are closed and tied together.

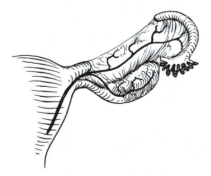

E. Blood supply continues normally between ovary and uterus. Hydrosalpinx or adhesion has not been noticed.

Figure 17–10. Uchida method of sterilization. (Reproduced, with permission, from Benson RC: *Handbook of Obstetrics & Gynecology,* 8th ed. Lange, 1983.)

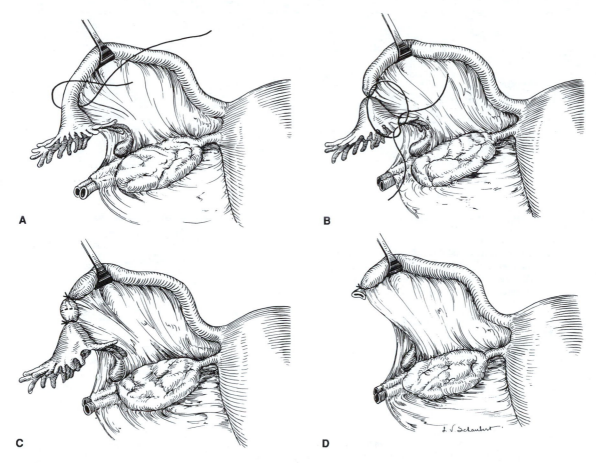

A

B

C

D

Figure 17–11. Sterilization by fimbriectomy. (Reproduced, with permission, from Benson RC: *Handbook of Obstetrics & Gynecology,* 8th ed. Lange, 1983.)

bladder catheter is usually placed at least overnight. This permits the patient to stay in bed immediately after operation and allows accurate instantaneous measurement of urine output during the critical hours just after surgery. As newer anesthetic agents are developed, postoperative somnolence will not occur, and the need for catheterization may decrease—especially for women undergoing vaginal hysterectomy. If the operation has included procedures to correct involuntary loss of urine (stress urinary incontinence), the bladder catheter is usually left in longer (up to 3 days). Some women cannot void spontaneously when the catheter is removed (transurethral) or clamped (suprapubic). If they have been counseled about this matter preoperatively, they will not be so hesitant about going home with a bladder catheter and a bed bag (for sleep) and a leg bag for daily use. It is rarely necessary to prolong hospitalization in order to remove a bladder catheter.

The postvoid urinary residual must be measured following catheter removal or clamping to make certain the bladder is functioning normally.

GASTROINTESTINAL TRACT

Any time the abdominal cavity is opened, the potential for altered bowel function exists. The more extensively the large and small bowel are manipulated, the greater the likelihood that return of normal function will be slow. Any patient undergoing general anesthesia should receive nothing by mouth (NPO) until fully awake and able to swallow. After abdominal surgery, the best guides to when oral intake can be started and with what foods are historical information (flatus) and physical examination (bowel sounds). Patients are not commonly hungry for several days, but they may be thirsty, starting with the first preoperative day. The mouth is dry, and water sips are appropriate, with a clear liquid diet on the first postoperative day. With return of normal bowel sounds and passage of flatus, progressive dietary advancement to a regular diet can occur. One must pay attention to fluids and electrolytes if the patient is not eating; low serum potassium (hypokalemia) can cause cessation of bowel activity (ileus), with abdominal distention.

Postoperative Order Guidelines

1. List surgical procedures performed.
2. Check vital signs:
   a. Blood pressure, pulse rate, and respiratory rate
      ____ q15min × 4
      ____ q30min until stable
      ____ q2h × 12 hours
      ____ q6–12h
   b. Temperature q4h
   c. Notify physician for:
      ____ BP ≥ 150 systolic or ≥ 100 diastolic
      ____ BP ≤ 100 systolic or ≤ 60 diastolic
      ____ PR ≥ 110
      ____ PR ≤ 60
      ____ T ≥ 38 °C
      ____ Difficulty breathing
      ____ Chest pain
3. Activity: Variable from bed rest to assist to bathroom first time.
4. Respiratory care:
   a. Turn, cough, and deep breathe q2h × 24 hours.
   b. Deep breathe q4h while awake.
5. Venous: Plantarflex, dorsiflex q4h.
6. Fluid intake and output:
   a. Every hour × 4
   b. Every 4 hours × 2
   c. Every 8 hours until discontinued
7. Current IV fluids:
   a. Run hanging fluids at _____ mL/h, then DC; or—
   b. Follow with 1 L ____ at _____ mL/h, then—
   c. Follow with 1 L ____ at ____mL/h.
8. Urinary system:
   a. Foley or suprapubic catheter to closed drainage, or—
   b. Catheterize if patient unable to void in 6 hours; leave indwelling catheter in place if bladder volume ≥ 150 mL.
9. Diet: Variable from NPO to regular diet, depending on surgical procedure performed.
10. Pain relief: Variable from oral medication PRN to parenteral medication q2h.

VENOUS SYSTEM

Early ambulation, support and/or pneumatic stockings, and prophylactic administration of heparin have greatly reduced symptomatic evidence of intravascular coagulation. Radioactive tagged fibrinogen studies demonstrate that clots do form in the deep veins of the lower extremities on the operating table. The incidence of clot formation after abdominal hysterectomy (15–50%) is about twice that observed after vaginal hysterectomy. Categories of patients at increased risk are those who are over 45 years old, obese patients, and those with diabetes, chronic pulmonary disease, large varicose veins, previous venous thrombosis, and heart failure.

Venous stasis is responsible for clot formation, and efforts should be directed at reducing known contributors to a minimum. Major contributing factors include prolonged bed confinement between admission and operation and delayed ambulation after the operation. Exercises to enhance blood return from the lower extremities can be performed while the patient is in bed, ie, plantar-flexing and then dorsiflexing the feet. These instructions should be given prior to the scheduled time of surgery so that the patient can practice.

Heparin, 5000 units subcutaneously every 8–12 hours, beginning several hours before surgery and continuing until the patient is ambulatory, has significantly reduced the incidence of significant venous thrombosis after major gynecologic surgery. It may be associated with increased bleeding, so many surgeons are utilizing pneumatic devices on the lower extremities until the patient is ambulatory.

POSTOPERATIVE ORDERS

The orders listed in the accompanying box are provided as a plan for patient care when the patient returns to her nursing unit. They must be modified to accommodate individual patients' needs.

The postoperative orders are written immediately after the operation. The patient will be in the recovery room until the anesthesiologist is satisfied that she is stable enough to return to stepped-down surveillance on the floor nursing unit or day surgery unit. She should be evaluated by the surgeon within the next several hours and at least twice daily thereafter while in the hospital. As the patient's condition improves and monitoring needs decrease, appropriate orders should be written so that nurses can focus attention in other areas.

DISCHARGE INSTRUCTIONS

Preferably before hospital admission, and at least the day before the hospitalized patient is to be discharged, the surgeon should review the surgical procedure, review the pathology laboratory results, and tell the patient what her medical and physical status will be at home. These matters should then be reviewed again on the day of discharge.

An instruction sheet should be prepared that deals with the patient's care after discharge and anticipates some common questions about how she will feel, coping with household duties, etc. Items to be covered should include at least the following:

Pain	Lifting
Vaginal discharge	Intercourse
Vaginal bleeding	Bath/shower
Temperature	Urinary symptoms
Activity	Whom to call with questions/problems

SELECTED READINGS

Thompson JD, Rock J: *TeLinde's Operative Gynecology,* 7th ed. Lippincott, 1991.

Wheeless CR Jr: *Atlas of Pelvic Surgery,* 2nd ed. Lea & Febiger, 1988.

18

Postoperative Complications

Postoperative complications significantly increase surgical morbidity rates, lengthen the hospital stay and increase costs of care, and in rare cases are a major factor in patient deaths. Women undergoing pelvic surgery are especially at risk for hemorrhagic or infectious complications. Complications may occur immediately after surgery or may not develop for days to weeks after the operation.

Hemorrhagic, pulmonary, and gastrointestinal tract complications and postoperative infections are the subjects of this chapter. Venous thrombosis is discussed in Chapters 17 and 50. It should be emphasized here, however, that venous thrombotic phenomena are most often seen in postoperative patients.

HEMORRHAGIC COMPLICATIONS

Hemorrhage is potentially one of the most serious of all postoperative complications. Acute hemorrhage occurring in the immediate postoperative period is frequently life-threatening. Bleeding of a less acute nature may not become clinically apparent until the first postoperative day or later and is generally manifested as a hematoma.

ACUTE HEMORRHAGE

Acute hemorrhage following pelvic surgery is initially manifested by a rapid pulse or tachycardia, a decrease in urine output, and soon thereafter by hypotension—the initial signs of hypovolemic shock. Since the patient is losing both plasma and red blood cells, the *initial* hematocrit may not reflect the true amount of blood loss. However, subsequent hematocrit determinations will generally reflect actual blood loss. Fortunately, signs of acute hypovolemia are almost always detected in the recovery room. Besides signs of hypovolemia, a patient with acute intra-abdominal hemorrhage may also have a markedly distended abdomen.

Treatment

Treatment of acute hemorrhage consists of fluid replacement and control of bleeding. The patient should be evaluated for possible coagulation defects. Fluid replacement should consist mainly of whole blood, which should be readily available for all patients undergoing major pelvic surgery. Rapid volume expansion with intravenous fluids such as lactated Ringer's injection should be accomplished to maintain blood pressure and urine output until blood is available. If whole blood is not available, packed red cells should be utilized along with crystalloid solutions.

One unit of whole blood or packed red blood cells will result in an increase in hematocrit of about 3–5%. Patients requiring massive transfusions of either whole blood or packed cells (ie, 10 units or more) or patients with coagulation defects may require several units of fresh frozen plasma and platelets. The composition of various blood fractions is set forth in Table 18–1.

Acute bleeding leading to hypovolemic shock in a patient without known bleeding dyscrasia is almost always associated with a poorly ligated or unligated pelvic vessel. Ligatures may occasionally be loosened or freed when abdominal packs are removed before closure of the incision. Control of hemorrhage for a major bleeder almost always requires surgical reexploration. A major bleeder at the vaginal cuff can occasionally be controlled with a single suture ligature.

HEMATOMA

Although hematomas may be acute and large enough to cause hypovolemic shock—especially those involving the retroperitoneal space—they most often evolve over a longer period of time, and the pressure resulting from their containment often is sufficient to tamponade bleeding vessels.

The signs and symptoms of hematoma depend chiefly

Table 18–1. Composition of blood fractions.[1]

	Volume (mL)	Composition	Comments
Whole blood	500	All components	Increase hematocrit 3–5%
Packed red cells	250–300	Red cells	Increase hematocrit 3–5%
Frozen plasma	200	Clotting factors	Increase fibrinogen by 10 mg/dL per unit
Platelets	20–50	Platelets	Increase platelets by 7500/mL per unit
Cryoprecipitate	40	I, V, VIII, XIII	Increase fibrinogen by 10 mg/dL per unit

[1]Adapted from ACOG: Blood component therapy. Tech Bull No. 78, July 1984.

on its size and location. The most common sites include the subfascial area of the surgical incision and the pelvic sidewalls. The patient may complain of pain and generally manifest a low-grade fever and a low or falling hematocrit. A wound hematoma is often readily palpable. However, a pelvic sidewall hematoma may or may not be palpable and requires other diagnostic techniques such as ultrasonography or CT scanning.

Treatment

For patients who manifest signs and symptoms of hypovolemic shock, treatment is generally the same as for any patient with hemorrhagic shock, ie, fluid and blood replacement and control of bleeding. However, the patient may not require surgery for control of bleeding if the bleeding site has been adequately tamponaded by the pressure of the hematoma.

Small to moderate-sized uninfected hematomas may require no specific therapy other than observation and perhaps transfusion. Large hematomas, especially if infected, often require surgical drainage. This is best accomplished retroperitoneally if possible.

PULMONARY COMPLICATIONS

A variety of pulmonary complications may occur following female pelvic surgery. The most common and least serious is atelectasis, and the most life-threatening is pulmonary embolism. Other pulmonary complications include pneumonia and aspiration.

ATELECTASIS

Pulmonary atelectasis is probably the single most common postoperative complication and results from inadequate expansion of the lungs, often as a result of incisional pain. It is generally evident in the early postoperative period (ie, after the first 24 hours) and is characterized by low-grade fever and decreased or absent breath sounds over the lung bases. The patient may have a few inspiratory rales. Chest x-ray is generally unremarkable and not

indicated for the more common milder forms of atelectasis.

Treatment

Treatment consists mainly of preventing the complication by having the patient breathe deeply and cough frequently in the postoperative period. Heavy smokers and patients with chronic lung disease may develop severe atelectasis requiring oxygen therapy and intermittent positive pressure breathing.

ASPIRATION PNEUMONITIS

Aspiration pneumonitis (Mendelson's syndrome) was first described by an obstetrician, Curtis Mendelson, in 1946. It is manifested by dyspnea, tachypnea, wheezing, rhonchi, bronchospasm, cyanosis, hypoxia, and tachycardia. The pulmonary insult is usually associated with aspiration of gastric contents with a pH of less than 2.5 but may occur also following aspiration of alkaline gastric contents. Aspiration of particulate matter is an important risk factor with regard to fatalities.

Treatment & Prognosis

Treatment consists chiefly of prevention by proper preparation of patients and by preanesthesia ingestion of antacids or H_2 inhibitors. If aspiration does occur, therapy consists of immediate suctioning and supplemental oxygen. Patients may also require positive-pressure ventilation with positive end-expiratory pressure (PEEP). Neither steroid therapy nor prophylactic antibiotics appear to improve the outcome for aspiration pneumonitis, but the preanesthetic administration of antacids has significantly reduced morbidity and mortality rates associated with this postoperative complication.

At one time, the mortality rate from aspiration pneumonitis in the general population was as high as 90%, but with prompt recognition and treatment the prognosis for relatively young women is much better than that.

PNEUMONIA

Bacterial or viral pneumonia is uncommon following pelvic surgery in women, but bacterial pneumonia may occur in patients with significant atelectasis or following aspiration of gastric contents. Viral pneumonia may occur in patients with viral syndromes who require emergency surgery. Obese patients or those with chronic debilitating diseases, those with chronic lung disease, and heavy smokers who do not ambulate are at greater risk of developing postoperative pneumonia.

The patient with pneumonia is much "sicker" than the patient with simple atelectasis. Temperature is generally higher, and there is often dyspnea, tachypnea, and a persistent cough. If sputum is produced, it should be gram-stained and cultured. Auscultation may reveal decreased breath sounds and rales. The chest x-ray may be unremarkable with early milder forms of pneumonia but generally reveals diffuse infiltrates.

Treatment

Treatment in most cases of postoperative pneumonia should be with penicillin or cephalosporins. For patients with suspected aspiration, therapy should be with a broad-spectrum cephalosporin (second- or third-generation) or one of the extended-spectrum penicillins, since these pneumonias may be associated with anaerobes and gram-negative aerobes in addition to the usual gram-positive organisms.

PULMONARY EMBOLISM

The risk of pulmonary embolism is increased in women undergoing pelvic surgery, especially if they remain immobile for significant periods of time. Obesity and older age probably are also risk factors. The classic triad of pulmonary embolism is chest pain, acute shortness of breath, and tachycardia. Other classic features and laboratory and other findings are summarized in Table 18–2. Although it has traditionally been taught that a Po_2 greater than 80 mm Hg on room air rules out pulmonary embolism, patients with this complication may occasionally have a normal

Po_2. It is not unusual for the chest x-ray and ECG to be normal also, especially with small emboli.

Since the pulmonary emboli may result in cardiac arrest and death in a relatively short period of time, it is imperative to confirm the diagnosis when it is clinically suspected. The patient should be anticoagulated with heparin until this can be accomplished. The diagnosis can generally be confirmed with either a perfusion lung scan or selective pulmonary arteriography.

Treatment

Treatment consists of full anticoagulation with heparin (partial thromboplastin time 1½–2½ times normal), which can usually be achieved with an intravenous infusion of approximately 1000 units/h. Some clinicians recommend an initial intravenous bolus injection of 5000–10,000 units. Heparin therapy is generally continued for 7 days, after which the patient is maintained on warfarin (to maintain a prothrombin time at ½ times the normal control) for 2–3 months.

GASTROINTESTINAL COMPLICATIONS

The two most common gastrointestinal complications associated with pelvic surgery in women are adynamic ileus and bowel obstruction.

ADYNAMIC ILEUS

Most women have some degree of small bowel hypofunction or ileus following abdominal or pelvic surgery. This is usually evident by 24–48 hours postoperatively. The chief signs and symptoms are abdominal distention and absence of bowel sounds. The patient may experience nausea and vomiting also. On auscultation, the bowel sounds will be absent or diminished. Abdominal radiographs often reveal dilated loops of small and large bowel, with gas in the lower colon and sometimes in the rectum. Air-fluid levels usually are not present.

Prolonged or severe ileus should raise the possibility of other complications such as pelvic infection, hematoma, or leakage of urine into the abdomen.

Treatment

Patients with adynamic ileus generally can be managed conservatively since most cases will resolve spontaneously. A nasogastric tube may relieve discomfort associated with distention. An enema or rectal suppository may be helpful.

Table 18–2. Clinical, laboratory, and imaging findings in women with pulmonary embolism.[1]

Clinical
- Dyspnea
- Chest pain
- Tachycardia
- Cough
- Hemoptysis
- Fever
- Rales
- Cyanosis
- Friction rub

Laboratory and imaging
- Low Po_2 (< 80 mm Hg on room air)
- X-ray changes: elevation of diaphragm, decreased vascular markings, pleural effusion
- ECG changes: tachycardia, right axis shift, T wave inversion
- Elevated white blood cell count, sedimentation rate, AST (SGOT), LDH, CPK

[1]Adapted from Rutherford SE, Phelan JP: Thromboembolic disease in pregnancy. Clin Perinatol 1986;13:719–739.

BOWEL OBSTRUCTION

Bowel obstruction is a serious complication of pelvic or abdominal surgery—if associated with strangulation and sepsis, it is life-threatening. Unlike ileus, which occurs in the early postoperative period, bowel obstruction usually becomes manifest in the late postoperative period and occasionally even after the patient has gone home (see Chapter 17).

Patients with bowel obstruction complain of colicky pain, nausea, and vomiting. Distention is generally more marked than with ileus, and bowel sounds are frequently hyperactive and "high-pitched." Radiographs of the abdomen generally reveal air-fluid levels in "stepladder" fashion and dilated loops of bowel proximal to the obstruction.

Treatment

Treatment consists of suction decompression of the bowel and fluid and electrolyte replacement. Operation is often necessary to relieve adhesions. Operation is mandatory if strangulation or sepsis is present.

INFECTIOUS COMPLICATIONS

Most infections involving the female pelvis are polymicrobial and arise from organisms indigenous to the female genital tract (Table 18–3). Other organisms such as *Chlamydia trachomatis, Mycoplasma, Candida albicans, Neisseria gonorrhoeae,* herpes simplex virus, and *Trichomonas vaginalis* may also inhabit the female genital tract without causing obvious clinical infection.

The pathogenesis of these infections involves contamination and colonization of the operative site with potential bacterial pathogens from the normal vaginal flora followed by surgical trauma. This along with foreign material (sutures) and serous drainage serve to establish a favorable milieu for the proliferation of microorganisms, especially anaerobes.

PELVIC INFECTIONS

The most common infectious complication of hysterectomy is infection of the vaginal cuff and operative pedicles ("cuff cellulitis"). Although this infection usually is localized, it may extend upward to cause pelvic cellulitis, which in turn may lead to cuff or pelvic abscess. An infected hematoma may also involve this area.

The diagnosis of cuff cellulitis is based primarily on the presence of fever (> 38 °C on at least two occasions excluding the first postoperative day) and exclusion of other causes such as pulmonary or urinary tract infections. On examination, patients generally have a tender indurated vaginal cuff. If a cuff abscess or hematoma is present, a mass will also be felt.

Treatment

Since these infections are polymicrobial in nature, with a mixture of aerobic and anaerobic bacteria, therapy should consist of an antibiotic that provides broad-spectrum coverage (see Table 18–4). Either single-agent or dual-agent therapy may be used. Triple-agent therapy should be reserved for patients with abscesses or those who do not respond to initial antibiotic therapy. The cuff should be opened and drained when an abscess or hematoma is present.

In patients who have no palpable mass but who worsen or fail to improve within 48–72 hours after antibiotics are started, ultrasonography or CT scan should be considered to rule out pelvic or abdominal abscess. Large abscesses often require surgical drainage.

Table 18–3. Normal vaginal bacterial flora.

Aerobes
  Gram-positive cocci
    Streptococci
    Enterococci
    Staphylococci
  Gram-negative bacilli
    Escherichia coli
    Klebsiella species
    Proteus mirabilis
Anaerobes
  Gram-negative cocci
    Peptococcus species
    Peptostreptococcus species
  Gram-positive rods
    Clostridium species
  Gram-negative rods
    Bacteroides species
    Fusobacterium species

Table 18–4. Antimicrobial therapy for postoperative female pelvic infection.

Single-agent therapy
  Cefoxitin
  Cefaperazone
  Ceftizoxime
  Cefotetan
  Cefotaxime
  Other second- and third-generation cephalosporins
  Piperacillin
  Mezlocillin
  Ticarcillin plus clavulanic acid
  Ampicillin plus sulbactam
Dual-agent therapy
  Clindamycin plus an aminoglycoside
Triple-agent therapy[1]
  Ampicillin plus clindamycin (or metronidazole) plus an
    aminoglycoside

[1]Primarily for treatment failures or abscesses.

WOUND INFECTIONS

Wound infections are relatively common, especially in obese patients, and may occur in 5–10% of women following abdominal hysterectomy. Diagnosis is based on the presence of fever and a red indurated wound.

Treatment

Primary treatment is to open, drain, and explore the wound. Antibiotics may be useful if there is significant induration or cellulitis, a subfascial abscess, or an infected hematoma. If an abscess or hematoma is present, it should be drained.

The fascia should be inspected closely to detect dehiscence. A large dehiscence calls for debridement and secondary closure with some type of retention suture technique. "Internal" retention closure of the Smead-Jones variety is often satisfactory, ie, closing the fascia and peritoneum in a single layer with interrupted sutures placed at the fascia edges and widely through both the fascia and peritoneum.

Uncomplicated superficial wound infections may be closed secondarily once the patient is afebrile and the wound is clean and free of induration and cellulitis.

OVARIAN ABSCESS

Ovarian abscess is an uncommon complication of pelvic surgery and usually results from bacterial contamination and colonization of a ruptured ovarian follicle or cyst at the time of vaginal (rarely abdominal) hysterectomy. These patients usually will have late-onset fevers and abdominal masses requiring ultrasound or CT scan for detection.

Treatment

Treatment consists of triple-agent antimicrobial therapy. Surgical drainage is often required as well.

URINARY TRACT INFECTION

Urinary tract infections are discussed in Chapter 16. It is important to recognize, however, that hospital-acquired infections (usually secondary to prolonged retention of a Foley catheter) may involve uncommon organisms such as *Citrobacter, Enterobacter,* or *Serratia.*

Foley catheters should be removed as soon as possible following surgery.

SUGGESTED READINGS

American College of Obstetricians and Gynecologists: Blood component therapy. ACOG Tech Bull No. 78, 1984.

Hankins GDV, Gilstrap LC: Postoperative anesthetic complications. Chapter 27 in: *Cesarean Delivery.* Phelan JP, Clark SL (editors). Elsevier, 1988.

Mendelson CL: The aspiration of stomach contents into the lungs during obstetric anesthesia. Am J Obstet Gynecol 1946; 52:191.

Rutherford SE, Phelan JP: Thromboembolic disease in pregnancy. Clin Perinatol 1986;13:719.

Schwartz DJ et al: The pulmonary consequences of aspiration of gastric contents at pH values greater than 2.5. Anesthesiology 1979;51:452.

Unit II

Reproductive Endocrinology

19

Reproductive Success & Failure: Ovulation & Fertilization

THE LIMITING RESOURCE IN HUMAN REPRODUCTION: OVARIAN FUNCTION

Notwithstanding the fact that many men are sterile or subfertile—thus contributing to less than optimal fecundity of the race—women are physiologically the limiting resource in human reproduction. One of the keys to the success of human development and reproduction is postponement of puberty until the second decade of life. At the completion of puberty, periodic release of germ cells is established. Indeed, the cyclic release (or surgical retrieval) of a mature ovum is necessary for reproduction. Ideally, reproduction involves the female's choice of the male sperm donor, but this is not a limiting physiologic factor. Accordingly, a comprehensive understanding of the development of the ovaries, including maturation of the oocytes and ovulation, is fundamental to the role of the obstetrician-gynecologist as a reproductive biologist.

Cyclic, Spontaneous, Predictable Menses

The occurrence of spontaneous, predictable menses at reasonable intervals is strong evidence for the occurrence of ovulation. Moreover, if such menses are associated with some degree of discomfort, which may vary from only a prodrome signifying impending menstruation to severe dysmenorrhea, the likelihood of cyclic ovulation is even greater. This is probably because menstruation induced by progesterone withdrawal—ie, that which is characteristic of ovulation—is associated with endometrial formation of $PGF_{2\alpha}$, which causes endometrial ischemia and myometrial contractions, the "parturition" of fertility failure.

Ovulation Equals Normal Sex Hormone Production

With the exception of those that are artificially produced by exogenous steroid compounds, regular menses do not occur with any frequency in anovulatory women. This being the case, two equations can be formulated: (1) cyclic, predictable, spontaneous menses = ovulation; and (2) ovulation = normal sex hormone production.

In ovulatory women, therefore, it can be assumed that the production of pituitary gonadotropins, both follicle-stimulating hormone (FSH) and luteinizing hormone (LH), as well as estrogens, androgens, and progesterone, is appropriate. One exception to this general rule may be the entity called **luteal phase deficiency** (see Chapter 24). But ordinarily, the history of cyclic, predictable, spontaneous menstruation is more valuable in an evaluation for infertility than hundreds of dollars worth of endocrine tests. For this reason, a carefully obtained menstrual history is the essential first step in the approach to investigation of fertility problems in gynecologic practice.

EMBRYOLOGY

The morphologic, physiologic, and anatomic events that lead to development of the mature graafian follicle and release of the mature ovum have their origin early in embryonic development. About 3 weeks after conception, the germ cells in the human fetus are localized in the epithelium of the yolk sac near the developing allantois (Figure 19–1). Thereafter, these germ cells migrate to the connective tissue of the hindgut and thence move progressively to the gonadal primordia or ridges. The number of germ cells is believed to increase by mitosis. There may be a substance (telopheron) that directs the anatomic migration of the germ cell to the genital ridge. The exact means by which germ cells migrate is not fully defined; ameboid activity, chemotactic substances, and lytic enzyme activities all may be involved. Even movement by

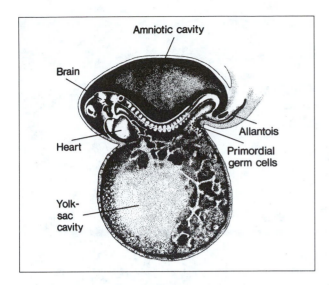

Figure 19–1. Reconstruction of 24-day human embryo in its amnion. The primordial germ cells (black dots) are grouped at the top of the yolk sac and in the ventral wall of the developing hindgut. (Reproduced, with permission, from Baker TG in: *Reproduction in Mammals. I. Germ Cells and Fertilization.* Austin CR, Short RV [editors]. Cambridge Univ Press, 1978.)

way of blood with "homing in" mechanisms to the gonad may be involved. Generally, the germ cells remain in the cortex if the presumptive gonad is destined to be an ovary. Differentiation of the fetal female gonad is later than that of the male. The number of germ cells in developing ovaries changes rapidly—by mitosis—during gestational development.

After a definitive number of mitoses, the oogonia are transformed into oocytes. At this time, prophase is entered—the first of two meiotic divisions; thereafter, no new oocytes are formed. Therefore, as oogonia are eliminated from the ovary—primarily before birth—the population of germ cells can only be reduced in number.

Prodigality is the main feature of the early history of the germ cells, ie, the oogonia. But if this is true of ova, consider the extraordinary prodigality in the case of spermatogonia—typically more than 200 million ejaculated in a single copulation.

There is no reliable evidence that ova normally are formed in the human after birth. It has been estimated that there are 600,000 oogonia in the ovaries of female fetuses at 2 months of gestation and 6,800,000 at 5 months. Degeneration occurs thereafter—2,000,000 at birth, but only 300,000 in prepubertal girls. Before puberty, mature graafian follicles are found only in the deeper portions of the cortex. Later, however, mature follicles also develop in the superficial portions of the ovary. During each cycle, one follicle makes its way to the surface, and there it appears as a transparent vesicle that may vary from 2 to 12 mm in diameter. As the follicle approaches the surface of the ovary, the wall becomes thinner and more abundantly supplied with vessels—except in the most prominent pro-jecting portion, which appears almost bloodless. This avascular locus is called the **follicular stigma,** the site on the follicle where rupture is to occur.

FOLLICULOGENESIS

After formation of the oocytes in the early primordial follicles, these cells are surrounded by flattened epithelium-like cells.

As folliculogenesis progresses, the follicular cells proliferate and become cuboidal and then commence to secrete a fluid that accumulates ultimately into one large pool, and an antrum is formed. Ovarian stromal cells differentiate to form the theca externa and theca interna (Figures 19–2 and 19–3). This stage of follicular development appears to proceed independently of gonadotropin action. Thereafter, an integrated set of metabolic events appears to be necessary for complete maturation of the follicle, ie, selection of the dominant follicle that will be the source of the ovum to be ovulated in a given cycle. Thereafter, as folliculogenesis proceeds, there is an orderly and progressive sequence of hormonally responsive and operative events that permit and facilitate the final stages in the maturation of the dominant follicle in preparation for ovulation.

During folliculogenesis, two major functions become active: (1) a gonadotropin hormone-receptor adenylyl cyclase coupling system and (2) a cell contact system for intercellular communication. Gonadotropins serve to stimulate and activate the enzymatic processes of the cells of the follicles, and as a consequence estradiol-17β is synthesized within the granulosa cells. The estradiol-17β acts in turn to alter gonadotropin receptor content and serves to stimulate growth and development of gap junctions in preantral follicles. The great majority of vesicular follicles, including all of those before puberty, undergo degeneration at various stages of formation.

As follicular maturation progresses, the order of events is as follows: (1) increase in size of the oocyte; (2) alteration in granulosa cells from flat to cuboidal, followed by replication; and (3) formation of the zona pellucida. The zona pellucida is a clear mucoid band that envelops the ovum and persists until after the fertilized ovum reaches the uterus. Thereafter, the theca interna is vascularized and is surrounded by the theca externa (Figures 19–2 and 19–3). The follicle increases in size disproportionately to the ovum.

During any ovarian cycle, 20 or more follicles may embark on processes that appear to be on the road to ovulation. We know nothing about how these few of so many thousand are chosen, let alone how one of these 20 or so follicles becomes the dominant or chosen one.

MATURE GRAAFIAN FOLLICLE

The mature follicle (folliculus ovaricus vesiculosus) is known as the **graafian follicle** after the 17th century

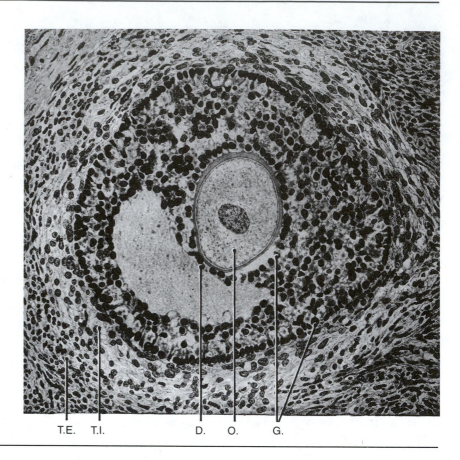

Figure 19–2. Graafian follicle approaching maturity. T.E., theca externa; T.I., theca interna; D., discus proligerus (cumulus oophorus); O., ovum; G., granulosa cell layer.

T.E.   T.I.   D.   O.   G.

Dutch amateur microscopist Reijnier de Graaf, who described the structure.

As the graafian follicle grows, the stromal cells that surround it enlarge and the capillary net about these cells becomes closer and forms the **theca interna** (Figure 19–3), which is the cellular site of synthesis of C_{19} steroids, and in particular androstenedione, which serves as the precursor for estradiol-17β formation in the granulosa cells. In the cells of the theca interna, lipid droplets develop; after ovulation, these cells persist and lie immediately adjacent to the enlarged follicular cells that are now called the granulosa lutein cells.

Measurements of ova in sections of a well-preserved ovary show that although the ovum grows slowly during development of the graafian follicle, the volume of the ovum increases about 40-fold before maturity is completed. The nucleus, however, increases in size only about three-fold during this period. The large increase in cytoplasm is accompanied by the accumulation of nutrients such as yolk granules.

From the outside inward, the mature graafian follicle is composed of (1) a layer of specialized connective tissue, the theca folliculi; (2) an epithelial lining, the membrana granulosa; (3) the ovum; and (4) the liquor folliculi. The theca folliculi is composed of an outer layer of cells, the theca externa; and an inner layer, the theca interna. The

theca externa is composed of ordinary ovarian stroma arranged concentrically about the follicle, but the connective tissue cells of the theca interna are modified greatly.

Almost as soon as the primordial follicle begins to develop, mitotic figures appear in the cells of the surrounding stroma, considerable multiplication of cells occurs, and these cells become distinctly larger than those of the surrounding connective tissue. As the follicle increases in size, these **theca lutein cells** accumulate lipid and a yellowish pigment, which gives rise to a granular appearance. Simultaneously, a striking increase develops in the vascularity and number of lymphatic spaces of the theca.

Before ovulation, the theca cells are separated from the granulosa cells by a highly polymerized membrane. It is possible that luteinizing hormone may act to depolymerize this membrane at about the time of ovulation and thus allow vascularization of the granulosa cells to take place.

The epithelial lining of the follicle, or membrana granulosa, is one that consists of several layers of small polygonal or cuboidal cells in which there are round, darkly staining nuclei; the larger the follicle, the fewer the number of layers. At any one time, the membrana granulosa is much thicker than elsewhere, and a mound is formed in which the ovum is included, ie, the cumulus oophorus (discus proligerus).

The follicle is filled with a clear, proteinaceous fluid,

Follicular fluid   Granulosa

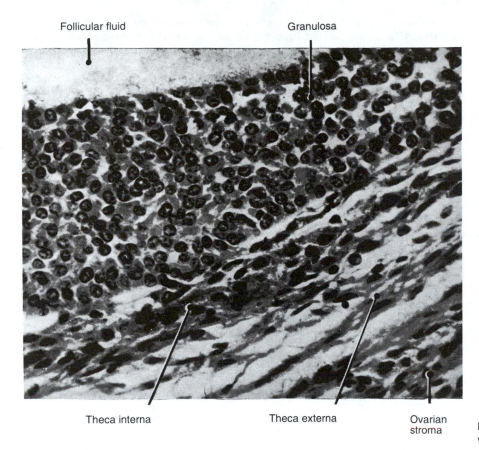

Theca interna   Theca externa   Ovarian stroma

Figure 19–3. Section through the wall of a mature graafian follicle.

the **liquor folliculi,** ie, the follicular fluid. The usual fat stains are not taken up by the granulosa cells until the stage of preovulatory swelling, a time of rapid growth that commences about 24 hours before ovulation and apparently is related to the onset of—or preparation for—the secretion of progesterone.

Ovarian follicles develop throughout childhood and occasionally attain considerable size, but they normally do not rupture at this time—instead, they undergo atresia in situ. The relative rates of increase in oocyte size and follicular size with maturation are greatly different. Even in adult women, many follicles that reach a diameter of 5 mm or more undergo atresia. Usually only one of a group of enlarging follicles continues to grow and to produce a normal mature egg that is extruded by ovulation.

THE MATURE OVUM

The human ovum, as it approaches maturity, is barely visible to the naked eye when brightly illuminated on a dark background. The average diameter of the mature human ovum is 0.133 mm.

If the nearly mature ovum is examined in the follicular fluid or in physiologic saline solution, the structures that can be distinguished in and about it are as follows: (1) a surrounding corona radiata; (2) a zona pellucida; (3) a perivitelline space; (4) a small clear zone of protoplasm; (5) a broad, finely granulated zone of protoplasm; (6) a central deutoplasmic zone; (7) the nucleus, or germinal vesicle, and within it a germinal spot; and, with appropriate staining, (8) many small spheroidal mitochondria. The ovum is free to rotate within the zona pellucida even though the outer vitelline membrane of the ovum appears to be applied closely to it. After fertilization, shrinkage of the ovum results in its complete separation from the zona pellucida as it floats in the perivitelline fluid. During growth, the oocyte accumulates deutoplasm (yolk granules). Before ovulation, the ovum, in the living state, is transparent, with a faint yellowish tinge. There are also larger lipoid granules, which in preserved material appear to surround the nucleus (germinal vesicle). Numerous mitochondria are distributed through the cytoplasm. The spherical nucleus is located near the center of the oocyte, and within it there is a large nucleolus and sparsely distributed chromatin. Shortly before ovulation, the nucleus migrates toward the periphery, and meiosis is reinitiated. At the completion of the first and second meiotic divisions, the number of chromosomes in the oocyte is halved, and two polar bodies are formed—the first before ovulation and the second after penetration of the oocyte by a spermatozoon. Both polar bodies are extruded into the perivitelline space.

GAMETOGENESIS

Primitive germ cells are present in the human embryo by the end of the third week of development. Both **oogenesis,** in the course of which mature ova are formed from primitive oogonia, and **spermatogenesis,** which results in the production of spermatids, share a basic biologic feature of maturation, ie, reduction and division (Figure 19–4). Such special cellular division, known as **meiosis,** is limited to germ cells. The process of meiosis is characterized by a long and unusual prophase and involves a process that provides for the exchange of genetic material between homologous chromosomes and reduction of the **diploid** number of chromosomes (46) to the **haploid** number (23). In humans, the diploid number of chromosomes is composed of 44 autosomes and two sex chromosomes; during meiosis, mature gametes are formed, in each of which there are 22 autosomes and one sex chromosome.

The diploid number of chromosomes is not restored until fertilization with the union of the ovum and sperm. Spermatogenesis encompasses the final maturational events that lead to production of mature male gametes and involves changes in the shape of the spermatids and transformation of these cells into spermatozoa. The fact that the mature germ cells are derived directly from primitive cells which may have migrated from the yolk sac to the developing gonads as early as the fifth week of embryonic life underlies the concept of continuity of the germ plasm. In the case of human ova, some germ cells may remain dormant for as long as 40 years.

Meiosis

In all primitive germ cells, ie, **oogonia** and **spermatogonia,** there are a diploid number of chromosomes (46). When these stem cells divide to produce primary oocytes and spermatocytes, each chromosome undergoes replication by splitting longitudinally to form a double-stranded structure. During this process of **mitosis,** one strand of each chromosome enters each daughter cell, and in this manner the identical chromosomal components of the parent cells are obtained.

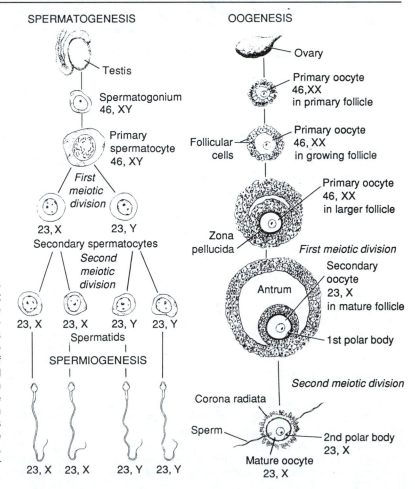

SPERMATOGENESIS

OOGENESIS

Testis

Spermatogonium
46, XY

Primary
spermatocyte
46, XY

First
meiotic
division

23, X   23, Y
Secondary spermatocytes

Second
meiotic
division

23, X   23, X   23, Y   23, Y
Spermatids

SPERMIOGENESIS

23, X   23, X   23, Y   23, Y

Ovary

Primary oocyte
46, XX
in primary follicle

Follicular
cells

Primary oocyte
46, XX
in growing follicle

Primary oocyte
46, XX
in larger follicle

Zona
pellucida

First meiotic division

Antrum

Secondary
oocyte
23, X
in mature follicle

1st polar body

Second meiotic division

Corona radiata

Sperm

2nd polar body
23, X

Mature oocyte
23, X

Figure 19–4. Comparison of spermatogenesis and oogenesis. The chromosome complement of the germ cells is shown at each stage. The numbers designate the total number of chromosomes, including the sex chromosomes shown after the comma. Note that (1) after the two meiotic divisions, the diploid number of chromosomes, 46, is reduced to the haploid number, 23; (2) four sperm are formed from one primary spermatocyte, whereas only one mature oocyte (ovum) results from maturation of a primary oocyte; and (3) the cytoplasm is conserved during oogenesis to form one large cell, the mature oocyte (ovum). (Reproduced, with permission, from Moore KL: *The Developing Human,* 2nd ed. Saunders, 1977.)

When the primary oocytes and spermatocytes continue maturation to form secondary oocytes and spermatocytes, however, the meiotic division that ensues is quite different: each of the newly formed cells receives only 23 chromosomes, the haploid number. The basic difference between meiosis and mitosis is the prolonged prophase in meiosis, in which there is preliminary pairing of homologous chromosomes before division. During the **leptotene stage** of meiotic prophase, the 46 chromosomes appear as single slender threads; in the ensuing **zygotene stage,** the homologous chromosomes are aligned in parallel fashion in **synapsis,** with the formation of 23 bivalent components. Each chromosome then divides longitudinally except at the **centromere,** and the ensuing **pachytene stage** is composed of **tetrads** of four chromatids whose shape is dependent upon the position of the centromere. At this stage, the chromatids break and then recombine with strands from the homologous chromosome to effect an exchange of genetic material. During the **diplotene stage** that follows, the homologous strands separate. During metaphase of the first meiotic division, the bivalents (two chromatids that comprise each chromosome) become oriented on the spindle; when the cell divides, the members of each pair move toward opposite poles into the daughter cells, which then contain the haploid number of chromosomes, still as chromatid pairs. *The individual chromosomes now are no longer genetically identical with those of the parent cell.* Each secondary oocyte will thus receive 22 autosomes and an X chromosome, and each secondary spermatocyte will receive 22 autosomes and either an X or a Y chromosome.

At the second meiotic division, the **dyad** splits at the centromere to form two **monads,** one of which becomes associated with each daughter cell, probably having already undergone a typical mitotic longitudinal replication. The mature ovum (23,X), if fertilized by a spermatocyte with a Y chromosome (23,Y), will produce a male zygote (46,XY), whereas if the ovum was fertilized by a spermatocyte with an X chromosome (23,X), the result will be a female (46,XX).

Biochemistry of Cellular Division

During mitotic interphase, duplication of the chromosomes is accomplished by replication of DNA. Autoradiographic studies of the incorporation of tritium-labeled thymidine into chromosomes show that duplication is accomplished by separation of the two original DNA strands of each chromosome and subsequent synthesis of two new DNA strands. At the next cellular division, each chromatid receives one original and one newly synthesized strand.

Oogenesis

In the first phase (migration) of human ovum development, the germ cells reach the medial slope of the mesonephric ridge where the gonads arise, divide rapidly, and become oogonia; in the second phase (division), the germ cells divide mitotically at a rate that is maximal during the eighth to 20th weeks, slows thereafter, and finally ceases at birth. In the third phase (maturation), the cells enter the prophase of the first meiotic division, acquire a ring of granulosa cells, and become definitive oocytes within the primary follicles.

All oocytes are derived from the primitive germ cells. Working with mice, Blandau and associates (1963) recorded cinematographically the ameboid-like migration of primitive germ cells from the yolk sac to the germinal ridges. The primitive oogonia, furthermore, continue movements locally within the developing ovary even after the pachytene stage of meiosis is reached.

The primary oocytes increase in size, and cuboidal follicular cells proliferate to form increasingly thick coverings around them (Figure 19–5). The follicular cells, furthermore, deposit on the surface of the oocyte an acellular glycoprotein mantle that gradually thickens to form the **zona pellucida** (Figures 19–5 and 19–6). Irregular fluid-filled spaces between the follicular cells then coalesce to form an antrum. The radially elongated follicular cells that surround the zona pellucida form the corona radiata (Figure 19–5). A solid mass of follicular cells, the cumulus oophorus, surrounds the ovum in the developing vesicular ovarian follicle (Figure 19–5). As the follicle nears maturity, the cumulus projects further into the antrum, and as a consequence the oocyte appears to be supported by this column of follicular cells. At this stage, the follicle may vary from 6 to 12 mm in diameter and lies immediately beneath the surface of the ovary.

The formation of the oocyte completes the first meiotic division, which was begun before birth, during the final stage of transformation of the primordial follicle into the mature graafian follicle. The important result is the formation of two daughter cells, each with 23 chromosomes but of greatly unequal size. One receives almost all of the cytoplasm of the mother cell and becomes a secondary oocyte; the other, the first polar body, receives very little cytoplasm. The polar body lies between the zona pellucida and the vitelline membrane of the secondary oocyte.

The Chosen Ovum

Not only is there a chosen (dominant) follicle, there is also a dominant oocyte, ie, the only oocyte in the preovulatory follicle that matures, whereas all others fail to develop beyond the immature dictyotene state (Figure 19–5).

It is believed that a compound known as **maturation inhibitor** may serve an important role in oocyte maturation. This substance appears to be present in all follicles except preovulatory ones. It seems clear that a substance in follicular fluid that arises from granulosa cells inhibits oocyte maturation.

There is in human and other mammalian follicular fluid an inhibitor of oocyte maturation (MW < 2000) that is probably a polypeptide secreted by granulosa cells. The action of oocyte maturation inhibitor is probably mediated by cells of the cumulus oophorus. LH in all likelihood acts on the chosen follicle to block the action of oocyte maturation inhibitor.

The first polar body is cast off while still in the ovary. A

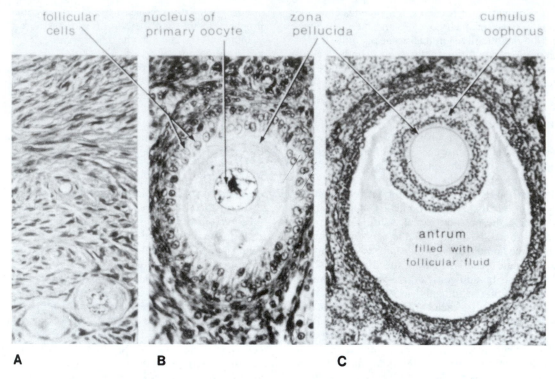

Figure 19–5. Photomicrographs of sections from adult human ovaries. **A:** Ovarian cortex showing two primordial follicles that contain primary oocytes which have completed the prophase of the first meiotic division and have entered the dictyotene state, a "resting" stage between prophase and metaphase (× 250). **B:** Growing follicle that contains a primary oocyte, surrounded by the zona pellucida and a stratified layer of follicular cells (× 250). **C:** An almost mature follicle with a large antrum. The oocyte, embedded in the cumulus oophorus, does not show a nucleus because it has been sectioned tangentially (× 100). (Reproduced, with permission, from Moore KL: *The Developing Human.* 3rd ed. Saunders, 1982.)

second division is consummated in the formation of the second polar body at about the moment the sperm penetrates the egg.

In human ova, the second maturation division is completed only if the ovum is fertilized. If penetration by a spermatozoon does not occur within a few hours after ovulation, the ovum begins to degenerate. Although it is not certain that the first polar body always undergoes subsequent division, fertilized ova have been found that were accompanied by three polar bodies. During maturation, the diameter of the human ovum increases from 19 μm in the original oocyte to 135 μm in the fully mature ovum, a seven-fold increase in size.

TRANSPORT OF OVA & SPERMATOZOA

Tubal Transport

In women, the ovaries normally lie free in the peritoneal cavity except for the supporting mesovarium and the ovarian ligament. About the time of ovulation, however, the fimbriae of the uterine tubes—perhaps as a consequence of hormonal and (doubtfully) neural regulation—are believed to completely cover the ovary at the site of ovula-

tion. Ovulation is not an explosive phenomenon; instead, as the follicular stigma is digested by proteolytic enzymes, there is a gentle outpouring of the contents of the follicle, which include the egg surrounded by the zona pellucida and the cumulus oophorus. The cumulus cells appear to be important for uptake and transport of the ovum by the oviduct. Because fertilization in mammals usually occurs in the ampulla—whatever the roles of the tubal cilia and peristalsis may be—an adequate theory must explain how movement of ova and spermatozoa in opposite directions can occur.

Migration of Fertilized Ovum

In most mammals, the fertilized ovum migrates through the uterine tube and reaches the cavity of the uterus about 3–4 days after ovulation. In women, the ovum is believed to be able to wander across the pelvis and then be taken up by the opposite tube **(external migration);** a theoretic alternative is that the ovum may cross inside the uterus and migrate up to the opposite tube **(internal migration).** Presumptive clinical evidence of migration of the ovum includes successful intrauterine pregnancies in women with only one tube and only the contralateral ovary.

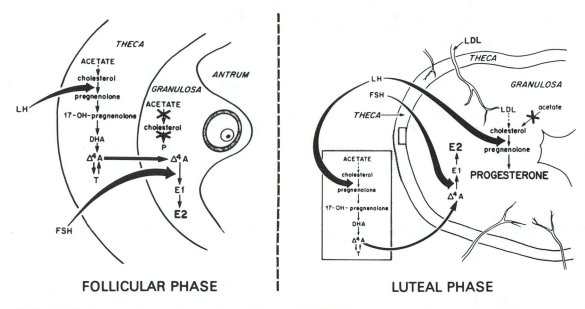

Figure 19–6. Relation between theca and granulosa cells in estradiol-17β (E_2) production. Androstenedione (Δ^4A) is synthesized by way of pregnenolone and dehydroepiandrosterone (DHA) formation in theca cells. Note that LH stimulates the formation of pregnenolone by increasing side-chain cleavage of cholesterol. Aromatization occurs in granulosa cells to give E_2 by way of estrone (E_1). The aromatization of androstenedione is stimulated by FSH. Progesterone synthesis from plasma low-density lipoprotein (LDL) occurs in luteinized granulosa cells. Testosterone (T) also is synthesized in the ovary.

Transport of Spermatozoa

Each ejaculate deposited in the vagina consists of an average volume of 2–5 mL of seminal fluid containing approximately 70 million sperm per milliliter. Of these 100 million spermatozoa or more, of which 80–90% are presumed to be normal forms, perhaps fewer than 200 actually reach the site of fertilization, the ampulla of the tube. Sperm reach the site of fertilization in the ampulla of the oviduct shortly—often only 5 minutes—after ejaculation, much faster than can be explained by the flagellar action of spermatozoa. For successful fertilization, only one spermatozoon must meet, in the upper portion of the uterine tube, the single mature ovum that is released during each ovulatory cycle.

Fertilization

As soon as the sperm penetrates the zona pellucida and comes in contact with the vitelline membrane, a second polar body is formed and the female pronucleus—as well as the male pronucleus—are evident in the ovum. Ordinarily, penetration of the zona pellucida and vitelline membrane by one sperm inhibits entry by others; at times, however, more than one sperm does enter. The mechanism by which the sperm penetrates the zona pellucida is not clearly defined but probably involves enzymatic action. Materials other than genetic material that are contained in the sperm degenerate within the ovum.

Zona Pellucida

The zona pellucida is shed from the blastocyst during

the fifth day after fertilization, apparently due to an intrinsic manifestation of growth and maturation of the blastocyst. The removal of the zona pellucida is a likely prerequisite for implantation.

In 1976, a test was developed to assess the capacity of human spermatozoa to fertilize the ovum. The test is dependent upon the capacity of the sperm of one species—humans—to penetrate the ovum of another species provided that the acellular, sperm-resistant zona pellucida (perhaps containing a specific antigen) of such ova are removed. It was demonstrated that capacitated human spermatozoa could penetrate zona-free hamster eggs. Thereafter, there was decondensation of the sperm chromatin and pronucleus formation—events analogous to those of fertilization. In some clinics, this test correlates reasonably well with male fertility. It is of great potential importance that there appear to be zona pellucida-specific antigens. Antibodies appear to react with these antigens in such a manner that binding receptors for sperm are masked, so that fertilization cannot take place. Indeed, there are reports of infertility due to the presence of circulating antizonal antibodies, but the status of this entity is as yet not clear. Nonetheless, the possibility is real that an antizonal antibody might produce passive and even temporary infertility in this day of monoclonal antibody technology.

Aging of Gametes

The increased incidence of the trisomy 21 variety of Down's syndrome late in reproductive life is well established. It may be related to an increased tendency toward nondisjunction in ova that have remained dormant in the ovary for 40 years or more. Although the incidence of this syndrome in the population as a whole is only three per 2000 live births, the incidence rises to about 1:100 in women by age 40. Gametes of aging males also exert deleterious effects on the embryo and fetus.

The risk of new autosomal dominant mutations in children is increased many times among the offspring of fathers who are 40 years of age or older. Indeed, the risk is similar to that of Down's syndrome in infants of 35- to 40-year-old mothers.

THECA-GRANULOSA CELL COOPERATIVITY & STEROIDOGENESIS

MOLECULAR EVENTS INVOLVED IN THE FINAL STAGES OF FOLLICULAR MATURATION & OVULATION

It now is clear that a variety of molecular events in the theca and granulosa cells of the ovaries are subject to regulatory processes that involve the actions of gonadotropins and of steroids as well. It is recognized that follicular maturation can proceed in the absence of pituitary hormone stimulation to the preantral stage of development and even to replication of granulosa cells to a finite point, ie, a thickness of four cell layers. Beyond this stage, however, gonadotropin and probably steroids produced in response to gonadotropin action are required for full expression of follicular maturation and responsiveness.

THE TWO-CELL HYPOTHESIS OF OVARIAN STEROIDOGENESIS

In the ovaries of young women, there is a characteristic cyclicity of secretion of estradiol-17β and progesterone and formation of the C_{19} steroids androstenedione, dehydroepiandrosterone, and testosterone. Regulation of C_{18} and C_{21} steroids (estrogen and progesterone) is by mechanisms that are considerably different from those responsible for formation of C_{19} steroids (androgen or androgen-like compounds).

FSH acts to increase the enzymatic activity in granulosa cells that catalyzes the aromatization of C_{19} steroids to produce estrogen. This activity is believed to be modulated by an increase in adenylyl cyclase activity and by "androgens" that act in an undefined manner to increase aromatase activity. Furthermore, estradiol-17β synthesized by the dominant follicle also appears to increase the follicular cell actions of FSH to enhance LH responsiveness. The stimulation of aromatase activity by cAMP is probably mediated by cAMP-dependent phosphorylation of a number of cellular proteins and by an increase in the

rate of transcription of the specific gene that encodes for the aromatase protein. It is only after FSH priming that cells become responsive to LH action. This is believed to be the result of FSH-induced LH receptors and, perhaps, FSH-induced prolactin receptors. Thus, FSH appears to induce an increase in aromatase activity (by way of synthesis of new enzyme) as well as LH receptors.

Approximately three decades ago, the **two-cell hypothesis** was put forward by Ryan and Smith (1959) to account for steroid production in the ovary and especially in the maturing follicle. The attempt is to describe the cooperativity between theca and granulosa cells in steroid formation.

LH is known to act in theca cells to increase cholesterol side chain cleavage enzyme activity (which is believed to be the rate-limiting step in steroidogenesis in many steroidogenic tissues) and to increase the activities of steroid 17α-hydroxylase/17,20-lyase, an enzyme that is crucial to the formation of C_{19} steroids, ie, androgen-like compounds such as dehydroepiandrosterone, androstenedione, and testosterone.

Androstenedione, formed in theca (Figure 19–6), diffuses into the follicular fluid and thereby becomes available to the granulosa cells for aromatization to form estrone and then estradiol-17β. Before ovulation, there is little or no de novo synthesis of steroids in granulosa cells because of the limited capacity for de novo synthesis of cholesterol.

STEROID PRODUCTION IN ISOLATED CELL TYPES

Granulosa cells can be isolated and maintained in culture, but strange events occur—most importantly, spontaneous luteinization. Before ovulation, granulosa cells do not produce steroids but are dependent upon preformed C_{19} steroids (from theca cells) for estradiol-17β formation. This is probably because human granulosa cells cannot form cholesterol de novo.

Source of Cholesterol for Steroidogenesis

It has long been known that cholesterol must be the ultimate precursor of all steroid hormones. What was not known until recently is that the sources of cholesterol for specific steroidogenic cells may differ. After Brown and associates (1979) demonstrated that many extrahepatic tissues assimilate cholesterol by uptake and processing of circulating lipoproteins, it became apparent that similar processes are applicable to the assimilation of cholesterol for steroidogenesis in endocrine glands and placenta. In women, there is little de novo synthesis of cholesterol in granulosa cells or in the corpus luteum. Low-density lipoprotein (LDL) is virtually the only form of cholesterol that can be used by the granulosa cells for progesterone biosynthesis. Bearing in mind that the molecular weight of LDL is approximately 3 million and that follicular granulosa cells are not vascularized, it is apparent that a precursor source of cholesterol is essential for full luteinization and optimal progesterone biosynthesis.

LDL Utilization by Granulosa Cells

There is a very limited capacity for synthesis of cholesterol in granulosa cells, and these cells do not utilize HDL as a source of cholesterol. Furthermore, in the follicular fluid that surrounds the avascular granulosa cells, there is little or no LDL. Thus, it is obvious that little or no steroidogenesis by utilization of LDL cholesterol could proceed in this unique environment. Therefore, before ovulation, little progesterone is produced by the granulosa cells. The steroid produced, estradiol-17β, is synthesized from androstenedione produced in the theca.

On the other hand, if granulosa cells obtained from the ovarian follicles are placed in culture, the cells luteinize and respond to appropriate trophic stimuli by producing progesterone in large amounts. It must be remembered, however, that the culture medium that bathes these cells usually contains serum—and thus LDL, a lipoprotein not present in follicular fluid but the one known to be used specifically as a source of cholesterol in human granulosa cells. Thus, the "spontaneous" luteinization of granulosa cells and therefore the biosynthesis of progesterone may be attributable, in part, to the addition of a utilizable source of cholesterol—specifically, LDL—to these cells.

OVULATION

As the graafian follicle grows to a size of 10–12 mm in diameter, it gradually reaches the surface of the ovary and ultimately protrudes above it. Necrobiosis of the overlying tissues—rather than pressure within the follicle—is the principal cause of follicular rupture. The cells at the exposed tip of the follicle float away at the site of the pale follicular stigma so that the region becomes transparent. The thinnest clear area then bursts, and the follicular liquid and the ovum, surrounded by the zona pellucida and corona radiata, are extruded at the time of ovulation. The actual rupture of the follicle is not explosive. The discharge of the ovum together with the zona pellucida and attached follicular cells takes not more than 2–3 minutes, and in the rabbit, at least, it is expedited by the separation, just before rupture, of the ovum with the surrounding granulosa cells (corona radiata) from the follicular wall as the result of accumulation of fluid in the cumulus oophorus. Thus, the ovum floats freely in the liquor folliculi.

TIME OF OVULATION

Although ovulation frequently occurs between the 12th and 16th days of the cycle, there is considerable variation in the timing of ovulation. It is not uncommon for ovulation to take place at any time between the 8th and 20th days. The time of ovulation bears a closer temporal relation to the onset of the next menstrual period than to the previous menses. Ovulation usually occurs approximately 14 days before the first day of the succeeding menstrual period.

SIGNS & SYMPTOMS OF OVULATION

On or about the day of ovulation, as many as 25% of women experience lower abdominal discomfort on the involved side. This so-called **mittelschmerz** is believed to be caused by peritoneal irritation by follicular fluid or blood that escapes from the ruptured follicle. It is rare for this phenomenon to occur during every cycle.

A useful means of detecting ovulation is by documentation of a shift in basal body temperature from a relatively constant lower level during the follicular or preovulatory phase to a somewhat higher level early in the luteal or postovulatory phase, as illustrated in Figure 19–7. Most likely, ovulation occurs just before or during the shift in temperature. The increase in the basal body temperature is believed to be caused by the thermogenic action of progesterone in the brain. Perhaps this is mediated by the progesterone-induced generation of the cytokine interleukin-1β (see Chapter 38).

CORPUS LUTEUM FORMATION

The corpus luteum ("yellow body") forms in the ovary at the site of the ruptured follicle immediately after ovulation. It is colored by a golden pigment from which it derives its name. Microscopic observation shows that the corpus luteum undergoes four stages of development and demise: proliferation, vascularization, maturity, and regression.

CORPUS LUTEUM OF PREGNANCY

The duration and function of the corpus luteum of pregnancy are the subjects of much speculation, and the scientific rationale of hormonal therapy in the prevention of early abortion after surgical removal of the corpus luteum derives from our understanding of the function of this structure.

The morphologic criteria of a very early corpus luteum of pregnancy include (1) a surge of cellular hyperplasia in the corpus luteum from the 23rd to the 28th days after the last menstrual period, which results presumably, at least in part, from the stimulus of chorionic gonadotropin; (2) an increasing number of K cells in the granulosa; and (3) the

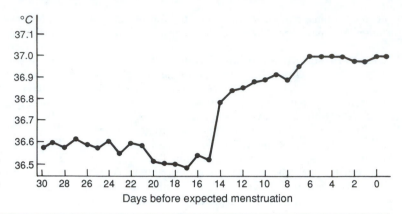

Figure 19–7. Basal temperature shift characteristic of rupture of follicle. (Reproduced, with permission, from Palmer R: Obstet Gynecol Surv 1979;4:1.)

absence of atrophic, ischemic, or regressive changes such as those that appear when menstruation is imminent. The degenerative changes in the corpus luteum are delayed for a variable time but occur most frequently at about 6 months of gestation—though corpora lutea that appear to be normal have been found at term.

Function of the Corpus Luteum in Pregnancy

The clinician must face certain therapeutic choices when obliged to remove the corpus luteum in early pregnancy from a woman who wishes to continue that pregnancy. Our choice is the use of a parenteral progestin, eg, hydroxyprogesterone caproate (125 mg) when the corpus luteum is removed prior to 10 weeks of gestation. We choose hydroxyprogesterone caproate because it has a predictable duration of action, rarely (if ever) leads to virilization of a female fetus, and can be given intramuscularly. After 8 weeks, we administer the progestin only at the time of surgery, if at all. Between 6 and 8 weeks, there may be some merit in a second injection 1 week after surgery.

CORPORA ALBICANTIA

In the absence of pregnancy, degenerated lutein cells are rapidly reabsorbed, and in a short time the corpus luteum is replaced by newly formed connective tissue closely resembling that of the surrounding ovarian stroma. The structures formed, called corpora albicantia, appear on cut section to be dull and white, somewhat like scar tissue. They are, however, gradually invaded by surrounding stroma and broken up into increasingly smaller hyaline masses that eventually are completely reabsorbed. Ultimately, the site of the original follicle is indicated only by an area of slightly thickened connective tissue. In older women, this process may be slower and less complete. In

women near the age of menopause, it is not uncommon to find that ovaries are almost filled by scars of various sizes.

ATRETIC FOLLICLES

Theca lutein cells are admixed somewhat with granulosa lutein cells, but for the most part the two cell types are distinctive in appearance. The granulosa lutein cells are larger and more highly vacuolated, with a smaller nucleus; the theca lutein cells are somewhat smaller, more deeply stained, and have a larger nucleus. The theca lutein cells serve a prominent role in the life history of follicles that degenerate without rupture. This process of **follicular atresia** is especially pronounced during pregnancy. In this circumstance, after the follicle has attained a certain size, the ovum undergoes cytolysis while the membrana granulosa degenerates, is cast off into the liquor folliculi, and eventually is reabsorbed. While these changes are in progress, the theca lutein cells proliferate to form, about the follicle, a tunic many layers thick that frequently becomes yellowish. Eventually, as the follicular fluid disappears, the walls of the follicle collapse, and in the theca cells that surround it there are fatty and hyaline changes. Finally, an irregular hyaline body results that cannot be distinguished from a similar structure that was derived from a corpus luteum.

Atresia is the fate of the vast majority of follicles that develop beyond the primordial stage; the process begins during intrauterine life and continues until after the menopause. Corpora lutea, however, always develop only from the comparatively few follicles—usually one in each ovarian cycle—that rupture after reaching maturity. It may be that one of the functions of the corpus luteum is obliteration of the spaces left by the ruptured follicles without the formation of cicatricial tissue; thus, conversion of the entire ovary to scar tissue is prevented.

SUGGESTED READINGS

Blandau RJ, White BJ, Rumery RE: Observations on the movements of the living primordial germ cells in the mouse. Fertil Steril 1963;14:482.

Brown MS, Kovanen PT, Goldstein JL: Receptor-mediated uptake of lipoprotein cholesterol and its utilization for steroid synthesis in the adrenal cortex. Recent Prog Horm Res 1979;35:215.

Friedman JM: Genetic disease in the offspring of older fathers. Obstet Gynecol 1981;57:745.

Pinkerton JHM, McKay DG, Adams EC, Hertig AT: Development of the human ovary: Study using histochemical technics. Obstet Gynecol 1961;18:152.

Ryan KJ, Smith OW: Biogenesis of estrogens by the human ovary: 1. Conversion of acetate-1-C14 to estrone and estradiol. J Biol Chem 1959;234:268.

Speroff L, Glass RH, Kase NG (editors). *Clinical Gynecologic Endocrinology and Fertility,* 4th ed. Williams & Wilkins, 1989.

Yanagimachi R, Yanagimachi H, Rogers BJ: The use of zona-free animal ova as a test-system for the assessment of the fertilizing capacity of human spermatozoa. Biol Reprod 1976;15:471.

20

Sexual Differentiation

The detection of sexual ambiguity in the newborn is a primary medical responsibility of the utmost seriousness, since incorrect assignment of sex may create grave psychologic and social problems for the baby and its family. Proper functional sex assignment can almost always be made at the time of delivery in newborns with ambiguous external genitalia.

Male phenotypic sexual differentiation is controlled by the fetal testis. In the absence of a fetal testis, female differentiation ensues irrespective of genetic sex.

SEXUAL DIFFERENTIATION

Chromosomal Sex

Genetic sex, XX or XY, is established at the time of fertilization of the ovum. Thereafter, for the first 8 weeks, the development of male and female embryos is identical. It is the differentiation of the primordial gonad into testis or ovary that heralds the establishment of gonadal sex (Figure 20–1).

Gonadal Sex

The Y chromosome is of paramount importance in gonadal differentiation into testes, but the precise mechanism is not known. Male-specific cell-surface proteins—eg, the H-Y antigens—are correlated with testicular development in many species. Recently, testicular determining factors, specifically the SR-Y locus on the short arm of the Y chromosome, appear to be the primary regulators of fetal testicular development. There probably are a number of male-specific antigens, and at present no constant relationship has been established between the presence of a given antigen and the development of a testis.

The contribution of chromosomal sex to gonadal sex is clarified by the apparent paradox presented by the XX male. The incidence of 46,XX phenotypic human males is estimated to be about 1:24,000–1:20,000 male births. Most cases seem to result from interchange of a Y chromosome fragment with the X chromosome. Translocation of a testis-determining region of the Y chromosome to the X chromosome during meiosis of male germ cells gives rise to this possibility.

Nonetheless, once gonadal sex is established, phenotypic sex develops rapidly.

Phenotypic Sex

The urogenital tract of the human fetus is identical in the two sexes before the eighth week of gestation. Thereafter, development of the internal and external genitalia of the male phenotype is dependent upon testicular function.

The basic experiments to determine the role of the testis in male sexual differentiation were conducted by a French anatomist, Alfred Jost, who ultimately demonstrated that the induced phenotype is male and that secretions from the gonad, including the ovary, are not necessary for female differentiation. Jost et al (1973) found that if castration of the rabbit fetus was done before differentiation of the genital anlagen, all newborns were phenotypic females with female external genitalia and the paramesonephric (müllerian) ducts developed into a uterus, uterine tubes, and upper vagina. If castration was done before differentiation of the genital anlagen and this was followed by implantation of a testis on one side, the phenotype of all fetuses was male; the external genitalia of such fetuses were masculinized; and on the side of the testicular implant, there was mesonephric (wolffian) duct development in that the vas deferens, epididymis, and seminal vesicle were formed. On the side of the testicular implant, müllerian structures, ie, uterine horn and uterine tube, were not present. On the other hand, the paramesonephric duct did develop on the side of castration where there was no testis graft.

Jost found also that if after castration of the fetus—at the sexually indifferent stage—a testosterone pellet was implanted on one side (in the site of a removed gonad), the external genitalia masculinized, as did the mesonephric duct, but the paramesonephric duct did not regress—ie, the uterine horn and uterine tubes did develop in spite of the "androgen" implant.

These fundamental observations, together with those of Wilson and coworkers, form the basis of our understanding of the mechanisms of sexual differentiation.

Testosterone Conversion to 5α-Dihydrotestosterone

Wilson and Gloyna (1971) demonstrated that in most androgen-responsive tissues, testosterone is converted to 5α-dihydrotestosterone in a reaction catalyzed by 5α-reductase. In these tissues, androgen action is expressed by way of this 5α-reduced metabolite. The 5α-dihydrotes-

154

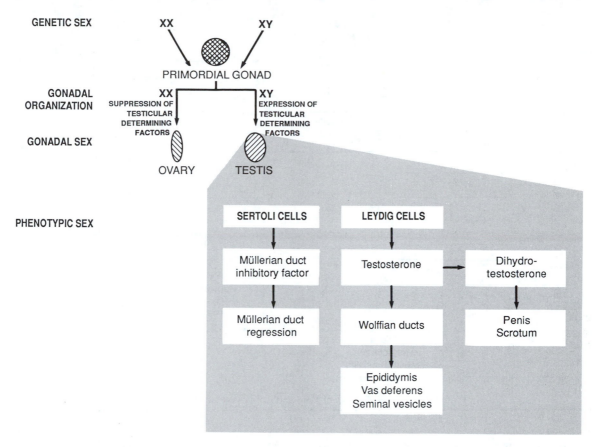

Figure 20–1. Sexual differentiation. Genetic sex is established at the time of fertilization of the ovum. At a time thereafter, the primordial gonad is acted upon by male-specific substances, eg, testicular determining factors that bring about the organization of the gonad as a testis whose secretions are responsible for male phenotypic sex differentiation.

tosterone is bound to an androgen-binding protein, and the steroid-receptor protein complex in the nucleus becomes associated with chromatin. Thus, in the genital tubercle and urogenital sinus, testosterone acts only after conversion to 5α-dihydrotestosterone.

There is a notable and important exception, however, to this generalization for testosterone action in genital tissues. Wilson and Lasnitzki (1971) also demonstrated that testosterone as such acts on the mesonephric duct of the embryo to cause development of the male ductal system; indeed, this action of testosterone is expressed before 5α-reductase activity is detectable in this tissue.

Physiologic & Biomolecular Basis of Sexual Differentiation

Based on these observations, the biochemical basis of sexual differentiation can be formulated as illustrated diagrammatically in Figure 20–2 and summarized as follows:

(1) Genetic sex is established at the time of fertilization of the ovum.

(2) Gonadal sex is determined by organizing factors that may arise on autosomes but by way of genetic action that is affected positively by factors encoded on loci on the Y chromosome or negatively by factors encoded on loci on the X chromosome. By way of these coordinated processes, differentiation of the primitive gonad as a testis is accomplished.

(3) The fetal testis secretes a proteinaceous substance called müllerian-inhibiting substance, a dimeric glycoprotein that acts locally (ie, not as a hormone) to cause regression of the paramesonephric duct—ie, it causes failure of development of a uterus, uterine tubes, and upper vagina. Müllerian-inhibiting substance is produced by the Sertoli cells of the seminiferous tubules; importantly, the seminiferous tubules appear in fetal gonads before the Leydig cells, the cellular site of origin of testosterone, and müllerian-inhibiting substance is produced by Sertoli cells even before differentiation of the seminiferous tubules. Therefore, regression of the paramesonephric ducts is initiated at a time in fetal development before testosterone secretion commences. Because müllerian-inhibiting substance acts locally, ie, near its site of formation, if a testis were absent on one side, the paramesonephric duct on that side would persist and the uterus and uterine tubes would develop from it. It may be the case also that müllerian-inhibiting substance is important in testicular descent be-

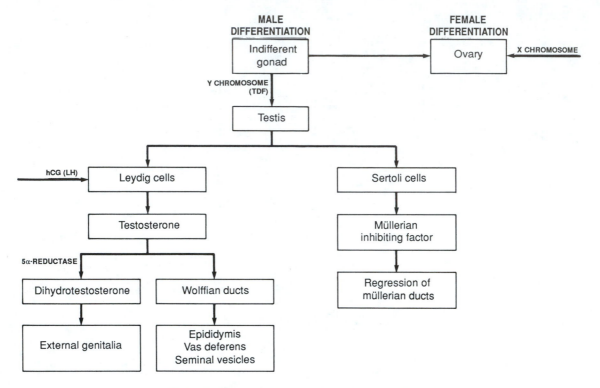

Figure 20–2. Flow diagram of male and female sexual differentiation.

cause the testes of newborn boys with cryptorchidism contain less of the glycoprotein than those of normal newborns (Figures 20–3 and 20–4).

(4) The fetal testis, initially under the influence of chorionic gonadotropin and thence fetal pituitary LH, secretes testosterone that acts directly on the mesonephric duct to give rise to development of the vas deferens, epididymides, and seminal vesicles. Testosterone of fetal testicular origin enters the blood, reaches the genital tubercle and urogenital sinus, and, in these tissues, is converted to 5α-dihydrotestosterone, the active androgen that brings about virilization of the external genitalia.

GENITAL AMBIGUITY OF THE NEWBORN

The development of ambiguous genitalia is invariably brought about by abnormal androgenic representation in utero. In simple terms, this means too much androgen for an embryo that was destined to be female or too little androgenic representation for an embryo or fetus that was destined to be male.

In the case of the fetus destined to be male, inadequate androgenic representation may be caused either by deficient fetal testicular secretion of testosterone or by a deficiency in responsiveness to testosterone or 5α-dihydrotestosterone in tissues that normally respond to androgen. Based on these premises, all abnormalities of sexual differentiation can be assigned to one of three general cate-

gories: female pseudohermaphroditism, male pseudohermaphroditism, or dysgenetic gonads and true hermaphroditism.

Category 1: Female Pseudohermaphroditism

The salient characteristics of female pseudohermaphroditism are the following: (1) müllerian-inhibiting substance is not produced; (2) androgen exposure of the embryo and fetus is variable; (3) karyotype is 46,XX; and (4) ovaries are present. All subjects in this category were destined to be female by virtue of genetic and gonadal sex.

Thus, the only abnormality that can occur is androgenic excess. Because müllerian-inhibiting substance was not produced (ovaries, not testes, are present), each affected individual will have a uterus, uterine tubes, and upper vagina. If such embryos were exposed to a small androgenic excess reasonably late in embryonic (early fetal) development, the only abnormality would be slight clitoral hypertrophy with an otherwise normal female phenotype. With somewhat greater androgenic excess, clitoral hypertrophy and posterior labial fusion may develop. With progressively increasing androgenic excess somewhat earlier in embryonic development, there is greater virilization. This process of virilization can proceed through the formation of labioscrotal folds, the development of a urogenital sinus (in which the vagina empties into the posterior urethra), and even to the development of a penile urethra with scrotal formation—the "empty scrotum" syndrome.

The cause of female pseudohermaphroditism is exces-

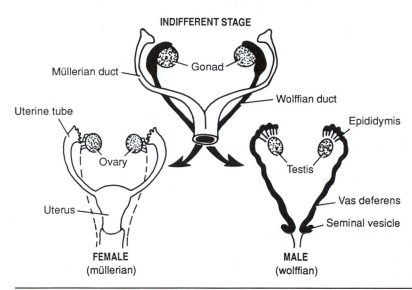

Figure 20–3. Paramesonephric (müllerian) or mesonephric (wolffian) duct development from indifferent ductal stage (see text).

sive androgen exposure of a fetus destined to be female. The androgenic excess most commonly arises by secretion from the fetal adrenal because of increased secretion of androgen or androgen prehormones as a result of enzymatic defects in the pathway to cortisol formation in the adrenal cortex, ie, congenital adrenal hyperplasia (most commonly 21-hydroxylase deficiency). With inadequate cortisol synthesis, it is assumed that ACTH secretion is elevated. Excessive stimulation of the adrenals leads to excessive secretion of precursors of cortisol and its metabolites, which include androgens or androgenic prehormones that can be converted to testosterone—principally by way of androstenedione—in extraglandular tissues. The enzyme deficiency may involve any of the five enzymatic reactions in the pathway to cortisol biosynthesis, ie, cholesterol side-chain cleavage, 3β-hydroxysteroid dehydrogenase, 17α-hydroxylase, 21-hydroxylase, or 11β-hydroxylase.

Another cause of female pseudohermaphroditism is androgen excess in the fetus that is caused by increased androgen formation in the maternal compartment. Excess androgen in the mother may arise by secretion from maternal ovaries, ie, hyperreactio lutealis, or from tumors of the maternal ovary, eg, luteomas, arrhenoblastomas, or hilar cell tumors. Most commonly, however, the female fetus of a pregnant woman with an androgen-secreting tumor is not virilized. During most—perhaps all—of pregnancy, the female fetus is protected from androgen excess in the mother because of the extraordinary capacity of the trophoblast to convert aromatizable C_{19} steroids (androgens) to estrogens (see Chapter 35).

In addition, if certain drugs—most commonly synthetic progestins—are given to pregnant women, virilization of their female fetuses may occur. It is not altogether clear how progestins have this effect. Some of the compounds—especially those of the 19-nortestosterone con-

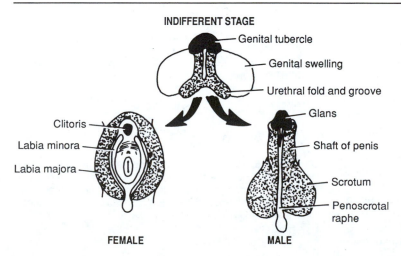

Figure 20–4. Feminization or masculinization of indifferent stage external genitalia.

figuration—may act on fetal tissues as androgens. Or the agents may act to inhibit aromatization in the placenta and thus allow transfer to the fetus of androgens that escape aromatization.

All female pseudohermaphrodites can become normal fertile women if the diagnosis is made early and appropriate therapy is initiated.

Category 2: Male Pseudohermaphroditism

This group has the following characteristics: (1) müllerian-inhibiting substance is produced; (2) androgenic representation is variable; (3) karyotype is 46,XY; and (4) testes—or no gonads—are present. All subjects in this category were destined to be male by virtue of genetic sex. Thus, the abnormalities in sexual differentiation are the result of incomplete virilization, ie, inadequate androgenic representation.

Incomplete masculinization of the fetus can be caused by inadequate production of testosterone by the fetal testis or by diminished responsiveness of the genital anlagen to normal quantities of androgen, including failure of in situ formation of 5α-dihydrotestosterone in tissues destined to form the external genitalia.

Because müllerian-inhibiting substance is produced during embryonic life in these subjects (testes present, at least at some time in embryonic life), there is no uterus, uterine tubes, or upper vagina.

A. Diminished Fetal Testicular Testosterone Secretion: Deficient fetal testicular testosterone production may occur if there is an enzymatic defect in the testis that involves any one of the four enzymes (which catalyze five enzymatic reactions) in the biosynthetic pathway to testosterone formation (Figure 20–5). Defects in each of these enzymatic reactions—as a cause of abnormal sex differentiation—have been described. Enzymatic defects in testicular testosterone biosynthesis give rise to decreased rates of fetal testosterone secretion, and incomplete masculinization of the external genitalia is the consequence. The phenotype of such newborns is variable in the degree of ambiguity because the degree of enzyme deficiency varies.

B. Embryonic Testicular Regression: Embryonic or fetal loss of testes gives rise to a phenotype that is dependent upon the time in embryonic life that the testes regress. If the testes regress during embryonic or fetal life, testosterone production will be deficient thereafter. Such an occurrence has been referred to as embryonic testicular regression.

Edman et al (1977) analyzed the phenotypes of reported cases of agonadism in 46,XY persons and in three of their own cases. They compared these findings with those that would be expected if the testes regressed at various stages of embryologic sexual differentiation. They found that a spectrum of phenotypes had been described, and among affected persons the phenotypes varied from normal female with absent uterus, uterine tubes, and upper vagina to that of a normal male but with anorchia. Because paramesonephric duct regression commences before virilization is initiated in embryonic life, such a spectrum of phe-

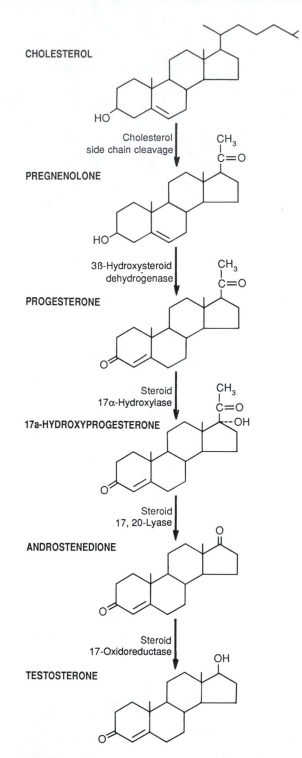

Figure 20–5. Biosynthetic pathway of testosterone formation in the testis. There are five enzymatic reactions involved in the conversion of cholesterol to testosterone. A defect in each of these enzymes has been identified as the cause of inadequate fetal testicular testosterone production.

notypes was to be expected if testicular regression were to occur at various times during the process of sexual differentiation.

C. Androgen Resistance: Deficiencies in androgen responsiveness are caused by inadequate or abnormal androgen receptor macromolecules in androgen-responsive tissues or may be due to failure of conversion of testosterone to 5α-dihydrotestosterone in such tissues because of deficient 5α-reductase enzyme activity (Wilson and MacDonald, 1978).

The most extreme form of the disorders of androgen resistance is testicular feminization. In this entity, there appears to be little or no tissue responsiveness to androgen. The phenotype is female but with a short, blind vagina, no uterus or uterine tubes, and no mesonephric duct structures. At the expected time of puberty, testosterone levels in such women rise to values similar to or greater than those found in normal adult men. Nonetheless, virilization does not occur, and even sexual hair (pubic and axillary) fails to develop because of end-organ resistance to androgen action. Presumably because of androgen resistance at the level of the brain and pituitary, LH levels are elevated in these women. In response to LH in high concentrations, there is also increased testicular secretion of estrogen compared with that found in normal men (MacDonald et al, 1979). The increased estrogen, together with the absence of androgen responsiveness, may act in concert to cause feminization, ie, breast development.

In the disorder known as incomplete testicular feminization, there appears to be slight androgen responsiveness. Affected individuals usually have modest clitoral hypertrophy at birth, but at the expected time of puberty, virilization does not occur and pubic and axillary hair do develop. These women also develop feminine breasts, presumably through the same endocrine mechanisms that are operative in women with the complete form of testicular feminization (Madden et al, 1975).

A third syndrome of androgen resistance has been called familial male pseudohermaphroditism type I (Walsh et al, 1974), also called Reifenstein's syndrome. Abnormalities of genital virilization vary from a phenotype similar to that of women with incomplete testicular feminization to that of a male phenotype with bifid scrotum, infertility, and gynecomastia. In these subjects, androgen resistance was established by the demonstration of diminished 5α-dihydrotestosterone-binding capacity in fibroblasts grown in culture from genital skin biopsies.

A fourth form of androgen resistance is caused by 5α-reductase deficiency in androgen-responsive tissues. Because androgen action in the genital tubercle and urogenital sinus is mediated by the action of 5α-dihydrotestosterone in persons with 5α-reductase deficiency, the external genitalia are female, modest clitoral hypertrophy. But because androgen action in the mesonephric duct of the embryo is mediated by testosterone per se, there are well-developed epididymides, seminal vesicles, and vasa deferentia, and the male ejaculatory ducts empty into the vagina (Walsh et al, 1974).

A composite photograph of the genitalia of subjects with each of the four types of androgen resistance is presented in Figure 20–6.

Category 3

This category includes individuals with the following abnormalities: (1) müllerian-inhibiting substance is not produced; (2) fetal androgen production among subjects is variable; (3) karyotype varies among subjects and commonly is abnormal; and (4) gonads are not present, neither ovaries nor testis. In all affected individuals, there is a uterus, uterine tubes, and upper vagina.

In most subjects in category 3, dysgenetic gonads are found. With the typical case of gonadal dysgenesis (eg, those with Turner's syndrome), there is a female phenotype; but at the time of expected puberty, sexual infantilism persists. In some persons with gonadal dysgenesis, there are ambiguous genitalia, implying that an abnormal gonad produced androgen, albeit in small amounts, during embryonic development. Generally in such subjects, one finds mixed gonadal dysgenesis, ie, a dysgenetic gonad on one side and an abnormal testis or dysontogenetic tumor on the other. Subjects with these disorders often have abnormal karyotypes, including mosaic (ie, 45,X and 46,XY). In most subjects with true hermaphroditism, the guidelines for this category are met. True hermaphrodites are persons in whom both ovarian and testicular tissues are present and in whom—most importantly—the germ cells (ova and sperm) of both sexes are formed.

PRELIMINARY DIAGNOSIS OF THE CAUSE OF GENITAL AMBIGUITY

A preliminary diagnosis of the cause of genital ambiguity can be made at delivery. By physical and ultrasonic examination of the newborn, the experienced examiner can ascertain whether the child has a uterus. If a uterus is present, the diagnosis must be female pseudohermaphroditism, testicular or gonadal dysgenesis, or true hermaphroditism. A family history of congenital adrenal hyperplasia is helpful. If a uterus is not present, the diagnosis is male pseudohermaphroditism. Androgen resistance and enzymatic defects in testicular testosterone biosynthesis are familial.

SEX ASSIGNMENT

The critical decision about sex assignment by the obstetrician is usually easy, though sometimes painful. In the author's judgment, any newborn with ambiguity of the genitalia so severe as to represent more than hypospadias should be designated a female. This conclusion is based on the following considerations:

(1) Individuals in category 1 (female pseudohermaphrodites) can become normal, fertile women.

(2) Individuals in category 2 (male pseudohermaphrodites) either cannot produce testosterone or are refractory to its action. Moreover, all will be infertile.

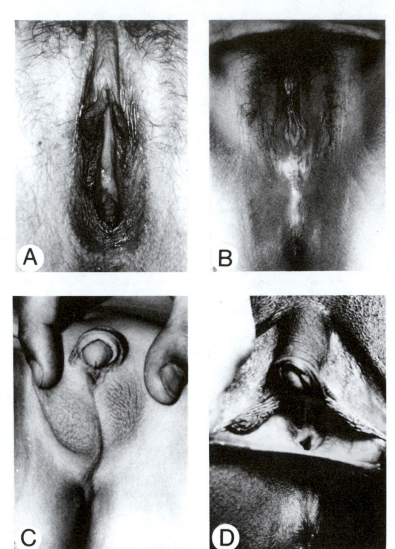

Figure 20–6. External genitalia of representative patients with male pseudohermaphroditism due to androgen resistance. **A:** Testicular feminization. **B:** Incomplete testicular feminization. **C:** Familial male pseudohermaphroditism, type I (Reifenstein's syndrome). **D:** 5α-Reductase deficiency. (Reproduced, with permission, from Wilson JD, MacDonald PC: Male pseudohermaphroditism due to androgen resistance: Testicular feminization and related syndromes. In: *The Metabolic Basis of Inherited Disease.* Stanbury JB, Wyngaarden JD, Frederickson DS (editors). Mc-Graw-Hill, 1978.)

(3) Currently, reconstruction of the penis in persons with androgen resistance is possible, but the achievement of male sexual function—let alone fertility—is not.

PRINCIPLES OF MANAGEMENT

Steps in the evaluation of a child born with ambiguous genitalia are outlined in Figure 20–7. It is of primary importance to rule out congenital adrenal hyperplasia, which is a life-threatening disorder. Gender assignment should be made in the delivery room if possible, but if the physician is uncertain, correct sex assignment should be made within a few days to weeks. In almost all cases, sex assignment is female; male gender assignment is made only if there is an adequate phallus (> 2 cm) with the presence of erectile tissue and no more than minimal to moderate hypospadias. The testes should be present in the scrotum or inguinal canal. All other patients are assigned a female gender role. Under extraordinary circumstances, the initial decision can be reversed up until about 18 months of age.

It is important to describe the defect to the parents as "incomplete" or "unfinished." One should avoid the use of terms such as "hermaphrodite" and, later, "chromosomal discrepancies." The parents should be encouraged to examine and hold the infant, as this may stimulate bonding and allay some of their fears. A family history of similar defects, unexplained death of a sibling in the newborn period, maternal drug exposure to progestins, androgens, danazol, or spironolactone, or a history of maternal virilization (suggestive of androgen exposure) during pregnancy can help in establishing the diagnosis and determining the cause of the defect.

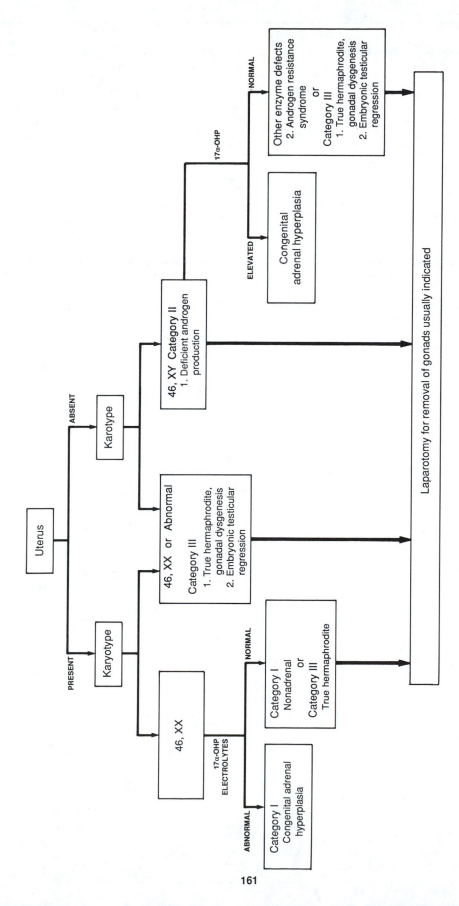

Figure 20–7. Flow diagram of steps in evaluation of a child with ambiguous genitalia. 17αOHP = 17α-hydroxyprogesterone.

Physical Examination of the Newborn With Ambiguous Genitalia

Physical examination of the infant should disclose the presence of extra-adrenal malformations such as cardiac, renal, or gastrointestinal anomalies. In evaluation of the phallus, it is important to document the degree of hypospadias and the length, width, and degree of erectile tissue. The degree of labial fusion and the presence of a palpable gonad in the scrotum or inguinal hernia or canal should be documented. The presence of a uterus is indicative of absence of müllerian-inhibiting substance, either due to absent testes (ie, the presence of ovaries) or embryonic testicular regression.The newborn uterus is usually palpable by rectal examination or can be distinguished by ultrasound, radiographic dye studies, or endoscopy. Laboratory tests should be started immediately and completed by 1 week. Preliminary results of chromosome analysis should be available in 5 days. The presence of a fluorescent Y body in a buccal smear upon quinacrine staining can speed the diagnosis of genetic sex. Serum electrolytes should be measured to look for salt wasting in congenital adrenal hyperplasia. 17α-Hydroxyprogesterone or urinary 17-ketosteroids and pregnanetriol will be elevated in cases of congenital adrenal hyperplasia. Other laboratory tests may be required to make the final diagnosis, such as a complete steroid hormonal profile associated with an hCG stimulation test, androgen receptor determination from sexual skin fibroblasts, or 5α-reductase determination, also from sexual skin fibroblasts.

Surgical Resources

Phallus reduction by an experienced operator should be done early. Vaginal and vulvar reconstruction is performed at about the age of puberty. Intra-abdominal streaks and gonads should be removed in all individuals with congenital sexual ambiguity with a Y chromosome before puberty, since there is a higher incidence of gonadal tumors in these patients.

SUGGESTED READINGS

Coulam CB: Testicular regression syndrome. Obstet Gynecol 1979;53:44.

Donahoe PK, Fuller AFJ, Scully RE: Müllerian inhibiting substance inhibits growth of human ovarian cancer in nude mice. Ann Surg 1981;194:472.

George FW, Wilson JD: Sex determination and differentiation. Page 3 in: *The Physiology of Reproduction.* Knobil E, Neill J (editors). Raven Press, 1988.

Griffin JE, Wilson JD: Disorders of sexual differentiation. Page 1819 in: *Campbell's Urology.* Walsh PC et al (editors). Saunders, 1986.

Jeffs RD, Gearhart JP: Reconstructive surgery of male external genitalia. Semin Reprod Endocrinol 1987;5:315.

Jones HW, Scott WW: *Hermaphroditism, Genital Anomalies, and Related Endocrine Disorders,* 2nd ed. Williams & Wilkins, 1971.

Jost A, Vigier B, Prepin J: Studies on sex differentiation in mammals. Recent Prog Horm Res 1973;29:1.

Madden JD et al: Clinical and endocrinological characterization of a patient with syndrome of incomplete testicular feminization. J Clin Endocrinol 1975;41:751.

Ohno S, Najai Y, Cicares S: Testicular cells lyso-stripped by H-Y antigen organize ovarian follicle-like aggregates. Cytogenet Cell Genet 1978;20:351.

Silvers WK, Glasser DL, Eicher EM: H-Y antigen, serologically detectable male antigen and sex determination. Cell 1982;28:439.

Simpson JL: Abnormal sexual differentiation in humans. Ann Rev Genet 16:193, 1982

Simpson JL: True hermaphroditism: Etiology and phenotypic considerations. Birth Defects 1978;14(6C):9.

Simpson JL et al: *Genetics in Obstetrics and Gynecology.* Grune & Stratton, 1982.

Wachtel SS: Errors of sexual determination. Proceedings of the Kroc Foundation Conference. Hum Genet 1981;58:1.

Walsh PC et al: Familial incomplete male pseudohermaphroditism, type 2: Decreased dihydrotestosterone formation in pseudovaginal perineoscrotal hypospades. N Engl J Med 1974;291:944.

White PC, New MI, DuPont B: Congenital adrenal hyperplasia. (Two parts.) N Engl J Med 1987;316:1519, 1580.

Wilson JD et al: The role of gonadal steroids in sexual differentiation. Recent Prog Hormone Res 1981;37:1.

21

Amenorrhea & Abnormal Uterine Bleeding

AMENORRHEA

Amenorrhea is defined as failure of menarche by age 16, irrespective of the presence or absence of secondary sexual characteristics; or the absence of menstruation for 3–6 months in a woman with previous periodic menses. By age 16, approximately 98% of all American girls have begun menstruating, with a cycle length ranging from 25 to 34 days. The incidence of nonphysiologic amenorrhea in women who previously menstruated remains 2–3%.

Young women should be evaluated for amenorrhea if they or their families are greatly concerned, if no maturation of secondary sexual characteristics (ie, breast development) has occurred by age 14, or if any sexual ambiguity or virilization is present (see accompanying box).

Amenorrhea is categorized as either **primary** (in a woman who has never menstruated) or **secondary** (in a woman who has previously menstruated but then ceases to do so). However, some disorders can cause either primary or secondary amenorrhea, so that categorization of amenorrhea as primary or secondary is less helpful in the differential diagnosis than one based upon the following major underlying physiologic derangements: (1) anatomic defects, (2) ovarian failure, and (3) chronic anovulation with or without the presence of estrogen. (See Figure 21–1.)

At least 80% of cases of amenorrhea are due to chronic anovulation. Anovulation resulting in amenorrhea occurs normally prior to puberty, during pregnancy and lactation, and following menopause. Treatment of women with certain medications that inhibit gonadotropins such as GnRH analogues, danocrine, and oral contraceptives can also cause amenorrhea. Pregnancy exclusion is an important first step in the evaluation of amenorrhea.

Evaluate Patients for Amenorrhea If—
1. Failure of menarche by age 16.
2. Absence of menses for 6 months.
3. Family and patient concern.
4. No breast development by age 15.
5. Sexual ambiguity or virilization.

AMENORRHEA DUE TO ANATOMIC DEFECTS

Abnormalities of the genital outflow tract are frequently identified during physical examination, but the diagnosis of some disorders requires additional testing. Anatomic or structural defects of the female genital tract can preclude menstrual bleeding.

Classification & Diagnosis

Starting from the lower end of the female genital tract, **labial agglutination or fusion** is often associated with disorders of sexual development, particularly female pseudohermaphroditism (congenital adrenal hyperplasia or exposure to maternal androgens in utero). Congenital defects of the vagina such as **imperforate hymen** and **transverse vaginal septa** can also cause amenorrhea. Patients with these disorders frequently have accumulation of menstrual blood behind the obstruction (hematocolpos, hematometra) and may have cyclic, predictable episodes of abdominal pain suggestive of intra-abdominal bleeding (Figure 21–2).

A. Müllerian Agenesis: More severe anomalies of the female genital tract include **absence of the uterus and vagina** (also called müllerian agenesis, or Mayer-Rokitansky-Küster-Hauser syndrome), second in frequency only to **gonadal dysgenesis** as a cause of primary amenorrhea. Women with this syndrome have a 46,XX karyotype, female secondary sex characteristics, and normal ovarian function, including cyclic ovulation, but absence of the vagina and severe hypoplasia of the uterus. The uterus usually consists only of rudimentary bicornu-

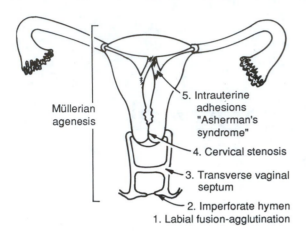

Müllerian
agenesis

5. Intrauterine
adhesions
"Asherman's
syndrome"

4. Cervical stenosis

3. Transverse vaginal
septum

2. Imperforate hymen

1. Labial fusion-agglutination

Figure 21–1. Flow diagram for the evaluation of women with amenorrhea. The most common diagnosis for each category is shown in parentheses. (Reproduced, with permission, from Carr BR, Wilson JD: Disorders of the ovary and female reproductive tract. Chap 118, pp 700–720, in: *Harrison's Principles of Internal Medicine,* 10th ed. Petersdorf RG et al [editors]. McGraw-Hill, 1983.)

ate cords, but if the uterus contains endometrium, cyclic abdominal pain and accumulation of blood may occur as in other forms of outlet obstruction. Urogenital tract and skeletal anomalies are frequently present in these cases.

B. Testicular Feminization: A major diagnostic problem is to distinguish müllerian agenesis from **complete testicular feminization** (androgen resistance), in which 46,XY genetic males with testes present clinically with a blind vaginal pouch and an absent uterus. Patients with androgen resistance have feminized breasts (gynecomastia) but a paucity of pubic and axillary hair. The disorder is due to abnormalities in the androgen receptor that results in profound resistance to the action of testosterone. Androgen resistance can be diagnosed by demonstrating a male level of serum testosterone or a 46,XY karyotype, whereas the diagnosis of müllerian agenesis is established by demonstrating a 46,XX karyotype, biphasic basal body temperature characteristic of ovulation, and elevated progesterone concentrations during the luteal phase.

C. Asherman's Syndrome: Other abnormalities of the uterus that cause amenorrhea include **obstruction** due to scarring or stenosis of the cervix, often resulting from surgery, electrocautery, or cryosurgery. Destruction of the endometrium (**Asherman's syndrome**) may follow vigorous curettage, usually in association with postpartum hemorrhage or therapeutic abortion complicated by infection. Tuberculous endometritis and uterine surgery are rare causes of Asherman's syndrome. The diagnosis is confirmed by the finding of filling defects and intrauterine synechiae during hysterosalpingography or by direct hysteroscopic inspection of the endometrial cavity.

Treatment

Treatment of disorders of the outflow tract is surgical. Repair of vaginal agenesis results in normal menstruation and potential fertility only if an intact uterus and cervix is present.

AMENORRHEA DUE TO OVARIAN FAILURE

Primary ovarian failure is uniformly associated with elevated plasma gonadotropins (FSH level greater than 40 mIU/mL—hypergonadotropic hypogonadism) and can result from several causes. The most frequent cause is gonadal dysgenesis, in which the germ cells are lacking and the ovary is replaced by a fibrous streak.

Classification & Clinical Findings

Individuals with **gonadal dysgenesis** may present with a variety of clinical features and can be divided into two broad groups on the basis of karyotype. The most common type is due to deletion of genetic material in the X chromosomes and accounts for about two-thirds of cases. A 45,X karyotype (Turner's syndrome) is found in about half, and most have associated somatic defects, including short stature, webbed neck, shield chest, and cardiovascular anomalies. The remainder of patients with gonadal dysgenesis have chromosomal mosaicism with or without associated structural abnormalities of the X chromosome. The most common form of mosaicism is 45,X/46,XX, yet mosaicism with Y chromosomes is also found. Gonadal tumors are rare in 45,X patients, but malignancies have been reported in several women with chromosomal mosaicism involving the Y chromosome. Therefore, chromosomal analysis should be obtained in all cases of amenorrhea associated with ovarian failure, and the streak gonad should be removed if a Y chromosome is present because of the increased incidence of gonadal tumors in these patients. Approximately 90% of individuals with gonadal dysgenesis associated with deletion of genetic material in the X chromosome never have menstrual bleeding, and the remainder have sufficient residual follicles to experience menses, breast development, and, rarely, fertility.

One-tenth of subjects with bilateral streak gonads have a normal 46,XX or 46,XY karyotype and are said to have pure gonadal dysgenesis. These individuals have either normal or above-average stature due to failure of estrogen-mediated epiphyseal closure in the presence of a normal chromosomal constitution. Pure gonadal dysgenesis does not constitute a phenotypic or chromosomally homogeneous disorder. Some are the result of X-linked or autosomal gene defects. Other possible causes include chromosomal mosaicism limited to gonadal tissue and destruction of germinal tissue in utero by environmental or infectious processes. About 10% of individuals with the 46,XY karyotype develop signs of virilization, including clitoromegaly, and have an increased incidence of tumors in the gonadal streaks; as a consequence, streak gonads should be removed prophylactically when a Y chromosome is present.

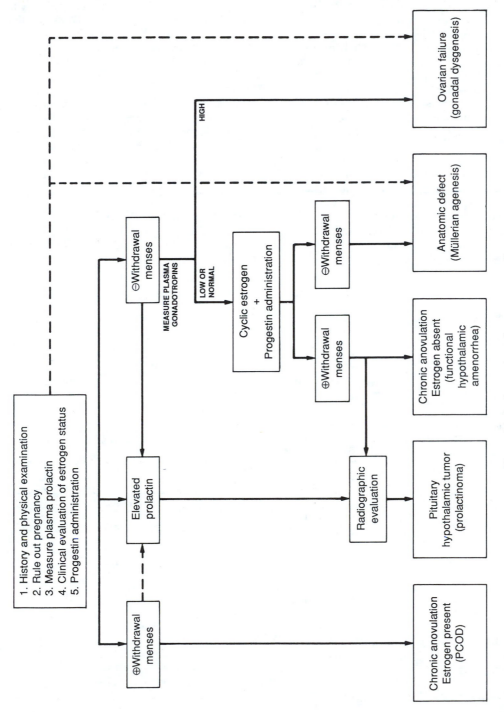

Figure 21–2. Anatomic outflow tract anomalies.

Other Causes of Ovarian Failure

Other causes of ovarian failure and amenorrhea include 17α-hydroxylase deficiency, 17,20-desmolase deficiency, premature ovarian failure, and the resistant ovary syndrome. **17α-Hydroxylase deficiency** is characterized by primary amenorrhea, sexual infantilism, and hypertension that is due to increased production of deoxycorticosterone (DOC), whereas **17,20-desmolase deficiency** is characterized only by primary amenorrhea and sexual infantilism (Figure 21–3). The diagnosis of **premature ovarian failure** or **premature menopause** is applied to women who cease menstruating prior to age 40. The ovaries are structurally similar to the ovaries of postmenopausal women, ie, with paucity or absence of follicles as the result of accelerated follicular atresia. Premature ovarian failure due to ovarian antibodies may be one component of polyglandular failure, together with adrenal insufficiency, hypothyroidism, or other autoimmune disorders.

A rare form of ovarian failure is the **resistant ovary syndrome,** in which the ovaries contain many follicles arrested in development prior to the antral stage, perhaps because of resistance to the action of FSH in the ovary. To differentiate this disorder from the 46,XX variety of pure gonadal dysgenesis—both of which are associated with sexual immaturity—it would be necessary to perform ovarian biopsy. However, such a distinction is not clinically useful, since the treatment of infertility in both conditions is usually unsuccessful.

Treatment

Women with ovarian failure can conceive if treatment with cyclic hormone therapy is followed by transfer of a fertilized donor egg. Treatment of ovarian failure is directed at estrogen-progesterone replacement to augment or maintain secondary sexual characteristics and prevent osteoporosis and lower the risk of cardiovascular disease.

CHRONIC ANOVULATION

Chronic anovulation is a disorder in which women fail to ovulate spontaneously but may ovulate if appropriate

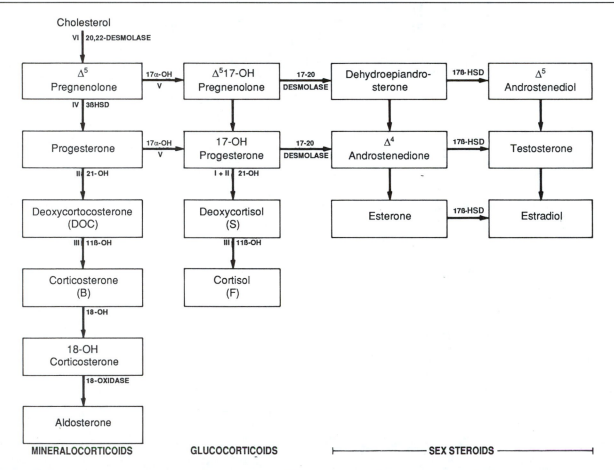

Figure 21–3. Diagram of steroid biosynthetic pathways depicting importance of 17 α-hydroxylase, 17,20 desmolase in production of glucocorticoids and sex steroids. (Reproduced, with permission, from Grumbach MM, Conte FA: Disorders of sexual differentiation. In: *Williams Textbook of Endocrinology,* 7th ed. Wilson JD, Foster DW [editors]. Saunders, 1985.)

therapy is given. The ovaries of women with chronic anovulation do not secrete estrogen in a normal cyclic pattern; it is clinically useful to attempt to separate these women into those who produce sufficient estrogen to have withdrawal bleeding after progesterone therapy and those who do not and who often have hypothalamic-pituitary dysfunction.

1. CHRONIC ANOVULATION WITH ESTROGEN PRESENT

Polycystic Ovarian Disease

Women with chronic anovulation who experience withdrawal bleeding after progesterone administration are said to be in a state of "estrus" due to the acyclic production of estrogen—largely estrone—by extraglandular aromatization of circulating androstenedione. The most common term for this disorder is polycystic ovarian disease. This disorder is frequently characterized by infertility, hirsutism, obesity, and amenorrhea or oligomenorrhea. When spontaneous uterine bleeding occurs in subjects with polycystic ovarian disease, it is unpredictable with respect to time of onset, duration, and amount, and on occasion the bleeding can be severe. The dysfunctional uterine bleeding in this disorder is usually due to estrogen breakthrough.

Polycystic ovarian disease was originally described by Stein and Leventhal in 1935 and may be transmitted as an autosomal dominant or X-linked trait. The syndrome and its accompanying endocrine abnormalities are now known to be associated with a variety of pathologic findings in the ovaries. The most common finding is a white, smooth, sclerotic ovary with a thickened capsule, multiple follicular cysts in various stages of atresia, and a hyperplastic theca and stroma with rare or absent corpora albicans. Other ovaries have the pattern of hyperthecosis, in which the ovarian stroma is hyperplastic and may contain lipid-laden luteal cells. Thus, the diagnosis of polycystic ovarian disease is a clinical one, based upon the presence of chronic anovulation and varying degrees of androgen excess. A subset of patients with polycystic ovarian disease also exhibit insulin resistance and acanthosis nigricans.

In most women with polycystic ovarian disease, menarche occurs at the expected time, but further uterine bleeding is usually unpredictable in onset, duration, and amount, and amenorrhea is often present. Occasionally, women with polycystic ovarian disease present with primary amenorrhea. Signs of androgen excess (hirsutism) usually become evident around the time of menarche. One theory suggests that this disorder originates as an exaggerated adrenarche in obese girls. The combination of elevated adrenal androgens and obesity results in increased formation of extraglandular estrogen and leads to acyclic positive feedback of LH secretion and negative feedback of FSH secretion, so that the LH/FSH ratios in plasma are greater than 2. The increased LH levels could then lead to hyperplasia of the ovarian stroma and theca cells and increased androgen production, which in turn would provide more substrate for peripheral aromatization and therefore perpetuation of the chronic anovulation. The ovary is the major site of androgen production, but the adrenal may continue to secrete excess androgen as well. The more severe the obesity, the more this cycle would be perpetuated, because fat stromal cells aromatize androgens to estrogens, which in turn exaggerates inappropriate LH release by positive feedback.

Thus, the fundamental defect in polycystic ovarian disease is viewed as one of inappropriate signals to the hypothalamus and pituitary. In fact, the hypothalamic-pituitary axis responds appropriately to high levels of estrogen, and ovulation can be induced with antiestrogens such as clomiphene citrate. The concept that the fundamental defect is one of inappropriate signals is supported by findings in the ovary itself. Ovarian follicles from women with polycystic ovarian disease have low aromatase activity, but normal aromatase can be induced when the follicles are treated in vitro with FSH.

Treatment of polycystic ovarian disease is directed toward interrupting this self-perpetuating cycle and can be accomplished in several ways, including decreasing ovarian androgen secretion (ovarian wedge resection or birth control pills), decreasing peripheral estrogen formation (weight reduction), or enhancing FSH secretion (administration of clomiphene citrate, human menopausal gonadotropin, or urofollitropin). The choice of therapy depends on the clinical findings and the needs of the individual patient. Attempt at weight reduction is appropriate in all who are obese. If the woman is not hirsute and does not desire pregnancy, periodic withdrawal menses can be induced with medroxyprogesterone acetate monthly or every 2 months; such treatment prevents development of endometrial hyperplasia. If the woman is hirsute but does not desire pregnancy, the ovarian (and possibly the adrenal) component of androgen production can be suppressed with the use of oral contraceptive pills.

Oral contraceptives are also indicated if prolonged or excessive menstrual bleeding is present in patients with polycystic ovaries. Once androgen excess is controlled, treatment of previously existing hair growth by shaving, depilatories, or electrolysis may be indicated. If the woman wants to become pregnant, induction of ovulation is necessary. The drug of choice for this purpose is clomiphene citrate, which promotes ovulation in three-fourths of cases, and treatment with HMG or wedge resection of the ovaries may be successful in the remainder.

Anovulation Due to Ovarian Tumors

Chronic anovulation with estrogen present may also occur with tumors of the ovary. These include granulosa-theca cell tumors, Brenner tumors, cystic teratomas, mucous cystadenomas, and foregut tumors metastatic to the ovary (ie, Krukenberg tumors). These tumors can either secrete excess estrogen themselves or produce androgens which can then be aromatized at extraglandular sites. As a result, chronic anovulation and the clinical features of polycystic ovarian disease are produced. Occasionally, areas of the ovary not involved with tumors show the characteristic histologic changes of polycystic ovarian disease. Other causes of chronic anovulation with estrogen present include adrenal production of excess androgen (adult-onset adrenal hyperplasia) and various thyroid disorders.

Treatment is by surgical removal of the tumor and is usually followed by resumption of ovulatory cycles. Tumors metastatic to the ovary are managed with surgical removal of the ovaries, possible total hysterectomy, and resection of primary tumor.

2. CHRONIC ANOVULATION WITH ESTROGEN ABSENT

Women with chronic anovulation who have low or absent estrogen production and do not experience withdrawal bleeding after progestin treatment usually have hypogonadotropic hypogonadism due either to pituitary disease or to organic or functional disorders of the central nervous system.

Hypogonadotropic Hypogonadism

Hypogonadotropic hypogonadism associated with defects of smell (olfactory bulb defects) is known as **Kallman's syndrome.** These women are sexually infantile with a eunuchoid habitus and appear to have a defect in either the synthesis or release of LHRH. A variety of rare hypothalamic lesions can also impair LHRH production and lead to the development of hypogonadotropic hypogonadism; these include craniopharyngioma, germinoma (pinealoma), glioma, Hand-Schüller-Christian disease, teratomas, endodermal-sinus tumors, tuberculosis, sarcoidosis, and metastatic tumors that cause suppression or destruction of the hypothalamus. Central nervous system trauma and radiation can also cause hypothalamic amenorrhea and deficiencies in secretion of growth hormone, ACTH, and thyroid hormone.

More commonly, gonadotropin deficiency leading to chronic anovulation is believed to arise from functional disorders of the hypothalamus or higher centers. A common presentation is a history of a stressful event in a young woman. Gonadotropin and estrogen levels are in the low to low normal range. In addition, rigorous exercise such as jogging or ballet or diets that can result in excessive weight loss may lead to the development of chronic anovulation. An extreme form of weight loss with chronic anovulation is seen in **anorexia nervosa.** In this condition, the hypothalamic dysfunction is severe and may involve other pituitary hormones as well. Anorexia nervosa is characterized by the development in a young woman of amenorrhea with associated severe weight loss, distorted attitudes toward eating and weight gain, self-induced vomiting, extreme emaciation, and distorted body image. Amenorrhea in anorexia nervosa can precede, follow, or appear coincidentally with the loss in body weight. During successful therapy, gonadotropin changes recapitulate those observed during normal puberty.

Chronic debilitating diseases such as end-stage kidney disease, cancer, or malabsorption syndrome are believed to lead to development of hypogonadotropic hypogonadism via a hypothalamic mechanism.

Treatment of chronic anovulation due to hypothalamic disorders includes reversal of the stressful situation or correction of weight loss if appropriate. Estrogen replacement therapy to induce and maintain normal secondary sexual characteristics and to prevent osteoporosis is recommended in women who do not desire pregnancy, and exogenous gonadotropin therapy is indicated when pregnancy is desired.

Pituitary Tumors

Disorders of the pituitary can lead to the estrogen-deficient form of chronic anovulation by at least two mechanisms—direct interference with gonadotropin secretion by lesions that either obliterate or interfere with the gonadotrope cells (chromophobe adenomas; Sheehan's syndrome) or inhibition of gonadotropin secretion in association with excess prolactin (prolactinoma). **Pituitary tumors** comprise approximately 10% of all intracranial tumors and may secrete no hormone or one or more hormones.

Prolactinomas can be divided into microadenomas (< 10 mm in diameter) and macroadenomas (> 10 mm). Prolactin excess is associated with low levels of LH and FSH and constitutes a specific subgroup of hypogonadotropic hypogonadism. One-tenth or more of amenorrheic women have increased levels of serum prolactin, and more than half of women with both galactorrhea and amenorrhea have elevated prolactin levels. The amenorrhea in this disorder is most often associated with decreased or absent estrogen production, but prolactin-secreting tumors may on occasion be associated with normal ovulatory menses or chronic anovulation with estrogen present. Most prolactin-secreting adenomas grow slowly, and some cease growth after attainment of a certain size. The increased frequency of diagnosis of prolactin-secreting adenomas is probably due to several factors, including increased awareness, improved radiographic detection methods, and the development of radioimmunoassays for prolactin. However, since in older autopsy series a 9–23% prevalence of pituitary adenomas was observed in asymptomatic women, the clinical and prognostic significance of small microadenomas remains to be established. When tumors of any size are associated with symptoms of amenorrhea or galactorrhea, however, therapy should be considered, and when visual field defects or severe headaches are present, neurosurgical evaluation is mandatory. In the latter half of pregnancy, prolactin-secreting tumors may expand, leading to headaches, compression of the optic chiasm, and blindness. Therefore, prior to induction of ovulation for the purposes of achieving pregnancy, it is mandatory to exclude the presence of a pituitary tumor by CT scanning or MRI.

Large pituitary tumors such as **chromophobe adenomas**—whether or not hyperprolactinemia is present—are likely to be associated with deficiency of hormones in addition to gonadotropins.

Craniopharyngiomas, thought to arise from remnants of Rathke's pouch, account for 3% of intracranial neoplasms, occur most frequently in the second decade of life, and may extend into the suprasellar region. A large percentage of these tumors calcify and can be diagnosed by conventional skull films. Patients often present with sexual infantilism, delayed puberty, and amenorrhea due to gonadotropin deficiency. Craniopharyngioma may also result in impaired secretion of TSH, ACTH, growth hormone, and vasopressin.

Panhypopituitarism may occur spontaneously, may result from surgical or radiation treatment of pituitary adenomas, or may develop after postpartum hemorrhage (Sheehan's syndrome). The latter patients exhibit characteristic clinical manifestations, including failure to lactate or ovulate, loss of sexual hair, hypothyroidism, and adrenal insufficiency.

EVALUATION OF AMENORRHEA

A general scheme for the evaluation of women with amenorrhea is presented in Figure 21–1. In the initial examination, special attention should be given to three features: (1) degree of maturation of the breasts, the pubic and axillary hair, and the external genitalia; (2) the current estrogen status; and (3) the presence or absence of a uterus. All women with amenorrhea should be assumed to be pregnant until proved not to be. Even when the history and physical examination are not suggestive of pregnancy, it is prudent to exclude pregnancy by measuring urinary hCG. Once this is done, the cause of amenorrhea can frequently be diagnosed on the basis of the history and physical examination.

For example, Asherman's syndrome is suggested by a history of prior curettage in a woman who previously menstruated. In women with clear-cut primary amenorrhea and sexual infantilism, the essential differential diagnosis is between gonadal dysgenesis and hypopituitarism. In addition, the diagnosis of gonadal dysgenesis (Turner's syndrome) or anatomic defects of the outflow tract (müllerian agenesis, testicular feminization, and cervical stenosis) is frequently suggested on the basis of physical findings. When a specific cause is suspected, it is appropriate to proceed directly to confirm the diagnosis (such as obtaining a chromosomal karyotype or measurement of plasma gonadotropins). It is also useful to measure serum prolactin levels during the initial evaluation.

Estrogen status is evaluated by determining whether the vaginal mucosa is moist and rugated and if the cervical mucus can be stretched and shown to "fern" upon drying. If these criteria are indeterminate, a progestational challenge is indicated—most often, administration of 10 mg of medroxyprogesterone acetate by mouth once or twice daily for 5 days or 100 mg of progesterone in oil intramuscularly. If estrogen levels are adequate (and the outflow tract is intact), menstrual bleeding should occur within 1 week after stopping the progestin. If withdrawal bleeding occurs, the diagnosis is chronic anovulation with estrogen present, usually due to polycystic ovarian disease.

If no withdrawal bleeding occurs, the nature of the subsequent workup is dependent on the results of the initial prolactin assay. If plasma prolactin is elevated or if galactorrhea is present, CT or MRI of the pituitary sella should be undertaken to screen for prolactin-producing micro- or macroadenomas.

When plasma prolactin is normal in the woman who does not develop withdrawal bleeding after progestin administration, measurement of plasma gonadotropins is required. If gonadotropin levels are elevated, the diagnosis is ovarian failure. If gonadotropins are in the low or normal range, the diagnosis is either hypothalamic-pituitary disorder or anatomic defect. As indicated previously, the diagnosis of anatomic defects of the outflow tract is usually suspected or established on the basis of the history and physical findings. When the physical findings are not clear-cut, it is useful to administer cyclic estrogen plus progestin (1.25 mg of oral conjugated estrogens per day for 3 weeks with 10 mg of medroxyprogesterone acetate added for the last 5–7 days of estrogen treatment) followed by 10 days of observation. If no bleeding occurs, the diagnosis of Asherman's syndrome or another anatomic defect of the outflow tract is confirmed. If withdrawal bleeding occurs following the estrogen-progestin combination, the diagnosis of chronic anovulation with estrogen absent (functional hypothalamic amenorrhea) is suggested. Radiologic evaluations of the pituitary and hypothalamus should be performed if the history or physical examination is suggestive—for fear of overlooking a pituitary-hypothalamic tumor, since the diagnosis of functional hypothalamic amenorrhea is one of exclusion.

ABNORMAL UTERINE BLEEDING

Abnormal uterine bleeding can frequently be evaluated and diagnosed with a thorough history and physical examination and minimal testing. Ovulatory cycles are characterized by regular, cyclic, predictable menses. Intervals range from 25 to 34 days, and most women bleed 3–8 days with a total blood loss of 30–80 mL. **Menorrhagia** is cyclic menstrual bleeding that is excessive in duration or amount. It may be secondary to anatomic uterine abnormalities such as leiomyoma or uterine polyps but may also be associated with endometrial hyperplasia due to the unopposed estrogen secretion associated with chronic anovulation.

Oligomenorrhea is bleeding or light spotting that occurs at intervals longer than 35 days. **Metrorrhagia (polymenorrhea)** is bleeding that occurs at irregular intervals, while **menometrorrhagia** is excessive and prolonged bleeding at frequent and irregular intervals.

In the evaluation of abnormal uterine bleeding, it is important to ascertain the sequence of bleeding intervals and in that way to determine if the patient is ovulatory. For example, a woman may bleed every 2 weeks and have ovulatory cycles. Upon careful questioning, she may describe uterine bleeding for 4–5 days every 28 days preceded by breast tenderness and dysmenorrhea and episodes of bleeding that occurs intermenstrually. This type of bleeding is probably due to uterine disease such as uterine polyps or leiomyoma. Oligomenorrhea or **polymenorrhea** (intervals of bleeding less than 21 days apart) are most often associated with anovulation.

The anovulatory endometrium (with absence of luteal progesterone) is in a chronically estrogen-stimulated proliferative state. This thickened tissue bleeds irregularly and sheds incompletely. A history of missed menses followed by spotting associated with the onset of lower quadrant pain is typical of ectopic pregnancy, and β-hCG measurement and vaginal sonography should confirm the diagnosis.

The physical examination must exclude chronic disease, the presence of thyroid abnormalities, obesity, hirsutism, or signs of Cushing's syndrome. A careful pelvic examination is done to exclude obvious sources of bleeding such as an incomplete abortion, endometrial polyp (Figure 21–4), leiomyoma, uterine or cervical cancer, foreign body, or vaginitis.

Appropriate laboratory testing includes sensitive pregnancy testing when indicated, a complete blood count to evaluate for anemia, and an endometrial biopsy to rule out endometrial carcinoma or hyperplasia. A recent Papanicolaou smear is essential to rule out cervical carcinoma. In certain circumstances with severe bleeding, coagulation or clotting studies may be indicated.

Treatment

Uterine leiomyomas or endocervical polyps are removed surgically. Polyps or small pedunculated submucosal leiomyomas can be located by hysteroscopy and removed. Large mural myomas are treated by hysterectomy or myomectomy in women who wish to preserve reproductive function (Figure 21–5).

In treating dysfunctional uterine bleeding due to anovulation, it is important to first stabilize the endometrium before allowing a controlled bleeding episode. This can be accomplished by several methods. On an outpatient basis, administration of high-dose combined estrogen-progestin

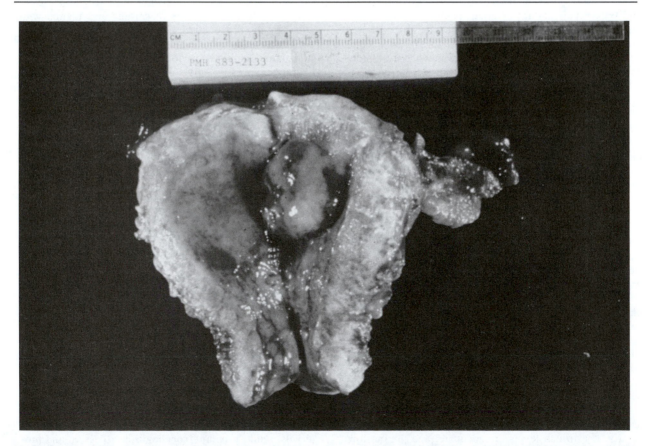

Figure 21–4. Hysterectomy specimen showing endometrial polyp in the fundus. (Courtesy of University of Texas Southwestern Pathology Department.)

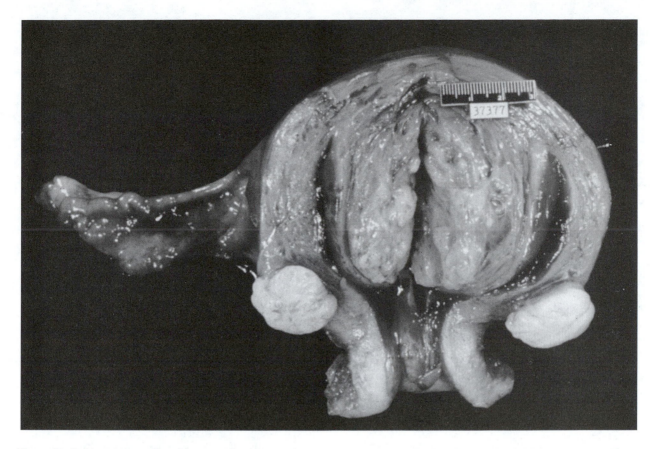

Figure 21–5. Hysterectomy specimen revealing large submucosal leiomyoma and smaller mural leiomyoma. (Courtesy of University of Texas Southwestern Pathology Department.)

oral contraceptives is usually successful in stopping bleeding. One pill is given 3 times daily for 7 days. Bleeding usually ceases, and then either withdrawal bleeding is allowed or the patient continues to take one oral contraceptive pill for 21 days and is then allowed to withdraw. Progestin therapy for 10 days will result in relatively complete sloughing of the endometrial lining and is useful in the estrogen-primed individual. For patients with severe bleeding, anemia, or other medical disorders, intravenous conjugated estrogens may be used to stabilize a denuded endometrium. Conjugated estrogens in a dose of 25 mg intravenously every 6 hours for up to 24 hours will cause

estrogen-stimulated growth and repair of a raw denuded lining. It is then necessary to allow for a controlled bleeding episode, as with the use of oral contraceptive pills. In patients who continue to bleed despite medical therapy, D&C is necessary to control bleeding and for tissue diagnosis.

Anovulation is frequently a chronic problem, and long-term therapy is essential. If contraception is not needed, cyclic medroxyprogesterone acetate, 10 mg daily for the first 10 days of each month, will allow for scheduled bleeding. Low-dose oral contraceptives provide both contraception and endometrial stabilization.

SUGGESTED READINGS

Carr BR, Wilson JD: Disorders of the ovary and female reproductive tract. Chapter 118 in: *Harrison's Principles of Internal Medicine,* 10th ed. Petersdorf RG et al (editors). McGraw-Hill, 1983.

Speroff L, et al: *Clinical Gynecologic Endocrinology and Infertility,* 3rd ed. Williams & Wilkins, 1983.

Yen SSC: Neuroendocrine regulation of the menstrual cycle. Hosp Pract (March) 1979;14:84.

Gold JJ, et al: *Gynecologic Endocrinology.* Harper & Row, 1980.

22

Hirsutism & Virilization

The clinical presentation of androgen excess in women can be highly variable. Patients may present with cosmetically disturbing hirsutism or acne, mild disturbances in menstrual function, infertility, dysfunctional uterine bleeding, or frank virilization.

Hirsutism in women is excessive growth of hair in specific androgen-sensitive areas of the body such as the face, lower back, chest, buttocks, areolae, inner thighs, linea alba, external genitalia, and pubis. It is usually a benign condition. **Hypertrichosis** is coarseness of the hair of the face, trunk, and extremities. This is non-sexual hair growth occurring with conditions such as anorexia nervosa, certain neoplastic conditions, or drug ingestion. **Virilization** is the combination of hirsutism plus clitoral enlargement, deepening of the voice, temporal hair loss, and loss of female body contour (Figure 22–1). Virilization is a more serious disorder and may indicate the presence of a tumor or steroidogenic enzyme deficiency (especially if congenital sexual ambiguity is present).

There is great racial variation in numbers of hair follicles present and thus amount of hair growth. The gynecologic patient from a Mediterranean background may have genetic influences for moustache and coarse leg hair growth. Treatment is the same as for hirsutism in general, yet results are frequently disappointing.

Factors influencing the presentation of androgen excess include (1) the amount and biologic activity of androgen production, (2) target tissue sensitivity, (3) the rate of androgen metabolism, and (4) the plasma concentration of androgen-binding proteins.

SOURCES OF ANDROGEN ACTION & METABOLISM

To understand the development of hirsutism and virilization, one must review androgen metabolism and action. Androgens are C_{19} steroids that stimulate male secondary sexual characteristics, promote masculinization of secondary sexual characteristics, promote nitrogen retention, and bind with high affinity to androgen receptors. Types of androgens and their relative potencies are listed in Table 22–1. Testosterone, androstenedione, and dehydroepiandrosterone are secreted in the female from ovarian and adrenal sources. The ovarian androgens are primarily androstenedione and testosterone, secreted by the ovarian stroma and theca cells. The principal androgens produced from the zona reticularis of the adrenal cortex are dehydroepiandrosterone (DHEA) and DHEAS, the sulfated form of DHEA. The relative contributions of androgens from the ovary and adrenal vary with the phase of the menstrual cycle or pathologic condition. Normally, about 250–300 μg of testosterone is produced per day in women (in contrast to 6000 μg/d in men). Approximately 50% of testosterone in the body is from glandular secretion and about 50% from peripheral conversion of androstenedione. Up to 3 mg/d of androstenedione is produced—half from the ovary and half from the adrenal—of which approximately 14% is converted to testosterone in the liver, skin, blood, and skeletal muscle by the action of 17-ketosteroid reductase. Androgen action in target tissue such as the hair follicle is mediated by dihydrotestosterone, which is derived from testosterone by the enzyme 5α-reductase. A major metabolite of dihydrotestosterone, androstanediol glucuronide, is also produced peripherally, and in one series of hirsute women it was the hormone most consistently elevated in the plasma. The total daily production of testosterone in normal women yields a plasma concentration of 30–35 ng/dL, which exists in bound and unbound (free) forms. Normally, about 1% of testosterone is free or unbound. About 80% is bound to testosterone-binding globulin (TeBG), also called sex hormone-binding globulin (SHBG); 20% to albumin; and 1% to transcortin. TeBG binding capacity can be decreased by elevated androgen levels or by obesity, which alters the hormone metabolic clearance rate. If one assumes that testosterone bound to TeBG is biologically inactive while free testosterone is active, a decreased TeBG concentration will result in an increased free testosterone level.

The clinical finding of androgen excess, with its resultant hirsutism or other manifestations, can be mediated by overproduction of androgens or androgen precursors, an decrease in TeBG, or an increase in enzymatic activity or androgen receptor in hormonally responsive tissues.

BIOLOGY OF HUMAN HAIR GROWTH

Embryonic hair follicles develop at about 8 weeks of gestation as derivatives of the epidermis. This solid col-

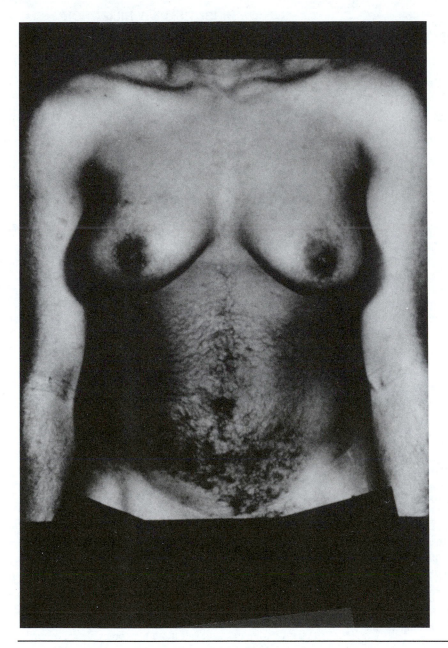

Figure 22–1. Loss of female body contour and severe hirsutism in female with virilizing tumor.

umn of cells proliferates downward, to be surrounded by a cluster of dermal cells, the dermal papilla. The number of hairs per unit area of skin is determined by genetic factors, with the number of hairs fixed in embryonic life. Men and women have about the same number of hairs. The three types of hair in humans are (1) lanugo—fine, short hairs covering the body of the fetus and newborn; 2) vellus—fine, short, nonpigmented "peach fuzz"; and (3) terminal—long, coarse, pigmented, and hormone-responsive hairs, like that found on the scalp and in stimulated sexual hair areas. Villus hair may be converted to terminal hair with androgen stimulation—an example is male beard growth at puberty.

Hair grows in cycles of alternating activity and inactivity, and this can account for the lengthy treatment times necessary in the treatment of hirsutism. The phases are **anagen** (growth), **catagen** (rapid involution), and **telogen** (resting or shedding).

Table 22–1. Relative potencies of androgens.

Types	Relative Potency
Preandrogens	
Dehydroepiandrosterone	3
Androstenedione	10
True androgens	
Testosterone	100
Dihydrotestosterone	200
Androgen metabolite	
Androstanediol glucuronide	0

CLINICAL EVALUATION OF ANDROGEN EXCESS

The goal of the physician in the evaluation of androgen excess is to rule out life-threatening disorders such as adrenal or ovarian neoplasms and to determine the source of excess androgen production as a guide to therapy. A history of pubertal onset of hirsutism and menstrual aberrations may be a clue to **polycystic ovarian disease** or adult-onset **congenital adrenal hyperplasia.** A family history of hirsutism may be indicative of ethnic or "idiopathic" hirsutism, with elevations of 5α-reductase or androgen receptors in the skin. Patients with congenital adrenal hyperplasia may also have a significant family history. A history of rapid onset and progression of hirsutism with the appearance of virilization may indicate tumor development.

Physical examination should be thorough, both to help quantitate the degree of hirsutism or virilization and to look for other clinical findings related to androgen excess. One should search for acanthosis nigricans associated with polycystic ovary disease; insulin resistance, abdominal striae, and truncal obesity associated with **Cushing's syndrome;** and galactorrhea associated with **hyperprolactinemia.** A careful abdominal and pelvic examination to palpate adrenal or adnexal masses is essential. Abdominal imaging by ultrasonography, CT scanning, or MRI is used to document palpable masses or to locate a mass when the index of suspicion is high.

Laboratory studies can aid in the diagnosis (Figure 22–2). Regardless of the plasma DHEAS or testosterone levels, a tumor must be ruled out if the history is one of rapid onset of symptoms. Other possible tests include 17α-hydroxyprogesterone and ACTH stimulation tests in patients with short stature, a family history of congenital adrenal hyperplasia, or severe hirsutism or in those who are unresponsive to standard therapy. A rapid rise in 17α-hydroxyprogesterone with ACTH stimulation is associated with 21-hydroxylase deficiency. The overnight dexamethasone suppression test is useful to rule out Cushing's syndrome.

CAUSES OF HIRSUTISM & VIRILIZATION

Idiopathic Hirsutism

In idiopathic hirsutism, excessive male pattern hair growth occurs in women who have normal ovulatory menstrual cycles and normal serum levels of androgens. However, when the production of androgens by peripheral tissues such as skin—hair follicles and sebaceous glands—is studied, there may appear to be increased activity of the enzymatic conversion of testosterone to dihydrotestosterone by the action of 5α-reductase (Figure 22–3). Investigators have measured distal metabolites of dihydrotestosterone formation in hirsute women and have found them to be significantly elevated. Serum androstanediol glucuronide was elevated in 86% of hirsute women with normal menses, and the degree of elevation correlated with the degree of hirsutism.

Polycystic Ovarian Disease

Polycystic ovarian disease is often associated with increased androstenedione and testosterone secretion from the ovary and is the most common cause of androgen excess. Patients with polycystic ovarian disease usually give a history of peripubertal onset of increased hair growth and irregularity of menses. The hirsutism may or may not be progressive, and in occasional cases some evidence of virilization may be present. This history of peripubertal onset is essential for the diagnosis of polycystic ovarian disease, since a recent rapid progression of hirsutism or virilization requires a more intensive search for other causes of androgen excess, such as tumor formation. An elevated LH/FSH ratio aids in the diagnosis of polycystic ovarian disease but may be found in other states of androgen excess as well. A subset of polycystic ovarian disease is associated with acanthosis nigricans and insulin resistance, manifested by elevated fasting insulin levels and an exaggerated insulin response to an oral glucose load. In these patients, insulin appears to act in the ovary through various mechanisms to stimulate androgen production.

Hyperthecosis

Islands of luteinized theca cells in the ovarian stroma are pathognomonic for hyperthecosis. Androgen levels are usually higher in these patients than in those with polycystic ovarian disease, and there may be evidence of virilization. The history is similar to that of patients with polycystic ovarian disease, with onset of symptoms of androgen excess at puberty. The LH/FSH ratio is typically 1.0, as compared to the elevated LH/FSH ratio in classic polycystic ovarian disease. Most patients are anovulatory and fail to respond to clomiphene citrate for ovulation induction. The diagnosis is based on the history, the degree of virilization, and microscopic findings of stromal hyperthecosis at wedge resection of the ovary or oophorectomy if clinically indicated.

Androgen Secretory Tumors of the Ovary

Any history of rapid onset or progression of hirsutism or virilization should alert the clinician to the possibility

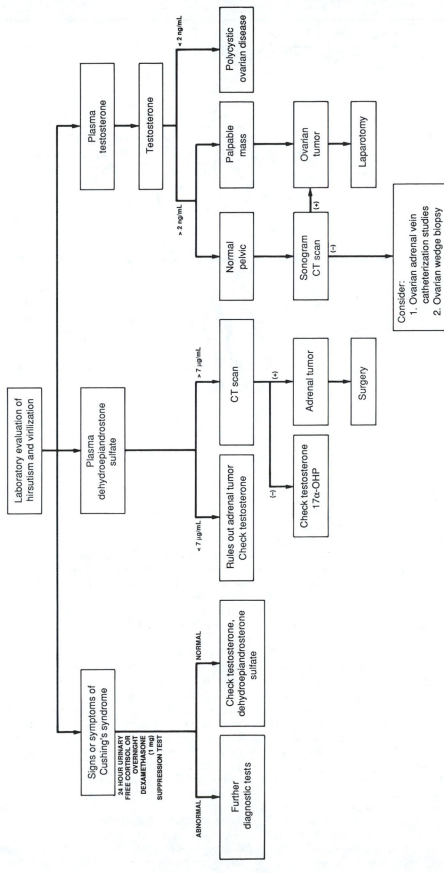

Figure 22–2. Flow chart for the evaluation of hirsutism and virilization. T = testosterone; DS = dehydroepiandrosterone sulfate; PCOD = polycystic ovarian disease; 17α-OHP = 17α-hydroxyprogesterone. (See text: adrenal androgen excess.)

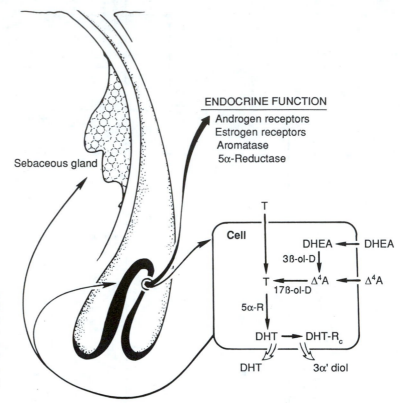

Figure 22–3. The pilosebaceous unit as an endocrine target as well as local modulation of endocrine micro-environments via enzymatic conversion of androgens to more potent androgen and to estrogens. Both DHEA and Δ^4 dione can be converted to testosterone within the hair follicle. 3β-ol-D, 3β-hydroxysteroid dehydrogenase; T, testosterone; 5α-R, 5α-reductase; DHT-r_c, dihydrotestosterone receptors.

of an ovarian tumor. Solid tumors of the ovary that have endocrine function occur infrequently, accounting for only about 3% of ovarian tumors, yet this figure may be due to underreporting or failure to account for the less than spectacular endocrine effects. It is difficult to attribute a specific endocrine activity to tumors of a particular cell type, as there may be great variations in the amount and type of hormone produced by a specific tumor. For instance, granulosa-theca cell tumors that usually secrete estrogens have been associated with virilization, and some Sertoli-Leydig cell tumors which usually secrete androgens have been associated with feminization.

Tumors of the ovary that are associated with hirsutism and virilization include thecoma, luteoma, hyperreactio luteinalis, Sertoli-Leydig cell tumors, hilar cell tumors, and, rarely, granulosa cell tumors. Hilar cell tumors are found in older women and may be small (1–3 cm) and not palpable. Lipoid cell tumors are thought to arise from adrenal rest cells, and some tumors are associated with clinical evidence of Cushing's syndrome. The incidence of malignancy is higher in this group and may range from 20% to 30%. Typically, these tumors are small.

Interestingly, after the primary androgen-secreting tumor has been removed, the masculine characteristics regress, except for voice changes, which remain deep and harsh. Some changes in body contour, clitoromegaly, and the degree of hirsutism will regress within months after

surgical removal of the tumor. Menstrual periods typically return within 3 months, and about 10% of patients become pregnant and deliver normal children.

Adrenal Enzyme Deficiencies

Congenital adrenal hyperplasia of adult onset (late-onset, "acquired") may be due either to 21-hydroxylase, 11β-hydroxylase, or 3β-hydroxysteroid dehydrogenase deficiency. In these deficiencies, reduction of cortisol production results in an increased release of ACTH from the pituitary, stimulation of adrenal steroidogenesis, and overproduction of C_{19} (androgenic) steroids. These autosomal recessive enzyme deficiencies may be difficult to distinguish from polycystic ovarian disease, since the clinical presentation is similar to that of polycystic ovarian disease, with postpubertal onset of hirsutism, menstrual dysfunction, and androgen excess. The prevalence of attenuated congenital adrenal hyperplasia among hirsute patients has been estimated to be 1.2–20%. Stimulation with ACTH results in measurable increases in 17α-hydroxyprogesterone levels and can help to distinguish these patients from those with polycystic ovarian disease.

Adrenal Androgen Excess

Clinical signs of androgen excess can occur with Cushing's syndrome. This may be due to central ACTH excess or pituitary adenoma (Cushing's disease). Other causes include ectopic ACTH production from tumors of the lung, thymus, or pancreas or ACTH-independent sources such as adrenal adenoma or carcinoma. Androgen excess results in glucocorticoid excess with concomitant increase in adrenal androgen production. Patients may present with obesity, menstrual disorders, hirsutism, virilization, or infertility and thus mimic the presentation of patients with polycystic ovarian disease. However, the onset and progression of symptoms may help to distinguish these patients from those with polycystic ovaries, as may the findings of "moon facies," abdominal striae, hypertension, and osteoporosis. Cortisol production is elevated in women with Cushing's syndrome, as evidenced by an elevated 24-hour urinary free cortisol test or failure of an 8 AM cortisol level to suppress after a 1 mg dose of dexamethasone given at 11 PM on the evening prior to the test.

Adrenal Adenoma or Carcinoma

Virilizing adrenal neoplasms in women are rare. The diagnosis of virilizing tumor is based on the clinical picture of hirsutism, amenorrhea, clitoromegaly (or other obvious signs of virilization), and markedly elevated serum levels of DHEA and DHEAS and elevation of urinary 17-ketosteroids. Cortisol and androstenedione may also be secreted in large amounts. Dexamethasone suppression usu-

ally fails to result in suppression of morning cortisol levels. CT or MRI scans usually detect clinically significant tumors (Figure 22–4). Only six rare cases of adrenal adenomas producing primarily testosterone have been reported. In these cases, urinary 17-ketosteroids were normal, testosterone levels were greatly elevated, and an adrenal tumor was confirmed on CT scan or at exploration.

Prolactin Excess

The association of galactorrhea with hirsutism and acne has been described. Hyperprolactinemia may be associated with elevations in DHEA and DHEAS, with peripheral conversion to biologically active androgens. Bromocriptine therapy may result in improvement of hirsutism in association with reduction of prolactin and androgen levels.

Drugs

Many drugs may induce increased hair growth, either hirsutism or hypertrichosis. Hirsutism is largely induced by drugs related to androgens or adrenal corticosteroids. Hypertrichosis is coarsening of hair on the face, trunk, and extremities and may be caused by phenytoin, diazoxide, minoxidil, streptomycin, hexachlorobenzene, cyclophosphamide, and danazol.

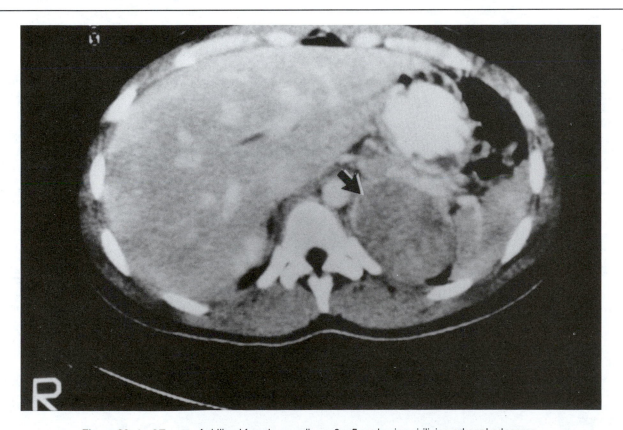

Figure 22–4. CT scan of virilized female revealing a 6 × 5 cm benign virilizing adrenal adenoma.

Alterations in Testosterone-Binding Globulin (TeBG)

Alterations in androgen levels and production can markedly change production levels of TeBG, resulting in higher levels of active androgens. Obesity and hyperthyroidism may also be associated with lowering of TeBG and hirsutism.

THERAPEUTIC APPROACHES TO ANDROGEN EXCESS

The therapeutic approach to androgen excess must be tailored to individual patients and etiologic origins. Adrenal and ovarian neoplasms are surgically removed, retaining reproductive integrity when possible. Thyroid disease and Cushing's syndrome are treated with appropriate therapy. Obesity is treated with simple weight loss programs, since a significant lowering in androgen levels following weight reduction has been documented. One must be aware, however, that transformation of vellus hair to terminal hair may be permanent, and hirsutism may be persistent despite resumption of ovulatory cycles.

Treatment of hirsutism falls into two main categories: medical and cosmetic. Medical therapy includes (1) therapy directed toward suppression of secretion of androgens by the ovary or adrenal, accomplished with oral contraceptives, glucocorticoids, and GnRH analogues; and (2) therapy with antiandrogenic agents that act at the level of the hair follicle or sebaceous glands. Cosmetic therapy such as plucking, waxing, shaving, depilatory creams, and electrolysis is frequently used in combination with medical therapy. Acne will often respond to a decrease in androgen levels with medical therapy and resultant decrease in androgen levels.

Medical Treatment

The ideal response to medical treatment is eradication of hirsutism, but alleviation of hirsutism is the more usual outcome. Treatment should be continued for 8–10 months before it is deemed ineffective. As the rate of hair growth increases in the summer, therapy may need to be continued longer before judgment is made. Electrolysis or depilatory therapy should be added to treatment regimens for patients who are quite concerned about their cosmetic appearance.

To adequately suppress ovarian sources of androgen production, as in polycystic ovarian disease, gonadotropin release must be inhibited. **Oral contraceptive pills** lower cyclic and basal levels of LH and cause an increase in TeBG, resulting in lower levels of biologically active testosterone. Oral contraceptives also increase the hepatic clearance of testosterone by inducing A-ring reductase ac-

tivity in the liver and are associated with a decline in DHEAS levels. One must be careful, however, not to select an oral contraceptive with an androgen-dominant progestational agent such as norgestrel in combination with a low dose of estrogen, as these pills have a higher androgenic potential than pills containing norethynodrel or ethynodiol diacetate.

Adrenal sources of androgen excess due to adult-onset adrenal hyperplasia are suppressed by glucocorticoid therapy to lower ACTH levels. **Prednisone,** 7.5–10 mg daily in divided doses, resulted in maximum suppression of androgens after 2 months of therapy. **Dexamethasone,** 0.5 mg at bedtime, inhibits nighttime surges of ACTH and is associated with less water retention than prednisone therapy. Morning cortisol levels should be maintained at about 2 μg/dL.

Antiandrogens are effective by interfering with androgen action at target sites. Drugs such as cyproterone acetate and spironolactone bind to the androgen receptor and competitively inhibit the binding of dihydrotestosterone. Because antiandrogens may in theory result in feminization of a male fetus, contraception is imperative during therapy.

Spironolactone is the major antiandrogen used in the United States. An aldosterone antagonist, spironolactone was originally used as a potassium-sparing diuretic for the treatment of mild hypertension. The main action of spironolactone is to compete with androgen for the androgen receptor. It also inhibits P-450 enzymes in steroid-producing cells, with a decrease in plasma androgens. Clinical response occurs with a dosage of 50–200 mg/d, and successful results are seen within 2–6 months. Following discontinuation of the medication, hirsutism may rapidly reappear. In patients who are unresponsive to spironolactone alone, the combination of spironolactone and oral contraceptives or dexamethasone may be useful.

Cosmetic Therapy

Depilatory creams may be superior to shaving as a mechanical method of hair removal, because the regrowing hair has a softer, subtle tip as opposed to the bristly stubble of shaven hairs. **Waxing** may allow a greater area of hair growth to be removed at one time, and, since regrowing hairs are in the anagen phase, no stubble results. Folliculitis and skin irritation may occur with these methods.

Electrolysis relies on destruction of the dermal papillae by electrical vibrations and effects permanent hair removal. This therapy should be delayed for 9–10 weeks following medical therapy to ensure synchronization of terminal hairs. Side effects include scarring, pigmentation, and the spread of condyloma and hepatitis with unsterilized instruments.

SUGGESTED READINGS

Abraham GE: Ovarian adrenal contribution to peripheral androgens during the menstrual cycle. J Clin Endocrinol Metabol 1974;39:430.

Knobil E et al: *The Physiology of Reproduction.* Raven Press, 1988.

Maroulis GB: Evaluation of hirsutism and hyperandrogenemia. Fertil Steril 1981;36:273.

Pittaway DE, Maxson WS, Wentz AC: Spironolactone in combination drug therapy for unresponsive hirsutism. Fertil Steril 1985;43:878.

Speroff L, Glass RH (editors): *Gynecologic Endocrinology and Infertility,* 4th ed. Williams & Wilkins, 1988.

Wiebe RH (editor): *Androgenology in Women. Seminars in Reproductive Endocrinology,* Vol 4, No. 2, 1986.

Yen SSC et al: *Reproductive Endocrinology, Physiology, Pathophysiology and Clinical Management,* 3rd ed. WB Saunders, 1991.

23

Endometriosis & Adenomyosis

ENDOMETRIOSIS

Endometriosis is a benign condition in which endometrial glands and stroma are found in extrauterine locations (Figure 23–1). The ovary is the most common primary site of endometriosis. The peritoneum of the posterior cul-de-sac, the uterosacral ligaments, the round ligaments, the oviducts and mesosalpinx, the peritoneum of the uterus, the anterior cul-de-sac, and the rectosigmoid colon are also frequently involved. Less commonly, the cecum, appendix, bladder, vagina, small bowel, lymph nodes, and omentum have foci of endometriosis. Endometriosis has rarely been seen in distant sites such as the umbilicus, laparotomy or episiotomy scars, the spinal canal, the lungs, and the heart. The incidence of endometriosis ranges from 5–15% of all premenopausal women. Endometriosis accounts for one-fourth of all gynecologic laparotomies and is present in 50% of women undergoing surgery for infertility. The average age is 28 years (range, 10–83 years), although 75% of cases occur in women between 25 and 50 years of age. There appears to be no racial preference.

Etiology

The etiology of endometriosis is not known. Sampson proposed a theory of transtubal regurgitation of menstrual blood and implantation of endometrium. Other theories have involved tissue metaplasia of coelomic epithelium and lymphatic or hematogenous spread of endometrium (extraperitoneal disease). Some investigators have suggested that endometriosis may be due to a decreased cellular immune response to endometrial antigens.

Association With Infertility

Endometriosis is often associated with infertility, but the mechanism is unclear. Possibilities include distortion of normal anatomy, adhesions involving the tubes and ovaries, and development of large ovarian endometriomas filled with bloody fluid ("chocolate cysts") that may destroy ovarian cortex. There is increased release or concentrations of prostanoids in the peritoneal fluid. Some investigators have reported increased concentrations of certain prostaglandins in the peritoneal fluid of women with endometriosis compared to control women. Prostaglandins may prevent conception by interfering with sperm and ovum transport, causing luteolysis, or by interfering with implantation. Cell-mediated cytotoxicity associated with an increased number of peritoneal macrophages in women with endometriosis may lead to increased destruction of sperm. Anovulation, a luteal phase defect, luteinized unruptured follicle syndrome, hyperprolactinemia, and increased pregnancy wastage have all been proposed to explain the association of infertility and endometriosis, but conclusive evidence has not been forthcoming.

Numerous classification schemes for endometriosis have been proposed. The recommended classification at present is that proposed by the American Fertility Society, revised in 1985 (Figure 23–2).

Clinical Findings

A. Symptoms and Signs: The history and physical examination frequently suggest the diagnosis. Patients complain of dysmenorrhea, dyspareunia (especially with deep penetration), infertility, rectal pain, premenstrual spotting, and backache. Pelvic tenderness with induration and nodularity of uterosacral ligaments is evident. The ovaries may be enlarged and tender. The uterus is frequently fixed in retroflexion. In patients with mild disease, the pelvic examination may be normal.

Laparoscopy has increased our ability to verify a suspected diagnosis of endometriosis. The usual findings are superficial brownish or blue-black raised lesions on the peritoneal surfaces. Older lesions are fibrosed and often puckered. Ovarian involvement includes endometriomas (chocolate cysts) or superficial surface involvement. Nonpigmented endometriotic lesions have recently been identified and characterized.

B. Laboratory Findings: Biopsy of the lesion confirms the diagnosis. A histologic finding of hemosiderin-laden macrophages is compatible with a diagnosis of endometriosis, which is confirmed by identifying the presence of endometrial glands and stroma. In the future, noninvasive diagnosis may be possible with the use of MRI or serum levels of CA-125.

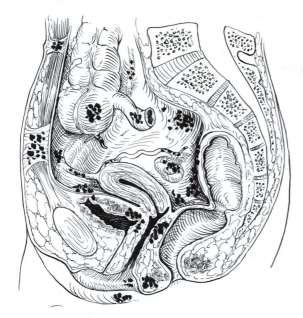

Figure 23–1. Common sites of endometriosis in decreasing order of frequency: (1) ovary, (2) cul-de-sac, (3) uterosacral ligaments, (4) broad ligaments, (5) uterine tubes, (6) uterovesical fold, (7) round ligaments, (8) vermiform appendix, (9) vagina, (10) rectovaginal septum, (11) rectosigmoid colon, (12) cecum, (13) ileum, (14) inguinal canals, (15) abdominal scars, (16) uterus, (17) urinary bladder, (18) umbilicus, (19) vulva, and (20) peripheral sites. (Reproduced, with permission, from Hacker NF, Moore JG: *Essentials of Obstetrics and Gynecology.* Saunders, 1986.)

Treatment
(Table 23–1)

It should be remembered that endometriosis is usually not "cured" until the menopause. Medical therapy or surgery should be considered suppressive or debulking procedures, since biopsy and electron microscopy of normal peritoneum often reveals evidence of endometriosis.

In the young, asymptomatic infertile patient with mild endometriosis, a period of observation or expectant therapy is indicated. During this time, a thorough evaluation of other causes of infertility is warranted. In a number of studies of infertile patients with mild endometriosis, pregnancy rates of up to 72% have been reported. Similar rates of conception with laser laparoscopy, conservative surgery at laparotomy, and medical therapy have been reported. If conception does not occur after a period of observation of 12–18 months, surgical therapy is then indicated. In the patient over 35 years of age, most investigators would proceed with medical or, more often, surgical therapy.

A. Medical Therapy: Pharmacologic suppression of ovulation may be indicated in the young symptomatic patient with mild to moderate endometriosis who does not desire pregnancy or in women who are also complaining of infertility. The purpose of pharmacologic therapy is to prevent ovulation and induce pseudomenopause, which results in temporary regression of endometriosis and atrophy of the lesions. There is usually a high rate of recurrence after treatment is stopped.

1. Estrogens–Continuous low-dose birth control pills or progestins may be the best therapy for mild to moderate endometriosis in women not desiring pregnancy. Most studies have not shown an increase in pregnancy rate with this treatment above that reported with expectant therapy alone. One of the side effects is breakthrough bleeding.

2. Danazol–Prior to the availability of the GnRH analogues (see below), danazol was the most commonly used form of medical therapy and is still an important mainstay of medical management. This isoxozole derivative of 17α-ethynyl testosterone has multiple sites of action, including the hypothalamus, pituitary gland, ovary, and endometrium, and results in anovulation, a reduced estrogenic environment, and atrophy and regression of foci of endometriosis. Danazol usually has a minimal effect on large endometriomas. The side effects include weight gain, edema, decreased breast size, acne, hirsutism, oily skin, and deepening of the voice. Following cessation of therapy, some symptoms may regress. Menorrhagia, headache, vaginitis, decreased libido, muscle cramps, and hot flashes may also occur. The optimal dosage is controversial, but most investigators recommend 800 mg/d (400 mg twice a day) for 6–9 months. Barrier contraception is usually recommended during therapy to protect against the rare occurrence of masculinization of a female fetus. Most patients report a significant decrease in pain during therapy. Some reports have indicated that 2 months of danazol therapy prior to conservative surgery simplifies the operation and is associated with an increased pregnancy rate. Danazol may be indicated postoperatively in patients with severe endometriosis if residual disease exists. The use of danazol as primary therapy in mild to severe disease results in pregnancy rates between 15% and 60%. In most studies comparing danazol therapy to surgical outcome, pregnancy rates are similar for mild to moderate endometriosis.

3. GnRH Analogues–These drugs, exemplified by leuprolide (Lupron), produce "medical oophorectomy" and have minimal side effects compared to danazol. They have been administered via subcutaneous, nasal, and depot injection routes in patients with mild to moderate endometriosis. Preliminary investigations suggest that this method of therapy causes regression of endometriosis, but it is too early to state that higher pregnancy rates can be expected.

B. Surgical Therapy:

1. Laparoscopy–Laparoscopic surgery for mild and occasionally moderate endometriosis is growing in popularity. Both unipolar and bipolar electrocautery techniques have been used. More recently, the CO_2, argon, and Nd:YAG lasers have been advocated because they offer increased flexibility with the potential of reduced tissue damage by vaporizing endometriotic lesions and adhesions. There are insufficient data to suggest that increased pregnancy rates occur following laser treatment when compared to electrocautery or medical therapy.

THE AMERICAN FERTILITY SOCIETY
REVISED CLASSIFICATION OF ENDOMETRIOSIS

Patient's Name _____ Date _____

Stage I   (Minimal) – 1-5
Stage II (Mild)   – 6-15
Stage III (Moderate) – 16-40
Stage IV (Severe)   – >40

Laparoscopy _____ Laparotomy _____ Photography _____

Recommended Treatment _____

_____

Total _____   Prognosis _____

	ENDOMETRIOSIS	<1 cm	1-3 cm	>3 cm
PERITONEUM	Superficial	1	2	4
	Deep	2	4	6
OVARY	R Superficial	1	2	4
	Deep	4	16	20
	L Superficial	1	2	4
	Deep	4	16	20

	POSTERIOR CULDESAC OBLITERATION	Partial	Complete
		4	40

	ADHESIONS	<1/3 Enclosure	1/3–2/3 Enclosure	>2/3 Enclosure
OVARY	R Filmy	1	2	4
	Dense	4	8	16
	L Filmy	1	2	4
	Dense	4	8	16
TUBE	R Filmy	1	2	4
	Dense	4*	8*	16
	L Filmy	1	2	4
	Dense	4*	8*	16

*If the fimbriated end of the fallopian tube is completely enclosed, change the point assignment to 16.

Figure 23–2. Revised American Fertility Society Classification of Endometriosis, 1985. Fertil Steril 1985;43:351, 1985. (Reproduced with permission of the publisher.)

Table 23–1. Treatment of endometriosis.
(AFS = classification of the American Fertility Society.)

A. Observation and expectant therapy (AFS mild)
B. Pharmacologic (AFS mild to moderate)
   1. Continuous low-dose contraceptives or progestins
   2. Danazol
   3. GnRH analogues
C. Surgical (AFS mild to severe)
   1. Laparoscopy (laser or electrocautery)
   2. Conservative laparotomy
   3. Radical laparotomy (total abdominal hysterectomy and
      bilateral salpingo-oophorectomy)
D. Treatment of infertility (AFS mild to severe)
   1. Intrauterine insemination (IUI)
   2. Gamete intrafallopian transfer (GIFT)
   3. In vitro fertilization and embryo transfer (IVF-ET)

2. Laparotomy–Laparotomy is indicated for patients with large adnexal masses; for women with symptoms refractory to medical management; for women with severe endometriosis not currently desiring pregnancy; and for endometriosis associated with significant pelvic adhesions, tubal obstruction, or leiomyomas. The patient's age and informed preference and the training of the surgeon are also important factors in the choice of medical versus surgical therapy.

The principles and goals of conservative surgery via laparotomy include gentle handling of tissue and use of microscopic technique when possible. Foci of endometriosis are removed by excision, fulguration (electrocautery), or vaporization (laser). As much ectopic tissue is removed as possible (debulking or cytoreduction). When ovarian involvement is present, it is important to excise and fulgurate the lesions, conserving as much ovarian cortex as possible and protecting the ovarian blood supply. With unilateral severe disease, unilateral oophorectomy may be indicated. Appendectomy should be performed if the appendix is involved. Presacral neurectomy is performed in patients with severe midline pain. Pre- and postoperative danazol or leuprolide may be indicated with severe endometriosis and where residual disease involves the ureters, bladder, and bowel.

Total abdominal hysterectomy and removal of both ovaries is usually indicated for debilitating, symptomatic endometriosis when childbearing is no longer desired. In most instances of severe endometriosis—and in all cases with residual disease—it is usually wise to remove both ovaries. The use of hormonal therapy after the procedure must be considered if significant residual disease exists: Continuous progestins for 6 months to 1 year will help control vasomotor symptoms and promotes the regression of endometriosis. Thereafter, estrogens may be substituted, though one must be alert to the possibility of recurrences. If all disease is removed, estrogen replacement may be started immediately postoperatively.

C. Management of Infertility: (See also Chapter 24.) For the treatment of infertility in patients with endometriosis, intrauterine insemination (IUI) has been advocated for patients with minimal to mild disease. There is no conclusive evidence that higher conception rates are achieved

by this method than those reported with expectant or medical therapy. Gamete intrafallopian transfer (GIFT) has been suggested for mild to moderate disease when the tubes are uninvolved. Not enough studies are available, however, to evaluate the effectiveness of this procedure. In vitro fertilization and embryo transfer (IVF-ET) has recently been proposed as therapy for infertility in endometriosis, usually when significant tubal disease exists. Rates of recovery of oocytes and fertilization are not affected by the presence or degree of endometriosis. However, the pregnancy rates of some groups are lower if moderate to severe endometriosis is present.

ADENOMYOSIS

Adenomyosis is the finding of endometrial glands and stroma within the myometrium on histologic examination of the uterus. Grossly, the uterus may appear enlarged, softened, and "boggy." The cut surface may reveal a loss of definition between the endometrial and myometrial borders. Small cystic lesions are frequently seen in the uterine wall.

Microscopically, islands of endometrial glands and stroma are found throughout the myometrium (Figure 23–3). These glands are hormonally responsive, with some degree of proliferative and secretory changes occurring with the menstrual cycle.

Hyperplastic changes are evident in the myometrium surrounding the ectopic islands. Bleeding may occur within the glands causing hemorrhagic cystic areas within the myometrium. Hemosiderin-laden macrophages are evident within the muscularis.

Clinical Findings

Patients with adenomyosis usually present with worsening dysmenorrhea or an increase in the amount of menstrual flow. Some patients may be relatively symptom-free, with adenomyosis as an incidental histologic finding on a hysterectomy specimen.

Adenomyosis should be suspected in women—primarily over age 30 years—who complain of menorrhagia and dysmenorrhea. Pelvic examination done premenstrually may reveal a tender, slightly enlarged and softened uterus. The examiner must also rule out pregnancy, the presence of submucosal myomas, endometrial hyperplasia or neoplasia, and the finding of pelvic endometriosis. MRI may prove to be a noninvasive means of diagnosing adenomyosis preoperatively, but the only certain means of diagnosis is by histologic examination of the uterus at hysterectomy.

Treatment

Numerous hormonal regimens have been tried for treatment of adenomyosis, but none have been successful. The use of oral contraceptives may even worsen the condition. Analgesics may be used to provide relief in patients desiring pregnancy or in women nearing the menopause. Hysterectomy is curative and is the treatment of choice in women who do not wish to preserve childbearing capacity.

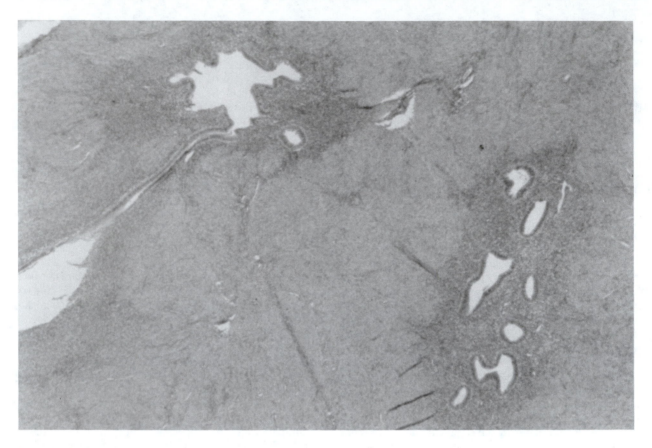

Figure 23–3. Photomicrograph of adenomyosis with islands of endometrial glands and stroma deep within the myometrium. (Courtesy of University of Texas Southwestern Pathology Department.)

SUGGESTED READINGS

Barbieri RL, Ryan KJ: Danazol: Endocrine pharmacology and therapeutic application. Am J Obstet Gynecol 1981;141:453.

Guzick DS, Rock JA: A comparison of danazol and conservative surgery for the treatment of infertility due to mild or moderate endometriosis. Fertil Steril 1983;40:580.

Malinak LR, Wheeler JM: Endometriosis. In: *Infertility: Diagnosis and Treatment.* Aimen J (editor): Springer-Verlag, 1984.

Management of endometriosis: ACOG Technical Bulletin No. 85, 1985.

Martin DC: CO_2 laser laparoscopy for the treatment of endometriosis associated with infertility. J Reprod Med 1985;30:409.

Meldrum DR: Management of endometriosis with gonadotropin-releasing hormone agonists. Fertil Steril 1985;44:581.

Olive DL, Haney AF: Endometriosis-associated infertility: A critical review of therapeutic approaches. Obstet Gynecol Surv 1986;41:538.

Pelvic endometriosis: Semin Reprod Endocrinol 1985;3:No. 4.

Pittaway DE, Fayez JA: The use of CA-125 in the diagnosis and management of endometriosis. Fertil Steril 1986;46:790.

Schmidt CL: Endometriosis: A reappraisal of pathogenesis and treatment. Fertil Steril 1985;44:157.

24

Female Infertility

Involuntary infertility affects about 15% of couples, or approximately 11 million reproductive-age people in the United States. Infertility is defined as the inability of a couple to conceive a child after 1 year of unprotected intercourse. Women who are over the age of 35 or who have a known cause for infertility are evaluated earlier. With the tendency of more couples to delay childbearing and the increasing incidence of sexually transmitted diseases and anovulation in older women, the true prevalence of infertility has increased. Infertility may have a profound emotional impact upon affected couples. Feelings of frustration, anger, depression, grief, and anxiety are common and should be dealt with appropriately. Referrals to psychologists or psychiatrists are sometimes necessary to help couples deal with the emotional aspects of infertility.

The most common causes of infertility are listed in Table 24–1. The basic infertility evaluation is aimed at evaluating couples for these disorders.

Thorough evaluation of the infertile couple should reveal one or more causes of failure to conceive in 90% of cases. Motivated couples who comply with therapeutic guidelines can expect a 50–60% chance of fertility.

THE BASIC INFERTILITY EVALUATION

The infertility evaluation serves to (1) determine the causes of infertility, (2) provide the couple with recommended treatment protocols, (3) assess the anticipated success rates of recommended therapy, and (4) educate the couple about their specific disorder and available alternatives of treatment or adoption. A certain percentage of patients are merely seeking diagnosis and do not intend to pursue therapy or cannot afford recommended diagnostic tests or therapy. Some couples proceed with adoption, while others comply with specific medical or surgical therapy.

History & Physical Examination

A thorough workup is based on an extensive history and physical examination. Both the woman and her partner should be present for the initial evaluation and consultation, so that the most accurate information can be obtained. The woman should be asked about the timing of her pubertal development and menarche. The menstrual history should include cycle length, duration and amount of bleeding, and associated dysmenorrhea or premenstrual symptoms. A history of regular, cyclic, predictable menses is consistent with ovulation, while a history of amenorrhea or menometrorrhagia may point toward anovulation or some uterine disorder. The patient should be asked about dyspareunia or severe dysmenorrhea that may be linked to endometriosis. A history of pelvic inflammatory disease, ruptured appendix or other abdominal surgical disease, or past use of an intrauterine device may be associated with tubal disease. A history of galactorrhea may be a clue to hyperprolactinemia, while a history of pubertal-onset hirsutism or rapidly worsening adult hirsutism may indicate polycystic ovarian disease or other disorders of androgen excess. A thorough past medical and family history should be obtained. Sexual, social, and psychologic issues should be explored. It is essential to obtain and interpret information about prior infertility evaluation and therapy.

A thorough physical examination is necessary to help define factors that may lead to infertility. Acne, oily skin, and hirsutism may be due to androgen excess. Thyroid enlargement, acanthosis nigricans, the presence of galactorrhea, skin pigmentation, abdominal striae, surgical scars, or abnormalities in body weight should be carefully sought. The degree of estrogenization of the vagina (the presence of pink, moist, rugose vaginal cells and the percentage of superficial cells on vaginal wall scrape) and the quality and quantity of cervical mucus should be noted. The cervix must be examined for exposure to diethylstilbestrol or prior cervical surgery, cryocautery, or laser treatment. On pelvic examination, one should search for the presence of cervical, uterine, or adnexal tenderness, masses, and mobility. The size and contour of the uterus and adnexa should be recorded.

Men should be questioned about prior fertility, general health, medications, and any history of genital surgery, trauma, or infection. Factors that may suggest lowering of sperm numbers and motility include a history of drug or alcohol abuse, frequent hot tub baths, constricting underwear or excessive physical or mental stress, chronic fatigue, or too-frequent coitus.

The physical examination of men should focus on the degree of secondary sexual development and the presence

Table 24–1. Common causes of infertility.

Factor	Incidence (%)	Basic Investigations
Male	40	Semen analysis, postcoital test
Ovulatory	15–20	Basal body temperature, serum progesterone, endometrial biopsy
Cervical	5–10	Postcoital test
Uterine tubal	30	Hysterosalpingography, laparoscopy
Peritoneal	40	Laparoscopy
Unexplained	10	All

of gynecomastia, hypospadias, cryptorchidism, varicocele, or hydrocele.

Documentation of Ovulation

A history of regular, cyclic, predictable menses with some degree of molimina is presumptive evidence of ovulation. Basic laboratory evaluation for documentation of ovulation begins with a menstrual chart that records the first day of menstrual bleeding as cycle day 1. This chart can be used to document the daily basal body temperature (BBT) (Figure 24–1). A special basal thermometer is designed for this purpose, with the ovulatory ranges of temperatures expanded for greater accuracy. The temperature is taken in bed each morning at approximately the same time before eating or drinking, smoking, or brushing the teeth. Episodes of fever or illness, coitus, vaginal spotting,

or bleeding should be recorded. The menstrual temperature charts are brought to the office at each visit so that copies can be kept in the patient's chart. The charts are interpreted as follows:

(1) Proliferative phase temperatures are usually less than 98 °F (36.7 °C).

(2) At the time of ovulation, some patients exhibit a slight decrease in temperature. (In a typical 28-day cycle, this generally occurs on cycle day 13 or 14.)

(3) Luteal phase temperatures rise 0.6–0.8 °F owing to the thermogenic effects of progesterone. The duration of the luteal phase is timed from the midcycle drop in temperature to the onset of the next menses. The luteal phase should last 11–16 days.

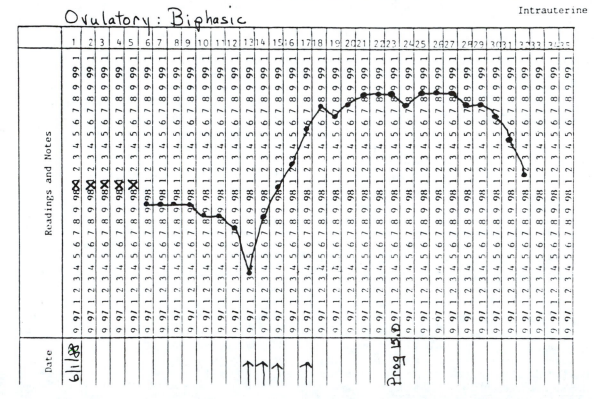

Figure 24–1. Typical ovulatory basal body temperature chart. Arrows denote timing of intercourse.

If an approximate time of ovulation can be predicted from the temperature charts, a schedule of coitus should be encouraged every 36–48 hours for 3–4 days prior to and 2–3 days after the temperature rise. More reliable methods of ovulation prediction are available. Commercial kits can be purchased without prescription to determine urinary luteinizing hormone and can be used to monitor the midcycle LH surge that triggers ovulation. Intercourse should occur 12–24 hours after the onset of an LH surge.

Progesterone is the main secretory product of corpus luteum. A luteal phase progesterone level of 3–4 ng/mL or higher is indicative of ovulation. However, levels at the middle of the luteal phase are ideally greater than 10 ng/mL. Levels below these figures may signify inadequate luteal phase or other hormonal abnormality.

Biopsy of the endometrium taken 2–3 days prior to the expected onset of menses can also be used as evidence of ovulation. Progesterone will stimulate secretory changes within the endometrium, and specific histologic criteria have been established to date the endometrium. Using these criteria, luteal phase insufficiency is said to exist if development of the endometrium lags behind the cycle day in relation to the onset of the LH surge or subsequent menstrual period by more than 2 days in at least two cycles.

Semen Analysis

A semen specimen should be examined in all couples presenting with a complaint of infertility. The specimen is obtained by masturbation into a sterile collection cup. Forty-eight to 72 hours of sexual abstinence is recommended prior to analysis. The sample should be delivered to the laboratory within 1 hour after collection. Normal values for semen analysis established by the World Health Organization are set out in Table 24–2.

Postcoital Test

The postcoital test can provide information about the quality and receptivity of ovulatory cervical mucus. Midcycle mucus should be watery, thin, clear, and acellular and should exhibit a phenomenon called spinnbarkeit, or stretchability. Owing to the increased estrogen levels at the time of ovulation, the salt content of cervical mucus is increased, and this leads to the development of a fern pattern when midcycle cervical mucus dries on a microscope slide.

The test should be scheduled for the expected date of ovulation, and cervical mucus is examined within 8 hours after coitus. Cervical mucus is removed from the cervix with an Angiocath or the hub of an insulin syringe and examined for spinnbarkeit, ferning, and the presence of progressive motile sperm. The finding of more than 20 motile sperm per high-power field usually correlates with a normal semen analysis and a pregnancy rate somewhat higher than if the count is less than that number; however, abnormal postcoital tests have been recorded in fertile patients, and recent studies have shown little predictive value of the test. The absence of sperm—or the presence of nonmotile or "quivering" sperm without progressive motility—is considered to be an abnormal test calling for further evaluation.

Hysterosalpingography

Tubal damage may occur secondary to pelvic inflammatory disease, septic abortion, IUD use, ruptured appendix, or uterine or tubal surgery. Hysterosalpingography, consisting of injection of a radiopaque dye into the uterus under fluoroscopic vision, is performed 3–6 days after cessation of menses. A normal examination performed under fluoroscopy demonstrates a normal uterine cavity and prompt filling and spill of contrast dye from the uterine tubes into the peritoneal cavity.

Diagnostic Laparoscopy

If the history suggests endometriosis or pelvic inflammatory disease—or if an abnormal hysterosalpingogram is obtained or if no cause for the infertility can be found—diagnostic laparoscopy can be performed to directly view the pelvic organs. Adhesions, endometriosis, distal tubal occlusion, and ovarian cysts are common findings in infertility patients. Chromotubation (injection of methylene blue dye through the cervix) may be performed to document tubal patency. Recent advances in operative laparoscopy have meant many surgical procedures for correction of infertility that were routinely done via exploratory laparotomy can now be successfully accomplished by laparoscopy.

MANAGEMENT OF INFERTILITY

Disorders of Ovulation

Disorders of ovulation account for 10–15% of all infertility problems. Pharmacologic therapy for anovulatory women has been a dramatic advance in reproductive endocrinology. The physician must first rule out disorders of the pituitary, ovary, uterus, adrenal, and thyroid. If lack of ovulation is the only problem causing infertility, persistent couples can now expect their chances of conceiving to almost match the rate found in the general population.

A. Clomiphene Citrate: The first ovulatory agent to become available for general clinical use was clomiphene citrate, which remains the safest, the most broadly effective, and the most widely used of several agents now available.

Clomiphene citrate is an oral nonsteroidal drug whose

Table 24–2. Classification of normal semen standards.[1]

Assay	Normal Values
Volume of ejaculate	≥ 2 mL
Sperm density	≥ 20 million/mL
Sperm motility	≥ 50% with forward progression
Total motile sperm	≥ 40 million
pH of seminal fluid	7.2–7.8
White cells in seminal fluid	None

[1]Data from World Health Organization.

structure resembles that of the synthetic drugs with estrogenic effects such as diethylstilbestrol (DES). Clomiphene citrate has only a weak estrogenic as well as an antiestrogenic effect, and it is thought to act by releasing pituitary FSH and LH. The rise in FSH and LH leads to the recruitment, growth, and maturation of ovarian follicles. Clomiphene citrate does not stimulate ovulation directly—it initiates a sequence of events that are physiologic features of a normal cycle. It is administered as a 50-mg tablet on cycle days 5 through 9, resulting in a rise in serum LH and FSH. Ovulation occurs between the 15th and 20th days in successful cycles.

Treatment is started with a dose of 50 mg and is increased—if ovulation does not occur—to a maximum of 200 mg/d.

The major indications for use of clomiphene citrate are infertility due to polycystic ovarian disease and luteal phase deficiency. The patients most likely to respond are those who display some evidence of endogenous estrogen activity, such as occasional spontaneous menses or withdrawal bleeding in response to a progestogen challenge such as medroxyprogesterone acetate. A hypoestrogenic patient usually will not ovulate following a trial of clomiphene citrate.

The timing of ovulation and the adequacy of response to clomiphene citrate are determined by midcycle evaluations of cervical mucus, monitoring with home urinary LH kits, or ultrasound documentation of follicular development and collapse of a dominant follicle. A midcycle serum progesterone level or endometrial biopsy done on the 27th or 28th day of the cycle may be used to document ovulation and to test the adequacy of the luteal phase. Failure to ovulate after adequate doses can occasionally be corrected by the addition of human chorionic gonadotropin (hCG), 5000–10,000 IU intramuscularly, following identification of a ripe follicle by ultrasound. Side effects of clomiphene citrate are listed in Table 24–3.

Seventy to 80 percent of properly selected anovulatory women will be made to ovulate with large enough doses of clomiphene. Pregnancy rates per cycle are similar to those of normal ovulatory women. As long as an adequate response occurs and there are no unusual side effects, clomiphene therapy is continued usually for 36 months. If pregnancy has not occurred by that time, other causes of infertility are reassessed.

B. Menotropins (Human Menopausal Gonadotropin, HMG): HMG is obtained by extraction from the urine of postmenopausal women. The commercial preparation (Pergonal) contains 75 IU of FSH and 75 IU of LH. The drug is inactive orally and must be given by intramuscular injection.

Because of the expense and the need for careful clinical and laboratory monitoring as well as the potential for serious side effects, patients should be properly selected for management with this drug. HMG is indicated to induce ovulation in patients who fail to ovulate with clomiphene, those with hypopituitarism, or those selected for "superovulation." Pregnancy rates with superovulation with hMG followed by insemination with washed husband's sperm may approach 20–30%.

Injections of hMG are typically begun on the third day of a spontaneous cycle or following withdrawal bleeding induced by medroxyprogesterone acetate, or at any time if the woman has hypogonadotropic hypogonadism and is amenorrheic. The initial dosage is one or two ampules (150–300 IU) per day until about the seventh day. Assessment is made of follicular size by ultrasound and serum estradiol levels, and the dosage of hMG is adjusted accordingly. Adequate follicular stimulation is achieved usually by 7–14 days of continuous administration of hMG. With the rising estradiol levels (produced by the developing follicles), cervical mucus will become abundant and clear, with spinnbarkeit and a fernlike pattern upon drying. At the time of follicular maturity, estradiol levels will approach 200–300 pg/mL per mature follicle, and ultrasound measurements of follicular diameter will reach about 16–20 mm. At this time, ovulation is initiated by an injection of 5000–10,000 IU of human chorionic gonadotropin (hCG) given 24–48 hours after the last hMG injection. HCG is biologically and structurally similar to LH and will simulate the midcycle LH ovulatory surge. Ovulation usually occurs 32–36 hours after hCG administration.

When the estradiol rises above 2000 pg/mL or when appreciable ovarian enlargement occurs, hCG should be withheld. This will prevent excessive ovarian hyperstimulation, and the woman usually will not ovulate. Hyperstimulation is associated with ovarian enlargement, abdominal distention, and weight gain. In severe cases, a critical condition develops with ascites, pleural effusion, electrolyte imbalance, and hypovolemia, with hypotension and oliguria. Treatment consists of hospitalization, bed rest, and intravenous fluids.

About 90% of properly selected women can be made to ovulate with hMG. The pregnancy rate is 25% per cycle of those who ovulate. The occurrence of multiple pregnancies averages about 20%, with 15% of those being twins and 5% triplets or more. HMG may be repeated for 3–6 cycles. If pregnancy does not occur by that time, treatment should be suspended for 2–3 months and the case carefully reviewed.

C. Combined Clomiphene and HMG: The combined use of clomiphene and hMG offers several advantages over the use of either drug alone. Clomiphene in doses of 100 mg daily on days 3–7 is followed by one to two ampules of hMG. Monitoring and timing of hCG injection is similar to that of hMG alone. Comparable results for hMG alone can be anticipated, but using smaller

Table 24–3. Side effects of clomiphene citrate.

Vasomotor flushes	10%
Multiple pregnancies	7%
Abdominal distention, bloating	5.5%
Breast discomfort	2%
Nausea and vomiting	2.2%
Headache	1.3%
Visual disturbances	1%
Dryness or loss of hair	0.3%

amounts of the latter drug materially reduces the cost of treatment. Although monitoring of the effects of the combined drugs must be just as stringent as with hMG, there seems to be less evidence of excessive stimulation.

D. Follicle-Stimulating Hormone (Urofollitropin): Women with polycystic ovary disease often exhibit high levels of LH while the level of FSH remains normal or slightly below normal. The treatment of choice for polycystic ovary disease is usually clomiphene; however, if ovulation or pregnancy has not occurred after an adequate clinical trial, an appropriate next choice of therapy is with hMG or with urofollitropin (FSH). Each ampule of urofollitropin contains 75 IU of FSH and less than 1 IU of LH. Urofollitropin is administered intramuscularly in doses of one or two ampules daily and monitored as described for hMG. About 80% of patients with polycystic ovary disease taking FSH will ovulate. It is estimated that 10–40% of patients receiving FSH will become pregnant as long as no other fertility factors are present. The risks, multiple pregnancy rates, and rate of hyperstimulation appear to be similar to those associated with hMG.

E. Gonadorelin (Gonadotropin-Releasing Hormone, GnRH; Factrel): Pulse administration of GnRH results in pituitary release of FSH and LH and results in ovulation in women with anovulation. The best candidates for GnRH therapy are women with hypogonadotropic hypogonadism. The advantage of GnRH over hMG is that ovarian hyperstimulation syndrome rarely, if ever, occurs with a dose of GnRH of 1–5 μg every 90 minutes. Multiple follicular development may be achieved by higher doses at more frequent intervals, eg, 10 μg every 60 minutes.

To accommodate to the short half-life and the physiologic pulsatile nature of its secretion, GnRH is best administered intravenously or subcutaneously by pulsatile infusion pumps. These computerized, programmable pumps deliver desired doses at predetermined intervals. Follicular development is monitored by ultrasound and is usually complete by 10–14 days. Ovulation occurs spontaneously as a result of endogenous LH surge.

F. Bromocriptine: Routine fertility evaluation should include serum prolactin measurement, since 10–15% of anovulatory women will be found to have excessive levels. No more than 50% of those will have galactorrhea. In women with elevations in serum prolactin and amenorrhea, bromocriptine in doses of 2.5–7.5 mg usually results in ovulatory cycles.

Cervical Factor

Cervical mucus can be a significant barrier to sperm penetration and should be assessed. In ovulatory women with abnormal cervical mucus manifested by an abnormal postcoital test, it is necessary to rule out "poor timing" by proper timing with LH urinary testing or careful review of the BBT. If a postcoital test is abnormal as a result of immobile or "quivering" sperm, antisperm antibody testing should be performed on both partners. Treatment for inadequate cervical mucus includes conjugated estrogens, 0.325 mg daily on cycle days 3–12, or bypassing the cer-

vix by treatment with intrauterine insemination (IUI) with the husband's sperm.

Tubal Factor

Thirty percent of women with infertility are found to have tubal disease by hysterosalpingography (Figure 24–2) or at the time of laparoscopy. Pelvic inflammatory disease or pelvic adhesions from prior surgery or endometriosis can cause impairment of uterine tube patency. Treatment of tubal factor infertility is primarily surgical. With severely damaged uterine tubes, therapy with in vitro fertilization may have a higher success rate than microsurgical repair of the tube. Tubal patency and the success of fertility treatment depend on the degree of tubal dilation, the thickness of the tubal wall, and the degree of intratubal damage. Pregnancy rates range from 15–40% depending on the severity of tubal damage.

Pelvic adhesions may interfere with fertility by obstructing ovum pickup or distorting ovarian-tubal proximity. Adhesions are carefully excised, using microsurgical techniques and meticulous hemostasis.

Endometriosis is thought to impair fertility by interfering with tubal motility or by causing macrophage activation, tubal obstruction, or a luteal phase defect. Therapy is individualized and consists of removal of peritoneal implants by excision, cautery, or laser, lysis of adhesions, and drainage of endometriomas. Medical therapy is used for patients with mild disease or following surgery for suppression of residual disease. Oral contraceptives, progestins, danocrine, and GnRH analogues have all been used with success.

Uterine Factors

Anatomic defects such as intrauterine adhesions (Asherman's syndrome), polyps, or submucosal leiomyomas may impair fertility. Treatment consists of hysteroscopic removal except for large submucosal leiomyomas, which need to be removed at laparatomy. Congenital uterine malformations such as a uterine septum may be more frequently associated with habitual abortion. Septa may be corrected hysteroscopically or by uterine metroplasty.

Male Factor

Selection of the appropriate therapy for male factor infertility depends on the cause of the defect. Azoospermia is often untreatable. An elevation in serum FSH signifies loss of functional germinal tissue, and artificial insemination by donor (AID), or adoption, is recommended. Obstruction of the ejaculatory ducts or retrograde ejaculation into the bladder is associated with normal FSH levels. Sperm are recovered from the urine in men with retrograde ejaculation.

Oligospermia is defined as less than 20 million sperm per milliliter and is usually idiopathic but may be associated with some form of testicular insult, such as trauma, infection, or varicocele. Varicocele is abnormal dilatation of the pampiniform plexus of the internal spermatic vein. Twenty to 40 percent of infertile men are found to have

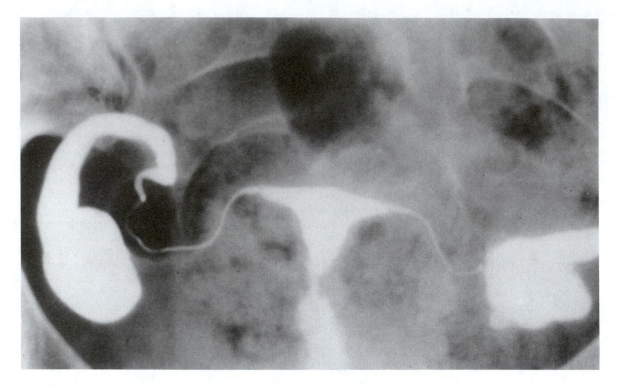

Figure 24–2. Hysterosalpingogram revealing severe bilateral hydrosalpinx.

some degree of varicocele. The mechanism of infertility is thought to be an elevation in testicular temperature or venostasis. Semen quality improves in 50–90% of men treated with surgical ligation or radiologic occlusion of the internal spermatic vein. However, conception rates are not higher than 25–50%, and more investigation is required before this therapy can be widely recommended.

Any acute or chronic illness or stress should be treated and semen analysis repeated to determine its accuracy. *The routine use of thyroid hormone, clomiphene citrate, or testosterone to improve oligospermia should be condemned, since paradoxic sperm suppression occurs.*

Unexplained Infertility

Approximately 10% of all couples presenting with infertility will have no identifiable cause for their inability to conceive. There is a substantial rate of treatment-independent conception in these couples (30% within the first year and a cumulative pregnancy rate of 60% at the end of 3 years). It is still important to review the initial evaluation and determine if additional studies should be done. If the couple remains infertile after a period of observation, empiric therapy with ovulation induction, intrauterine insemination, or assisted reproductive technologies may be instituted.

Assisted Reproductive Technologies

Women with damaged or occluded uterine tubes and couples with long-standing infertility who have failed by other methods can be helped by in vitro fertilization (IVF) (Figure 24–3), gamete intrafallopian transfer (GIFT), zygote intrafallopian transfer (ZIFT), or tubal embryo transfer (TET). Ovum retrieval is performed after hormonal stimulation of the ovaries with hMG and a GnRH agonist, so that multiple oocytes can be obtained for fertilization. Most IVF groups obtain oocytes by transvaginal ultrasound-guided oocyte aspiration. Rarely is laparoscopy or mini-laparotomy used nowadays for ovum retrieval for IVF. Oocytes are incubated with sperm, and after fertilization occurs embryos are transferred into the uterus—approximately 48 hours after aspiration (Figure 24–3).

In the GIFT procedure, oocytes are retrieved either transvaginally or via laparoscopy. The ova and sperm are then injected directly into the uterine tubes via a catheter placed laparoscopically. ZIFT and TET are a combination procedure in which oocytes are aspirated transvaginally, fertilized, and the zygotes or embryos placed within the tubes at time of laparoscopy—usually 24–48 hours after aspiration.

Success rates vary with these techniques and range from 10–33%.

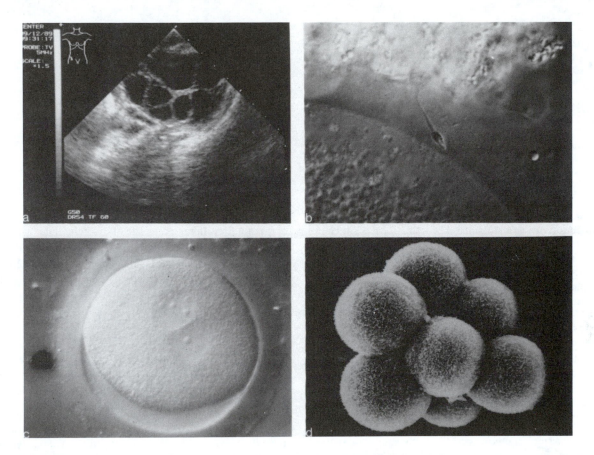

Figure 24–3. Sequence of events in in vitro fertilization. **A:** Ultrasound guided aspiration of gonadotropin stimulated ovaries. **B:** Fertilization of aspirated ovum with sperm. **C:** Pronuclei stage of embryo. **D:** Eight-cell stage prior to uterine embryo transfer.

SELECTED READINGS

Abraham GE: Ovarian adrenal contribution to peripheral androgens during the menstrual cycle. J Clin Endocrinol Metabol 1974;39:430.

Knobil E et al: *The Physiology of Reproduction.* Raven Press, 1988.

Maroulis GB: Evaluation of hirsutism and hyperandrogenemia. Fertil Steril 1981;36:273.

Pittaway DE, Maxson WS, Wentz AC: Spironolactone in combination drug therapy for unresponsive hirsutism. Fertil Steril 1985;43:878.

Wiebe RH (editor): Androgenology in women. Semin Reprod Endocrinol 1986;4:No. 2.

Yen SSC, Jaffe RB: *Reproductive Endocrinology: Physiology, Pathophysiology, and Clinical Management,* 2nd ed. Saunders, 1986.

25

Menopause

Menopause is the cessation of menses, or the last menstrual period in a woman's life. The transitional period between ovulatory cycles and the menopause, during which progressive loss of ovarian function occurs, is known as the **climacteric,** or **perimenopausal period.** The term "postmenopausal" or "menopausal" refers to the time after the menopause. During this time, a woman usually experiences various endocrine, somatic, and psychologic changes.

The median age at menopause is 50–51 years, and the average life expectancy of women in the USA at birth is 79 years; therefore, approximately one-third of a woman's life is spent after the menopause. The average age at menopause does not appear to be related to the age at onset of menarche, social or economic conditions, race, parity, height, or weight. The age at menopause may be affected by smoking, however. Cigarette smokers experience earlier spontaneous menopause than do nonsmokers.

ENDOCRINE CHANGES ASSOCIATED WITH AGING

Endocrine changes characteristic of the female climacteric are caused primarily by decreased ovarian estrogen secretion. This cessation of ovarian estrogen secretion is caused, in turn, by a loss of ova and associated follicles, mainly by atresia, a process that begins in fetal life at about 20 weeks of gestation and continues until menopause. The ovary of the postmenopausal woman is reduced in size, weighing less than 2.5 g, and is wrinkled ("prunelike"). The cortical area is reduced in size because of loss of ova and follicular cells, and the stromal cells thus predominate. After menopause, the levels of plasma gonadotropins increase, with levels of FSH rising to a greater extent than those of LH. The higher concentration of FSH than of LH in postmenopausal women may be due to loss of suppression of FSH by follicular inhibin (a small protein hormone), or it may be that FSH is cleared less rapidly than LH because of the higher sialic acid content of FSH. Estrogen and C_{19} steroid levels are significantly lower in the postmenopausal years than during reproductive life. After menopause, extraglandular formation of estrone becomes the dominant pathway for estrogen synthesis. The principal sites of extraglandular aromatization of androstenedione are adipose tissue, bone, muscle, skin, and brain. Because a major site of extraglandular estrogen synthesis is adipose tissue, the rate of conversion or extent of aromatization increases with obesity as well as with age, liver disease, and hyperthyroidism.

CLINICAL SYMPTOMATOLOGY OF THE MENOPAUSE

The term "menopausal syndrome" denotes a spectrum of symptoms that may occur during the 4- to 6-year period surrounding menopause. These symptoms include hot flushes or flashes (vasomotor instability), dryness and atrophy of the urogenital epithelium and vagina, and probably other related symptoms including psychologic changes such as insomnia, mood shifts, irritability, and nervousness. Vasomotor symptoms and urogenital atrophy are clearly related to the deficiency of estrogen.

Hot Flushes

It is estimated that 30–80% of perimenopausal and postmenopausal women experience hot flushes. Approximately 40% of these women suffer symptoms severe enough to cause them to seek medical care. Hot flushes are characterized by a sensation of warmth and heat followed by profuse sweating. The frequency, duration, and intensity of vasomotor symptoms vary widely, but in most cases they begin to subside 4–6 years after menopause.

The pathogenesis of hot flushes is unclear. Recent studies suggest a close relationship between the hot flush and pulses of LH secretion (Figure 25–1). Hot flushes do occur in some women after hypophysectomy, however, and in women treated with GnRH analogues, suggesting that the menopausal syndrome is not due solely to increased levels or pulses of gonadotropin. Furthermore, estrogen replacement, which alleviates these symptoms, does not fully suppress gonadotropin levels. Interestingly, women with primary ovarian failure (eg, gonadal dysgenesis), in whom gonadotropin levels are high, do not experience hot flushes unless they are first treated with estrogens and estrogen therapy is then withdrawn. Thus, it appears that central nervous centers, such as the hypothalamus, are more likely to be the site for the trigger of vasomotor symptoms. Although estrogen treatment of hot

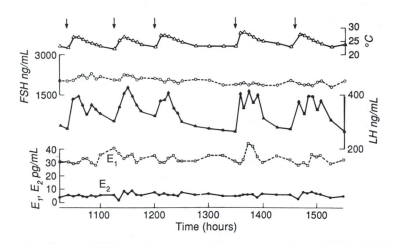

Figure 25–1. Skin temperature of the finger and serum gonadotropin, estrone (E_1) and estradiol (E_2) levels in a woman with frequent hot flushes. Note the close correlation of skin temperature rises and pulsatile LH release with the occurrence of subjectively experienced hot flushes (arrows). (Reproduced, with permission, from Meldrum DR et al: Gonadotropins, estrogens, and adrenal steroids during menopausal hot flash. J Clin Endocrinol Metab 1980;50:687.)

flushes usually is effective and relief is prompt, not all women are relieved of these symptoms by estrogen. Furthermore, in all investigations in which the effectiveness of estrogen to relieve vasomotor symptoms was evaluated, a high degree (25%) of relief of symptoms was found also with placebo therapy. Thus, some of these symptoms may not be due to estrogen deficiency alone.

Genitourinary Atrophy

Diminished estrogen production also leads to atrophy of the vagina and symptoms of atrophic vaginitis. Atrophic vaginitis is characterized by itching, discomfort, burning, dyspareunia, and sometimes vaginal bleeding as the epithelium thins. Estrogen deficiency may also lead to loss of uterine support, with subsequent uterine descensus. Other symptoms of estrogen deficiency include urinary urgency and stress incontinence, dysuria, and urinary frequency. Estrogen treatment is effective in relieving the symptoms of atrophic vaginitis and other symptoms of estrogen deficiency of the lower urinary tract.

Other Symptoms

After the menopause, symptoms such as depression, anxiety, fatigue, and irritability appear to increase. It is not certainly known whether treatment with estrogen affects these symptoms directly or whether estrogen therapy prevents hot flushes and promotes improved sleeping patterns. Others have found that administration of estrogen to women with severe hot flushes was associated with a significant reduction in the symptoms of anxiety, irritability, and insomnia and improvement in memory when compared to control subjects. It is suggested that reduction of hot flushes during sleep results in an improvement in sleep quality and thus prevents symptoms of chronic sleep disturbances. Other investigators have observed a decrease in sleep latency and an increase in rapid eye movement sleep with estrogen therapy.

OSTEOPOROSIS

Osteoporosis is the most important health hazard associated with postmenopausal hypoestrogenism. Osteoporosis is defined as loss of structural support in trabecular bone, chiefly of the axial skeleton. Bone loss after the menopause appears to proceed at a rate of 1–2% per year. In Caucasian women, there is an estimated loss of 50% of bone mass by the age of 80 years. Thus, if left untreated, osteoporosis is one of the most devastating diseases of aged women. It has been estimated that 25% of all women over age 60 years have radiologic evidence of vertebral crush fractures. Such fractures (and their complications) in the elderly are a major cause of death and disability (Figure 25–2).

Estrogen deficiency is believed to be a major cause of bone loss in women. Estrogen treatment attenuates height loss, improves calcium balance and bone density, and reduces the number of vertebral, wrist, and hip fractures in young castrated and postmenopausal women. Dual-photon absorptiometry and CT scanning of bone density are used most commonly to evaluate vertebral bone mass.

The major factors known to increase the risk of osteoporosis include white or Oriental race, low body weight, hypoestrogenism, early menopause, a positive family history for osteoporosis, diet low in calcium and vitamin D, diet high in caffeine, phosphate, alcohol and protein, cigarette smoking, and a sedentary life style. Postmenopausal women require a daily intake of 1500 mg of elemental calcium to maintain calcium balance. This requirement is usually not met in the average American diet. It has been demonstrated that reduced amounts of endogenous estrogen levels are correlated with increased urinary calcium excretion. Estrogen is believed to increase bone turnover, though the mechanism is not clear. Estrogen receptors have been found in bone, and estrogen may therefore act directly. Estrogen deficiency may also lead to increased sensitivity to parathyroid hormone in bone, whereas the sensitivity in other organs such as the kidney and intestine remains the same. The end result would be increased bone

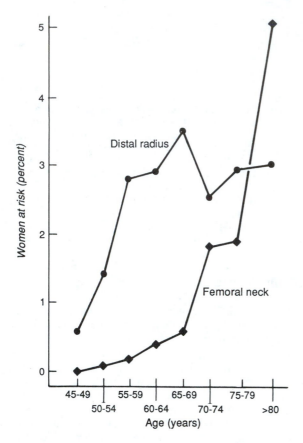

Figure 25–2. Relationship between the incidence of fractures of the distal radius and femoral neck and the ages of women. (Reproduced, with permission, from Aitken JM: Bone metabolism in postmenopausal women. Page 99 in: Beard RJ [editor]: *The Menopause: A Guide to Current Research and Practice.* MTP Press, 1976.)

resorption and mobilization of calcium without increased urinary or intestinal excretion of calcium.

Recent studies indicate that early and long-term estrogen replacement in women undergoing early menopause (due to surgical or natural causes) is beneficial. Bone loss, as measured by bone biopsy and indirect techniques, was prevented by a delay in bone resorption, and an actual decrease in the rate of development of fractures was reported in women who ingested estrogens. Thus, it appears that if estrogen replacement is to be of greatest benefit, replacement should be initiated before serious loss of bone density occurs.

RISKS & BENEFITS OF ESTROGEN REPLACEMENT

Cardiovascular Effects

There appears to be no evidence for an increased incidence of thromboembolism or stroke in women receiving estrogen replacement therapy, nor does there appear to be an increase in blood pressure. The evidence favors the view that estrogen therapy reduces the risk of coronary heart disease. The mechanism whereby coronary heart disease is reduced in women taking estrogen is by a favorable lipoprotein pattern, ie, a lowering of cholesterol, lowering of low-density lipoproteins (LDL), and elevation of high-density lipoproteins (HDL). Both increased levels of LDL and decreased levels of HDL correlate positively with the risk for coronary heart disease—the opposite of what is seen in estrogen users.

Gallbladder Disease

Investigators with the Boston Collaborative Drug Surveillance Study reported a slight increase in the development of gallbladder disease in postmenopausal women taking conjugated estrogens. Because estrogen therapy causes an increase in cholesterol concentration in bile, this relationship most likely is the cause of the increased predisposition for development of gallstones in these women.

Breast Disease

The breast is a target organ of estrogen, and some breast tumors are found to be estrogen-responsive. For these and other reasons, there has been great concern that estrogen treatment of postmenopausal women might contribute to the development of benign and malignant breast disease. In most studies of the literature pertaining to the relationship between breast cancer and estrogen use, there are reports both for and against a relationship between dose and duration of estrogen therapy and the development of breast cancer. Based on currently available data, it appears that long-term use of estrogen in small doses does not increase the risk of breast cancer. Even so, however, estrogen therapy should not be instituted if there is preexisting malignant breast disease and should be discontinued if breast cancer develops.

Endometrial Cancer

Evidence exists that estrogen treatment or increased amounts of endogenously produced estrogen in postmenopausal women are associated with an increased incidence of endometrial adenocarcinoma (see Chapter 30). It is now known that postmenopausal women with the constitutional features commonly associated with endometrial cancer—ie, aging and obesity—are those who produce the most estrogen in extraglandular sites. Increased endogenous estrogen formation occurs in these women because the extent of conversion of plasma androstenedione to estrone in extraglandular sites increases with aging, obesity, and liver disease.

Numerous studies have concluded that the risk of developing endometrial cancer in unopposed estrogen use is seven times higher and the risk is both dose-related and increases with duration of treatment. However, there is no evidence of increased mortality—probably because the added cancers are of low-grade malignancy and perhaps because it is difficult to separate low-grade endometrial adenocarcinoma from various forms of endometrial hyperplasia.

Because unopposed estrogen use in the postmenopausal woman has clearly been associated with an increased incidence of endometrial hyperplasia and endometrial cancer, many investigators and physicians have advocated that women in whom the uterus is present should also receive 10–13 days of progestogen to oppose the effect of estrogen on the uterus. The addition of progestogens to both continuous and cyclic estrogen regimens is associated with a decreased incidence of endometrial hyperplasia and endometrial cancer. With loss of ovarian function, there is a decrease in HDL cholesterol and an increase in LDL cholesterol, and estrogen treatment tends to reverse this trend. In contrast, progestogen treatment also leads to increased LDL and decreased HDL, both of which are definite risk factors for coronary heart disease. This effect appears to be dependent upon the potency, dose, and duration of therapy of the progestin. Addition of oral micronized natural progesterone in a dosage of 200 mg/d for 10 days of each treatment cycle does not appear to influence HDL cholesterol or its subfractions. Micronized progesterone may be an alternative to the synthetic progestins used currently. Continuous daily treatment with both an estrogen and a progestogen has also been advocated by some, though the alterations in lipids need to be addressed more closely.

Other Cancers

There appears to be no increased risk of developing cancer of the ovary, cervix, uterine tubes, vagina, or vulva in women receiving long-term postmenopausal estrogen replacement therapy.

THERAPEUTIC RECOMMENDATIONS

The estrogen preparations recommended for oral use are natural estrogens, eg, conjugated estrogens prepared from pregnant mares' urine or micronized 17β-estradiol. Estrogen acts on target tissues after the free hormone enters the cell by simple diffusion and thence becomes bound to a specific receptor in the nucleus. Thereafter, the estrogen-receptor complex binds with nuclear chromatin and directs messenger RNA synthesis and eventually protein synthesis. The metabolic fate of the estrogens is variable—eg, 17β-estradiol in micronized form is converted largely to estrone before reaching target tissues. But the primary hormone ultimately associated with the estrogen receptor is a potent one, 17β-estradiol.

Currently, estrogen therapy is recommended for all estrogen-deficient women unless there is some contraindication. The most commonly used treatment regimen in the United States is 0.625 mg of conjugated equine estrogens or estrone sulfate or 1 mg of micronized estradiol for the first 25 days of each month. Another popular means of administration is transdermal delivery of estradiol. A 4-cm patch (containing 0.05 mg) can produce constant blood levels of estradiol of approximately 72 pg/mL and of estrone of 37 pg/mL. With this route of administration, hepatic effects are limited, but the patch must be replaced every 3–4 days. Subcutaneous implants of hormone, while effective, do not permit easy discontinuance of treatment if complications develop. Various estrogen-containing vaginal creams offer an effective alternative to oral replacement therapy.

In women without a uterus, estrogens used alone are sufficient and progestogens are not recommended.

SELECTED READINGS

Boston Collaborative Drug Surveillance Program, Boston University Medical Center: Surgically confirmed gallbladder disease, venous thromboembolism, and breast tumors in relation to postmenopausal estrogen therapy. N Engl J Med 1974; 290:15.

Carr BR, MacDonald PC: Estrogen treatment of postmenopausal women. Adv Intern Med 1983;28:491.

Dennerstein L, Burrows GD: A review of studies of the psychological symptoms found at the menopause. Maturitas 1978; 1:55.

Droegemueller W et al: *Comprehensive Gynecology*. Mosby, 1987.

Estrogen replacement therapy: ACOG Tech Bull No. 93, 1986.

Judd HC et al: Estrogen replacement therapy. Obstet Gynecol 1981;58:267.

Mishell DR Jr: *Menopause: Physiology and Pharmacology*. Year Book, 1987.

Riggs BW, Melton LJ III: Involutional osteoporosis. N Engl J Med 1986;314:1676.

Smith DC et al: Association of exogenous estrogens and endometrial carcinoma. N Engl J Med 1975;293:1164.

Ziel HK, Finkle WB: Increased risk of endometrial carcinoma among users of conjugated estrogens. N Engl J Med 1975;293:1167.

26

Family Planning

When no contraception is used by presumably fertile sex partners, about 90% of the women will conceive within 1 year. Women who do not want to become pregnant are best advised to use contraception whenever they become sexually active, no matter how young. At least some girls—perhaps the majority—ovulate before their first menstrual period. For older women aged 40–50, ovulation was shown in one study to be more closely related to regularity of menstruation than to age. When menstruation remained regular, there was evidence of ovulation in almost every cycle. A recent history of oligomenorrhea or of increasing length of the cycle was associated with diminished frequency but not complete absence of ovulation. Even the presence of hot flashes, amenorrhea, and elevated plasma or urine FSH does not guarantee against subsequent ovulation.

COMMONLY EMPLOYED CONTRACEPTIVE TECHNIQUES (Figure 26–1)

Current methods of contraception include (1) oral steroidal contraceptives, (2) injected or implanted steroidal contraceptives, (3) intrauterine devices, (4) physical and chemical barrier techniques, (5) withdrawal, (6) sexual abstinence during ovulation, (7) breast feeding, and (8) permanent surgical sterilization.

Oral steroidal contraceptives are the method of birth control most commonly used by American women. Results of a 1992 survey indicated that in about 15 million couples, one partner had been sterilized; about 18 million women used oral contraceptives; and 12 million couples relied on condoms for birth control.

Estimates of the failure rate with each of these techniques during the first year of use are presented in Table 26–1. It is emphasized that failures from improper use are included, which means that education and motivational reinforcement would reduce the failure rate appreciably.

Elective abortion is not strictly speaking a contraceptive technique, though it serves at times as a means of preventing the birth of unwanted children (see Chapter 9). The synthetic progesterone antagonist mifepristone (RU 486) is an oral abortifacient that may in the future provide an alternative to surgical sterilization. In preliminary studies, oral administration of epostane, a 3β-hydroxysteroid dehydrogenase inhibitor, induced early pregnancy termination in 84% of women.

ESTROGEN PLUS PROGESTIN CONTRACEPTIVES

Over 18 million women in the United States use one of the several hormonal contraceptives available for fertility control. The oral contraceptives most often employed now consist of a combination of an estrogen and a progestational agent taken daily for 3 weeks and omitted for 1 week, during which time withdrawal uterine bleeding normally occurs. In the United States, the estrogen is ethinyl estradiol or its 3-methyl ether (mestranol), which is promptly metabolized to ethinyl estradiol. A great variety of compounds with progestational activity are used, including norethindrone, norgestrel, ethynodiol diacetate, norethindrone acetate, norgestimate, and desogestrel.

Mechanisms of Action

The combined estrogen-progestin steroidal pills act in more than one way to prevent conception. Prevention of ovulation is almost certainly achieved by suppression of hypothalamic releasing factors, which in turn leads to inappropriate secretion by the pituitary of FSH and LH. Other contraceptive effects induced by the combined steroids include altered maturation of the endometrium, rendering it inappropriate for successful implantation if a blastocyst were to develop, and the production of cervical mucus hostile to penetration by sperm. The possible role, if any, of altered tubal and uterine motility induced by the hormones is not clear. As a consequence of these actions, combined estrogen-progestin oral contraceptives, if taken daily for 3 weeks out of every 4, provide virtually absolute protection against conception.

Dosage & Administration

To prevent induction of ovulation as well as to help in recognizing preexisting early pregnancy, it is generally

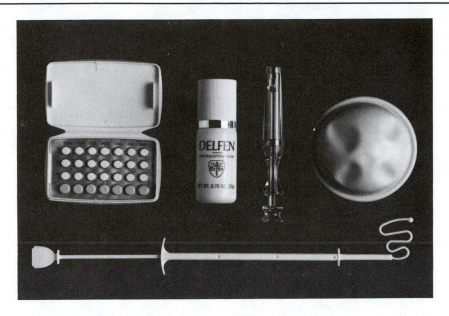

Figure 26–1. Shown left to right are oral contraceptive tablets in a container, a tube of vaginal contraceptive cream plus applicator, a diaphragm, and, below, a Lippes Loop intrauterine device and inserter. Just before insertion, the rod is withdrawn until all of the device is pulled into the inserter tube.

recommended that women begin the use of oral contraceptives on one of the first 7 days of the menstrual cycle. Many women, however, start use after delivery or abortion, before the return of spontaneous menses. If contraception is to be initiated at any time other than during or immediately after a normal menstrual cycle or within 3 weeks after delivery, another method should be used throughout the first week to avoid the risk of induced ovulation.

To help achieve regular administration of the combined oral contraceptive and thus obtain maximum protection, several suppliers offer dispensers that provide in packaged sequence 21 individually wrapped, color-coded tablets that contain hormones, followed by seven inert tablets of another color. Many of these dispenser packages come with the day of the week imprinted next to each tablet or with a variable calendar that can be affixed to the dispenser.

It is important for maximum contraceptive efficiency and for peace of mind that the woman adopt an effective scheme for assuring daily (or nightly) dosage. If one dose is missed, nothing serious will happen, though it may be desirable to double the next dose to minimize breakthrough bleeding and to "stay on schedule." If several doses are missed, another form of effective contraception (a barrier technique) should be used when intercourse is anticipated. The pill can then be restarted after withdrawal bleeding occurs. If bleeding does not occur, the possibility of pregnancy must be considered.

Since oral contraceptives first came into use, the amounts of estrogen and progestational agent contained in each tablet have been reduced considerably. The amount of estrogen most commonly administered daily is 30–50 μg of either ethinyl estradiol or mestranol.

Phasic pills were developed in an effort to reduce the amount of total progestin ingested in a single cycle without sacrificing contraceptive efficacy or cycle control. Reduction of the progestin dose is achieved by beginning the contraceptive cycle with a low dose of progestin and increasing the dose later in the cycle. The theoretic advantage of reduction in dose is that it minimizes some of the metabolic changes discussed below that are attributable to the progestin—bearing in mind that beneficial effects attributable to progestins may also be reduced. The triphasic oral contraceptives initially marketed in 1984 in the United States now account for most new oral contraceptive prescriptions. Estrogen dose may be kept constant or may be increased temporarily later in the cycle, but in all preparations it is kept low, with only 30–40 μg of ethinyl estradiol.

Beneficial & Adverse Effects

A. Beneficial Effects: The combined estrogen-progestin pill taken 3 weeks out of every 4 is the most effective reversible form of contraception available. Failure rates of 0.32 per 100 woman-years or lower have been documented. Reported beneficial effects other than contraception include less menstrual blood loss, fewer premenstrual complaints, and a lower incidence of dysmenorrhea, functional ovarian cysts, salpingitis, rheumatoid arthritis, endometrial and ovarian cancer, and various benign breast diseases, and perhaps breast cancer.

B. Adverse Effects: The possibility of adverse effects from oral contraceptives has received so much attention for so long that the major adverse effect among users may be the anxiety thus generated. Prior to prescribing these agents, a careful history is taken with special attention given to those disorders listed in Table 26–2.

Table 26–1. Failure rates during the first year of attempted use of contraceptives.[1]

Methods	Lowest Observed Failure Rate (%)	Failure Rate in Typical Users (%)
Injectable progestin	0.25	0.25
Combination birth control pills	0.5	2.0
Progestin-only pills	1.0	2.5
Intrauterine device	1.5	5.0
Condom	2.0	10
Diaphragm (with spermatocide)	2.0	19
Sponge (with spermatocide)	9–11	10–20
Foams, creams, jellies, and vaginal suppositories	3–5	18
Withdrawal	16	23
Periodic rhythmic abstinence	2–20	24
Douche	—	40
Chance (no method)	90	90

[1]Adapted from Williams NB: *Contraceptive Technology 1986–1987.* Irvington, 1986.

1. Metabolic changes–A variety of metabolic changes, often qualitatively similar to those of pregnancy, have been identified in women taking oral contraceptives. For example, plasma thyroxine and thyroid-binding proteins are elevated appreciably, whereas triiodothyronine uptake by resin is lowered. Another change similar to that induced by normal pregnancy is elevation of plasma cortisol concentration, with a nearly comparable increase in transcortin. Laboratory test results should therefore be interpreted in light of whether or not the patient is using an estrogen-containing oral contraceptive. The estrogen in a combined pill appears to decrease serum LDL cholesterol and increase HDL cholesterol, but some progestins have the reverse effect.

The contraceptive steroids may intensify preexisting diabetes or may prove sufficiently diabetogenic to induce clinically apparent disease in women prone to develop diabetes. Cholestasis and cholestatic jaundice are uncommon complications in users of oral contraceptives; the signs and symptoms clear when the medication is stopped.

A somewhat increased risk of surgically identified gallstones and gallbladder disease was reported for users of oral contraceptives.

Some important contraindications to this method of contraception are summarized in Table 26–2.

2. Neoplasia–The role of hormonal contraception in tumor formation is not clear. Reports can be cited suggesting that the risk of malignant and premalignant change in the cervix and breast is increased—or that it is decreased—or that it is unchanged. If there is an increased risk, it must be slight. Recent data from the CDC Cancer and Steroid Hormone Study (see Suggested Readings) provide evidence that oral contraceptive use protects against endometrial and ovarian cancers. Use of estrogen-progestin contraceptives has been linked circumstantially with the development of hepatic focal nodular hyperplasia and actual tumor formation that is usually but not always benign. Recent studies support the conclusion that the risk of breast cancer is not increased.

C. Cardiovascular Effects: The risk of deep vein thrombosis and pulmonary embolism has been estimated to be 3–11 times greater in women who have used oral contraceptives than in apparently similar women who have not. Moreover, the use of oral contraceptives during the month before an operative procedure appears to increase the risk of postoperative thromboembolism significantly. Pills that contain less estrogen appear to be associated with a smaller increase in risk of venous thrombosis and thromboembolism. In 1988, all manufacturers of oral contraceptives stopped production of preparations containing more than 50 μg of estrogen. The enhanced risk of thromboembolism appears to decrease rapidly once the oral contraceptive is stopped.

An association between oral contraceptives and hypertension became apparent in the late 1960s, when several reports appeared of the occasional woman who became

Table 26–2. Some important contraindications to use of estrogen plus progestin contraceptives.

1. Thromboembolism, current or past
2. Cerebrovascular accident, current or past
3. Coronary artery disease
4. Impaired liver function
5. Liver adenoma, current or past
6. Breast cancer
7. Hypertension
8. Diabetes
9. Gallbladder disease
10. Cholestatic jaundice during pregnancy
11. Sickle cell hemoglobinopathy
12. Surgery contemplated within 4 weeks
13. Major surgery on or immobilization of lower extremity
14. Smoke heavily
15. Familial hyperlipidemia
16. Antiphospholipid antibodies

overtly hypertensive while using estrogen-progestin contraceptives. The women usually became normotensive when the medication was stopped. The oral contraceptives—presumably in response chiefly to the estrogen component—were shown to increase markedly the plasma level of renin substrate and, to a lesser degree, renin, almost to the levels that occur in normal pregnancy. The great majority of women using oral contraceptives demonstrate these changes, as in pregnancy, yet do not become hypertensive. The progestin appears to contribute to the hypertension that develops in some women. Unfortunately, normotensive women who become hypertensive in response to oral contraceptives usually cannot be identified in advance. The development of hypertension during pregnancy does not preclude subsequent use of oral contraceptives.

Several epidemiologic studies strongly imply that use of estrogen-progestin oral contraceptives increases the risk of myocardial infarction. The frequency and intensity of attacks of migraine headaches may be enhanced also.

3. Risk of death–A number of adverse effects have been identified for users of oral contraceptives. The risk of death from the use of an oral contraceptive is very low if the woman is under 35, has no systemic illness, and does not smoke. The mortality risk from oral contraceptives is certainly less than that associated with pregnancy.

4. Effects on reproduction and nursing–Ovulation usually returns promptly when the estrogen-progestin contraceptive is discontinued. Within 3 months after discontinuance, at least 90% of women who previously ovulated regularly will have done so again. Postpill amenorrhea poses no long-term threat to fertility.

Use of contraceptive hormones by nursing mothers tends to reduce the amount of breast milk, but only very small quantities of the hormones are excreted in the milk.

PROGESTATIONAL AGENTS ALONE

ORAL PROGESTINS ALONE

The so-called minipill, consisting solely of 0.5 mg or less of a progestational agent daily, has not achieved widespread popularity because of a much higher associated incidence of irregular bleeding and a higher failure rate (Table 26–1). The progestational agent alone presumably impairs fertility—without necessarily inhibiting ovulation—by causing formation of cervical mucus that impedes sperm penetration and by altering endometrial maturation sufficiently to thwart successful implantation of a blastocyst.

INJECTABLE HORMONAL CONTRACEPTIVES

The advantages of injected medroxyprogesterone acetate (Depo-Provera) are a contraceptive effectiveness comparable to the combined oral contraceptives; long-lasting action, with injections required only two to four times a year, and lactation not likely to be impaired. The mechanisms of action appear to be multiple and include inhibition of ovulation, increased viscosity of cervical mucus, and an endometrium unfavorable to ovum implantation.

The disadvantages are prolonged amenorrhea or uterine bleeding—or both—during and after use and prolonged anovulation after discontinuation. The risk of venous thrombosis and thromboembolism appears to be increased, as with estrogen-progestin oral contraceptives.

Hormonal Implants

Progestin-containing implants have been studied in several countries and one of these remarkably effective contraceptive systems, Norplant, has been approved recently for use in the United States. Six silastic capsules, each containing 36 mg of L-norgestrel, are implanted beneath the skin of the upper arm. The slowly released progesterone analog prevents pregnancy by ovulation inhibition and thickening of cervical mucus. Implants are removed when fertility is desired again; they are changed at 5-year intervals. Although the one-year pregnancy rate of 0.2% (Table 26–1) is very low, the manufacturer reports a 5-year cumulative pregnancy rate of nearly 4%.

POSTCOITAL CONTRACEPTION

Diethylstilbestrol administered after intercourse to prevent unwanted pregnancy has come to be known as the "morning-after pill." In one study, there were no pregnancies in 1000 women who had inadequate contraceptive protection at the time of intercourse but within 3 days began to take diethylstilbestrol, 25 mg twice daily for the 5 days. The mechanism of action is not fully understood, but implantation is very likely interfered with in some way. Nausea and vomiting are common side effects. The possible teratogenic effect of the drug must be kept in mind if pregnancy does occur (Chapter 54).

Prevention of pregnancy has also been reported using large doses of either ethinyl estradiol or conjugated equine estrogens (Premarin) for several days after unprotected intercourse.

INTRAUTERINE CONTRACEPTIVE DEVICES

Since early in this century, attempts have been made—sporadically at first but intensely since 1960—to design a device that when inserted into the uterus would prevent pregnancy without causing adverse effects. An interesting anecdote describes the first successful experience to have been the insertion of small stones into the camel uterus to prevent pregnancy during long caravan journeys.

At one time, it was estimated that in the United States 6–7% of sexually active women of reproductive age used an intrauterine device for contraception. Some of the devices are shown in Figure 26–2. The pregnancy rates in

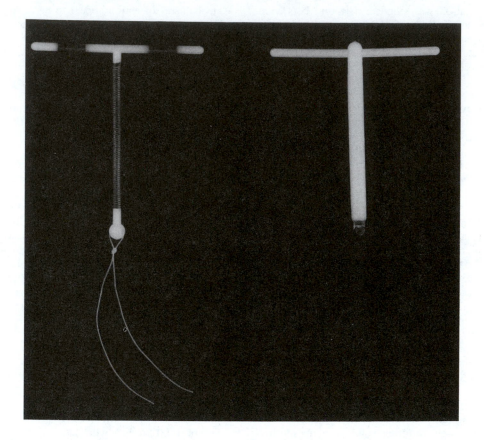

Figure 26–2. Intrauterine contraceptive devices available in 1989. *Left:* Copper T 380A (Courtesy of GynoPharma, Inc., Somerville, New Jersey). *Right:* Progestasert (Courtesy of Alza Corp., Palo Alto, California).

larger studies generally vary from 0.5 to 5 per 100 woman-years.

In general, devices are of two types: (1) those that appear to be chemically inert in that they are made of a nonabsorbable material, most often polyethylene impregnated with barium sulfate for radiopacity; and (2) those in which there is more or less continuous elution from the device of a chemically active substance such as copper or a progestational agent.

Of the chemically inert devices, the Lippes Loop was quite popular before it was withdrawn from the market in 1985. Many American women still have these devices in place.

Mechanisms of Action

The mechanisms of action of the chemically inert devices have not been defined precisely, but interference with implantation of the fertilized ovum may result from induction of a local inflammatory response that leads in turn to lysosomal action on the blastocyst and perhaps phagocytosis of spermatozoa. The contraceptive effec-

tiveness of the chemically inert devices generally increases with the size and extent of contact with the endometrium.

Certain metals, especially copper, greatly enhance the contraceptive action of inert devices of equal size and shape. A local rather than systemic effect of copper must be assumed, since metallic copper placed in one horn of the rabbit uterus prevents blastocyst implantation there but not in the other horn.

Adverse Effects

A variety of complications have been described, but for the most part the common complications have not been serious and the serious ones have not been common. Perforation of the uterus—which may be clinically silent—may occur while sounding the uterus or during insertion. Insertion may also interrupt an unsuspected pregnancy. The frequency of these mishaps will depend upon the skill of the operator and the precautions taken to identify pregnancy beforehand. Although devices may migrate spontaneously into and through the uterine wall at any time, most perforations occur—or at least begin—at the time of insertion.

Uterine cramping and some bleeding are likely to develop soon after insertion and to persist for variable periods. Considering inert devices only, the smaller the device, the less the likelihood of cramping and bleeding but the greater the likelihood of conception with the device in situ or—and especially—after spontaneous expulsion. Conversely, the larger and more rigid the device, the lower the probability of expulsion and pregnancy but the greater the likelihood of troublesome cramping and bleeding.

Blood loss with menstruation is commonly increased by a factor of about 2 but may be so great as to cause severe iron deficiency anemia

Pelvic infections, including septic abortion, have been reported, as well as tubo-ovarian abscesses, which may be unilateral. When infection is suspected, the device should be removed and antibiotics administered. Careful observation is essential, since there have been deaths from sepsis. Epidemiologists continue to argue the question of whether there is an increased risk of pelvic infection associated with wearing these devices.

Because of the presumed risk of salpingitis, pelvic peritonitis, pelvic abscess, and resulting sterility, use of an intrauterine device is discouraged for women under age 25 of no or low parity as well as for women who appear to be at increased risk of developing pelvic infection (eg, multiple partners).

Pregnancy with a Device in Utero

A device within the pregnant uterus is risky for both the mother and the fetus. When pregnancy is recognized and the tail of the device is visible through the cervix, removing the device will help minimize the occurrence of late abortion, sepsis, and preterm birth. The abortion rate is about 50% with the device left in, compared to 25% if it is promptly removed. If the tail is not visible, attempts to locate and remove the device by instrumentation may lead to abortion.

A device in the abdominal cavity may be risky for the mother. Appropriate steps are taken at delivery to identify and assure removal of the device.

Extrauterine Pregnancies

Although most intrauterine pregnancies are prevented, the device provides less protection against nidation in other locations. There has been concern that use of an intrauterine device greatly increases the risk of ectopic pregnancy, but the risk remains rather constant with duration of use at 1.2 per 1000 women per year. However, since the device does not prevent extrauterine pregnancy reliably, women already at high risk for ectopic pregnancy (previous salpingitis, ectopic pregnancy, or tubal surgery) are poor candidates for an intrauterine contraceptive device.

LOCAL BARRIER METHODS

CONDOMS

Condoms can provide effective contraception. Their failure rate with experienced and strongly motivated couples has been as low as 3 or 4 per 100 couple-years of exposure. Generally—and especially during the first year of use—the failure rate is much higher (Table 26–1).

The use of condoms has increased exponentially in recent years, though not necessarily for contraception. When used properly, condoms provide effective but not absolute protection against a broad range of sexually transmitted diseases, including gonorrhea, syphilis, herpes simplex, chlamydiosis, trichomoniasis, and HIV infection. They may give some protection against premalignant changes in the cervix.

INTRAVAGINAL CONTRACEPTIVES

Intravaginal contraceptive agents are widely used as alternatives to other methods or for temporary protection, eg, during the first week after starting oral contraceptives or while nursing. They are available as creams, jellies, suppositories, films, sponges, and foam in aerosol container.

Such agents can be purchased over-the-counter (without prescription). Typically, they work by providing a physical barrier to sperm penetration as well as chemical spermatocidal action. The active spermatocidal ingredient is nonoxynol-9. To be highly effective, the spermatocide must be deposited high in the vagina and in contact with the cervix shortly before intercourse. The duration of maximal spermatocidal effectiveness is usually no more than 1 hour, which means that insertion must be repeated before intercourse is repeated. Douching should be avoided for at least 6 hours after intercourse.

DIAPHRAGM PLUS SPERMATOCIDAL AGENT

The vaginal diaphragm, consisting of a circular rubber dome supported by a metal spring, has long been used for contraception in combination with spermatocidal jelly or cream. The spermatocidal agent is applied to the superior surface both along the rim and centrally. The device is then placed in the vagina so that the cervix, vaginal fornices, and anterior vaginal wall are effectively partitioned from the rest of the vagina and the penis. At the same time, the centrally placed spermatocidal agent is held against the cervix by the diaphragm.

The diaphragm and spermatocidal agent can be inserted hours before intercourse, but if more than 2 hours elapse, additional spermatocide should be placed in the upper vagina for maximum protection and reapplied before a subsequent exposure. The diaphragm should be left in place for a least 6 hours after intercourse.

PERIODIC (RHYTHMIC) ABSTINENCE

The pregnancy rate with the various methods for application of periodic abstinence (rhythm methods, "natural" family planning) has been estimated to be 5–40 per 100 woman-years.

Ovulation most often occurs about 14 days before onset of the next menstrual period but—unfortunately—not necessarily 14 days after the onset of the last menstrual period. Therefore, calendar rhythm is not reliable. In 1982, the International Planned Parenthood Federation concluded that, "Couples electing to use periodic abstinence should . . . be clearly informed that the method is not considered an effective method of family planning."

BREAST FEEDING

Breast feeding is important to infant health and to child-spacing. For mothers who are fully nursing their infants, ovulation during the first 10 weeks after delivery is very unlikely. However, breast feeding is not a reliable method of family planning for women whose infants are on a 3-to 4-hour, daytime-only feeding schedule and are receiving other nourishment. Waiting for the first menses to resume contraception involves a risk of pregnancy because ovulation may antedate menstruation. After the first menses, contraception is essential unless the woman desires another pregnancy soon after her last one.

SURGICAL CONTRACEPTION

Surgical sterilization of one or both sexual partners is the most popular form of contraception among couples of reproductive age. In 1981, according to the Association for Voluntary Sterilization, nearly 900,000 sterilization procedures were performed in the United States; 52% were performed on women.

TUBAL STERILIZATION

Over 5 million women underwent tubal sterilization in the United States during the 1970s. The operation can be performed at any time, but many are done at cesarean section. For women who deliver vaginally, the early puerperium is a convenient time. Because the fundus is near the umbilicus and the oviducts are readily accessible directly beneath the abdominal wall for several days after delivery, the operation is technically simple and hospitalization need not be prolonged.

For women not recently pregnant, tubal sterilization is accomplished by laparotomy, transvaginal tubal ligation, or laparoscopy.

VASECTOMY

It is estimated that one-half million men undergo vasectomy annually in the United States. Through a small incision in the scrotum, the lumen of the vas deferens is disrupted to block the passage of sperm from the testes.

Vasectomy is usually performed in 20 minutes or so on an outpatient basis under local analgesia. The procedure is associated with less morbidity and fewer deaths and is less expensive than female sterilization.

SUGGESTED READINGS

American College of Obstetricians and Gynecologists: Sterilization. ACOG Tech Bull No. 113, 1988.

Cancer and Steroid Hormone Study of the Centers for Disease Control and the National Institute of Child Health and Development: Oral-contraceptive use and the risk of breast cancer. N Engl J Med 1986;315:405.

Cancer and Steroid Hormone Study of the Centers for Disease Control and the National Institute of Child Health and Development: The reduction in risk associated with oral-contraceptive use. N Engl J Med 1987;316:650.

Daling JR et al: Primary tubal infertility in relation to the use of an intrauterine device. N Engl J Med 1985;312:937.

Kronmal RA, Whitney CW, Mumford SD: The intrauterine device and pelvic inflammatory disease: The women's health study reanalyzed. J Clin Epidemiol 1991;44:109. (See also the response to this article on p 123 of the same issue.)

Mishell DR: Contraception. N Engl J Med 1989;320:777.

Vessey MP et al: Tubal sterilization: Findings in a large prospective study. Br J Obstet Gynaecol 1983;90:203.

Unit III

Gynecologic Oncology

27

Principles of Gynecologic Oncology

Treatment of gynecologic cancer requires the carefully planned use of surgery, radiation, and chemotherapy, singly or in combination. A successful treatment plan calls upon the oncologist's knowledge of carcinogenesis, pathology, and the biologic behavior of specific tumors.

CARCINOGENESIS

VIRUSES

Evidence continues to accrue that human papillomavirus (HPV) infection is a promoter or cofactor in the development of preinvasive and invasive carcinoma of cervical, vaginal, and perineal (vulvar, perianal) tissues. With the use of DNA hybridization techniques, over 50 HPV types have been identified. Several types have been characterized as specific for female and male genital infections, which may occur alone or as mixed infections. HPV types 16, 18, 31, and 33 are associated with the development of cervical dysplasia and carcinoma. In fact, the field effect of these viruses is such that patients with preinvasive disease of the vulva have a 60% chance of harboring a warty or preinvasive lesion on the cervix or in the vagina.

CHEMICAL EXPOSURES

Information concerning environmental exposure to chemicals that affect the occurrence of female pelvic malignancies is sparse. Arsenic, talc, and asbestos are frequently implicated, but definite proof is lacking.

Itinerant farmers exposed to Paris green—an arsenical insecticide shown to be mitogenic in laboratory animals—were noted to have an increased incidence of vulvar and perianal dysplasias. Ovarian epithelial carcinomas are causally associated with talc crystals and asbestos parti-

cles. Talc particles from hygienic products have been seen in histologic preparations of ovarian cancer and are in that way implicated as a potential carcinogen. Because nonovarian papillary serous tumors of the peritoneal cavity resemble lung mesotheliomas (thought to be due to asbestos contamination), the transcervical migration of asbestos is a possible cause of peritoneal papillary serous tumors.

HEREDITY

Hereditary transmission of ovarian carcinoma conforms to mendelian genetic patterns. Familial ovarian carcinoma, ovarian carcinoma associated with endometrial and colon carcinoma, and ovarian carcinoma associated with breast cancer are all reported to be autosomal dominant traits. A careful history of maternal and paternal pedigrees is required, because some tumor types such as colonic carcinoma in males may impose a risk of ovarian, endometrial, colonic, or breast cancer to female offspring.

SPECIFIC TYPES OF ANTICANCER THERAPY

PRINCIPLES OF CANCER CHEMOTHERAPY

Like solid tumors generally, gynecologic tumors go through a cell cycle with both predictable and unpredictable phases. The first phase (G_1) is an unpredictable or variable phase in which synthesis of protein and RNA occurs in preparation for synthesis of DNA (Figure 27–1). The S phase of DNA synthesis is predictable, lasting approximately 10–30 hours. The G_2 phase, during which the diploid DNA is present, is a predictably short interval preceding mitosis. The active mitotic (M) phase is very short. During the resting (G_0) phase, there is little metabolic activity, and cells may move freely in and out of the cycle

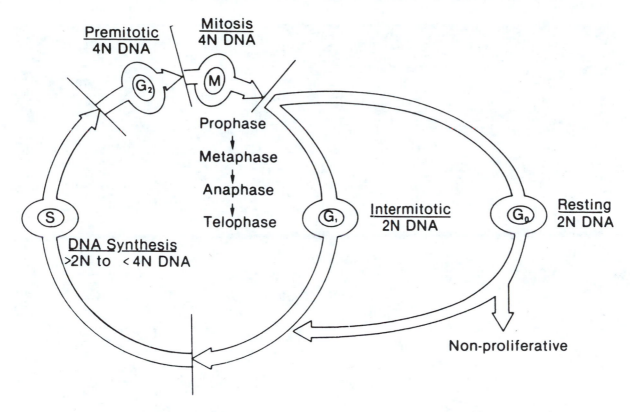

Figure 27–1. Cell cycles. All cells enter the cell cycle via G_1 into the predictable S, G_2, and M phases that are relatively short-lived. Cells either die or go into the G_0 resting stage to be recruited back into the cell cycle only if conditions such as high oxygen tension exist. (Reproduced, with permission, from Deppe G: *Chemotherapy of Gynecologic Cancer.* A.R. Liss, 1984.)

depending on oxygenation status. Most chemotherapeutic drugs are either cell cycle-specific, ie, they kill cells in a specific phase of the cell cycle; or cell cycle-nonspecific, ie, they kill cells in all phases with the possible exception of G_0. The rational use of chemotherapeutic agents depends upon knowing their cell cycle specificity.

Some important aspects of cancer chemotherapy can be set forth as follows:

(1) Kinetics of cellular action, or the so-called growth fraction of the cell cycle: When cells are actively replicating—in the S, G_2, or M phases—they are most vulnerable to chemotherapeutic agents.

(2) First-order kinetics of cell kill: A given fraction of the cell burden rather than an absolute number of cells is eradicated with each course of treatment, thus making repeated well-timed doses crucial for curative effect.

(3) Spontaneous mutation rate: The mutation rate dictates the resistance of tumor cells to chemotherapy. According to the Goldie-Codman hypothesis, the greater the tumor volume, the greater the probability of mutation. Large tumor volume—irrespective of prior chemotherapy—implies a poor outcome unless the volume is somehow reduced ("debulking"), usually by surgery.

(4) Exposure of agent to cancer cell: Antitumor effectiveness is increased by exposure of the cancer cell to

greater concentrations of drug for longer periods (C × T effect). Intraperitoneal administration greatly prolongs the exposure time and concentration over what can be achieved by oral, intravenous, intramuscular, or intra-arterial administration.

(5) Combination chemotherapy: Administration of two or more agents at the same time may have an additive or synergistic effect on cell kill. Furthermore, using agents with different cell cycle specificities reduces the chances for emergence of resistance. Using drugs with different toxicities often permits maximal dosage without overlapping side effects.

RADIATION THERAPY

The amount of radiation absorbed can be measured from two sources of radioactivity. For example, external radiation for cervical cancer is usually from an external x-ray source (Figure 27–2) and is intended both to treat the lymph nodes along the pelvic sidewall and to shrink the primary tumor. Internal radiation, or intracavitary radiation, whose energy is derived from isotope decay—usually radium, cesium, iridium, or iodine—is intended to radiate the primary tumor. As shown in Figure 27–3, the

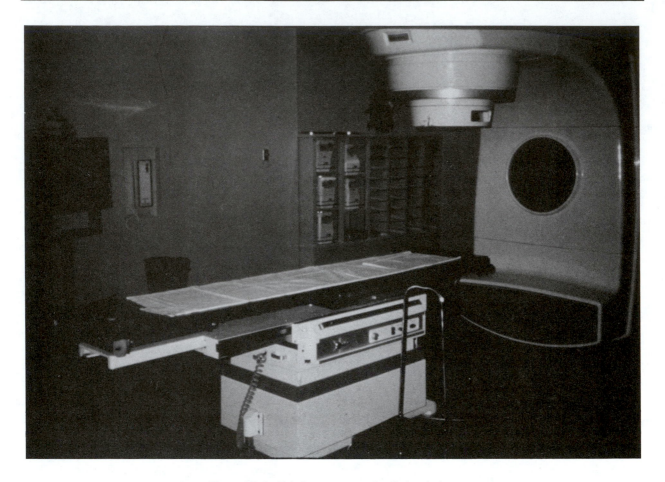

Figure 27–2. Teletherapy external radiation devise.

amount of radioactivity in this isodose curve drops off rapidly. The **inverse square law** states that as the distance from the source increases, the amount of energy at that point is inversely proportionate to the square of the distance. Hence, radioactivity drops precipitously as the distance from the source increases. Standard sources of reference are point A, where the uterine artery crosses over the ureter—also considered the most proximal portion of the cervix—and point B is located by a horizontal line extending laterally from point A to the sidewall, where the pelvic lymph nodes are located.

Biology of Radiation Therapy

The radiation sensitivity of any tumor depends on many factors. Factors that tend to shift the cell-surviving fraction curve to the left (Figure 27–4) are listed below.

A. Repair and Regrowth of Tumor Cells: The amount of sublethal damage from fractional radiation—represented as D_q, or the shoulder of the curve, is determined by various factors.

B. Oxic Effect: The more aerated the tumor, the better the response to radiation therapy. Slope D_0 is a good measure of this effect.

C. Effect of Temperature: Hyperthermia of tumor cells favorably affects the shoulder and slope of the survival curve.

D. Synergism of Chemotherapy and Radiation: The interaction of chemotherapy and radiation therapy results in greater cell kill than can be achieved with either modality used alone. An example is the use of fluorouracil and radiation therapy in the treatment of advanced tumors of the cervix. Theoretically, both the shoulder and the slope of the curve shown in Figure 27–4 are affected.

Complications of Radiation Therapy

A. Acute Complications: Acute complications most often occur during treatment and subside after the course of therapy is completed.

1. Abdominal skin–Desquamation is more common with orthovoltage doses. It is treated with applications of

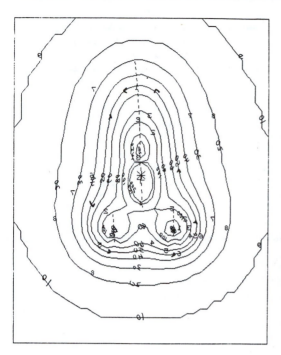

Figure 27–3. Brachytherapy. Intracavitary radium or cesium loading device for treatment of cervical cancer and isodose distribution.

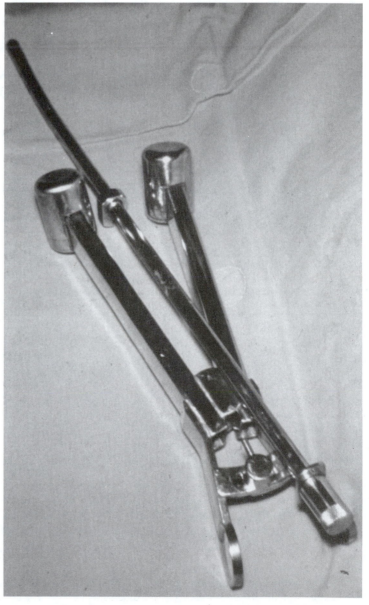

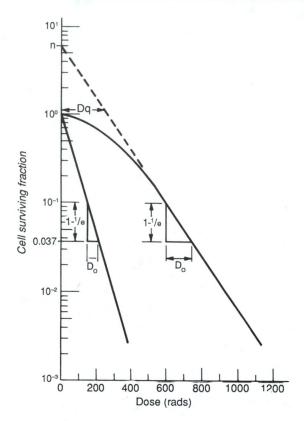

Figure 27–4. Cell survival curve. D_q represents the shoulder of the curve, where sublethal damage occurs with fractional radiation therapy. D_o represents the slope of the curve affected by relative degrees of oxygen tensions. (Reproduced, with permission, from Berek JS, Hacker NF: *Practical Gynecologic Oncology.* Williams & Wilkins, 1989.)

B. Chronic Complications: Chronic complications usually appear 6 months to 2 years after radiation therapy and occur in about 5% of all patients.

1. Large bowel and rectal complications–Chronic bleeding (causing anemia), bowel stricture, and rectovaginal fistula formation may occur. Severe complications often require colostomy or resection. About one-fourth of patients who develop severe complications involving the rectum or sigmoid colon will also have bladder complications.

2. Severe bladder complications–Hematuria, decreased bladder capacity, and vesicovaginal fistula may occur. Hematuria may require bladder irrigation and cystoscopically directed fulguration of bleeding sites. Occasionally, instillation of 4% formalin solution to chemically cauterize the bladder mucosa may be required. Rarely, bleeding must be controlled by partial or complete cystectomy. Small-capacity bladder due to fibrosis can be treated by augmentation techniques or by construction of diverting conduits. Small fistulas can be surgically corrected via a transvaginal approach utilizing the Martius bulbocavernosus fat pad interposition procedure or via a transvesical approach utilizing omentum as a vascular patch.

3. Small bowel complications–Obstruction and perforation most often occur in the terminal ileum. This complication requires bypass surgical procedures, often with construction of a mucosal fistula.

ointment and can be prevented by megavoltage therapy. Perianal skin desquamation during standard pelvic radiation protocols can also be treated with ointments.

2. Proctosigmoiditis, manifested by tenesmus and diarrhea and occasionally by bloody mucous rectal discharge, occurs in virtually all patients receiving pelvic radiation therapy. These complications are treated by a combination of antidiarrheal and antispasmodic drugs along with low-residue diets.

3. Cystitis–Patients complain of frequency, urgency, and dysuria similar to the symptoms of urinary tract infection. Occasionally, there is minimal bleeding and bladder spasm. Treatment is with antibiotics and antispasmodic drugs.

4. Enteritis occurs more commonly in cancer patients with a history of pelvic surgery and pelvic inflammatory disease. The terminal ileum is more commonly involved, since it is the fixed portion of the distal small bowel. The hallmark of this complication is abdominal pain and diarrhea. These symptoms can limit the total dose of medication. Treatment is with antidiarrheal and antispasmodic drugs.

SURGICAL THERAPY

COMMON SURGICAL MODALITIES

Preinvasive Disease

A. Cervix, Vagina, and Vulva: In preinvasive disease of the cervix, vagina, and vulva, laser vaporization may be utilized. Cone biopsy (Figure 27–5) utilizing surgical or laser resection may be used to diagnose the extent of dysplastic changes in the cervix. CO_2 laser vaporization and cone biopsy are both used for treatment of preinvasive disease of the cervix. Laser surgery has the advantage of sparing normal tissue, which is especially desirable in women of childbearing age. This tool is popular also for treatment of high-grade cervical dysplasia. The objectives of both cold-knife conization and CO_2 laser ablation are essentially the same—to remove the entire transformation zone and destroy enough tissue to minimize recurrence of dysplasia and prevent invasive squamous cell carcinoma. Excessive bleeding is more common with cold-knife conization.

For preinvasive disease of the vagina and vulva, the CO_2 laser is the mainstay of treatment. Minimal normal tissue destruction is a cosmetic advantage.

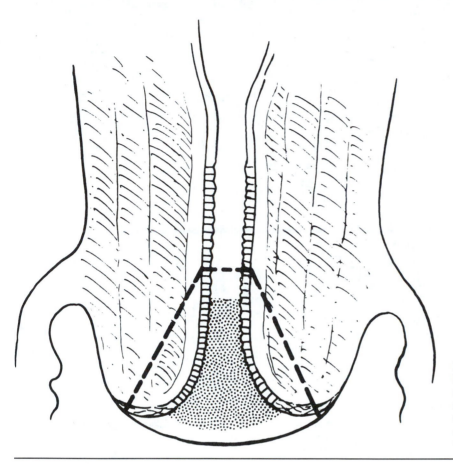

Figure 27–5. Cone biopsy and CO_2 laser ablative procedure for preinvasive disease of the cervix with removal of entire transformation zone. (Reproduced, with permission, from Berek JS, Hacker NF: *Practical Gynecologic Oncology.* Williams & Wilkins, 1989.)

Radical Vulvectomy & Inguinal Femoral Lymphadenectomy

Vulvar carcinoma is treated mainly by radical surgical ablation with concomitant inguinal and femoral lymphadenectomy (Figure 27–6). This radical mutilating approach is associated with dreadful long-term complications, such as chronic lymphedema of the lower extremities (> 70% of cases). Immediate postoperative complications are generally wound infection and suture line breakdown, since reapproximated surgical edges are under considerable tension. The anatomic location and the advanced age of most patients do not lend themselves to rapid recovery. The incidence of major postoperative wound breakdown has been reduced from 30% to 14% by utilization of separate groin incisions, leaving a skin bridge between the excised vulva and the groin.

Radical Hysterectomy & Pelvic Lymphadenectomy

In young women, the treatment of choice for small (< 3 cm) carcinomas confined to the cervix is radical hysterectomy and bilateral pelvic lymph node dissection (Figure 27–7). The extent of extirpation of parametrial tissue laterally toward the sidewall varies depending upon the size and depth of invasion of the primary lesion. Denervation of autonomic fibers to the bladder causes bladder atony of various degrees in virtually all patients. Rapid recovery is the rule except for older patients with underlying neurogenic bladder complications, in whom recovery is delayed if it occurs at all. Ureteral, vaginal, and vesicovaginal fistulas occur in about 1% of cases. Five percent of patients undergo chronic lymphocele formation in the retroperitoneum requiring intermittent drainage.

Ovarian Carcinoma

The debulking operations often required when ovarian carcinoma has spread toward the pelvic sidewalls and onto the sigmoid colon require an indirect retroperitoneal approach. Occasionally, a portion of colon and rectum is removed to allow optimal reduction of the cell burden. A stapler device is ideal for rectocolon reanastomosis, thus avoiding colostomy in most cases (Figure 27–8).

COMBINATION TREATMENTS UTILIZING SURGERY

Bulky Cervical & Vulvar Lesions

In the recent past, bulky cervical lesions were treated exclusively with radiation therapy and bulky vulvar le-

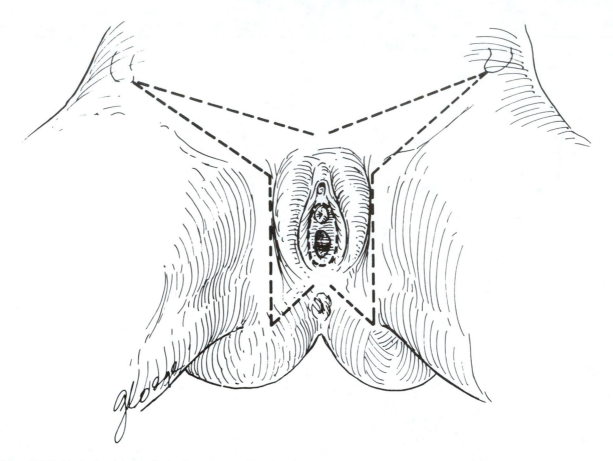

Figure 27–6. Typical en bloc radical vulvectomy and inguinal femoral lymphadenectomy. The surgical line of excision extends from the anterior superior iliac crest to the pubic symphysis and down through the labiocrural fold to the ischiorectal area posteriorly, with removal of part or all of the mons pubis anteriorly. (Reproduced, with permission, from Berek JS, Hacker NF: *Practical Gynecologic Oncology.* Williams & Wilkins, 1989.)

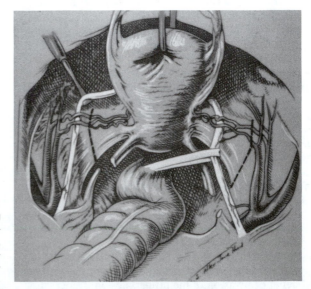

Figure 27–7. Radical hysterectomy specimen, showing removing of uterosacral ligaments. The line of dissection of the cardinal ligament is of varying degrees of thickness toward the sidewalls, with complete unroofing of the ureter through the cardinal ligament toward its insertion into the bladder. Tape is around the ureter, and clamps are on the uterosacral ligaments.

Table 27–1. Agents commonly used in gynecologic oncology.[1]

Drug	Common Treatment Schedules	Common Toxicities	Indications
Alkylating agents			
Mechlorethamine (nitrogen mustard, HN2, Mustargen)	0.4 mg IV as single dose or 0.1 mg/kg daily for 4 days; 0.2–0.4 mg/kg by intracavitary injection	Nausea and vomiting, myelosuppression	Cancer of ovary; malignant pleural or pericardial effusions
Cyclophosphamide (Cytoxan)	1.5–3 mg/kg/d orally; 10–50 mg/kg IV every 1–4 weeks	Myelosuppression, cystitis with or without bladder fibrosis, alopecia, hepatitis, amenorrhea, azoospermia	Breast, ovary, soft tissue sarcomas
Chlorambucil (Leukeran)	0.03–1.0 mg/kg/d orally	Myelosuppression, gastrointestinal distress, dermatitis, hepatotoxicity	Cancer of ovary
Melphalan (Alkeran)	0.2 mg/kg/d orally for 5 days every 4–6 weeks	Myelosuppression, nausea and vomiting (rare), mucosal ulceration (rare), second malignancies	Cancer of ovary, cancer of breast
Thiotepa	0.8 mg/kg IV every 4–6 weeks; 45–60 mg by intracavitary injection	Myelosuppression, nausea and vomiting, headaches, fever (rare)	Cancer of ovary, cancer of breast; intracavitary for malignant effusions
Alkylating-like agents			
Cisplatin (Platinol)	10–20 mg/m² IV daily for 5 days every 3 weeks or 50–75 mg/m² IV every 1–3 weeks	Nephrotoxicity, tinnitus and hearing loss, nausea and vomiting, myelosuppression, peripheral neuropathy	Ovarian and germ cell carcinoma, cervical cancer
Dacarbazine	2–4.5 mg/kg/d IV daily for 10 days every 4 weeks	Myelosuppression, nausea and vomiting, flu-like syndrome, hepatotoxicity	Uterine sarcomas, soft tissue sarcomas
Dactinomycin (Cosmegen)	0.3–0.5 mg/m² IV daily for 5 days every 3–4 weeks	Nausea and vomiting, skin necrosis, mucosal ulceration, myelosuppression	Germ cell ovarian tumors, choriocarcinoma, soft tissue sarcoma
Bleomycin (Blenoxane)	10–20 units/m² IV, SC, or IM once or twice weekly to a total dose of 400 units; for effusions, 60–120 units by intrapleural infusion	Fever, dermatologic reactions, pulmonary toxicity, anaphylactic reactions	Cancer of the cervix, germ cell ovarian tumors, malignant effusions
Mitomycin (Mutamycin)	10–20 mg/m² IV every 6–8 weeks	Myelosuppression, local vesicant action, nausea and vomiting, mucosal ulcerations, nephrotoxicity	Cancer of the breast, cervix, and ovary
Doxorubicin (Adriamycin)	60–90 mg/m² IV every 3 weeks or 20–35 mg/m² IV daily for 3 days every 3 weeks	Myelosuppression, alopecia, cardiotoxicity, local vesicant action, nausea and vomiting, mucosal ulcerations	Cancer of the ovary, breast, and endometrium
Mithramycin (Mithracin)	20–50 mg/kg/d IV every 4–6 weeks; for hypercalcemia: 25 mg/kg IV every 3–4 days	Nausea and vomiting, hemorrhagic diathesis, hepatotoxicity, nephrotoxicity, fever, myelosuppression, facial flushing	Hypercalcemia of cancer
Antimetabolites			
Fluorouracil	10–15 mg/kg/wk IV	Myelosuppression, nausea and vomiting, anorexia, alopecia	Cancer of breast, ovary
Methotrexate	15–40 mg/d orally for 5 days; 240 mg/m² IV with Leukovorin rescue; 12–15 mg/m²/wk by intrathecal injection	Mucosal ulceration, myelosuppression, hepatotoxicity, allergic pneumonitis; meningeal irritation with intracavitary	Choriocarcinoma; cancer of breast, ovary
Hydroxyurea (Hydrea)	1–2 g/m²/d orally or IV for 2–6 weeks	Myelosuppression, nausea and vomiting, anorexia	Cancer of cervix
Plant alkaloids			
Vincristine (Oncovin)	0.01–0.03 mg/kg/wk IV	Neurotoxicity, alopecia, myelosuppression, cranial nerve palsies, gastrointestinal upset	Ovarian germ cell carcinomas, sarcomas, cancer of cervix
Vinblastine (Velban)	5–6 mg/m² IV every 1–2 weeks	Myelosuppression, alopecia, nausea and vomiting, neurotoxicity	Ovarian germ cell carcinomas, choriocarcinoma
Etoposide (Vepesid)	300–600 mg/m² IV in divided doses over 3–4 days every 3–4 weeks	Myelosuppression, alopecia, hypotension	Ovarian germ cell carcinomas, choriocarcinoma

[1]Modified from Berek JS, Hacker NF: *Practical Gynecologic Oncology.* Williams & Wilkins, 1989.

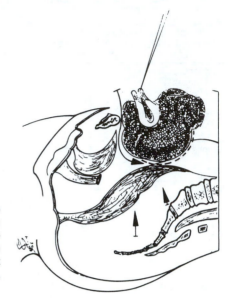

Figure 27–8. **A:** Tumor debulking via a retroperitoneal approach, starting from the pelvic sidewalls and often requiring dissection via the presacral space and resection of sigmoid colon and rectum for optimal cytoreduction. **B:** Reapproximation of the proximal sigmoid to the distal rectum can be done, with avoidance of colostomy in many instances using a stapler device. (Reproduced, with permission, from Heintz APM: *Advanced Ovarian Carcinoma: Surgical Treatment and Prognosis.* Noordwijk, 1985.)

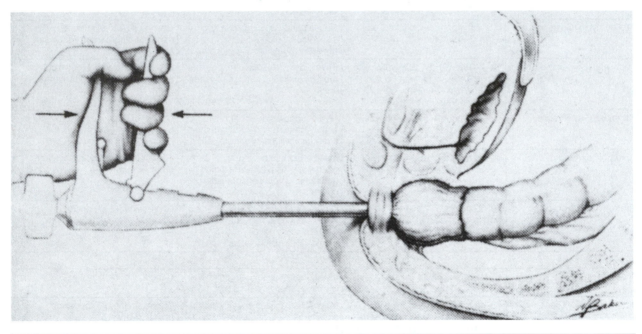

sions by radical surgery. The overall local control rates were only about 40%. Response rates of 60–65% can be achieved by combined chemotherapy plus radiation for carcinoma of the cervix and by radiation therapy preceding surgical resection of vulvar lesions. Bulky cancers confined to the cervix (barrel-shaped lesions) are better treated with a combination of sequential radiation therapy followed by hysterectomy.

Ovarian Cancer

Ovarian carcinoma widely metastatic to the upper abdomen and pelvis is best treated first with a debulking operation and then chemotherapy.

SUGGESTED READINGS

Berek JS, Hacker NF: *Practical Gynecologic Oncology.* Williams & Wilkins, 1989.

Deppe G: *Chemotherapy of Gynecologic Cancer.* A.R. Liss, 1984.

Fletcher GH: *Textbook of Radiotherapy.* Lea & Febiger, 1980.

Heintz APM: *Advanced Ovarian Carcinoma: Surgical Treatment and Prognosis.* Noordwijk, 1985.

Morrow CP, Townsend DE: *Synopsis of Gynecologic Oncology,* 3rd ed. Wiley, 1987.

Vulvar & Vaginal Cancer

CANCER OF THE VULVA & VAGINA

Vulvar cancer accounts for about 4% of all female genital malignant neoplastic diseases in the United States and is the fourth most common gynecologic cancer. Women with a history of preinvasive or invasive carcinoma of the cervix are at increased risk of developing vulvar neoplasias, suggesting a "field" effect of a common causative agent. Premalignant changes of the vulvar skin, such as vulvar dystrophies and intraepithelial neoplasia, often precede or coexist with vulvar cancer. The cause is unknown, but there is evidence of an association with sexually transmitted diseases—especially those caused by the human papillomavirus (HPV). In a recent study, evidence of viral infection was found in 84% of cases of vulvar intraepithelial neoplasias and in 58% of cases of invasive carcinomas.

The predominant histologic type of vulvar cancer is epidermoid or squamous carcinoma (90%). Less commonly encountered are melanomas, sarcomas, adenocarcinomas, and basal cell carcinomas (Table 28–1).

VULVAR INTRAEPITHELIAL NEOPLASIA

There is disagreement about both the terminology and the malignant potential of several vulvar skin lesions that have long been thought to precede the development of vulvar cancer. The most relevant of these conditions is squamous vulvar intraepithelial neoplasia, which has been classified based solely on histologic criteria. It is characterized by atypical cytologic features and disorientation of epithelial architecture that may be classified as mild, moderate, or severe (carcinoma in situ) according to extension of tumor through the epithelium. These abnormal cells do not invade the stroma, and the basal membrane remains intact. Carcinoma in situ is considered a preinvasive disease, though its progression rate to frankly invasive cancer is uncertain. Paget's disease of the vulva is a less common form of intraepithelial neoplasia and consists of proliferation of large pale cells of unclear origin. Although the invasive potential of Paget's disease is almost negligible, it may coexist with an underlying cutaneous adnexal adenocarcinoma or with another primary cancer in one or more genital locations.

In contrast with invasive neoplasia, vulvar intraepithelial neoplasia is seen in a younger population, with a median age of 35 years. In fact, at least 75% of patients with severe vulvar intraepithelial neoplasia are premenopausal.

Clinical Findings

A. Symptoms and Signs: About two-thirds of patients present with a history of long-standing pruritus or of a small vulvar lesion; the remainder are asymptomatic. On physical examination, a wide variety of unifocal or multifocal changes may be found, most often a well-demarcated macule or papule, which may be white (leukoplakia), red (erythroplakia), hyperpigmented, or warty in appearance.

Inspection of the vulva under adequate light is necessary to identify small lesions. Suspicious areas should be biopsied under local anesthesia as an office procedure using the Keyes punch (Figure 28–1) or excisional biopsy. A magnifying glass is an excellent aid. Colposcopy after application of 3% acetic acid is useful for detection of concealed and multiple lesions. Staining the vulva with toluidine blue is recommended for symptomatic patients with no obvious lesions. Retention of the stain after washing with 1% acetic acid is indicative of increased nuclear activity, which may be due to malignancy. Biopsy specimens should be taken from these suspicious areas. The rate of progression of untreated intraepithelial neoplasia into invasive carcinoma is unknown, but it seems to be uncommon. Despite the usually slow progression of this disease, treatment is recommended for all patients.

Treatment

The goal of therapy is to eradicate the lesion and diminish the risk of recurrence while preserving the anatomic integrity and physiologic functions of the vulva. The choice of treatment is based on the patient's age, the severity of the lesion, its "centricity" (unifocal or multifocal), and its location.

A. Local Excision: For unifocal disease, wide local excision under local anesthesia allows a more complete histologic assessment and an accurate estimation of surgical margins, which is essential in predicting recurrences.

Table 28–1. Cancer of the vulva by histologic type.[1,2]

Tumor Type	Percentage
Epidermoid carcinoma	86.2
Melanoma	4.8
Sarcoma	2.2
Basal cell carcinoma	1.4
Bartholin gland	
Squamous carcinoma	0.4
Adenocarcinoma	0.6
Adenocarcinoma	0.6
Undifferentiated	3.9

[1]Based on 1378 reported cases.
[2]Modified from Plentl AA and associates: *Lymphatic System of the Female Genitalia.* Saunders, 1971.

B. Laser Therapy: For unifocal or multifocal lesions, CO_2 laser vaporization under local or general anesthesia provides effective therapy, with vulvar conservation and minimal scarring. Two or more sessions may be required.

C. Vulvectomy and Skin Grafting: Skinning vulvectomy with split-thickness skin grafting has been replaced in many institutions by laser surgery, which seems to be equally effective and cosmetically more acceptable to young patients. Skinning vulvectomy may still be applicable for selected cases of multifocal or recurrent disease.

D. Chemotherapy: Topical fluorouracil 5% cream may be effective in up to one-half of patients, but it is in most cases poorly tolerated because of its necrotizing effect on the epithelium. It should be reserved for recurrent cases.

INVASIVE CARCINOMA

Invasive cancer is usually diagnosed in women between the ages of 60 and 70 (Figure 28–2).

Clinical Findings

A. Symptoms and Signs: Most patients detect the presence of a vulvar mass on self-examination, and there is often a long history of pruritus and chronic irritating vulvar skin conditions. Bleeding and perineal pain are generally associated with large tumors and extensive disease. Rarely, in very advanced cases, dysuria secondary to urethral involvement may be the presenting symptom.

Findings on pelvic examination are usually confined to the external genitalia. The vulvar tumor may be exophytic, endophytic, ulcerative, or verrucous. It most frequently arises from the labia majora, followed by labia minora, clitoris, vestibule, and occasionally multicentric locations. It may extend into the vagina, perineal skin, anus, and urethra. Careful palpation of groin nodes is important to detect enlargement or fixation suggestive of metastatic spread to the inguinal areas. In advanced cases, unilateral or bilateral leg lymphedema may be found.

B. Laboratory Findings: Tissue biopsy is required for diagnosis and can usually be performed in the office under local anesthesia either by excisional biopsy of small

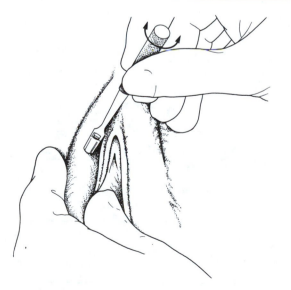

Figure 28–1. Vulvar biopsy with Keyes dermatologic punch instrument.

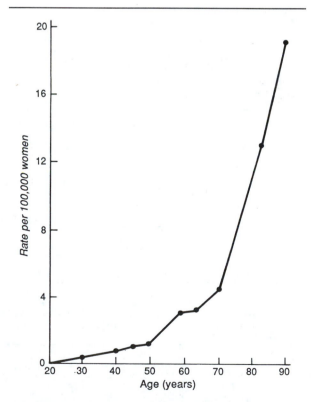

Figure 28–2. Age incidence curve for carcinoma of vulva in white women in the United States. (Adapted from Menczer J and associates: Am J Obstet Gynecol 143:893, 1982.)

lesions or representative biopsy of an area of viable tumor. Fine-needle aspiration of suspicious inguinal nodes is useful in cases where surgical excision is not contemplated and for formulating a more rational approach to therapy.

Staging & Patterns of Spread

Squamous cell carcinoma spreads to adjacent organs by continuous growth, particularly to the vagina, perineal skin and anus, urethra, bladder, and rectum. Lymphatic spread is via the superficial and deep inguinal and femoral nodes and then to the pelvic lymph nodes. Contralateral inguinal involvement in the absence of ipsilateral spread is extremely rare.

Staging is based on examination of the primary lesion and spread to adjacent organs and inguinal lymph nodes. The accepted staging system is that of the International Federation of Gynecology and Obstetrics (FIGO), modified in October 1988. The system is based upon the TNM (tumor, node, metastasis) classification (Table 28–2). Over 50% of cases are stages I or II at diagnosis. Prognosis and survival correlate well with stage. A thorough physical examination with emphasis on palpation of inguinal nodes must be performed in order to detect regional or distant extension. Additional procedures employed for staging purposes in advanced disease include chest x-rays, intravenous pyelography, cystoscopy, barium enema, and proctosigmoidoscopy.

Prognostic Factors

A. Stage of Disease: The stage of disease at diagnosis is an important indicator of outcome. The chances for cure diminish significantly when the neoplasm extends to adjacent structures and regional nodes. Other factors have been identified as having prognostic significance, particularly in stage I disease.

B. Grade of Disease: The significance of tumor grade has been controversial. Recent studies conducted by the Gynecologic Oncology Group are consistent with the view that there is some correlation between grade and lymphatic spread and ultimately prognosis.

C. Size of the Lesion: This is an important risk factor for groin lymph node metastases. The incidence of inguinal node involvement increases in tumors measuring 3 cm or more.

D. Depth of Invasion or Tumor Thickness: This is one of the most important prognostic indicators since it correlates well with the potential for lymphatic involvement (Table 28–3). The concept of microinvasive carcinoma of the vulva has been debated in the literature for the past decade. Because it is not defined in the FIGO staging system, the International Society for the Study of Vulvar Disease (ISSVD) has defined it as "a single lesion measuring 2 cm or less in diameter and with a depth of invasion of 1 mm or less." This substaging has important therapeutic implications because microinvasive disease usually will not spread to inguinal nodes, which means that patients may be treated with less than radical procedures.

E. Lymph Node Status: This is the most important prognostic factor. Documentation of spread to the inguinal, femoral, and pelvic lymph nodes significantly influences prognosis, treatment planning, and survival. Involvement of pelvic nodes in the absence of groin node disease is quite rare. Not only the number of positive nodes but also whether the nodes are involved bilaterally are important prognostic factors (Figure 28–3).

F. Vascular Space Involvement: According to several investigators, this factor correlates with groin node metastatic disease.

Treatment

A. Surgical Treatment: Microinvasive cancer as defined in the preceding section is adequately treated with wide local resection; however, care must be taken to include a margin of at least 1 cm of normal tissue in order to

---

Table 28–2. FIGO staging system for carcinoma of the vulva. (Modified October, 1988.)

Stage 0 Tis	Carcinoma in situ, intraepithelial carcinoma.
Stage I T1 N0 M0	Tumor confined to the vulva and/or perineum, 2 cm or less in greatest dimension. No nodal metastasis.
Stage II T2 N0 M0	Tumor confined to the vulva and/or perineum, more than 2 cm in greatest dimension. No nodal metastasis.
Stage III T3 N0 M0 T3 N1 M0 T1 N1 M0 T2 N1 M0	Tumor of any size with: (1) Adjacent spread to the lower urethra and/or the vagina, or the anus, and/or (2) Unilateral regional lymph node metastasis.
Stage IVA T1 N2 M0 T2 N2 M0 T3 N2 M0 T4, any N, M0	Tumor invades any of the following: Upper urethra, bladder mucosa, rectal mucosa, pelvic bone, and/or regional node metastasis.
Stage IVB Any T, any N, M1	Any distant metastasis, including pelvic lymph nodes.

Table 28–3. Relationship between tumor thickness and positive groin nodes.[1]

Tumor Thickness (mm)	Positive Nodes (%)
< 1	3.1
2	8.9
3	18.6
4	30.9
5	33.3

[1]Modified from Sedlis AS and associates: Positive groin lymph nodes in superficial squamous cell vulvar cancer: A Gynecologic Oncology Group study. Am J Obstet Gynecol 1987;156:1159.

decrease the chances of local recurrence. Depending on the size of the lesion, the operative field may be closed either primarily or secondarily with skin grafts.

Stage I invasive carcinoma traditionally has been treated by en bloc radical vulvectomy and bilateral inguinal femoral lymphadenectomy. However, treatment planning should include other factors such as the size of the lesion and the depth of invasion. There is a subset of patients with early invasive carcinoma of the vulva who are characterized as presenting with a small unifocal lesion, invading less than 3 mm, who have an incidence of lymph node involvement in the vicinity of 3%. In these cases, performance of wide local vulvar resection or a partial radical vulvectomy with "sentinel" ipsilateral lymph node

sampling seems acceptable. If the vulvar specimen reveals deeper invasion or if the nodes show microscopic spread, classic radical vulvectomy with bilateral inguinofemoral lymphadenectomy should follow. Radical vulvectomy and bilateral inguinal femoral lymphadenectomy should be the treatment of choice for all patients with invasion deeper than 3 mm or for those patients with more advanced stages (II, III, IV). Rarely, selected patients presenting with stage IV disease may be treated by pelvic exenteration in addition to radical vulvectomy and lymphadenectomy. The place of pelvic lymphadenectomy in the surgical treatment of this disease is controversial. A finding of positive pelvic nodes carries a very ominous prognosis and the benefit of pelvic lymphadenectomy remains unproved, but most gynecologic oncologists would rather irradiate the pelvis in cases with suspicious pelvic nodes.

Radical surgical treatment is complicated in over half of cases by wound breakdown and infection at the perineal and inguinal incisions, resulting in delayed healing. Chronic complications such as leg lymphedema, recurrent cellulitis, and psychosexual dysfunction are common also.

B. Radiation: Radiation therapy to the inguinal and pelvic areas usually is reserved as adjuvant treatment for patients with documented inguinal femoral lymph node involvement. Primary radiation to the vulvar tumor may

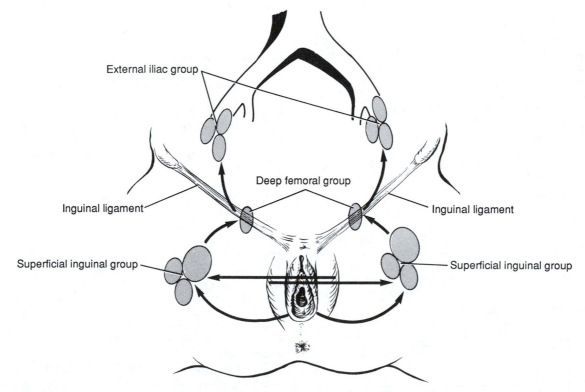

Figure 28–3. Diagram of lymphatic drainage of vulva, showing capacity for bilateral node involvement. (From Way S: Carcinoma of the vulva. In: *Progress in Gynecology,* Meigs JV, Sturgis SS [editors]. Vol 3, Grune & Stratton, 1957.)

be selectively indicated in patients in which reducing the size of the primary lesion before surgery is desirable, thus sparing them from ultraradical procedures such as exenteration. Combination therapy consisting of wide local resection (or radical vulvectomy) for the central tumor with radiation therapy to inguinal nodes (instead of lymphadenectomy) has been proposed by some surgeons. Whether node irradiation eliminates subclinical nodal disease is difficult to prove.

C. Chemotherapy: Chemotherapy is indicated in patients with distant metastatic disease and in those with regional or local recurrences not amenable to surgery or radiation therapy. The response of squamous cell carcinoma to chemotherapy is generally poor—in the range of 25%—without a clear survival benefit. Most regimens employ platinum-based combination therapy.

Survival & Prognosis

In all stages, the recurrence rate after therapy is about 30–40%. The prognosis for stage I and stage II patients with negative nodes is excellent, with an 85–90% survival rate at 5 years. The survival rate drops to about 50% when inguinofemoral nodes are involved and to 20% with metastases to the pelvic nodes.

OTHER VULVAR TUMORS

Melanoma

Melanoma is the second most common cancer of the vulva and accounts for about 5% of vulvar cancers. It usually presents as a pigmented lesion and rarely as an amelanotic melanoma. Although the FIGO staging system is used, the depth of penetration seems to be particularly relevant as a prognostic indicator. Therefore, the Breslow classification of melanoma, which is based on the thickness of the lesion measured from the surface epithelium to the deepest tumor penetration, has proved to be of value in prediction of survival.

Treatment is based on factors such as lesion size, location, and depth of invasion. Radical surgery does not significantly improve survival over what can be achieved with wide local excision.

Adenocarcinoma

Vulvar adenocarcinoma is a rare tumor that usually arises from Bartholin's gland, presenting as a palpable mass at that site. Treatment follows the same guidelines as for invasive squamous cell carcinoma of the vulva.

Basal Cell Carcinoma

Basal cell carcinoma of the vulva is rare and characterized by a lesion with advancing borders and minimal invasive potential. Treatment is by wide local excision.

Verrucous Carcinoma

Verrucous carcinoma of the vulva is a variant of squamous cell cancer, characterized by an exophytic papillary growth, locally aggressive but with a very low potential for metastatic spread. Treatment is by wide local excision.

Sarcoma

Sarcoma of the vulva is extremely rare but very aggressive; distant metastases are common. Treatment is as for squamous cell carcinoma.

VAGINAL CANCER

Vaginal cancer constitutes less than 2% of female genital tract cancers and is typically a disease of postmenopausal women. The peak incidence is in women over age 60. There are similarities in the etiologic and epidemiologic features of women with cervical and vaginal cancer, particularly with respect to sexually transmitted disease and the increased risk of developing vulvar neoplasias.

The most common histologic type is squamous cell carcinoma, seen in over 90% of the women. Other less common varieties include adenocarcinoma, melanoma, embryonal rhabdomyosarcoma (sarcoma botryoides), and endodermal sinus tumors. Secondary (metastatic) involvement of the vagina in malignant pelvic tumors is more frequent than primary carcinoma of the vagina, particularly in tumors arising from the cervix and corpus.

INTRAEPITHELIAL NEOPLASIAS

Vaginal intraepithelial neoplasia (dysplasia, carcinoma in situ) arises from the vaginal squamous epithelium and is more often seen in women with a history of cervical intraepithelial neoplasias; however, it is far less common than the cervical counterpart. Infection by human papillomavirus may also be an important cofactor. The lesion is characterized by atypical cytologic features and loss of normal epithelial architecture, usually involving its full thickness. A full-thickness epithelial change is considered preinvasive disease, though the progression rate to invasive cancer is uncertain.

Clinical Findings

A. Symptoms and Signs: Most patients are asymptomatic, and the diagnosis is suggested by Papanicolaou smear. Inspection of the vagina may disclose the presence of raised or warty lesions. In most cases, however, colposcopic examination is required in order to identify the abnormal area, usually a white lesion with or without punctation.

B. Laboratory Findings: Staining the vagina with Lugol's solution may be helpful. The lesion will stain lighter than the normal vaginal mucosa. Representative areas of these abnormal lesions can then be biopsied in the office with a punch biopsy forceps with minimal patient discomfort.

Treatment

There are several treatment options for this condition, including local surgical resection, laser vaporization, and intravaginal application of 5% fluorouracil cream. The choice of treatment depends on the location of the lesions and their number. A well-localized and accessible unifocal lesion is best treated by wide local resection, bearing in mind the possibility of vaginal scarring in young and sexually active patients. Lesions in inaccessible areas may be treated by laser vaporization under local or general anesthesia. Multifocal disease is best treated either by laser vaporization or topical application of fluorouracil cream. Total vaginectomy with skin grafting is occasionally required. Radiation therapy is rarely required.

INVASIVE CARCINOMA

Clinical Findings

A. Symptoms and Signs: Routine cytologic examination may detect carcinoma in up to 20% of asymptomatic women, but most patients will present with vaginal bleeding or a blood-stained vaginal discharge. Pelvic pain usually is indicative of advanced disease. Findings on pelvic examination usually are confined to the vagina. The lesion itself usually is exophytic, friable, and most frequently located on the posterior vaginal wall in the upper third of the vagina. The next most common location is on the lower anterior wall. The cervix must be uninvolved in order to establish the lesion as a vaginal primary. By convention, if the cervix is involved, it is classified as primary cervical cancer. The vaginal lesions can be exophytic, ulcerative, or infiltrative. Bimanual and particularly rectovaginal examination must be done in order to assess submucosal or paravaginal extension of the tumor. This is essential for staging purposes. If the histologic diagnosis is adenocarcinoma, endometrial curettage is mandatory in order to rule out an undiagnosed endometrial primary. Careful palpation of groin nodes is important, particularly in lesions arising from the lower third of the vagina. The presence of vesicovaginal or rectovaginal fistulas is indicative of transmural invasion to these organs.

B. Laboratory Findings: Tissue biopsy is required for diagnosis and can usually be done in the office by means of punch biopsy; anesthesia is not required.

Staging & Patterns of Spread

The International Federation of Gynecology and Obstetrics (FIGO) staging system for vaginal cancer is presented in Table 28–4. A thorough physical examination must be performed to detect regional or distant extension. The routine procedures employed for staging purposes include chest x-rays, intravenous pyelography, cystoscopy, barium enema, and proctosigmoidoscopy. CT scanning may give useful information about pelvic and retroperitoneal spread. Tumor dissemination occurs by direct exten-

Table 28–4. FIGO staging of vaginal cancer.

Stage 0	Intraepithelial carcinoma.
Stage I	Carcinoma is limited to the vaginal mucosa.
Stage II	Carcinoma has involved the subvaginal tissue but has not extended onto the pelvic wall.
Stage III	Carcinoma has extended onto the pelvic wall or pubic symphysis.
Stage IV	Carcinoma has extended beyond the true pelvis or has involved the mucosa of the bladder or rectum. Bullous edema or tumor bulge into the bladder or rectum is not acceptable evidence of invasion of these organs.

sion to pelvic structures and by lymphatic spread. Direct extension usually involves the bladder, rectum, urethra, or paravaginal pelvic tissues. Lymphatic spread varies according to the location of the tumor. Lesions arising from the lower third of the vaginal tube most frequently spread to the inguinofemoral nodes, while those arising from the upper third will extend preferentially toward the deep pelvic lymph nodes (obturator, external iliac, and internal iliac).

Prognostic Factors

The stage of disease at the time of diagnosis is the most important indicator of outcome. The chances for cure diminish significantly when the neoplasm extends to adjacent structures and regional nodes. Other factors such as grade, tumor size, or location have not been shown to influence the prognosis; however, lymph node spread significantly reduces the survival rate. Unfortunately, lymph node status rarely is assessed because initial therapy usually is with radiation.

Treatment

A. Radiation Therapy: Radiation therapy is the treatment of choice for most lesions. A combination of external pelvic radiation for the pelvic lymph nodes and intracavitary or interstitial implants for the vaginal tumor is most commonly required. For small stage I lesions, brachytherapy alone may be considered. Radiation to the inguinal lymph nodes should be considered for lesions localized in the lower third of the vagina.

B. Surgery: Surgery may be used in selected cases. For example, radical hysterectomy with partial or total vaginectomy and bilateral pelvic lymph node dissection is preferred for patients presenting with small stage I lesions located on the upper third of the vagina. Selected patients with early lesions localized close to the introitus may be treated by lower vaginectomy, vulvectomy, and inguinal lymphadenectomy. Patients with vaginal cancer and a history of previous pelvic irradiation must be treated by surgery and often require ultraradical surgery such as pelvic exenteration.

C. Chemotherapy: Chemotherapy may be indicated in cases of distant metastatic disease and in those with regional or local recurrences not amenable to further surgery or radiation therapy; however, the response of squamous cell carcinoma to chemotherapy is poor and without clear survival benefit. Most chemotherapy regimens employ platinum-based combination therapy.

Prognosis

Including all stages, recurrences or local failures are seen in about 50% of patients. The 5-year survival for stage I patients is about 80%, for stage II 50%, for stage III 30%, and for stage IV nil to 10%.

OTHER VAGINAL TUMORS

Adenocarcinoma

Adenocarcinomas of the vagina are more often metastases from other sites in the genital tract (cervix, endometrium, ovary) or from extragenital sites (breast, colon, kidney) than primary tumors. Primary vaginal adenocarcinoma accounts for about 15% of vaginal cancers. Clear cell adenocarcinomas are seen in adolescents and young adult women exposed in utero to diethylstilbestrol.

Treatment for this condition follows the guidelines described for squamous carcinoma.

Sarcoma

Sarcomas of the vagina occur almost exclusively in infants and adolescents (sarcoma botryoides). Spread is early and often hematogenous. These lesions appear as multiple grapelike polyps in the vagina.

For localized cases, the preferred treatment is a combination of surgery and chemotherapy; but even with localized disease, the prognosis is poor. A multimodality approach combining conservative surgery, radiation, and chemotherapy has been reported to be equally successful and much less mutilating than the traditional surgical procedures.

Melanoma

Melanomas are highly malignant tumors that carry a very poor prognosis. Most occur in the lower third of the vagina and particularly on the posterior wall. Treatment depends on the location and size of the lesion.

SUGGESTED READINGS

Dancuart F et al: Primary squamous cell carcinoma of the vagina treated by radiotherapy: A failures analysis: The M.D. Anderson Hospital experience 1955–1982. Int J Radiation Oncol Biol Phys 1988;14:745.

DiSaia P: Management of superficially invasive vulvar carcinoma. Clin Obstet Gynecol 1985;28:196.

Hoffman MS et al: Recent modifications in the treatment of invasive squamous cell carcinoma of the vulva. Obstet Gynecol Surv 1989;44:227.

Homesley HD et al: Radiation therapy versus pelvic node resection for carcinoma of the vulva with positive groin nodes. Obstet Gynecol 1986;68:733.

Rose PG et al: Conservative therapy for melanoma of the vulva. Am J Obstet Gynecol 1988;159:52.

Sedlis A et al: Positive groin lymph nodes in superficial squamous cell vulvar cancer: A Gynecologic Oncology Group study. Am J Obstet Gynecol 1987;156:1159.

Shimm DS et al: Prognostic variables in the treatment of squamous cell carcinoma of the vulva. Gynecol Oncol 1986; 24:343.

Spirtos NM et al: Radiation therapy for primary squamous cell carcinoma of the vagina: Stanford University experience. Gynecol Oncol 1989;35:20.

Sulak P et al: Nonsquamous cancer of the vagina. Gynecol Oncol 1988;29:309.

Zucker PK, Berkowitz RS: The issue of microinvasive squamous cell carcinoma of the vulva: An evaluation of the criteria of diagnosis and methods of therapy. Obstet Gynecol Surv 1985;40:136.

29

Cervical Intraepithelial Neoplasia & Cancer

Carcinoma of the cervix is the most commonly diagnosed gynecologic cancer worldwide. In the United States, however, a steady decline in incidence and a 70% decrease in death rate has occurred over the last 40 years. This is due to early detection of preinvasive cervical lesions in asymptomatic women by the use of exfoliative cytologic studies (Papanicolaou smear). In no other gynecologic cancer do patient education and physician intervention have such an impact on the incidence and severity of a disease.

EPIDEMIOLOGY & ETIOLOGY

Incidence

Cervical cancer is the sixth most common cancer in American women. It is the third most common malignancy of the female genital tract, after endometrial and ovarian cancer. Approximately 13,500 new cases of invasive cervical carcinoma are estimated for 1993. The mean age for patients with invasive cancer is between 45 and 50 years, with intraepithelial preinvasive disease preceding invasive cancer by more than 20 years.

Etiology & Risk Factors

The cause of carcinoma of the cervix remains conjectural, but most epidemiologic data include factors associated with sexual behavior. A reasonable hypothesis is that a sexually transmitted agent may act on the most susceptible area in the cervix, the transformation zone, which consists of columnar epithelium that undergoes continuous replacement by squamous epithelium through a metaplastic process. Most cervical neoplasias arise in this area (squamocolumnar junction). Identifying the woman at high risk based on known epidemiologic factors is critical to the success of screening efforts in the general population. The most important risk factors are listed in Table 29–1.

Oncogenic transformation as the result of integration of viral genetic information into cellular DNA is a sound theory that is being investigated.

SCREENING

Cervical cytologic examination (Papanicolaou smear) was introduced in 1941 and has been instrumental in reducing the incidence and mortality rates for cervical cancer. This simple and painless procedure is performed by inserting a dry speculum (no lubrication) into the vagina and exposing the cervix, then scraping the exocervix in an arc of 360 degrees with a wooden (Ayre) or plastic spatula and introducing a cotton-tipped applicator stick into the endocervix and rotating it also 360 degrees. The two samples containing the scraped material are then spread on a glass slide and fixed in alcohol-ether solution prior to staining. Abnormal epithelial features can be divided into those that are definitely benign and those believed to have neoplastic potential (Table 29–2). Viral cytopathic effects, particularly of HPV (koilocytic atypia; see Chapter 6), should be distinguished from cytologic evidence of cervical intraepithelial neoplasia, though they frequently coexist. The accuracy of a Papanicolaou smear in detecting preinvasive and early invasive lesions is about 85%. The ideal frequency of screening has been disputed by various health organizations. The recommendation most often accepted is that of the American Cancer Society (1987), which states that "all women who are, or who have been, sexually active, or have reached age 18 years, [should] have an annual Pap test and pelvic examination. After a woman has had three or more consecutive satisfactory normal annual examinations, the Pap test may be performed less frequently at the discretion of her physician". This recommendation seems to be acceptable to other organizations.

Table 29–1. Epidemiologic risk factors for cervical cancer.

Risk Factor	Risk Ratio
Age at first intercourse (< 17 years)	1.9–5
Number of sexual partners (> 6 vs 1)	2.8–6
High risk male partner	2.7–6.8
Herpes simplex virus type 2	2.8 to > 10
Papillomavirus infection	3.0 to > 10
Cigarette smoking	4

CERVICAL INTRAEPITHELIAL NEOPLASIA (CIN)

The term "cervical intraepithelial neoplasia" replaces the earlier "cervical dysplasia" and "carcinoma in situ," though the latter terms are both still in use. The terms essentially refer to the same process, ie, proliferation of neoplastic cells within the epithelium to various levels but with no invasion into the stroma. Lack of invasiveness and therefore of metastatic potential is what makes possible conservative treatment, in contrast to that required for invasive disease. The rationale for grading intraepithelial disease is based on the different progression rate of untreated cervical intraepithelial neoplasia to invasive carcinoma, which varies from 10% in CIN I to 30% in cases with CIN III.

PATHOLOGY

Squamous cell intraepithelial neoplasia typically arises from the transformation zone as a unifocal or multifocal lesion. Cervical intraepithelial neoplasia is characterized by abnormal maturation of the epithelium, abnormal mitotic figures, and nuclear aneuploidy. The extent to which the neoplastic cells replace the normal epithelium determines the severity of the disease. For example, in CIN I (mild dysplasia), one-third of the thickness of the epithelium is involved; in CIN II (moderate dysplasia), one-half to two-thirds of the epithelium is involved; and in CIN III

Table 29–2. Classification systems for Papanicolaou smears.

Classification	Dysplasia	Cervical Intraepithelial Neoplasia (CIN)
1	Benign	Benign
2	Benign with inflammation	Benign with inflammation
3	Mild dysplasia	CIN I
3	Moderate dysplasia	CIN II
3	Severe dysplasia	CIN III
4	Carcinoma in situ	CIN III
5	Invasive cancer	Invasive cancer

(severe dysplasia, or carcinoma in situ), the full thickness of the epithelium is involved. The basal membrane in all cases remains intact; therefore, no invasion is found in the underlying stroma.

DIAGNOSTIC EVALUATION

With the appropriate use of the five interrelated technical modalities described below, the diagnosis of preinvasive disease can be accurately made in virtually every case (Figure 29–1). A retrospective review of patients whose invasive cancer was missed after outpatient evaluation revealed that in most instances one or more of these techniques were omitted or not utilized properly.

Cytologic Examination

Because most patients are asymptomatic, the diagnosis of cervical intraepithelial neoplasia is usually made after routine cervical smear detects atypical cells compatible with that condition. There are two circumstances under which the Papanicolaou smear may be misleading: false-negative results are reported in 10–20% of cases—either due to errors in sampling and smearing techniques or in laboratory evaluation; and smears may be reported as "atypical" but not "dysplastic." Atypical cell morphology may result from vaginitis, cervicitis, or coexistent papillomavirus infections. If, however, there is no other clinical or cytologic evidence of inflammation to justify this report, these patients require further evaluation. It is important to emphasize that *a Papanicolaou smear is only a screening technique*—the definitive diagnosis is made by tissue biopsy. It must be stressed also that in the presence of a visible cervical lesion, biopsy always should be performed regardless of the cytologic findings. Complete evaluation of the cervix in a patient with abnormal cervical cell morphology consists of colposcopy, cervical biopsies, and endocervical curettage; in selected cases, cone biopsy may be required.

Colposcopy

The colposcope is a stereoscopic binocular microscope of low magnification power which is used to identify epithelial and vascular changes indicative of preinvasive or early invasive cancer. Colposcopy is indicated in all cases in which cytology is suggestive of cervical intraepithelial neoplasia or in which there are atypical noninflammatory features. The technique consists of careful visualization of the epithelial surface before and after application of 3% acetic acid. The purpose of the acetic acid is to accentuate the vascular alterations characteristic of neoplasia (Table 29–3). The expertise needed to visually "grade" the lesion is not as important as the ability to determine if the evaluation is satisfactory (ie, by identification of the transformation zone, ascertaining the extent of the entire lesion, and performing multiple biopsies in the presence of multifocal disease).

Under colposcopic guidance, a punch biopsy of one or more abnormal areas is performed with a cervical biopsy

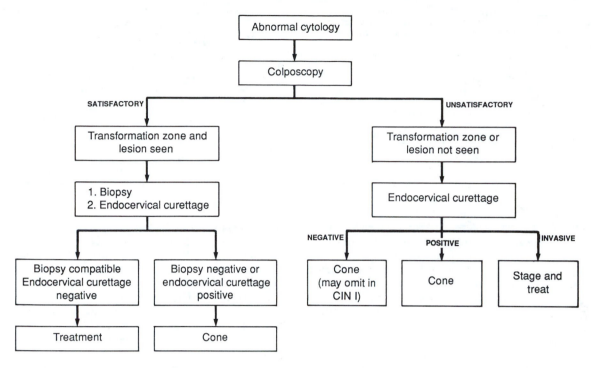

Figure 29–1. Diagnostic evaluation of a suspicious Papanicolaou smear.

instrument (Kevorkian-Younge). If the transformation zone is not entirely visualized, the colposcopic examination is considered unsatisfactory, and most of these patients will require diagnostic conization if there is cytologic evidence of CIN.

Endocervical Curettage

This procedure is designed to evaluate the portion of the endocervical canal that cannot be visualized by colposcopic examination. The endocervical canal is scraped with a small square curette and the specimen placed on a piece of filter paper before fixation. The procedure usually is well tolerated, and bleeding is minimal. Endocervical curettage is recommended in all cases and is mandatory in

Table 29–3. Colposcopic classification

A. Normal colposcopic findings
  1. Original squamous epithelium
  2. Columnar epithelium
  3. Transformation zone
B. Abnormal colposcopic findings
  1. Atypical transformation zone
    a. Leukoplakia
    b. Aceto-white epithelium
    c. Mosaic
    d. Punctation
    e. Atypical vascular pattern
  2. Suspect invasive carcinoma
C. Unsatisfactory colposcopy (squamocolumnar junction not entirely visible)
D. Miscellaneous colposcopic findings (inflammatory changes, atrophic changes, true erosion, condyloma, etc)

those where colposcopy is unsatisfactory (transformation zone not entirely visualized) or when there are no visible lesions. A recent study (Hatch and colleagues) reported that endocervical curettage was more accurate than cervical biopsy in 1% of patients with satisfactory colposcopy, 16% of those with unsatisfactory colposcopy, and 30% of those with no visible lesions. If the endocervical sample reveals abnormal cells, diagnostic conization is indicated.

Cone Biopsy (Conization)

Cone biopsy consists of surgical excision of that portion of the cervix which contains the transformation zone—the area at risk. It usually is indicated for diagnostic purposes; however it may be considered therapeutic when the surgical margins are free of disease. Although colposcopy has significantly decreased the number of cone biopsies being performed, its indications are valid and very well established (Table 29–4). The histopathologic evaluation must be thorough. The material obtained, therefore, must be sectioned at frequent intervals throughout the entire specimen.

CERVICAL INTRAEPITHELIAL NEOPLASIA DURING PREGNANCY

The full diagnostic evaluation of an abnormal Papanicolaou smear must be performed regardless of pregnancy and with only minor modifications. Colposcopic examination is easier to perform because the transformation zone is better exposed by the physiologic eversion of the

Table 29–4. Indications for cone biopsy.

1. Lesion not colposcopically visible in the presence of positive cytology
2. Unsatisfactory colposcopy in the presence of biopsy or cytology suggestive of CIN
3. CIN on endocervical curettage
4. Discrepancy between cytology and histology, with a higher grade cytology report than seen on biopsy specimens
5. Microinvasion or "suspicion" of invasion seen on the biopsy specimen
6. Biopsy-proven in-situ adenocarcinoma of the cervix

Table 29–5. Prerequisites for local treatment of cervical intraepithelial neoplasia.

1. Colposcopic examination must be satisfactory, with visualization of the entire transformation zone.
2. Margins of the lesion must be well defined and visible.
3. Endocervical curettage must not disclose atypical cells.
4. Correlation between cytology and histology must be adequate.

squamocolumnar junction during pregnancy. Punch biopsy sites may bleed actively because of the concomitant hyperemia. The bleeding can easily be arrested by the use of a vaginal pack or a suture. Curetting the endocervix should be omitted in order to avoid risks of hemorrhage and rupture of the membranes. Cone biopsy should be performed only if it is mandatory to exclude invasive cancer. It is best to avoid cone biopsy because of a 15–30% incidence of hemorrhage, abortion, and premature labor. Patients with a histologic diagnosis of cervical intraepithelial neoplasia can be followed by cytology and colposcopically directed biopsies, allowed to deliver vaginally, and then treated definitively after delivery. Because of the slow progression of disease, these intraepithelial lesions usually do not require immediate treatment when detected during pregnancy.

TREATMENT

Conservative local therapy usually is successful in eradicating intraepithelial disease and is appropriate for young women with cervical intraepithelial neoplasia. Before treatment is started, it is imperative to ascertain the severity of the lesion and its extent. Factors other than the histologic features of the lesion are important also in specific patients. For example, treatment selection must take into account the patient's age, menopausal status, fertility status, and reliability for follow-up and the presence or absence of coexisting benign disease. Treatment options include superficial ablative methods such as electrocoagulation, cryotherapy, and laser vaporization and excisional methods such as conization and hysterectomy. The preferred treatment in younger women with low-grade lesions is cryosurgery or laser vaporization in an office setting; if properly applied, an 85–90% success rate can be obtained after one application. However, certain prerequisites are mandatory before conservative local procedures are chosen. These prerequisites are listed in Table 29–5. If any of these prerequisites are not satisfied, local therapy should not be considered. Cone biopsy for diagnostic purposes may also serve the purpose of definite therapy in women whose biopsy specimens have clear surgical margins.

Electrocoagulation

Electrocoagulation consists of thermic destruction of

cervical tissue; it must be deep enough to destroy disease that may be present in the cervical glands. Although still used and considered effective, this procedure has been replaced by methods that are better tolerated.

Cryotherapy

Cryotherapy is the most cost-effective outpatient treatment modality. The procedure consists of freezing the cervix with a cervical probe at −50 °C, causing cell death. The ice ball that forms on the cervix should extend about 4 mm beyond the lesion. A 3-minute freeze, 5-minute thaw, and 3-minute refreeze technique is recommended. The method requires no anesthesia and is well tolerated. Side effects consist mainly of profuse watery vaginal discharge. Cure rates approach 90%. Treatment failures correlate with the extent of cervical involvement, higher grades of cervical intraepithelial neoplasia, and technical expertise of the operator.

Laser Surgery

Laser surgery is the most recently introduced treatment for cervical intraepithelial neoplasia. It acts by boiling the intracellular water and vaporizing the cell. The lesions and the entire transformation zone can be uniformly vaporized to a depth of 5–7 mm. Because laser surgery is more painful and less well tolerated than cryotherapy, many patients require either local infiltration of the cervix or some form of regional or general anesthesia. Postoperative healing is rapid, and complications such as bleeding or discharge are seen rarely. The cure rate is approximately 90%, which is similar to that of cryotherapy. Unfortunately, the laser procedure is much more costly because of the expense of laser equipment. The laser is better than cryotherapy in the treatment of large lesions, advanced grades, and lesions with glandular involvement.

Conization

Conization is more often indicated as a diagnostic than as a therapeutic procedure. It may be chosen, however, as a primary treatment option in cases of multifocal CIN III, in patients with recurrent cervical intraepithelial neoplasia, and in those who are unreliable for follow-up. Complications associated with this procedure occur in less than 10% of patients and include bleeding, cervical incompetence, infection, and cervical stenosis. The cure rate ranges from 50% to over 90% depending on the presence or absence of disease at the margins of the specimen. Management of the patient whose cone biopsy reveals positive margins must be individualized, and basically this depends on the grade of the lesion, whether the endocervix or exocervix is involved, and the patient's desire to maintain reproductive function. The actual management options vary from observation to reconization or hysterectomy.

Hysterectomy

In most instances less invasive procedures than hysterectomy are used to treat cervical intraepithelial neoplasia. Hysterectomy is a treatment option, however, in patients with CIN III who have completed their childbearing. Such an option is also a reasonable choice for women with a coexisting benign condition that may benefit from the surgical procedure, eg, uterine prolapse associated with urinary stress incontinence.

INVASIVE CERVICAL CANCER

PATHOLOGY

Histology

A. Microinvasive Carcinoma: Invasive squamous cell carcinoma of the cervix is the end point of a spectrum of disease beginning with intraepithelial neoplasia. The earliest manifestation of stromal invasion is termed microinvasion. Defining this term has been a matter of controversy; the official definition remains with the FIGO staging classification (see Staging, below). For practical purposes, however, the most accepted definition and one considered to be most helpful from a therapeutic standpoint is that proposed by the Society of Gynecologic Oncologists in 1974, which defines the entity as "stromal invasion to a depth of 3 mm or less below the base of the epithelium and in which lymphatic or vascular involvement is not demonstrated." The purpose of establishing such an entity is to identify a subset of patients in whom metastatic disease and recurrence are unlikely to occur. In such patients, treatment can be less radical than what is required to treat invasive disease.

B. Invasive Carcinoma (Table 29–6): Histologically, 90% of invasive cervical tumors are squamous (epidermoid) carcinomas. The lesions basically resemble their cell of origin and are arranged in sheets and cords having all the features of malignancy. These cancers are subdivided into three subtypes according to cell size and the presence of keratinization: (1) large cell keratinizing, (2) large cell nonkeratinizing, and (3) small cell carcinoma. Attempts to correlate cell type with prognosis have not met with success. The conventional system of tumor grading (well, moderately, and poorly differentiated) is utilized also, and some institutions report good correlation of these descriptive terms with clinical outcomes.

About 10% of invasive cervical cancers are adenocarcinomas or combined adenosquamous carcinomas. Adeno-

Table 29–6. Histologic classification of invasive cervical cancer.

A. Squamous cell carcinoma (epidermoid)
   1. Large cell keratinizing
   2. Large cell nonkeratinizing
   3. Small cell
B. Adenocarcinoma
   1. Pure endocervical adenocarcinoma
   2. Endometrioid
   3. Clear cell
   4. Adenoma malignum
   5. Papillary
C. Mixed carcinoma
   1. Adenosquamous carcinoma
   2. Adenoid cystic
   3. Glassy cell
   4. Adenoid basal
D. Sarcoma
   1. Leiomyosarcoma
   2. Endocervical stromal sarcoma
   3. Mixed mesodermal tumor
   4. Adenosarcoma
E. Lymphoma
F. Melanoma
G. Carcinoid
H. Secondary tumors

carcinomas of the cervix arise from the endocervical glands. Cervical adenocarcinomas must be differentiated from primary endometrial adenocarcinoma because therapy and prognosis are different for these two separate and distinct entities.

Other rare histologic varieties of cervical cancer are listed in Table 29–6.

Macroscopic Appearance

The macroscopic appearance of cervical cancer is variable. The lesions may be exophytic, endophytic, or ulcerative. Exophytic tumors are the most common; they arise on the exocervix and grow toward the vaginal canal. These lesions are usually squamous cell in origin. Endophytic tumors arise in the endocervix, are most often adenocarcinomas, and tend to distend the cervix and the endocervical canal. A third variety is the ulcerative type, which replaces the cervix and the upper third of the vagina with a necrotic crater.

CLINICAL FEATURES

Symptoms & Signs

Early invasive carcinoma of the cervix usually does not produce symptoms. After the tumor has attained a considerable size, the most frequently encountered symptoms are abnormal vaginal bleeding and vaginal discharge. The vaginal bleeding is often described as postcoital; however it may take any form of abnormal menstrual or intermenstrual bleeding. The discharge is usually bloodstained and malodorous. Other symptoms such as pelvic pain and leg edema are seen with pelvic sidewall involvement. Incontinence of urine or feces is suggestive of vesicovaginal or rectovaginal fistula, and these signs are late manifestations of advanced disease. Physical examination should include a careful search for lymph nodes in the supraclavicular and inguinal areas, evidence of pleural effusions, and the presence of abdominal masses. The pelvic examination is crucial for staging purposes. *The following should be accurately recorded: the size of the cervical tumor, extension of tumor into the vaginal mucosa, induration or nodularity of the parametrial areas, uterine size, and adnexal enlargement.* Accurate assessment of these features requires careful rectovaginal examination.

Diagnosis

Biopsy of the cervix is required for diagnosis and consists of sampling one or more representative areas of viable tumor. A biopsy specimen usually can be obtained in the office without anesthesia. Occasionally, in clinically occult lesions, it may be necessary to perform a cone biopsy in order to arrive at a definitive diagnosis. Cone biopsy is always required when the usual less invasive techniques have not excluded invasive disease and in all cases of suspected microinvasive carcinoma. Some cases may require histologic documentation of spread to the parametrium or lymph nodes. Such biopsies may be obtained by transvaginal or percutaneous fine-needle aspiration (or needle biopsy).

Staging

A. Clinical Staging (Table 29–7): The International Federation of Gynecology and Obstetrics (FIGO) staging system for cancer of the cervix is essentially based on clinical assessment and selected endoscopic and imaging techniques—with the exception of very early invasive cancer (microinvasion), in which staging is based on histologic findings. The pelvic examination is the basis for the staging procedure and consists of determining cancer spread beyond the cervix into the vagina and parametrium. Rectovaginal examination is essential for this purpose (Figure 29–2). Technical procedures accepted by FIGO for staging purposes include routine radiographs (chest, bones), colposcopy, intravenous pyelography, cystoscopy, barium enema, and proctosigmoidoscopy. Pelvic and abdominal CT scanning, MRI, and lymphangiography are helpful and often used, but they are not considered part of the routine staging procedure.

B. Surgical Staging: Although not officially recognized or routinely employed, pretherapy surgical staging has been used extensively. It consists of selective lymphadenectomy of the pelvic and periaortic areas in order to detect microscopic lymphatic spread. Treatment may be tailored to surgical findings by employing extended field radiation to involved areas with the purpose of improving survival. This approach remains controversial, and the survival benefit is seen mostly in patients with curable pelvic tumors and microscopic lymph node metastases.

Spread Pattern

The tumor spreads by continuity to the vagina, corpus, and parametrium and via lymphatic channels to the pelvic lymph nodes (external iliac, internal iliac, and obturator nodes). Further extension is toward the common iliac, periaortic, and pericaval lymph nodes. Hematogenous metastases and intra-abdominal extension are encountered less frequently.

Prognostic Factors

A. Stage of Disease: The stage of disease as determined clinically at the time of diagnosis correlates with outcome; cure rates decrease significantly when there is tumor extension beyond the cervix.

B. Tumor Size: Tumor size seems to be an independent prognostic factor. Large tumors usually are associated with advanced stages of disease, and even within the same stage (eg, stage I), the potential for lymphatic spread

Table 29–7. FIGO (1986) staging of cancer of the cervix.

Stage 0	Carcinoma in situ, intraepithelial carcinoma.
Stage I	Carcinoma strictly confined to the cervix (extension to the corpus should be disregarded).
Ia	Preclinical carcinomas of the cervix, ie, those diagnosed only by microscopy.
	Ia1 Minimal microscopically evident stromal invasion.
	Ia2 Lesions detected microscopically that can be measured. The upper limits of the measurement should not show a depth of invasion of > 5 mm taken from the base of the epithelium, either surface or glandular, from which it originates; and a second dimension, the horizontal spread, must not exceed 7 mm. Larger lesions should be staged as Ib.
Ib	Lesions of greater dimensions than stage Ia2, whether seen clinically or not. Preformed space involvement should not alter the staging but should be specifically recorded so as to determine whether it should affect treatment decisions in the future.
Stage II	Carcinoma extends beyond the cervix but has not extended onto the pelvic wall. Carcinoma involves the vagina, but not the lower third.
IIa	No obvious parametrial involvement. The vagina has been invaded, but not the lower third.
IIb	Obvious parametrial involvement.
Stage III	Carcinoma has extended onto the pelvic wall. On rectal examination, there is no cancer-free space between the tumor and the pelvic wall. The tumor involves the lower third of the vagina. All cases with hydronephrosis or nonfunctioning kidney should be included unless known to be due to other causes.
IIIa	No extension onto the pelvic wall but involvement of the lower third of the vagina.
IIIb	Extension onto the pelvic wall and/or hydronephrosis or nonfunctioning kidney.
Stage IV	Carcinoma extending beyond the true pelvis or clinically involving the mucosa of the bladder or rectum. Do not allow a case of bullous edema as such to be allotted to stage IV.
IVa	Spread to adjacent organs (ie, rectum or bladder, with positive biopsy from these organs).
IVb	Spread to distant organs.

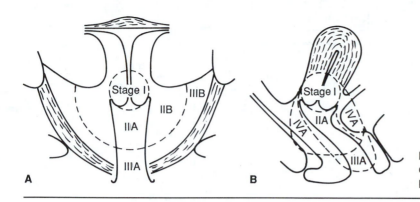

Figure 29–2. Schematic representation of the clinical stages of cervical cancer. **A:** Anterior projection. **B:** Lateral projection.

and local recurrence increases proportionately with tumor size.

C. Invasion: Depth of invasion into the stroma correlates well with the potential for lymphatic involvement. In fact, the entire concept of microinvasive carcinoma of the cervix is based on the depth of invasion. The purpose of defining microinvasive disease is that it has important therapeutic implications; such cases usually will not spread or recur. Therefore, these patients may be treated with less radical procedures.

D. Lymph Node Metastases: Lymph node metastasis is an important indicator of outcome. Survival rates correlate well with pelvic and aortic area lymph node status.

E. Vascular Involvement: Vascular space involvement may correlate with an increased probability of pelvic node metastatic disease.

F. Cell Differentiation: The grade of cellular differentiation of the tumor has been a controversial prognostic feature. Some evidence suggests that there is a correlation with lymphatic spread and recurrence, but this is not always the case.

TREATMENT

Microinvasive Disease

Early stromal invasion, defined as invasion less than 3 mm from the basement membrane and with no vascular space invasion, is best treated with simple hysterectomy. Young patients who wish to preserve childbearing function may be treated with conization as long as the margins are clear, careful follow-up is assured, and the patient understands that this course of action is not considered standard therapy.

Invasive Disease

A. Surgery: Definitive surgical therapy is an option in selected patients with stage I invasive carcinoma. With a depth of tumor invasion of over 3 mm, the procedure of choice is radical abdominal hysterectomy and bilateral pelvic lymphadenectomy. This is the treatment of choice also in those who present with small cervical lesions (< 3

cm in diameter). If the pelvic nodes reveal unexpected metastatic disease, postoperative radiation therapy is recommended, though its benefit remains unproved (Figure 29–3). Complications particular to this surgery are related to the urinary tract (postoperative bladder dysfunction and ureterovaginal fistulas). The incidence of these serious complications has decreased steadily with technical improvements and better-trained gynecologists.

B. Radiation Therapy: Radiation is standard therapy for invasive cervical carcinoma stages IIb through IVa. It consists of various combinations of external radiation to the pelvis and intracavitary implants (brachytherapy) of radioactive isotopes. External pelvic radiation treats the central lesion and the pelvic sites of potential dissemination (parametrium and pelvic lymph nodes) by delivering 4000–5000 cGy to the pelvis. Intracavitary treatment uses either cesium, radium, or cobalt as radioactive sources delivering a high dose to the centrally located tumor.

Complications are related to radiation injury to adjacent organs, particularly the rectum and bladder. Radiation injuries may be acute, subacute, or chronic and of various degrees. The combination of radiotherapy and adjunctive extrafascial hysterectomy is recommended in selected patients with barrel-shaped endophytic stage Ib tumors. In these cases, combined therapy appears to decrease the incidence of central recurrences. Extended field radiation to periaortic metastatic lymph nodes may be indicated and beneficial for selected patients with microscopically involved nodes and potentially curable pelvic disease.

RECURRENT CARCINOMA

Diagnosis

The symptoms and signs of recurrence are listed in Table 29–8. Approximately 40–50% of patients with cervical cancer develop recurrences following primary surgery or radiotherapy; most will be diagnosed within the first 2 years after treatment and will require further therapy. Central recurrence may involve the cervix, vaginal apex, bladder base, or anterior rectal wall, usually presenting with bleeding or vaginal discharge. Occasionally, tumor recurrence is detected in asymptomatic patients as a

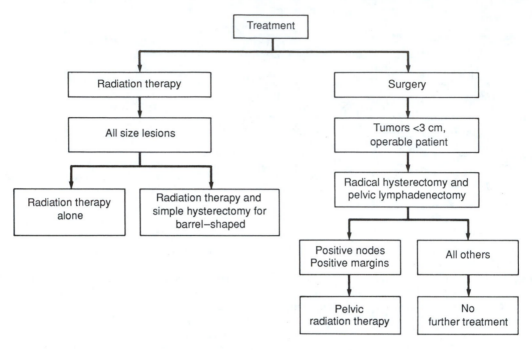

Figure 29–3. Treatment of cervical cancer: Selected stages Ia2, Ib, and IIa.

centrally located exophytic or infiltrative tumor. Regional recurrence is defined as tumor involving the pelvic sidewall, and it usually presents with symptoms and signs of pelvic or leg pain, leg edema, and ureteral obstruction. Distant recurrences result in symptoms unique to the metastatic sites. Although histologic documentation of recurrence is always desirable, it is not always practical. A major advance in this field has been the use of fine-needle aspiration cytology; most metastatic sites can be reached and the diagnosis confirmed using this procedure.

Treatment

The choice of therapy for recurrent cervical cancer depends of the site of recurrence and type of primary treatment delivered.

A. Radiation Therapy: Radiation therapy for pelvic recurrences is a treatment option for patients previously treated with surgery. Repeat irradiation of recurrences in previously irradiated fields is associated with high morbidity and low cure rates and is not recommended. Radiation of isolated distant metastases (eg, bone) may benefit selected patients.

B. Surgery: Pelvic exenteration is indicated in isolated central recurrences in patients primarily treated with radiation therapy. It consists of removing the involved pelvic organs (uterus, vagina), including the bladder (anterior exenteration), the rectosigmoid (posterior exenteration), or both (total exenteration). A cure rate of up to 50% may be expected in selected patients. The short- and long-term morbidity of this procedure is significant and only justified if indicated for cure and not for palliation. This operation requires diversion of the urinary stream by implantation of the ureters into an isolated segment of intestine (ileal or colon conduit) and of the fecal stream by a permanent colostomy. Innovative surgical techniques allow vaginal reconstruction by the use of myocutaneous flaps, end-to-end low rectal anastomosis by use of staplers (sparing a permanent colostomy), and construction of a continent urinary pouch.

C. Chemotherapy: Chemotherapy is considered in cases of distant metastatic disease and in those with regional or local recurrences not amenable to surgery or radiation therapy. Although the response of squamous cell tumors to chemotherapy averages 25%, there is no clear proof of prolongation of survival or in improvement in the quality of life. Most regimens employ cisplatin-based combination therapy.

Table 29–8. Symptoms and signs of recurrent cervical cancer.

Symptoms
Vaginal discharge or bleeding
Pelvic, back, hip, or knee pain
Weight loss
Edema of lower extremities
Signs
Central necrosis of cervix and vagina
Pelvic induration or mass
Leg edema
Enlarged nodes on physical or radiologic examination
Evidence of ureteral obstruction

SURVIVAL

Survival outcome depends on various factors, mainly stage, tumor volume, and lymphatic spread. Close to 100% survival may be expected for microinvasive carcinoma (as previously defined). For stage Ib tumors, a survival rate of 85% may be expected with either surgery or radiation therapy. Survival drops to 65% for stage IIb, 35% for stage IIIb, 16% for stage IVa, and nil for stage IVb. This decrease in survival with later stages is partly due to the increased incidence of metastasis to the pelvic and aortic nodes with advancing stages.

SPECIAL SITUATIONS

Pregnancy

The incidence of cervical cancer in pregnancy is about 1:2000. The most common symptom is vaginal bleeding; however, 20% will be asymptomatic and detected at the time of a routine visit. Diagnostic evaluation, including biopsies, should be performed as if there were no pregnancy, except for endocervical curettage. Accurate staging by pelvic examination may be more difficult to assess during the latter half of pregnancy. To avoid ionizing radiation, MRI is useful for determining the extent of disease and urinary tract involvement.

There is no evidence that pregnancy has a detrimental effect on the 5-year survival rates of appropriately treated patients. Similarly, the route of delivery does not seem to affect survival, though experience is limited because most patients are delivered by hysterotomy or cesarean section. Deciding whether treatment should be instituted immediately rather than waiting for fetal viability essentially depends on the gestational age at the time of diagnosis. Prior to 24 weeks of gestation, disease should be treated stage by stage as in the nonpregnant patient, with the understanding that fetal demise will occur as part of therapy. The treatment of choice for young women with early stage cancer is radical hysterectomy and pelvic lymphadenectomy. Pelvic radiation followed by intrauterine and vaginal cesium is used in all other cases. If radiation therapy is chosen, the uterine products usually will be expelled spontaneously during treatment. Occasionally during the second trimester, it may become necessary to perform hysterotomy for uterine evacuation. During the late second and early third trimesters, awaiting fetal viability becomes a reasonable option and delivery should be planned as soon as feasible. Treatment should be started approximately 1 week to 10 days after delivery to allow for uterine involution.

Carcinoma of the Cervical Stump

Although supracervical hysterectomy rarely is performed, patients with carcinoma of the cervical stump are still occasionally seen. There are no major differences in the diagnostic evaluation, staging, and principles of treatment as compared to those with an intact uterus. If radiation therapy is chosen, difficulties may be encountered in placing intracavitary tandems because of the absence of a uterine cavity. In these cases, the use of a higher dose of external pelvic radiation or a transperineal placement of a template may be adequate treatment. The 5-year survival rates are equal to those for cancer of the intact uterus.

Invasive Cancer in the Uterus Removed for Benign Condition

Occasionally, the pathologist may report an unexpected invasive cervical cancer in a hysterectomy specimen removed for a benign indication. Most of these cases consist of small early invasive lesions in patients in whom cervical disease was not suspected or not properly evaluated. These patients are treated with external pelvic radiation and local vaginal irradiation. The 5-year survival rate ranges from 96% to 37% depending on the status of margins in the hysterectomy specimen and the presence of residual disease.

OTHER HISTOLOGIC VARIETIES OF CERVICAL CANCER

Adenocarcinoma

Adenocarcinoma accounts for about 10% of cervical cancers, and according to some authors its frequency is increasing. It arises from the cervical mucus-producing glandular elements. It does not have the same epidemiologic risk factors as those described for squamous cell carcinoma.

Besides the more common pure form of endocervical adenocarcinoma, other histologic subtypes include adenosquamous carcinoma, clear cell adenocarcinoma, adenoid cystic carcinoma, and endometrioid adenocarcinoma. Age at presentation, spread pattern, and clinical symptoms are similar to those associated with the squamous variety. Screening by cervical cytologic testing may have a lower yield because most cases arise in the endocervix. Characteristic pelvic findings include the presence of a bulky endophytic growth with a barrel-shaped cervix. Some authors have suggested a worse prognosis for these patients, but the evidence indicates that stage by stage and for equivalent tumor size, the 5-year survival rates are comparable. Treatment guidelines are similar to those described for the squamous variety. Because of the increased volume of disease seen in some of these endophytic lesions, radiation therapy has been chosen as primary treatment followed by extrafascial hysterectomy.

Adenosquamous carcinoma is a mixture of malignant squamous and glandular elements, comprising 5–25% of cervical adenocarcinomas. Although there is conflict in the literature regarding the prognosis in these patients, it does not appear to be any different from the more common varieties. The most poorly differentiated variety of adenosquamous carcinoma is the glassy cell carcinoma. This lesion has well-defined histologic features and the worse prognosis in these patients is most likely related to the poor differentiation of the tumor.

Clear cell adenocarcinoma is characterized by clear

and hobnail-shaped tumor cells; it has been detected primarily but not exclusively in women exposed in utero to diethylstilbestrol. Both surgery and radiation have been effective in treating this condition, following the same guidelines as for other cervical malignancies.

Adenoid cystic carcinoma is an unusual gynecologic tumor. Such tumors are more frequently seen in the respiratory tract, salivary glands, and breast. The lesion is characterized by small cells with hyperchromatic nuclei and minimal cytoplasm. The prognosis is poor because of the known potential of this tumor for early metastatic spread.

Verrucous Carcinoma

Verrucous carcinoma is a variant of squamous cell carcinoma characterized by an exophytic growth which resembles that seen in condyloma acuminatum. Cervical cytologic tests and superficial biopsies may be deceptive, not indicating its malignant nature. The cells are usually well-differentiated. Verrucous carcinoma is locally invasive, tends not to invade underlying stroma, and seldom metastasizes to lymph nodes. Preferential therapy for stage I is surgery; radiation therapy is reserved for more advanced stages.

Small Cell Cancer

Small cell cancer has been considered traditionally to be a histologic subtype of squamous cell carcinoma; however, recent studies using the electron microscope have resulted in the recognition of other variants of small cell cancer that do not qualify as squamous. Neuroendocrine carcinoma is a variant characterized by the presence of neurosecretory granules, some showing argyrophilic staining. Characteristically, these cancers tend toward early and widespread dissemination. Combination radiation therapy and chemotherapy is often used, though the latter is as yet poorly evaluated. Carcinoid tumor of the cervix is another variant; it is a rare neoplasm of endocrine origin arising from argyrophil cells in the cervix. Oat cell carcinoma of the cervix is also a rare neoplasm very similar to bronchogenic oat cell carcinoma and has a very poor prognosis.

Other Tumors

Sarcomas of the cervix are rare; these lesions include leiomyosarcomas, stromal cell sarcomas, embryonal rhabdomyosarcomas (sarcoma botryoides), adenosarcomas, and mixed müllerian sarcomas. In general, the prognosis is very poor regardless of what treatment is provided.

Lymphomas arising in the cervix are also rarely seen. A malignant lymphoma presenting initially as a cervical tumor must be considered as an exceptional possibility. Radiation therapy seems to be adequate treatment for lymphomas originating in the cervix.

Melanomas of the cervix have been reported rarely. Surgery is the treatment of choice, but the prognosis is generally poor.

Secondary carcinomas of the cervix occur as extensions of endometrial cancer. Metastases to the cervix from extrapelvic sites are rare. Most are from the breast, gastrointestinal tract, lung, and urinary tract. Such occurrences are rare, but metastases may occasionally occur from clinically undetected primary tumors.

SUGGESTED READINGS

Brinton LA et al: Sexual and reproductive risk factors for invasive squamous cell cervical cancer. JNCI 1987;79:23.

Hacker NF et al: Carcinoma of the cervix associated with pregnancy. Obstet Gynecol 1982;59:735.

Hatch KD et al: Role of endocervical curettage in colposcopy. Obstet Gynecol 1985;65:403.

La Polla JP et al: The influence of surgical staging on the evaluation and treatment of patients with cervical carcinoma. Gynecol Oncol 1986;24:194.

Morley GW et al: Pelvic exenteration, University of Michigan: 100 patients at 5 years. Obstet Gynecol 1989;74:934.

Noguchi H et al: Pelvic lymph node metastasis of uterine cervical cancer. Gynecol Oncol 1987;27:150.

Yazigi R et al: Adenosquamous carcinoma of the cervix: Prognosis in stage IB. Obstet Gynecol 1990;75:1012.

zur Hausen H: Papillomaviruses in anogenital cancer as a model to understand the role of viruses in human cancers. Cancer Research 1989;49:4677.

30

Uterine Corpus Cancer

ENDOMETRIAL CARCINOMA

In the United States, endometrial carcinoma is the most common cancer of the female genital tract followed by ovarian and cervical cancer. Approximately 31,000 new cases are estimated for 1993, which makes this the fourth most common cancer in women after cancer of the breast, colon, rectum, and lung. About 80% of cases are seen in postmenopausal women, the diagnosis usually being made between the ages of 55 and 69. Fewer than 5% of cases occur in women under the age of 40.

Etiology & Risk Factors

The cause of endometrial carcinoma remains unknown, though the evidence points toward endocrine-related factors, particularly unopposed estrogenic stimulation of the endometrium from endogenous or exogenous sources. Factors that place certain women at high risk for developing this disease are listed in Table 30–1.

A. Obesity: Almost half of patients with endometrial cancer are obese. It has been postulated that the peripheral conversion of weak androgens normally secreted by the adrenals (eg, Δ^4-androstenedione) into estrogen (estrone) in adipose tissue would result in constant estrogenic stimulation of the endometrium, with the outcome being endometrial proliferation and carcinoma.

B. Diabetes and Hypertension: These conditions are present in 30–35% of patients with endometrial cancer. The relationship to cancer remains unclear except for the association of these diseases with obesity.

C. Chronic Anovulation: This condition is responsible for the association of endometrial cancer with nulliparity and with polycystic ovarian syndrome. The few cases seen in women under age 35 usually involve these features. Absence of a monthly corpus luteum and ensuing progesterone production makes the estrogenic stimulation constant and unopposed.

D. Estrogen-Producing Ovarian Tumors: Sex cord stromal ovarian tumors such as thecomas and granulosa-theca cell tumors are strongly associated with endometrial hyperplasias and carcinoma.

E. Estrogen Replacement Therapy: Postmeno-pausal patients receiving estrogen replacement therapy have an increased incidence of endometrial cancer that is apparently related to dosage and duration of exposure. Similar observations were made in patients using sequential oral contraceptives (now withdrawn from the market). A protective effect is achieved by adding cyclic progesterone to the regimens of estrogen-treated postmenopausal women, making the use of estrogen replacement therapy acceptable for most patients. Similarly, the use of combination contraceptives has resulted in a 50% reduction in cancer risk for women taking the pill.

F. Miscellaneous Conditions: Liver dysfunction, late menopause, and breast and colon cancer may also be associated with a higher incidence of endometrial carcinoma.

Premalignant Lesions

Endometrial hyperplasia and, rarely, endometrial polyps may eventually progress to endometrial adenocarcinoma. Endometrial hyperplasia is characterized by a proliferative response of the endometrium to the unopposed stimulation of estrogens (endogenous or exogenous) and is classified by the International Society of Gynecologic Pathologists and the World Health Organization (WHO) as cystic (simple), adenomatous (complex), or atypical hyperplasia. Simple or complex hyperplasia is commonly encountered in association with physiologic anovulation at menarche and perimenopausally, when progesterone production is either intermittent or absent. Hyperplasia is also frequently associated with the presence of estrogen-producing ovarian tumors (thecomas and granulosa-theca cell tumors), polycystic ovarian syndrome, and adrenocortical hyperplasia. Neither simple nor complex hyperplasia presents atypical cytologic features, and the differences between them are based on the complexity of the architectural pattern. Under these circumstances, they are not considered premalignant lesions and are usually treated successfully by cyclic supplementation of progesterone.

These lesions' potential for malignant transformation ranges between 1% and 4%. However, with the addition of atypical cytologic features (atypical endometrial hyperplasia), the potential for malignant transformation in

Table 30–1. Distribution of patients with carcinoma of the endometrium according to reported histories of risk factors.[1]

Risk Factors	Number	Percentage
Oligomenorrhea	382	5.5
Obesity	2971	43.0
Diabetes mellitus	1746	25.2
Hypertension	3048	44.1
Polycystic ovarian syndrome	80	1.2
Carcinoma of the ovaries	90	1.3
Carcinoma of the breast	211	3.1
Carcinoma of the colon and rectum	88	1.3
All other malignant diseases	136	2.0

[1]From Wharton JT and associates: Risk factors and current management in carcinoma of the endometrium. Surg Gynecol Obstet 1986;162:515. (A report of the Cancer Commission of the American College of Surgeons.)

postmenopausal women may approach 23% without treatment (Table 30–2). While this transformation process may take several years, some pathologists consider severe atypical hyperplasia to be carcinoma in situ of the endometrium. The main symptom of hyperplasia is abnormal vaginal bleeding, and the diagnosis is established by histologic sampling of the endometrium. If endometrial biopsy reveals hyperplasia with atypical features, curettage should follow to rule out invasive carcinoma.

Management varies according to the age of the patient and the histologic features of the hyperplasia. Simple or complex hyperplasia with no atypical features diagnosed in the teenager or perimenopausal woman can be adequately treated with cyclic progestational therapy, and the patient can be followed by means of serial biopsies. Atypical hyperplasia should be treated more aggressively, especially in the postmenopausal woman. Hysterectomy and bilateral salpingo-oophorectomy is the treatment of choice in those who have completed childbearing. Otherwise, progesterone therapy or induction of ovulation followed by serial histologic sampling of the endometrium is recommended.

Screening Methods: Endometrial Cytology

Screening the general population for endometrial cancer is not widely practiced because of the difficulties of sampling a postmenopausal endometrial cavity and the discomfort of dilating an atrophic and frequently stenotic endocervical canal. Nevertheless, several methods are available for cytologic or histologic sampling: endometrial lavage, brush biopsy, saline irrigation, vacuum aspiration, jet washing, endocyte, and the more accurate and reliable endometrial biopsy (Table 30–3). The sensitivity of these techniques ranges from 60–90%. The main drawback of the cytologic methods is their inaccuracy for diagnosis of hyperplasia; however, they are applicable in the group of patients at high risk for endometrial cancer.

Pathology

The vast majority of malignant tumors of the uterine endometrium are adenocarcinomas (95%) with differentiation toward endometrium-like glands (endometrioid), sometimes in combination with other histologic features such as benign (adenoacanthoma) or malignant squamous elements (adenosquamous carcinoma). Less commonly seen are clear-cell, mucinous, serous papillary, secretory, ciliated, and primary squamous cell carcinomas (Table 30–4). The prognostic significance of the histologic type is controversial. Some authors suggest that adenoacanthomas have a more favorable biologic behavior than the pure adenocarcinomas—and, conversely, that adenosquamous carcinoma would imply a worse prognosis than the pure form. Others have based their estimates of outcome on the grade of the lesion, which appears to be more often well-differentiated in adenosquamous tumors and poorly differentiated in pure adenocarcinomas.

According to FIGO, carcinoma of the uterine corpus should be classified as follows according to the degree of differentiation of the adenocarcinoma: **Grade 1:** 5% or less of a nonsquamous or nonmorular solid growth pattern. **Grade 2:** 6–50% of a nonsquamous or nonmorular solid growth pattern. **Grade 3:** more than 50% of a nonsquamous or nonmorular solid growth pattern.

Table 30–2. Classification of preinvasive lesions.[1]

Term	Features	Malignant Potential
Metaplasia	Replacement of usual gland cells by cells having cilia, eosinophilic cytoplasm, squamous metaplasia, or mucinous differentiation.	Little or none
Simple hyperplasia	Glands irregular, cells individually enlarged, some minor budding or outpouching	1–3% over 15 years
Complex hyperplasia	Back-to-back glands, budding, papillary processes, bridges, minor stratification, cells individually enlarged.	3–4% over 13 years
Atypical hyperplasia	Cytologic atypia with enlarged nuclei, enlarged nucleoli, hyperchromatism, stratification, dispolarity.	23% over 11 years

[1]From Norris HJ and colleagues: Preinvasive lesions of the endometrium. Clin Obstet Gynecol 1986;13:725.

Table 30–3. Office procedures for diagnosis of uterine carcinoma.

Technique	Unsatisfactory (%)	Sensitivity (%)
Papanicolaou smear	—	50
Saline irrigation	17	70
Brush cytology	32	64
Vacuum aspiration	25	50
Jet washer	21	60
Isaacs cell sampler	4	83
MiMark cell sampler	—	66
Endocyte (instrument)	6	83
Endometrial biopsy (Novak or Randall curette)	3	96

Clinical Findings

A. Symptoms and Signs: Ninety percent of postmenopausal women with endometrial carcinoma present with vaginal bleeding. In premenopausal or perimenopausal women, the main complaint is menometrorrhagia. Although endometrial cancer is rare in young patients, when it does occur it most often afflicts overweight women with a history of anovulatory cycles. The bleeding in postmenopausal women has no distinctive features—it may vary from bright red to dark brown staining or to a blood-tinged vaginal discharge. Differentiation from other causes of postmenopausal bleeding is of urgent concern (Table 30–5). Menopause is defined as absence of menses for 1 year or more. Any postmenopausal patient presenting with vaginal bleeding requires careful evaluation; roughly one out of five patients (20%) presenting with postmenopausal bleeding will prove to have endometrial cancer. This risk increases with age from a low of 15% in the immediate postmenopausal period to almost 50% in patients 80 years of age or older.

Findings on pelvic examination are usually unremarkable when the disease is confined to the corpus—in fact, the uterus may be normal in size or only slightly enlarged. Extension to the cervix, vagina, or parametrium, if present, should be readily apparent on careful pelvic examination. Occasionally, in the presence of cervical involvement, differentiation must be made from primary adenocarcinoma arising in the cervix. Associated abnor-

Table 30–4. Histologic classification of endometrial carcinoma by the International Society of Gynecologic Pathologists.

```
I.   Endometrioid
        A. Ciliated
        B. Secretory
        C. Papillary
        D. Adenoacanthoma
        E. Adenosquamous
II.  Papillary serous
III. Mucinous
IV.  Clear cell
V.   Squamous
VI.  Mixed
```

Table 30–5. Causes of postmenopausal bleeding.

```
Atrophic endometrium
Withdrawal to exogenous estrogens
Endometrial cancer
Endometrial hyperplasia
Endometrial or endocervical polyps
Other gynecologic malignancies
    Cancer of the cervix
    Cancer of the vagina
    Uterine sarcoma
```

mal findings such as lymph node enlargement, pleural effusion, abdominal masses, and ascites are indicative of advanced disease.

B. Laboratory Findings: Histologic specimens (required for diagnosis) are obtained either by endometrial biopsy as an office procedure or in the operating room by dilation and curettage (D&C), the choice depending on the patient's tolerance and the physician's ability to sample a postmenopausal uterus in an ambulatory setting. An unsatisfactory or negative endometrial biopsy performed for postmenopausal bleeding does not exclude the possibility of cancer. In this case, D&C should follow.

No matter which method is employed, the endometrial cavity must be sounded and its length documented. It is useful also to curette the endocervix separately (fractional curettage) in order to assess endocervical involvement. Both of these determinations were customary for proper staging when the staging system was based on clinical examination. With the newly developed primary surgical staging, these procedures become less important for staging unless the patient is not a candidate for primary surgical treatment, in which case she would be staged clinically.

C. Imaging: Sonography and other uterine imaging techniques may suggest an endometrial tumor. This may be an important incidental finding in patients who have these tests performed for diverse indications. Sonography is helpful also in visualizing the ovaries and other pelvic structures. Hysterosalpingography and hysteroscopy impose a theoretic risk of cell dissemination and are not routinely used. Hysteroscopy would be of benefit in cases with recurrent bleeding and nondiagnostic curettage. CT scan may be helpful for localizing spread to other intraperitoneal or retroperitoneal structures. MRI is helpful for the preoperative determination of myometrial invasion and involvement of the lower uterine segment.

Differential Diagnosis

Differential diagnosis almost always requires histologic sampling of the endometrium and should include all other possible causes of postmenopausal and perimenopausal bleeding. These are due most frequently to atrophic endometrium, endometrial polyps, benign or malignant myometrial tumors, endometrial hyperplasias, and other gynecologic malignancies.

Staging

The International Federation of Gynecology and Obstetrics (FIGO) staging for endometrial cancer was modified in October, 1988 and is presented in Table 30–6. The principal difference introduced by the new staging system is that it is based on surgical pathologic findings, which means that most patients must undergo primary surgical evaluation for this purpose unless there is a clear surgical contraindication or unless the patient has advanced disease. Fortunately, approximately 75% of cases are stage I at the time of diagnosis. The distinction between stages I and II is based upon histologic involvement of the endocervix. Unequivocal invasion into the endocervical stroma or endocervical glands is required in order to qualify as true cervical involvement.

In addition to a thorough physical examination, other procedures employed for staging purposes are chest x-rays, intravenous pyelography, cystoscopy, barium enema, and proctosigmoidoscopy.

Spread Pattern

Endometrial cancer spreads by various pathways—but most commonly by contiguity to the cervix, vagina, and myometrium; by lymphatic dissemination to the pelvic and periaortic nodes; by transluminal spread through the uterine tubes, reaching the peritoneal cavity; and finally by hematogenous spread to distant sites, especially the lungs, liver, and bone (Table 30–7). A Gynecologic Oncology Group study has clearly demonstrated that lymphatic spread is a preferential route of spread in cases characterized by poorly differentiated cells or deep myometrial invasion (Table 30–8).

Prognostic Factors

A. Stage: The extent of disease at the time of diagnosis is an important indicator of outcome. The chances for cure diminish significantly when the neoplasm leaves the confines of the corpus. Several other factors have been identified as having prognostic significance, particularly in stage I disease.

B. Grade: The potential for myometrial invasion,

Table 30–7. Spread pattern of endometrial carcinoma.

A. Direct
    Endometrial surface
    Myometrium
    Endocervix
    Uterine tubes
B. Lymphatic
    Pelvic nodes
    Aortic nodes
C. Hematogenous
    Lung
    Bone
    Liver

spread to pelvic and aortic lymph nodes, recurrence, metastasis, and fatal outcome correlates with histologic grade of differentiation. Well-differentiated (G1) tumors have the best prognosis, and poorly differentiated ones (G3) account for most cases with poor outcomes. This information can usually be obtained preoperatively at the time of diagnostic endometrial curettage and confirmed with the uterine specimen. In some cases, it may significantly influence the choice of therapy.

C. Myometrial Invasion: The depth of invasion into the myometrium is one of the most important prognostic indicators. Generally, tumors confined to the endometrium or invading the inner third of the myometrium have a very low incidence of lymphatic spread. Those that invade the middle third and especially the outer third have up to a 30% chance of containing occult metastatic cells. This information can be accurately obtained only by examining the uterine specimen; therefore, it is useful to have the pathologist open the specimen and assess the depth of invasion. There is an 80% correlation between preoperative determination of myometrial invasion by MRI and what is seen in the uterine specimen (Figure 30–1). This technique deserves further evaluation.

D. Lymph Node Metastasis: Documentation of microscopic spread to pelvic and aortic lymph nodes significantly influences therapeutic planning and the cure rate. It thus becomes imperative to perform selective lymphadenectomy in all patients at high risk for nodal metastasis, ie, those with poorly differentiated tumors and those with deep myometrial invasion. This is probably the most predictive indicator of the patient's chances for cure and correlates with the prognostic indicators listed above.

Table 30–6. Corpus cancer staging (FIGO, 1988).

Stage	Grade	
IA	G123	Tumor limited to endometrium
IB	G123	Invasion to < one-half of myometrium
IC	G123	Invasion to > one-half of myometrium
IIA	G123	Endocervical glandular involvement only
IIB	G123	Cervical stromal invasion
IIIA	G123	Tumor invades serosa and/or adnexa and/or positive peritoneal cytology
IIIB	G123	Vaginal metastases
IIIC	G123	Metastases to pelvic and/or para-aortic lymph nodes
IVA	G123	Tumor invasion of bladder and/or bowel mucosa
IVB		Distant metastases, including intra-abdominal and/or inguinal lymph nodes

Table 30–8. Depth of invasion, grade, and pelvic lymph node metastasis.[1]

Depth of Invasion	Grade		
	G1 (N = 180)	G2 (N = 288)	G3 (N = 153)
Endometrium only (N = 86)	0 (0%)	1 (3%)	0 (0%)
Inner myometrium (N = 281)	3 (3%)	7 (5%)	5 (9%)
Middle myometrium (N = 115)	0 (0%)	6 (9%)	1 (4%)
Deep myometrium (N = 139)	2 (11%)	11 (19%)	22 (34%)

[1]Modified from Creasman WT et al: Surgical pathologic spread patterns of endometrial cancer: A Gynecologic Oncology Group Study. Cancer 1987;60:2035.

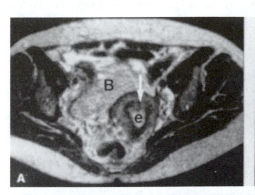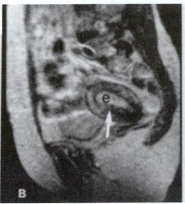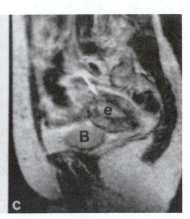

Figure 30–1. Endometrial carcinoma with superficial myometrial invasion. **A,** Transaxial and **B,** sagittal images (T_R 2.0, T_E 80) demonstrate a prominent irregular endometrial cavity (e). Loss of the low-signal junctional zone *(arrows)* corresponds with regions of histologically confirmed superficial infiltration of the myometrium (*B,* urinary bladder). (Reproduced, with permission, from Yazigi R and associates: Magnetic resonance imaging determination of myometrial invasion in endometrial carcinoma. Gynecol Oncol 1989;34:94.)

E. Peritoneal Cytology: A finding of freely floating cancer cells in peritoneal lavage fluid presents a controversial issue. Positive peritoneal cytology is seen more often in advanced stages of disease and in those cases apparently confined to the uterus with unexpected intraperitoneal or retroperitoneal spread. In cases judged to be stage I at surgical pathologic examination, its significance as an independent prognostic indicator remains uncertain.

F. Other Conditions: Capillary-like space involvement has been associated with an increased incidence of lymph node metastases and recurrence. Cytosol progesterone receptor levels seem to correlate with tumor differentiation, being highest in well-differentiated tumors and lowest in poorly differentiated ones. Progesterone receptor levels also are predictive of tumor response to hormone therapy. Tumor size has been implicated as an independent prognostic factor. The incidence of lymph node involvement correlates with the size of the tumor.

Treatment

A. Stage I: In the absence of contraindications to surgery, operation is the primary treatment for all cases. Surgery permits accurate estimation of the extent of disease (staging) and a more rational plan for therapy. The procedure of choice is abdominal extrafascial hysterectomy and bilateral salpingo-oophorectomy. Peritoneal washings should be taken in all cases for cytologic examination, and inspection and palpation of the subdiaphragmatic surfaces, liver, omentum, peritoneal surfaces, gastrointestinal tract, pelvis, and retroperitoneum should be performed. Biopsy samples should be obtained from any suspicious areas, and representative pelvic and aortic lymph node sampling should be done in all cases at high risk for occult metastatic spread (ie, high grade and deep invasion). If intraperitoneal spread is found unexpectedly at surgery, a maximal tumor reductive procedure should be performed.

Postoperative external radiation to the pelvis or extended field radiation to the aortic area is indicated in all cases in which lymph node involvement is documented. Such therapy should be considered also in those cases defined as high risk by virtue of advanced grade, deep invasion, or occult microscopic cervical spread when lymph node sampling was not performed.

B. Stage II: Patients with cervical involvement have a greater propensity for lymphatic spread and recurrence; therefore, these cases have usually been managed with combined pelvic radiation and surgery. Patients with gross cervical involvement on pelvic examination are best treated with preoperative radiation therapy to the pelvis followed by extrafascial hysterectomy. Those with unexpected microscopic occult cervical involvement noted in the hysterectomy specimen may be adequately treated following the guidelines described for stage I disease, adding postoperative radiation according to findings (ie, nodal status). This approach may spare patients the ordeal of being irradiated without benefit. Radical hysterectomy and pelvic lymphadenectomy may be considered as alternative treatment for selected patients with cervical involvement; however, most of these patients are not good candidates for radical surgery because of advanced age, obesity, and other medical conditions.

C. Stage III: Only a minority of patients are initially suspected on clinical grounds of having stage III disease, and these usually are identified by virtue of vaginal or parametrial spread. Following a negative metastatic workup, these patients are best treated with primary external radiation therapy followed by reductive tumor surgery in selected cases. If patients are found to have surgical stage III disease by virtue of unexpected ovarian or lymph node involvement, therapy should be tailored to the location of the intraperitoneal or retroperitoneal spread. Microscopic ovarian involvement does not necessarily carry an ominous prognosis; additional radiation therapy is recommended. Retroperitoneal lymph node involvement will require radiation therapy to the pelvis and periaortic area if these areas are involved. The treatment of positive peritoneal cytology remains as controversial as the issue itself; most gynecologic oncologists recommend avoiding aggressive therapy that could cause significant morbidity.

D. Stage IV and Recurrent Tumors: Stage IVa patients who present with bladder or rectal mucosal involvement are treated with primary external radiation therapy to the pelvis followed either by intracavitary cesium or radium. In selected patients with no spread to the sidewalls, curative exenteration could be considered. Patients with stage IVb disease and those with recurrent tumors need to be treated with systemic chemotherapy or hormonal therapy. Knowledge of the patient's progesterone receptor status may help in determining therapy. Progesterone receptor levels are significantly higher for well-differentiated tumors than for poorly differentiated ones. Parenteral medroxyprogesterone acetate (Provera) or oral megestrol acetate may be used initially for receptor-positive patients. Chemotherapy is considered for receptor-negative patients and for those whose disease progresses while they are receiving progestins. A 30% response rate may be expected with cisplatin- or doxorubicin-based combinations. Unfortunately, responses have been short-lasting. Isolated localized recurrences may be managed by radiation therapy.

Survival & Prognosis

Survival and prognosis correlate with the stage of disease at the time of diagnosis. Five-year survival figures based on collected series range from 90% to 60% for stages I and II and from 30% to nil for stages III and IV.

UTERINE SARCOMAS

Uterine sarcomas are relatively rare tumors, accounting for less than 4% of cases of corpus cancer. Even though they arise in the same organ as endometrial adenocarcinoma, their histologic features, clinical presentation, spread pattern, biologic behavior, and clinical outcome are entirely different. Sarcoma of the uterus is one of the most lethal gynecologic cancers even when apparently confined to the corpus.

The cause is unknown. Although at times uterine sarcoma is associated with the same high-risk epidemiologic factors seen with endometrial cancer (eg, obesity and hypertension), these associations are not consistent. Some authors have reported an increased incidence of uterine sarcoma in patients previously irradiated for other pelvic malignant tumors. Malignant degeneration of a uterine leiomyoma is always a concern, particularly when it rapidly increases in size during clinical observation; however, this is a rare eventuality, occurring in less than 1% of cases.

Histopathology

Several classifications have been proposed, but the most commonly used is that of Kempson and Bari (Table 30–9). Pure sarcomas differ from mixed sarcomas in that the former are composed of one cell type only. Homologous tumors are those that contain malignant elements arising in native uterine tissues (ie, smooth muscle, endometrial stroma); heterologous tumors arise from tissues not normally present in the uterus (ie, bone, fat). Mixed mesodermal tumors (or mixed müllerian tumors) present a combination of sarcomatous and carcinomatous elements, the former either of the homologous or heterologous type. The most frequently seen tumors are leiomyosarcoma, endometrial stromal sarcoma, and mixed mesodermal tumors.

A. Leiomyosarcoma: This lesion—the second most common uterine sarcoma—is a pure sarcoma that is most frequently intramural, though it may also be submucosal or subserosal. The number of mitoses per 10 high-power fields and the presence of cellular atypia are critical determinants of prognosis. Leiomyosarcoma must be differentiated from cellular leiomyoma and bizarre leiomyoma, which are considered to be benign and typically have less than 5 mitoses per 10 high-power fields. Besides the mitotic count, good prognostic indicators appear to be the premenopausal status of the patient, tumor confinement within a myoma, and absence of necrosis. Other rare entities that may be confused with leiomyosarcoma are intravenous leiomyomatosis, metastatic uterine leiomyoma, and disseminated intraperitoneal leiomyomatosis, all of which have a relatively benign biologic behavior.

B. Endometrial Stromal Sarcoma: These tumors are subdivided on the basis of their mitotic count and tumor borders. Those with more than 10 mitoses per 10

Table 30–9. Classification of uterine sarcomas.[1]

Pure sarcomas
  Pure homologous sarcomas
    Leiomyosarcoma
    Stromal sarcoma
    Endolymphatic stromal myosis
    Angiosarcoma
    Fibrosarcoma
  Pure heterologous sarcomas
    Rhabdomyosarcoma (including sarcoma botryoides)
    Chondrosarcoma
    Osteosarcoma
    Liposarcoma
Mixed sarcomas
  Mixed homologous sarcomas
  Mixed heterologous sarcomas
  Mixed heterologous sarcomas with or without homologous elements
Malignant mixed müllerian tumors (mixed mesodermal tumors)
  Malignant mixed müllerian tumor, homologous type; carcinoma plus leiomyosarcoma, stromal sarcoma, or fibrosarcoma, or mixtures of these sarcomas
  Malignant mixed müllerian tumor, heterologous type; carcinoma plus heterologous sarcoma with or without homologous sarcoma
Sarcoma unclassified
Malignant lymphoma

[1]From Kempson RL and associates: Uterine sarcomas: Classification, diagnosis and prognosis. Hum Pathol 1970;1:331.

high-power fields are high-grade endometrial stromal sarcomas, whereas those with less than 10 mitoses are low-grade endometrial stromal sarcomas (endolymphatic stromal myosis) or endometrial stromal nodules. The latter lesion has noninfiltrating tumor borders. The malignant behavior of these lesions correlates well with their mitotic count.

C. Malignant Mixed Mesodermal Tumor: This tumor usually develops as a polypoid mass distending the uterine cavity. Invasion into the myometrium is common, and the depth of invasion correlates well with the incidence of lymph node metastases. Some investigators have reported that homologous tumors have a better prognosis than heterologous ones.

Clinical Findings

The mean age of women with leiomyosarcoma is approximately 55, which is about 10 years younger than that of women presenting with mixed mesodermal tumors and endometrial stromal sarcoma. Uterine bleeding and pelvic pain are the most common presenting symptoms. On physical examination, an abdominal mass or uterine enlargement is often found, and a polypoid mass may occasionally be seen protruding through the cervix. Sampling of the endometrial cavity either by biopsy or D&C is diagnostic in less than 50% of cases owing to the fact that many of these tumors are intramural and thus without endometrial extension. This is particularly true of leiomyosarcomas. In the presence of cervical involvement, biopsy can be obtained readily. In many cases, the diagnosis is an unexpected finding at the time of hysterectomy done for other indications. The staging workup is similar to that described for endometrial carcinoma; uterine sarcomas are staged according to the FIGO system for corpus cancer. About half of all cases present with stage I disease.

The preferential route of spread is via the bloodstream. Over 90% of cases that recur do so at distant sites, especially the lung. Other less frequent routes of spread are via the lymph nodes and by contiguity.

Treatment & Prognosis

A. Surgical Treatment: The preferred treatment is total abdominal hysterectomy and bilateral salpingo-oophorectomy. Careful intraperitoneal and retroperitoneal exploration is performed, and biopsy specimens are taken from any suspicious areas. Unexpected lymph node metastatic disease has been found in up to 35% of apparently stage I cases. Negative surgical staging, however, does not ensure that recurrence will not follow. Approximately 50% of stage I cases will eventually develop distant metastatic spread. The role of cytoreductive surgery for extrauterine disease is not well established; however, it is of doubtful value in high-grade tumors because of their aggressiveness.

Leiomyosarcomas unexpectedly found in a myomectomy specimen have occasionally been treated conservatively without hysterectomy. Most of these cases have presented well-delimited and encapsulated tumors. This treatment is not recommended as primary therapy because the local recurrence rate is unknown.

B. Radiotherapy: Primary radiation therapy is not indicated unless there is a surgical contraindication. Adjuvant radiotherapy after surgery for stage I disease has been advocated in several series. Although radiotherapy confers no proven survival benefit, it appears to decrease the incidence of local pelvic recurrence. If tumors recur, they will do so at extrapelvic sites; therefore, regional treatment would not be expected to prevent this eventuality. Radiotherapy is indicated for patients presenting with advanced pelvic disease, though cures are rare.

C. Chemotherapy: Chemotherapy is indicated for palliation of patients presenting with distant metastases or recurrences. Doxorubicin, cisplatin, dacarbazine, and, more recently, ifosfamide—alone or in various combinations—have produced response rates of less than 30% and no apparent increases in survival time. Adjuvant chemotherapy for prevention of recurrences in stage I and II disease has not proven to be advantageous. High-dose progesterone therapy has produced objective responses in cases of endolymphatic stromal myosis.

Survival

The best 5-year survival rate has been achieved with stage I disease, in which it approaches 50%. The rate diminishes significantly as stage advances, with 0–10% survival for stages III and IV. Stage by stage, survival is not influenced by histologic type. Although some series have reported a worse prognosis for patients with mixed mesodermal tumors, this may be because they are diagnosed at later stages.

SUGGESTED READINGS

Creasman WT et al: Surgical pathological spread patterns of endometrial cancer. Cancer 1987;60:2035.

Edmonson JH et al: Randomized phase II studies of cisplatin and a combination of cyclophosphamide-doxorubicin-cisplatin (CAP) in patients with progestin-refractory advanced endometrial carcinoma. Gynecol Oncol 1987;28:20.

Feuer GA, Calanog A: Endometrial carcinoma: Treatment of positive para-aortic nodes. Gynecol Oncol 1987;27:104.

Grigsby PW et al: Stage II carcinoma of the endometrium: Results of therapy and prognostic factors. Int J Rad Oncol Biol Phys 1985;11:1915.

Silverberg SG et al: Carcinosarcoma (malignant mixed mesodermal tumor) of the uterus. Int J Gynecol Pathol 1990;9:1.

Norris HJ, Connor MP, Kurman RJ: Preinvasive lesions of the endometrium. Clin Obstet Gynecol 1986;13:725.

Wharton JT et al: Risk factors and current management in carcinoma of the endometrium. Surg Gynecol Obstet 1986;162: 515.

Yazigi R, Piver MS, Blumenson L: Malignant peritoneal cytology as prognostic indicator in stage I endometrial cancer. Obstet Gynecol 1983;62:359.

Yazigi R et al: Magnetic resonance determination of myometrial invasion in endometrial carcinoma. Gynecol Oncol 1989; 34:94.

31

Ovarian & Fallopian Tube Cancer

OVARIAN CANCER

Ovarian cancer is the second most common gynecologic malignancy in the United States, with approximately 19,000 new cases being reported every year. It is in fact the most lethal of all gynecologic cancers, accounting for an estimated 12,000 deaths annually. The mortality rate is high, probably because no effective screening devices are available for early detection. By the time the diagnosis is made, well over 70% of patients have disease that has spread beyond the ovaries and pelvis.

Risk Factors

The risk factors associated with ovarian carcinoma are listed in Table 31–1. Familial ovarian cancer (affecting more than one first-degree relative) occurs in younger women and is particularly lethal. Any patient with a history of familial ovarian carcinoma who is concerned about the development of cancer should have prophylactic oophorectomy after the age of 35. A family history of breast, endometrial, or colon cancer also implies an increased risk of ovarian cancer. Another risk factor—low parity in the absence of anovulation—suggests that constant disruption of the ovarian surface by ovulatory mechanisms may be a predisposing cause. The long-term use of oral contraceptives has a protective effect—the only known means of prevention other than oophorectomy.

Pathology & Classification

The WHO classification of ovarian tumors is presented in Table 31–2. Epithelial tumors make up the overwhelming majority—about 85%—of primary ovarian cancers. Germ cell tumors constitute approximately 8% to 10% and stromal tumors 4%.

The ovaries are sites of metastasis from other gynecologic and nongynecologic tumors, most commonly those of the breast, endometrium, colon, and stomach. Meta-

static carcinoma accounts for about 15% of all ovarian cancers.

Fifty percent of epithelial tumors are papillary serous tumors and are usually metastatic to the upper abdomen when diagnosed (Table 31–3). Mucinous tumors, which constitute 15% of epithelial tumors, have a histologic appearance resembling that of colonic and endocervical adenocarcinomas. These tumors generally are confined to the pelvis when discovered and are the largest primary epithelial carcinomas. Endometrioid ovarian carcinomas resemble endometrial carcinoma histologically and account for about 15% of epithelial tumors. Concomitant double primary carcinomas of the endometrium and ovaries are reported in 20% of cases of endometrial carcinoma. Infrequently, endometrioid ovarian carcinoma is associated with endometriosis of the ovary. Clear-cell tumors are associated with endometriosis of the ovary and constitute 5% of epithelial tumors. They are typically bilateral and often associated with primary endometrial carcinoma as well.

Histologic morphology is of secondary importance once ovarian carcinoma has metastasized to the upper abdomen, since all histologic types behave in a similar manner in terms of pattern of spread, response to chemotherapy, and survival. From a prognostic or survival standpoint, however, tumor grade remains a most important factor for all cell types, along with stage and the presence of residual disease. One classification system of epithelial tumors lists a separate type of tumor—the so-called tumor of low malignant potential, with an intermediary histologic presentation and a distinct pathologic and clinical identity. These ovarian tumors are described as being of low malignant potential and account for 12% of all ovarian malignancies. They are considered to behave "more benignly" than typically overt ovarian carcinomas, as reflected by survival data.

Staging

Ovarian cancer is the only gynecologic cancer exclusively staged surgically. The FIGO surgical staging scheme for stage III ovarian carcinoma addresses the pres-

Table 31–1. Risk factors associated with ovarian carcinoma.[1]

Risk Factor	Relative Risk	Risk Factor	Relative Risk
Positive family history	17–50	Use of talc	3
Number of pregnancies (vs 5)		Oral contraceptives used > 3 years	0.5
0	4–5		
1 or 2	3	Obesity	2
3 or 4	1.5	Blood type A	1.8
		White vs black race	1.5
Age at first pregnancy (vs < 20 years)		Gallbladder disease, cervical polyps, or intolerance to oral contraceptives	3–5
20–24	1.75		
≥ 25	3	Endometriosis, fibroids	?
Age at first marriage (> 30 years vs < 30 years)	2		

[1]From Morrow CP, Townsend DE: *Synopsis of Gynecologic Oncology.* Wiley, 1987.

ence of grossly visible disease and its dimensions in the upper abdomen (Table 31–4). Furthermore, the presence of retroperitoneal disease is predictive of survival and is very likely a poorer prognostic factor when compared to intra-abdominal disease alone. Stage III cancers constitute about 70% of all diagnosed cases.

Clinical Findings

A. Symptoms and Signs: Ovarian carcinoma for the most part is insidious in onset, giving rise to few early symptoms. As mentioned above, over 70% of cases are not diagnosed until spread beyond the pelvis has become apparent. Only occasionally do these early-stage malignancies result in menstrual irregularities. Even less frequently noted are symptoms due to pressure on contiguous structures, resulting in urinary frequency or constipation. Extensive upper abdominal disease most often causes abdominal distention due to ascites. Early satiety, peripheral weight loss, and gastrointestinal obstructive symptoms are noted also. The most common symptom of spread beyond the abdomen is shortness of breath. Stage IV disease often presents as right-sided pleural effusion.

The presence of ascitic fluid and a pelvic mass on physical examination is advanced ovarian carcinoma until proved otherwise. Occasionally, ascites may be present with normal-appearing ovaries on CT scan or MRI and no evidence of another primary. Under such circumstances, a papillary serous carcinoma arising from the peritoneum may be discovered. The culprit—a tumor similar in histologic appearance to ovarian papillary serous carcinoma—usually arises in the pelvis and may spread in much the same way as primary ovarian carcinoma.

B. Approach to Diagnosis: The diagnosis of ovarian enlargement is based upon the age of the patient and associated symptoms. Except in rare circumstances, all ovarian enlargements call for surgical exploration.

In menstruating women, cystic enlargements less than 7 or 8 cm and confirmed by sonography are considered functional cysts and treated expectantly or suppressed with oral contraceptives for 2 months, after which time surgical exploration is required if no involution takes place.

Table 31–2. Ovarian tumors: WHO classification.[1]

I. Common "epithelial" tumors (may be benign, borderline, or malignant)
    Serous
    Mucinous
    Endometrioid
    Clear cell
    Brenner
    Mixed epithelial
    Undifferentiated
    Mixed mesodermal tumors
    Unclassified
II. Sex cord stromal tumors
    A. Granulosa stromal cell
        1. Granulosa cell
        2. Thecoma-fibroma
    B. Androblastomas; Sertoli-Leydig cell tumors
        1. Well-differentiated (Pick's adenoma, Sertoli cell tumor)
        2. Intermediate differentiation
        3. Poorly differentiated
        4. With heterologous elements
    C. Lipid cell tumors
    D. Gynandroblastoma
    E. Unclassified
III. Germ cell tumors
    A. Dysgerminoma
    B. Endodermal sinus tumor
    C. Embryonal carcinoma
    D. Polyembryoma
    E. Choriocarcinoma
    F. Teratomas
        1. Immature
        2. Mature (dermoid cyst)
        3. Monodermal (struma ovarii, carcinoid)
    G. Mixed forms
    H. Gonadoblastoma
IV. Soft tissue tumors not specific to the ovary
V. Unclassified tumors
VI. Secondary (metastatic) tumors
VII. Tumor-like conditions (pregnancy, luteoma, etc)

[1]Modified from Morrow CP, Townsend DE: *Synopsis of Gynecologic Oncology.* Wiley, 1987.

Table 31–3. Epithelial ovarian cancers and their relative frequencies.

Cell Type	Percentage
Serous	50
Mucinous	15
Endometrioid	15
Undifferentiated	15
Clear cell	5

In perimenarcheal women, cystic ovarian enlargements may occur as a result of alterations in the pituitary-ovarian axis. The result of chronic anovulation is the appearance of multiple cystic structures on both ovaries. Once ovulation is regulated, the cystic ovaries regress.

C. Tumor Markers: Owing to the high frequency of malignant germ cell tumors that occur in the premenarcheal teens and early twenties, tumor marker levels (α-fetoprotein, βhCG, and lactic dehydrogenase) should be determined. CA-125 is an antigenic determinant for ovarian carcinoma which, unfortunately, lacks both the sensitivity and the specificity that would make it a good screening marker for epithelial ovarian carcinomas. Plasma CA-125 measurement does have clinical use, however, in following patients already diagnosed as having ovarian carcinoma. The test can be used to monitor the patient's relative responsiveness to chemotherapy. Unfortunately, however, even if CA-125 levels disappear with treatment, it is not certain that residual carcinoma does not still exist. This is because the marker may be present in plasma at levels too low for detection with currently available methods.

D. Imaging: Routine barium enema is recommended in patients over 50 years of age to rule out colonic carcinoma presenting as a pelvic mass. It is recommended also in any patient with symptoms of colonic obstruction. An upper gastrointestinal series is recommended for patients who present with symptoms of small bowel obstruction.

An intravenous pyelogram is necessary in all cases presenting with complex pelvic masses to rule out ureteral obstruction, especially if retroperitoneal exploration is necessary for pelvic tumor removal. *Routine mammography should be performed as well, since breast cancer has a strong tendency to metastasize to the ovaries.* Such metastases are often bilateral and rarely exceed 10 cm. Breast metastases to the ovaries are commonly associated with other metastatic sites as well. By and large, sonography is unnecessary if surgery is anticipated, since little is added to the overall patient evaluation.

Routes of Spread

Ovarian carcinoma spreads by three routes:

(1) The most common route is transcelomic, with a rather predictable pattern of spread along the normal flow route of peritoneal fluid, ie, along bilateral pericolic gutters, along the small bowel mesentery, and eventually up to the diaphragm, especially to the right side. Because omentum, small bowel, and large bowel may become seeded with tumor, these areas must be carefully inspected and sampled.

(2) Ovarian cancer can spread retroperitoneally not only directly to the periaortic lymph nodes but to the pelvic nodes as well. Lymph node sampling in both areas is imperative.

(3) Rarely, spread may be by hematogenous dissemination. Parenchymal lung, liver, and bone are common sites for distant metastasis by this route. Diagnostic evaluation of these areas is not done routinely owing to the rarity of this spread pattern.

Treatment of Epithelial Tumors

A. Stage I Tumors: Stage I ovarian carcinoma is diagnosed in only 15% of cases. However, even when ovarian cancer seemingly is confined to one or both ovaries, careful exploration will reveal disease in the upper abdomen or retroperitoneum in about 30% of cases. If proper

Table 31–4. FIGO staging system for ovarian carcinoma (December, 1985).

Stage I	Growth limited to the ovaries.
Stage IA	Growth limited to one ovary; no ascites. No tumor on the external surface; capsule intact.
Stage IB	Growth limited to both ovaries; no ascites. No tumor on the external surfaces; capsule intact.
Stage IC	Tumor either stage IA or IB but with tumor on surface of one or both ovaries; or with capsule ruptured; or with ascites fluid present containing malignant cells or with positive peritoneal washings.
Stage II	Growth involving one or both ovaries with pelvic extension.
Stage IIA	Extension and/or metastases to the uterus and/or tubes.
Stage IIB	Extension to other pelvic tissues.
Stage IIC	Tumor either stage IIA or IIB, but with tumor on surface of one or both ovaries; or with capsule(s) ruptured; or with ascites fluid present containing malignant cells or with positive peritoneal washings.
Stage III	Tumor involving one or both ovaries with peritoneal implants outside the pelvis and/or positive retroperitoneal or inguinal nodes. Superficial liver metastasis equals stage III. Tumor is limited to the true pelvis but with histologically proved malignant extension to small bowel or omentum.
Stage IIIA	Tumor grossly limited to the true pelvis with negative nodes but with histologically confirmed microscopic seeding of abdominal peritoneal surfaces.
Stage IIIB	Tumor of one or both ovaries with histologically confirmed implants of abdominal peritoneal surfaces, none > 2 cm in diameter. Nodes are negative.
Stage IIIC	Abdominal implants > 2 cm in diameter and/or positive retroperitoneal or inguinal nodes.
Stage IV	Growth involving one or both ovaries, with distant metastases. If pleural effusion is present, there must be positive cytology to allot a case to stage IV. Parenchymal liver metastases equal stage IV.

staging is accomplished and the patient truly has stage I disease, tumor grade becomes another important prognostic factor. (Grade 1 = well-differentiated; grade 2 = moderately well differentiated; grade 3 = poorly differentiated.) Well-differentiated (grade 1) lesions with disease confined to one ovary require no further treatment. In fact, in young women wishing to preserve childbearing potential, unilateral oophorectomy with wedge biopsy of the contralateral ovary is recommended after surgical staging. Once childbearing potential is completed, hysterectomy and removal of the contralateral ovary is recommended. Total abdominal hysterectomy and bilateral salpingo-oophorectomy is recommended for tumors of grades 2 or 3 and all tumors of stage IC and higher.

Controversy exists concerning adjuvant treatment in stage I cases. Most authorities recommend some form of therapy, but no prospective randomized trials have been conducted. The current trend is to treat patients with stage I, grades 2 and 3, disease with melphalan or a combination of cisplatin and cyclophosphamide, whereas stage IC cases can be treated with either ^{32}P (intraperitoneal radioactive phosphate), whole abdominal radiation, or combination chemotherapy (Chapter 27). All patients should be followed with serial CA-125 determinations if the levels are high at the beginning of therapy.

B. Low Malignant Potential Tumors: Since tumors of low malignant potential are usually (60% of cases) stage IA, conservation treatment is the rule for women who wish to preserve reproductive function; for those who do not, total abdominal hysterectomy and bilateral salpingo-oophorectomy is recommended. Generally speaking, surgical staging is not recommended for tumors of low malignant potential, and no adjuvant treatment is recommended. Five-year survival rates for stage I tumors are approximately 90%.

C. Advanced Epithelial Tumors: The primary objective for stage II and III ovarian epithelial carcinoma is to remove as much tumor as possible (Figure 31–1). Most patients undergo total abdominal hysterectomy with bilateral salpingo-oophorectomy, omentectomy, removal of peritoneal and retroperitoneal implants, and perhaps even extensive bowel resection. In many cases, the largest residual volume represents disease confined to the pelvic peritoneum and rectosigmoid. A retroperitoneal approach to "debulking" is necessary to remove bulky tumor. This may require resection of portions of the sigmoid colon and

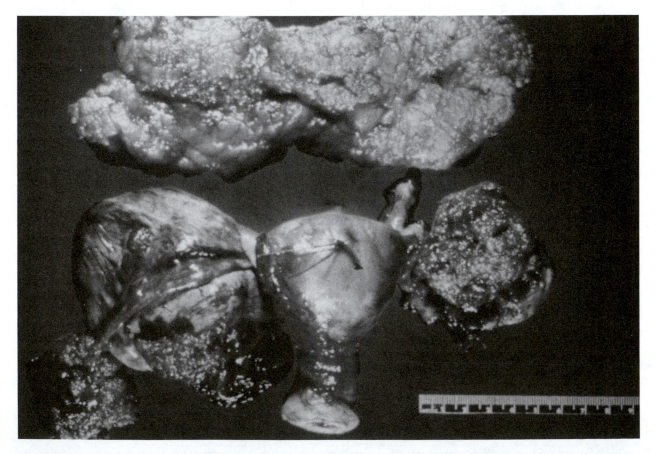

Figure 31–1. Stage III ovarian carcinoma. Papillary serous adenocarcinoma with bilateral ovarian involvement and metastasis to the omentum.

rectum and occasionally even entangled small bowel segments.

The concept of "debulking" or cytoreduction has resulted in significant benefit from the standpoint of palliating ascites, alleviating bowel obstruction, relieving ureteral obstruction, or a combination of these factors. Cytoreduction also theoretically increases the growth factor of cells—the number of cells actively replicating—thus making cancer cells more vulnerable to chemotherapeutic agents or radiation therapy. Finally, cytoreduction reduces the number of courses of chemotherapy the patient must endure.

D. Chemotherapy: Once surgery is completed, combination chemotherapy then follows. The most efficacious agents used are cisplatin and carboplatin. Both have been shown to have the highest overall response rates of any of the active agents. Cisplatin or carboplatin in combination with cyclophosphamide or doxorubicin is the combination usually given. It should not be necessary to give more than six to eight courses if cytoreduction therapy has been successful. In patients who are not successfully cytoreduced, three initial courses of PAC (platinum [cisplatin or carboplatin], Adriamycin [doxorubicin], and cyclophosphamide) or PC (platinum and cyclophosphamide) are given, and the patients are reexplored for a second try at cytoreduction. This often proves to be as effective as successful cytoreduction on initial exploration. For the rare patient with parenchymal liver or lung metastasis, surgical exploration is recommended only for palliative reasons such as relief of bowel obstruction (Figure 31–2).

E. Radiation Therapy: Radiation therapy is very limited and has never been compared with systemic combination chemotherapy as primary treatment. The only possible situation in which radiation therapy should be used primarily is stage IC, IIC, and perhaps IIIA disease with no visible residual disease in the pelvis (Figure 31–2).

F. Second-Look Operation: Upon completion of chemotherapy, a second-look operation is offered to the patient who has no clinical evidence of disease. This includes patients with CA-125 levels of less than 35 IU per mL, negative chest x-ray, negative CT scan of the abdomen and pelvis, and negative physical examination. The purpose of second-look operations is to spare the patient further chemotherapy if there is no pathologic evidence of disease and to offer the patient with residual carcinoma salvage treatment. To date, no single type of treatment has been shown to be superior to any other (see below). Unfortunately, second-look operations have not improved 5-year survival rates in epithelial ovarian carcinomas.

During a second-look operation, extensive surgical exploration is done to reinspect the sites previously explored for stage I or stage II disease—ie, careful inspection is done of the pelvis, upper abdomen, and retroperitoneum, and multiple biopsy specimens are taken from areas of known residual disease and potential target areas for cancer spread. Omentum, diaphragm, pericolic gutters, and bowel mesentery all are biopsied. If no residual disease is found in the specimens submitted, no further treatment is required.

Residual disease discovered at a second-look operation may be macroscopic or microscopic. For the most part, gross macroscopic residual disease that failed detection by CT scan, physical examination, or CA-125 measurement is probably not curable. In contrast, patients with microscopic residual disease or even small (< 0.5 cm) macroscopic residual disease may have prolonged survival times with the use of any of a number of salvage protocols. To date, no randomized prospective studies have been conducted, and there is no specific superior treatment regimen—ie, recommendations are for the most part based on anecdotal evidence (Figure 31–3). Listed below are the common salvage regimens used:

(1) Intraperitoneal chemotherapy.

(2) Whole abdominal radiation therapy.

(3) Dose intensification, ie, a doubling of the drug (eg, from 50 mg/m^2 to 100 mg/m^2 of cisplatin).

(4) Second-line systemic chemotherapy, ie, agents showing activity to ovarian carcinoma but not used as first-line therapy.

(5) Immune modifying agents such as interferon, BCG, *Corynebacterium parvum,* and interleukin-2 with natural killer cells.

(6) Drugs being evaluated in experimental protocols.

Prognosis

Although absolute cure rates have not significantly improved in epithelial ovarian cancer, survival times and disease-free intervals have increased following aggressive use of multiple chemotherapy regimens.

GERM CELL TUMORS

Germ cell tumors constitute approximately 10% of primary ovarian malignancies. Fortunately, they are usually stage I when detected.

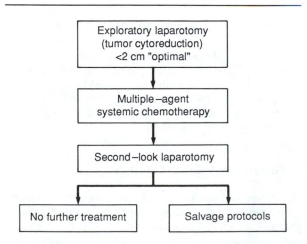

Figure 31–2. Algorithm for the treatment of advanced epithelial ovarian carcinoma.

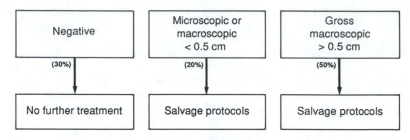

Figure 31–3. Algorithm of second-look operation.

1. DYSGERMINOMA

Dysgerminomas account for about 50% of all germ cell tumors and are bilateral in 15% of cases. Of all the germ cell tumors, dysgerminomas have the greatest proclivity to spread to the retroperitoneal lymph nodes. Because such spread occurs in approximately 30% of cases, the retroperitoneum must be explored at operation.

The peak incidence for dysgerminomas is the late teens and early 20s. There are no specific tumor markers for dysgerminomas, but mild elevations in β-hCG may occasionally be noted along with elevated levels of serum lactic dehydrogenase.

Treatment

A conservative operative approach is employed for dysgerminomas. This includes a unilateral salpingo-oophorectomy, wedge biopsy of the contralateral ovary, and retroperitoneal exploration of the pelvic and periaortic lymph nodes. Radiation therapy in a dosage no greater than 3000 cGy is the treatment of choice for positive lymph nodes. In addition, multiple-agent chemotherapy in the form of VAC (vincristine, actinomycin D [dactinomycin], and cyclophosphamide) has been shown to be very efficacious in cases where intraperitoneal spread has occurred. No adjuvant therapy is recommended if the tumor is confined to one ovary.

2. ENDODERMAL SINUS TUMORS

Endodermal sinus tumors are the most malignant of the germ cell tumors. Even with stage I tumors, the death rate is approximately 60%. These cancers are usually unilateral and are confined to the ovaries in over 70% of cases. Unfortunately, they are insensitive to radiation therapy. The hallmark of these tumors is production of α-fetoprotein, which is the tumor marker used in following response to chemotherapy.

Treatment

All patients with endodermal sinus tumors are treated adjuvantly with multiple-agent chemotherapy in the form of bleomycin, etoposide, and cisplatin or carboplatin.

3. IMMATURE TERATOMAS

Most immature teratomas are confined to one ovary, but upper abdominal metastases are present in 20% of cases. A benign dermoid cyst may exist in the contralateral ovary. The grading of immature teratomas is based upon the immaturity of the germ cell elements in the ovary.

Treatment

These tumors are very sensitive to vincristine, dactinomycin, and cyclophosphamide combination chemotherapy. Second-look procedures are generally recommended in immature teratomas that are stage III. Other combination therapy regimens, such as bleomycin, etoposide, and platinum, are recommended when first line agents result in no response.

4. MIXED GERM CELL TUMORS

Mixed germ cell tumors are a combination of several germ cell elements—dysgerminomas, endodermal sinus tumors, and immature teratomas—often all admixed. Treatment is directed at the worst-appearing histologic tumor—ie, if endodermal sinus tumors are present, the primary therapeutic regimen should be bleomycin, etoposide, and cisplatin or carboplatin.

TUMORS OF OVARIAN STROMAL ORIGIN

Tumors of ovarian stromal origin usually are unilateral when first discovered. They have a strong tendency to rupture and often produce symptoms related to excess hormone production. They are generally considered to be of low malignant potential, requiring for the most part no chemotherapy or radiation therapy.

1. GRANULOSA CELL TUMORS

Granulosa cell tumors occur most frequently in women in the fourth and fifth decades and are confined to one ovary in over 85% of cases. These hormonally active tumors produce symptoms of estrogen excess. In postmenopausal women, resumption of vaginal bleeding may occur; in menstruating women, irregular bleeding may be the only symptom. Adenocarcinomas and hyperplasias of the endometrium are seen in 25% of cases associated with granulosa cell tumors of the ovary. A variant of granulosa cell tumor, the so-called "juvenile" granulosa cell tumor, is seen more commonly in prepubertal females. The overall prognosis is generally the same as that associated with the "adult" granulosa cell tumor.

The presence of Call-Exner bodies on histologic specimens, while not pathognomonic, is presumptive evidence that an ovarian tumor is a granulosa cell tumor.

Treatment

Treatment for the most part consists of total abdominal hysterectomy with bilateral salpingo-oophorectomy. In the very young patient, conservative surgery is standard care. In the rare patient with intra-abdominal spread or with a tumor containing a high mitotic count, combination chemotherapeutic agents are used. The agents employed are similar to those used with germ cell tumors.

2. SERTOLI-LEYDIG CELL TUMOR

The Sertoli-Leydig cell tumor, a virilizing tumor, is encountered in patients in their 20s and 30s. Virilizing symptoms consist of increasing acne, clitoromegaly, hoarseness, and frontal baldness. Most tumors are unilateral (95%), and removal of the ovary is adequate treatment except in rare instances of intraperitoneal spread or in cases with poorly differentiated lesions (50% of cases). With such poorly differentiated tumors, treatment should consist of multiple-agent chemotherapy similar to that used to treat germ cell tumors.

FALLOPIAN TUBE CARCINOMA

Most "tumors" of the fallopian tubes represent either an ectopic pregnancy or pelvic inflammatory disease. Primary adenocarcinomas of the fallopian tube account for approximately 0.3% of all gynecologic malignancies. The mean age at diagnosis is approximately 58 years, but the range is extremely wide. The classically described **hydrops tubae profluens,** manifested by colicky lower abdominal pain relieved by discharge of urine-like fluid from the vagina, occurs only rarely in patients with fallopian tube carcinoma. These adenocarcinomas are histologically identical to primary ovarian serous carcinomas and very difficult to distinguish. Criteria for the diagnosis of a primary fallopian tube carcinoma include the histologic identification of a transition zone between benign and malignant tubal epithelium and tumor confined to the fallopian tube.

There is no official FIGO staging classification for fallopian tube carcinoma. Unlike ovarian carcinomas, however, over 70% of fallopian tube carcinomas are confined to the fallopian tube when first diagnosed as opposed to being in other parts of the abdomen. When metastases do occur, the pattern is identical to that of ovarian adenocarcinomas.

Treatment of fallopian tube carcinomas is identical to that of ovarian adenocarcinoma. Cytoreduction and combination chemotherapeutic agents (cisplatin and cyclophosphamide) are the preferred treatment.

SUGGESTED READINGS

Berek JS, Hacker NF: *Practical Gynecologic Oncology.* Williams & Wilkins, 1989.

Deppe G: *Chemotherapy of Gynecologic Cancer.* A.R. Liss, 1984.

Heintz APM: *Advanced Ovarian Carcinoma: Surgical Treatment and Prognosis.* Noordwijk, The Netherlands, 1985.

Morrow CP, Townsend DE: *Synopsis of Gynecologic Oncology,* 3rd ed. Wiley, 1987.

Piver MS: *Ovarian Malignancies: Diagnostic and Therapeutic Advances.* Churchill Livingstone, 1987.

32

Gestational Trophoblastic Disease

The term "gestational trophoblastic disease" denotes a spectrum of pregnancy-related trophoblastic proliferative abnormalities whose classification for many years was based principally on histologic criteria and included hydatidiform mole, chorioadenoma destruens, and choriocarcinoma. A clinical diagnostic classification was proposed in 1973, based principally upon clinical findings and serial determinations of chorionic gonadotropin, which is secreted by the abnormal tissue. Although these two classifications have caused some confusion, the clinical one is now accepted (Table 32–1).

Hydatidiform mole—also commonly referred to as molar pregnancy—is diagnosed when hydropic villi are identified grossly. The histologic term "choriocarcinoma" is still used to denote the extremely malignant variant of trophoblastic disease that frequently metastasizes and formerly was almost invariably fatal.

The diagnosis of these disorders is arrived at by clinical examination, which must include an assessment for extrauterine metastases. Initial evaluation of molar pregnancy includes chest x-ray, and classification is based upon trends in serum levels of chorionic gonadotropin measured by sensitive assay of the β subunit.

The term "gestational trophoblastic neoplasia" refers to persistent trophoblastic tissue that is presumably malignant and is identified by its continued secretion of chorionic gonadotropin. Clinical evaluation may demonstrate that the tissue is confined to the uterus, and thus nonmetastatic, or that it has metastasized to any of several organs.

HYDATIDIFORM MOLE (Molar Pregnancy)

Histologically, hydatidiform moles are characterized by abnormalities of the chorionic villi, consisting of varying degrees of trophoblastic proliferation and edema of villous stroma. Moles usually occupy the uterine cavity; however, they may rarely be located in the oviduct and even the ovary. As shown in Table 32–2, the presence or absence of fetal tissues allows classification in complete (classic) and partial (incomplete) moles. With complete mole, the chorionic villi are converted into a mass of clear vesicles (Figure 32–1). The vesicles vary in size from barely visible to a few centimeters in diameter and often hang in clusters from thin pedicles. The mass may become large enough to fill the uterus to the size occupied by an advanced normal pregnancy. The risk of trophoblastic neoplasia developing from a complete mole is approximately 20%.

When the hydatidiform changes are focal and less advanced and there is a fetus or at least an amnionic sac, the condition has been classified as partial hydatidiform mole. There is slowly progressing hydatidiform swelling of some usually avascular villi, while other vascular villi with a functioning fetal-placental circulation are spared (Figure 32–2). The risk of choriocarcinoma arising from a partial hydatidiform mole is slight; however, nonmetastatic gestational trophoblastic neoplasia may follow in 4–8% of partial moles.

In many cases of hydatidiform mole, the ovaries contain multiple **theca-lutein cysts** (Figure 32–1), which may vary from microscopic to 10 cm or more in diameter. The surfaces of the cysts are smooth, often yellowish, and lined with lutein cells. The incidence of obvious cysts in association with mole is reported to be 25–60%.

Theca-lutein cysts of the ovaries are thought to result from overstimulation of lutein elements by large amounts of chorionic gonadotropin secreted by proliferating trophoblast. In general, extensive cystic change is usually associated with larger hydatidiform moles and a long period of stimulation. Theca-lutein cysts are not limited to cases of hydatidiform mole, and they may be associated with placental hypertrophy with fetal hydrops or multifetal pregnancy.

Incidence & Epidemiology

Hydatidiform mole develops in approximately one in every 2000 pregnancies in the United States and Europe but much more frequently in other countries—especially

Table 32–1. Clinical classification of gestational trophoblastic disease.

Hydatidiform mole (molar pregnancy)
    Complete, or classic
    Incomplete, or partial
Gestational trophoblastic neoplasia
    Nonmetastatic
    Metastatic
        Low-risk (good prognosis)
        High-risk (poor prognosis)

in parts of Asia, where the frequency is at least 10 times that in the United States. A very high incidence is reported also in Mexico and among native Alaskans.

Hydatidiform mole is more common toward the beginning or end of the childbearing years. It is most commonly reported in women over 45 years of age, when the relative frequency of the lesion is more than 10 times greater than at ages 20–40. There are numerous authenticated cases of hydatidiform mole in women 50 years of age and older, whereas normal pregnancy at such advanced ages is practically unknown.

Clinical Findings

Persistent bleeding and a uterus larger than expected should suggest the possible presence of a mole. Consideration must be given to an error in menstrual data or a pregnant uterus further enlarged by myomas, hydramnios, or—especially—multiple fetuses.

A. Symptoms and Signs: In the very early stages of development, there is little to distinguish molar from normal pregnancy; later in the first trimester and during the second trimester, the changes described below are often evident. Symptoms are more likely to be dramatic with classic (complete) mole.

1. Bleeding–Uterine bleeding is the outstanding sign and may vary from spotting to profuse hemorrhage. It may begin just before abortion but usually occurs intermittently for weeks or even months. Anemia is common, and a dilutional effect from appreciable hypervolemia has been demonstrated in some women with large moles. Large amounts of blood may at times be sequestered within the uterus. Iron deficiency anemia is common and megaloblastic erythropoiesis uncommon, the latter occur-

ring presumably as a result of poor dietary intake because of nausea and vomiting coupled with the increased folate requirement imposed by rapidly proliferating trophoblast.

2. Uterine size–The growing uterus often (not always) enlarges more rapidly than usual. In about half of cases, uterine size clearly exceeds that expected from the duration of gestation. The uterus may be difficult to identify precisely by palpation especially in nulliparous women, because of its soft consistency beneath a firm abdominal wall. Ovaries that are appreciably enlarged by multiple theca-lutein cysts may be difficult to distinguish from the enlarged uterus. The ovaries are likely to be tender.

3. Pregnancy-induced hypertension–Of special importance is the frequent association of preeclampsia with molar pregnancies that persist into the second trimester. Since pregnancy-induced hypertension is rarely seen before 24 weeks, preeclampsia before this time strongly suggests hydatidiform mole or extensive molar change.

4. Thyroid dysfunction–Plasma thyroxine levels in women with molar pregnancy are usually appreciably elevated, but clinically apparent hyperthyroidism is identified in only about 2% of cases.

5. Spontaneous expulsion–Occasionally, grapelike hydatid vesicles are passed before the mole is aborted spontaneously or removed by operation. Spontaneous expulsion is most likely to occur at about 16 weeks and is rarely delayed beyond 28 weeks.

B. Imaging: The greatest diagnostic accuracy is obtained from the characteristic ultrasonic appearance of hydatidiform mole (Figure 32–3). The safety and precision of sonography make it the technique of choice. However, it must be kept in mind that other tissues may have an appearance similar to that of a mole, including uterine myoma with early pregnancy and pregnancies with multiple fetuses. A careful review of the history—coupled with careful sonographic evaluation repeated in 1 or 2 weeks when necessary—should help prevent an incorrect diagnosis of hydatidiform mole when the pregnancy is actually normal.

Treatment

Treatment consists of immediate evacuation of the mole (or hysterectomy) and later follow-up for detection of persistent trophoblastic proliferation or malignant

Table 32–2. Characteristics of partial and complete hydatiform moles.[1]

Feature	Partial (Incomplete) Mole	Complete (Classic) Mole
Embryonic or fetal tissue	Present	Absent
Hydatidiform swelling of villi	Focal	Diffuse
Trophoblastic hyperplasia	Focal	Diffuse
Stromal inclusions	Present	Absent
Villous scalloping	Present	Absent
Karyotype	Paternal and maternal 69,XXY or 69,XYY	Paternal 46,XX (96%) or 46,XY (4%)
Trophoblastic neoplasia	~5% (choriocarcinoma rare)	~20%

[1]From Berkowitz RS et al: Contemp Ob/Gyn 1986;27:77.

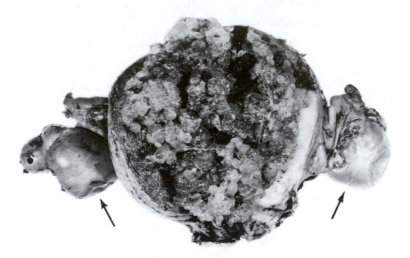

Figure 32–1. A complete (classic) hydatidiform mole, characterized grossly by an abundance of edematous enlarged chorionic villi but no fetus or fetal membranes. Note theca-lutein cysts in each ovary *(arrows)*.

change. Initial evaluation prior to evacuation or hysterectomy includes at least a cursory search for metastatic disease. A chest radiograph should be done to look for pulmonary lesions. Unless there is other evidence of extrauterine disease, CT scan or MRI of the liver or brain is not indicated.

A. Vacuum Aspiration: If the mole is large, at least two and preferably four units of compatible whole blood are made ready, and an intravenous system is established for rapid infusion in case of need. Unless the cervix is long, very firm, and closed, which is unlikely, dilatation can be safely accomplished under general anesthesia to a diameter sufficient to allow insertion of a plastic suction curette. Anesthetic agents that relax the uterus, such as

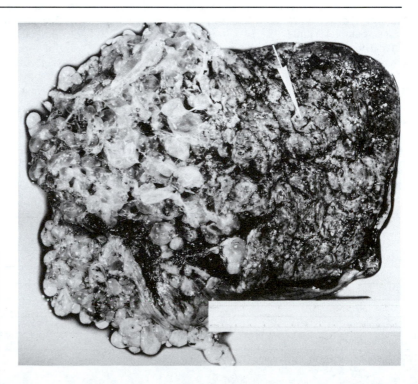

Figure 32–2. Molar placenta on the left and normal placenta *(white arrow)* on the right. The molar placenta was identified by sonography late in pregnancy when the mother developed preeclampsia. A healthy fetus was delivered near term by cesarean section. Most likely, this is a case of twins consisting of a placenta with a fetus from one ovum and a complete mole developing from the other ovum.

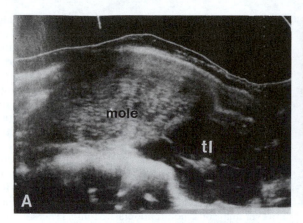
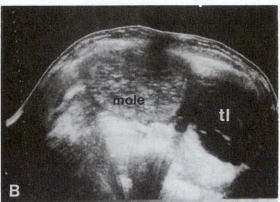

Figure 32–3. **A:** Longitudinal sonogram demonstrating a complete hydatidiform mole that fills a uterus enlarged to well above the umbilicus. A large theca-lutein cyst (tl) is seen above the uterus. **B:** Transverse sonogram of the same patient. (Courtesy of R Santos.)

halothane, should not be used. Throughout the procedure, oxytocin is infused to contract the uterus as its contents are being evacuated. This decreases bleeding from the implantation site, and as the myometrium retracts the uterine wall thickens, thus reducing the risk of perforation of the uterus.

After the great bulk of the mole has been removed by aspiration and the myometrium has contracted and retracted, thorough but gentle curettage with a large sharp curette is usually performed. The tissue obtained by sharp curettage should be so labeled and submitted separately for histologic examination.

B. Hysterectomy: If no further pregnancies are desired, hysterectomy may be preferred to suction curettage. Hysterectomy is a logical election in women age 40 or older because of the frequency with which malignant trophoblastic disease ensues in this age group.

C. Follow-Up Procedures: If the following procedures are not adhered to carefully, some women will die needlessly of malignant trophoblastic neoplasia. The objective of follow-up is prompt detection of any change suggestive of malignancy.

1. Prevent pregnancy during the follow-up period—at least for 1 year.

2. Measure serum chorionic gonadotropin levels every 2 weeks, using sensitive radioimmunoassay techniques. Although weekly assays are sometimes recommended, no distinct benefit has been demonstrated.

3. Withhold therapy as long as the serum chorionic gonadotropin levels continue to regress. A rise or persistent plateau in the serum level is an indication for chemotherapy.

4. Once the serum chorionic gonadotropin level is normal—ie, when it has reached the lower limit of measurability—test once a month for 6 months and then once every 2 months for a total of 1 year.

5. Follow-up may be discontinued and pregnancy allowed after 1 year.

Since follow-up depends on serial measurement of

serum chorionic gonadotropin levels to detect persistent trophoblastic neoplasia, the test must be sensitive enough to detect very low levels. Estrogen-progestin contraceptives have been used both to prevent subsequent pregnancy and to suppress pituitary luteinizing hormone, which cross-reacts with some tests for chorionic gonadotropin.

Chorionic gonadotropin levels should fall progressively to undetectable levels—otherwise, trophoblast persists. An increase signifies proliferation of trophoblast that is most likely malignant unless the woman is again pregnant. Treatment of suspected persistent trophoblastic disease is discussed separately below.

Chest x-ray is obtained at the first follow-up examination for comparison with the preevacuation film and to serve as a baseline in case further x-ray studies become necessary.

Treatment of Persistent Trophoblastic Disease

Following evacuation of a hydatidiform mole, about 20% of women subsequently undergo further treatment for suspected persistent gestational trophoblastic disease. If serum chorionic gonadotropin values have plateaued or are rising and there is no evidence for disease beyond the uterus, then—if the uterus is not important for future reproduction—hysterectomy will effect cure in some cases. Chorionic gonadotropin will often disappear and the woman will remain well. However, if the uterus is to be preserved or if there is radiographic evidence of lung lesions—or if there are vaginal metastases—chemotherapy is started with or without curettage. Therapy with methotrexate or dactinomycin, singly or in combination with other chemotherapeutic agents, is usually effective.

Prognosis

Nearly 20% of moles and about 5% of incomplete moles progress to gestational trophoblastic neoplasia. Rarely, years may intervene between molar pregnancy and the development of choriocarcinoma. Despite this, in recent surveys, the mortality rate for molar pregnancy is very low. Advanced molar pregnancies frequently are complicated by anemia and intrauterine infection and sepsis.

GESTATIONAL TROPHOBLASTIC NEOPLASIA

Gestational trophoblastic neoplasia is persistent trophoblastic proliferation that is considered malignant. It may follow molar pregnancy or normal pregnancy or may develop after abortive outcomes, including ectopic pregnancy. Gestational trophoblastic neoplasms are divided into two clinical categories: nonmetastatic and metastatic; the latter is further divided into those with good and poor prognoses (Table 32–1).

Clinical Findings

A. Symptoms and Signs: The most common—though inconstant—sign is irregular bleeding after the immediate puerperium in association with uterine subinvolution. The bleeding may be continuous or intermittent, with sudden and sometimes massive hemorrhages. Perforation of the uterus by the growth may cause intraperitoneal hemorrhage. Extension into the parametrium may cause pain and fixation that is suggestive of inflammatory disease.

In many cases, the first indication of the condition may be the metastatic lesions. Vaginal or vulvar tumors may be found. The woman may complain of cough and may produce bloody sputum from pulmonary metastases. In a few cases, it has been impossible to find choriocarcinoma in the uterus or pelvis because the original lesion has disappeared, leaving only distant metastases growing actively.

B. Approach to Diagnosis: Recognition of the possibility of the lesion is the most important factor in diagnosis. All women with hydatidiform mole are at risk and need to be followed as described in the preceding section. Any case of unusual bleeding after term pregnancy or abortion should be investigated by curettage—but especially by measurements of chorionic gonadotropin, since absolute reliance cannot be placed on the findings of examination of curettings. Malignant tissue may be buried within the myometrium, inaccessible to the curette, or hidden in a distant metastasis.

Solitary or multiple nodules present in the chest radiograph that cannot be otherwise explained are suggestive of the possibility of choriocarcinoma and warrant an assay for chorionic gonadotropin. It should be kept in mind, however, that some nontrophoblastic tumors secrete small amounts of chorionic gonadotropin.

Persistent or rising gonadotropin titers in the absence of pregnancy are indicative of trophoblastic neoplasia. Results of assays should be confirmed before beginning medical or surgical therapy.

Treatment & Prognosis

Treatment for gestational trophoblastic neoplasia is much more successful today than in the past. At one time, the only hope for cure was hysterectomy or resection of a metastatic lesion. With the advent of methotrexate and other antitumor agents—especially dactinomycin—the overall cure rate in recent years has been about 90%. Virtually all patients classified as having a good prognosis can now be cured.

Women with low-risk metastatic gestational neoplasia who are treated aggressively with single- or multi-agent chemotherapy do almost as well as those with nonmetastatic disease. Women with high-risk metastatic disease have an appreciable mortality risk that depends on what factors were considered "high-risk."

If unmodified by treatment, the course of choriocarcinoma is rapidly progressive, and death usually follows within a few months. The usual cause of death is hemorrhage in various locations.

SELECTED READINGS

Berkowitz RS, Goldstein DP, Bernstein MR: Management of partial molar pregnancy. Contemp Ob/Gyn 1986;27:77.

Cunningham FG, MacDonald PC, Gant NF, Leveno KJ, and Gilstrap LC, III (editors): Diseases and Abnormalities of the Placenta. Chapter 35 in *Williams Obstetrics,* 19th ed., Appleton & Lange, 1993.

Shane JM, Naftolin F: Aberrant hormone activity by tumors of gynecologic importance. Am J Obstet Gynecol 1975;121:133.

The Physiology of Pregnancy

33

Obstetrics in Broad Perspective

Obstetrics is the branch of medicine that deals with parturition, its antecedents, and its sequels. It is concerned principally with the phenomena of pregnancy, labor, and the puerperium and their management in both normal and abnormal circumstances. In a broader sense, obstetrics is concerned with the reproduction of societies. Obstetric care should promote health and well-being, both physical and mental, among couples and their offspring and help them develop healthy attitudes toward sex, family life, and the place of the family in society. Obstetrics is concerned with all the physiologic, psychologic, and social factors that influence both the quantity and the quality of human reproduction. The problems of population growth are a natural concern of this specialty. The vital statistics of the nation, published monthly by the National Center for Health Statistics, attest to society's concern with the charge of this specialty.

AIMS OF OBSTETRICS

The transcendent objective of obstetrics is that every pregnancy be wanted and that it culminate in a healthy mother and a healthy baby. Obstetrics strives to minimize the number of women and infants who die as a result of the reproductive process or who are physically, intellectually, or emotionally injured by it. Obstetrics is concerned further with the number and spacing of children, so that both the mother and the offspring—indeed, all the family—may enjoy optimal physical and emotional well-being. Finally, obstetrics strives to analyze and influence the social factors that influence reproductive efficiency.

VITAL STATISTICS

To help reduce the number of mothers and infants who die as a result of pregnancy and labor, it is important to know how many such deaths there are in the United States each year and in what circumstances they have occurred. To evaluate these data correctly, a variety of events concerned with pregnancy outcomes have been defined by various agencies:

Birth: The complete expulsion or extraction from the mother of a fetus, irrespective of whether the umbilical cord has been cut or whether the placenta is attached. Expulsion or extraction of a fetus weighing less than 500 g usually is not considered a birth but rather an abortion for purposes of prenatal statistics. In the absence of a birth weight, a body length (crown-heel) of 25 cm is usually equated with 500 g. Approximately 20 weeks of gestational age is commonly considered to be equivalent to 500 g of fetal weight; however, a 500-g fetus is more likely to be 22 (menstrual) weeks of gestational age.

Birth rate (crude): The number of births per 1000 population. The birth rate in the United States for the year ending May 1991 was 16.5 (National Center for Health Statistics, 1991).

Fertility rate: The number of live births per 1000 female population aged 15–44 years. In 1991, the fertility rate was 70.9.

Live birth: Expulsion or extraction of an infant which at or after birth breathes spontaneously or shows other signs of life such as heartbeat or spontaneous movements of the voluntary muscles.

Neonatal death: Death of a liveborn infant either early, during the first 7 days after birth; or late, after 7 days but before 29 days.

Neonatal death rate: Infant deaths per 1000 live births at less than 29 days.

Stillbirth: One in which none of the signs of life are present at or after birth.

Stillbirth (fetal death) rate: The number of stillborn infants per 1000 births.

Prenatal mortality rate: The number of stillbirths plus neonatal deaths at less than 28 days per 1000 births.

Low birth weight: A weight less than 2500 g at first weighing after delivery.

Term infant: An infant born after 37 completed (menstrual) weeks of gestation through 42 completed weeks of gestation (260–294 days).

Preterm or premature infant: An infant born before 37 completed weeks.

Postterm infant: An infant born after completion of the 42nd week.

Abortus: A fetus or embryo removed or expelled from the uterus during the first half of gestation (20 weeks or less), or weighing less than 500 g, or measuring (crown-heel) less than 25 cm.

Direct maternal death: Death of the mother resulting from obstetric complications of pregnancy, labor, or the puerperal and from interventions, omissions, incorrect treatment, or a chain of events resulting from any of the above. An example is maternal death from exsanguination resulting from rupture of the uterus.

Indirect maternal death: Death of the mother not directly due to obstetric causes but resulting from previously existing disease—or a disease that developed during pregnancy, labor, or the puerperal—but which was aggravated by the physiologic adaptation to pregnancy. An example is maternal death from complications of mitral stenosis.

Nonmaternal death: Death of the mother resulting from accidental or incidental causes unrelated to the pregnancy. An example is death from an automobile accident.

Maternal death rate or mortality rate: The number of maternal deaths per 100,000 live births that result from the reproductive process. (See Figure 33–1.)

MATERNAL MORTALITY RATE

The number of maternal deaths per 100,000 live births has decreased remarkably in the past half century. Only 295 maternal deaths were reported in the United States in 1985, or 7.8 per 100,000 live births. By way of comparison, in 1935 there were 12,544 maternal deaths, or 582.1 per 100,000 live births.

The maternal mortality rate is influenced by many factors. For example, in 1985 there was a fourfold greater difference in maternal deaths in black women as compared to white women. This difference results primarily from social and economic factors. Maternal mortality rates increase with the age of the mother, and a common contributing factor to excessive maternal deaths in older women is underlying hypertension.

Common Causes of Maternal Deaths

Hemorrhage, hypertension that is either induced or aggravated by pregnancy, and infection still account for half of the maternal deaths in the United States (Figure 33–2). The causes of obstetric hemorrhage are multiple and include postpartum hemorrhage, bleeding in association with abortion, bleeding from ectopic pregnancy, bleeding as a result of abnormal placental location or separation (placenta previa and abruptio placentae), and bleeding from a ruptured uterus. Hypertension induced or aggravated by pregnancy complicates about 6–7% of pregnancies and is commonly accompanied by edema and proteinuria (preeclampsia) and in some severe cases by convulsions and coma (eclampsia). Puerperal infection, or postpartum pelvic infection, usually begins as uterine and parametrial infection but sometimes undergoes extension to cause peritonitis, thrombophlebitis, and bacteremia. Details of the origin, prevention, and treatment of these conditions form a considerable portion of the subject matter of obstetrics.

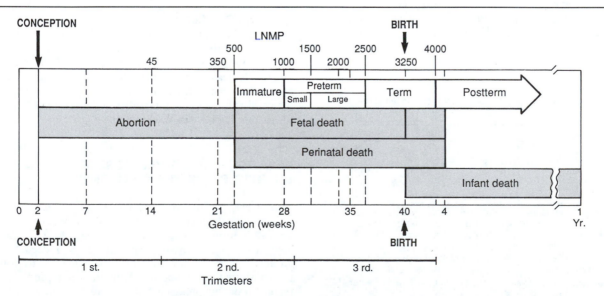

Figure 33–1. Graphic display of perinatal nomenclature.

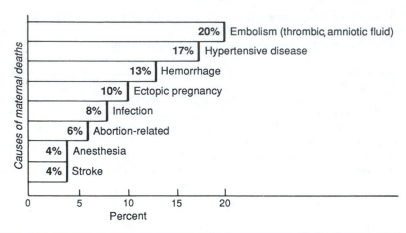

Figure 33–2. Selected distribution of 2475 maternal deaths from direct causes in the United States from 1974 to 1978. (Data from Kaunitz AM et al: Obstet Gynecol 1985; 65:605).

PERINATAL MORTALITY RATE

The sum of stillbirths and neonatal deaths is the perinatal mortality rate. The perinatal death rate has fallen by nearly 50% in the past 25 years (Table 33–1). Currently, there are about 180 prenatal deaths for every maternal death. With the current very low incidence of maternal deaths, perinatal loss rates not only are a better index of the level of obstetric care but also give a more valid indication of an equally important statistic, infant *morbidity*. To some extent, total perinatal loss is correlated with the age and parity of the mother. The rates tend to be highest for the firstborn of very young women and for births of the order of six and over.

Factors Affecting the Stillbirth Rate

Nearly half of perinatal deaths are stillbirths. Stillbirths tend to decline as the quality of care during and throughout pregnancy improves. With improvement in prenatal care and proper hospitalization, some of these deaths are preventable. In a large proportion of fetal deaths, there is no obvious explanation.

Table 33–1. Infant mortality rates in the United States, 1950–1985.[1]

Year	Perinatal[2]	Fetal[3]	Neonatal[4]
1950	39.0	18.8	20.5
1960	34.3	15.8	18.7
1970	28.9	14.0	15.1
1980	17.5	9.1	8.5
1985	14.7	7.8	7.0

[1]From National Center for Health Statistics: *Vital Statistics of the United States,* vol II: *Mortality,* 1985, and unpublished data courtesy of Dr Harry Rosenberg and Dr Manan MacDorman of the National Center for Health Statistics.
[2]Deaths at 20 weeks of gestation or older and infant deaths at less than 28 days. Rates are per 1000 live births and fetal deaths.
[3]Fetal deaths at 20 weeks of gestation or older. Rates are per 1000 live births and fetal deaths.
[4]Infant deaths at less than 29 days. Rates are per 1000 live births.

Neonatal Deaths

In 1977, for the first time in the United States, there were fewer neonatal deaths than fetal deaths (stillbirths). Nearly half of the neonatal deaths occur in the first 24 hours of life. The number of deaths during this time exceeds the number occurring from the second month to 1 year. The causes of this huge wastage during the neonatal period are numerous, but the most important is low birth weight, usually as a consequence of delivery long before term. The proportion of low-birth-weight infants differs among ethnic groups, ranging from about 60 per 1000 for white mothers to about 120 per 1000 for black mothers.

The second most common cause of neonatal deaths is injury to the central nervous system. Here the word "injury" is used in its broad sense to indicate both cerebral injury resulting from hypoxia in utero and traumatic injury to the brain during labor and delivery. Another important cause of neonatal death is congenital malformation.

The Birth Certificate

Statutes in all 50 states and the District of Columbia require that a birth certificate be submitted promptly to the local registrar of births. An extensively revised document was implemented in January 1989. After the birth has been duly registered, notification is sent to the parents of the child and a copy is forwarded to the National Center for Health Statistics in Washington.

RELATIONSHIP BETWEEN OBSTETRICS & OTHER BRANCHES OF MEDICINE

Obstetrics is a multifaceted discipline with many close relationships to other branches of medicine. It is related so intimately to gynecology that obstetrics and gynecology are generally regarded as one specialty—and, indeed, both are taught in residency training. Gynecology deals with the physiology and pathology of the female reproductive organs in the nonpregnant state, whereas obstetrics deals with the pregnant state and its sequelae. Correct differential diagnosis in either obstetrics or gynecology entails an intimate acquaintance with the clinical syndromes met in both, and the methods of examination and many operative techniques are common to both disciplines. It is obligatory, therefore, that every obstetrician have extensive experience in gynecology and vice versa.

Because pregnant and nonpregnant women are subject to the same diseases, the obstetrician commonly encounters and therefore must be knowledgeable about a variety of diseases in pregnant women. As emphasized in Chapter 60, the clinical picture presented by some of these disorders may be greatly altered during pregnancy and the immediate puerperal; conversely, these diseases may affect the course of gestation.

34

Diagnosis of Pregnancy

OVERVIEW OF REPRODUCTIVE FUNCTION IN WOMEN

Estrogen formation is confined largely to one ovary at a time and to the granulosa cells of a single follicle—the follicle destined for ovulation during the approaching ovarian cycle. The rate of formation and secretion of estradiol-17β by the granulosa cells of the chosen follicle corresponds to the rate of maturation and development of that follicle. Indeed, when the follicular apparatus of the ovaries is depleted, ovarian endocrine function diminishes and menopause occurs.

After ovulation, the corpus luteum produces prodigious amounts of progesterone. It is generally accepted that progesterone is essential to the maintenance of pregnancy in most mammalian species, and progesterone withdrawal—by removal of the corpus luteum before 8 weeks of human pregnancy—results in abortion.

ROLE OF THE FETUS

The fetus and extraembryonic fetal tissues are the source of bioactive agents that serve as the driving force in pregnancy. From the time of conception, a molecular dialogue is established between fetal and maternal tissues; some of the signal transmission systems no doubt are operative even before the time of blastocyst implantation.

The impetus for implantation is derived from the blastocyst and blastocyst products; invasion of the maternal decidua and blood vessels in the establishment of the implantation site and subsequent development of the placenta are under the active direction of bioactive products of fetal tissues; the maternal recognition of pregnancy is brought about by signals generated by the blastocyst; the maintenance of pregnancy is orchestrated by fetal contributions; the endocrine changes of pregnancy derive from products formed and secreted by fetal placenta; and, finally, it is probable that fetal retreat from the maintenance of pregnancy is the final event in the spontaneous initiation of parturition at term.

At about the time of implantation or just afterward, there is suppression of HLA antigen formation in extraembryonic fetal tissues (trophoblasts), ie, in tissues that embrace maternal tissues; this may be a fundamental mechanism by which the developing fetus gains immunologic acceptance during blastocyst implantation.

Almost without exception, the endocrine changes of human pregnancy are the consequence of fetal-placental function, either directly or indirectly. Thus, the fetus also is the prime contributor to the endocrine alterations of pregnancy (Chapter 35).

LACTATION & MILK LET-DOWN

During pregnancy, estrogen and progesterone, together with prolactin, act on maternal mammary tissue to induce optimal morphologic and biochemical maturation preparatory to lactation. Progesterone also acts to prevent lactogenesis, but with progesterone withdrawal after delivery of the placenta, lactogenesis promptly commences. Thereafter, suckling induces the secretion of oxytocin in the mother; oxytocin acts on the myoepithelial cells of the breast ducts to cause milk let-down and thus ensures the success of breast feeding.

PLACENTAL SEQUESTRATION OF NUTRIENTS

Fetal villous trophoblasts are remarkably efficient in extracting or sequestering essential nutrients from the maternal circulation. For example, in women with profound iron-deficiency anemia during pregnancy, the iron stores of the fetus are normal; in women with severe folic acid deficiency during pregnancy causing severe anemia, the fetal hematocrit is normal (Chapter 36). The fetus is a demanding and efficient parasite.

DIAGNOSIS OF PREGNANCY

For both men and women, few diagnoses are more important than that of pregnancy. For the woman, a diagnosis of pregnancy can evoke emotions of great joy or equally great despair. Because knowledge of the existence of pregnancy is important for proper management, every physician approaching a patient in the reproductive age range must always ponder the question, "Is she pregnant?" Failure to consider that possibility in appropriate cases often leads to incorrect diagnosis, inappropriate treatment, and, in some cases, medicolegal complications.

Most pregnant women are aware of their condition when consulting a physician, though the information may not be volunteered unless the right question is asked. Mistakes in diagnosis are made most frequently in the first several weeks of pregnancy, while the uterus is still a pelvic organ.

The diagnosis of pregnancy is based upon symptoms and signs elicited by history taking and examination and upon the results of laboratory tests. The symptoms and signs of pregnancy are classified into three groups: presumptive evidence, probable signs, and positive signs.

PRESUMPTIVE EVIDENCE OF PREGNANCY

Presumptive evidence of pregnancy is based largely on subjective symptoms that include (1) nausea with or without vomiting, (2) disturbances in urination, (3) fatigue, and (4) the perception of fetal movement. The signs include (1) cessation of menses, (2) anatomic changes in the breasts, (3) discoloration of the vaginal mucosa, (4) increased skin pigmentation and the development of abdominal striae, and (5) especially important, the patient's belief that she is pregnant.

1. SYMPTOMS OF PREGNANCY

Pregnancy is commonly characterized by disturbances of the digestive system, manifested particularly by **nausea and vomiting.** This so-called morning sickness of pregnancy usually commences during the early part of the day but passes in a few hours—though occasionally it persists longer and may occur at other times. Vomiting does not always occur. This disturbing symptom usually appears about 6 weeks after onset of the last menstrual period and ordinarily disappears spontaneously 6–12 weeks later.

During the first trimester of pregnancy, the enlarging uterus, by exerting pressure on the urinary bladder, may cause **frequent micturition.** The frequency of urination gradually diminishes as pregnancy progresses and the uterus rises up into the abdomen. This symptom reappears near the end of pregnancy, however, when the fetal head descends into the maternal pelvis.

Fetal activity usually is first recognized by the pregnant woman between 16 and 20 weeks of gestation and is designated as quickening, or the perception of life. This sign provides only corroborative evidence of pregnancy and in itself is of little diagnostic value. It is, however, a milestone of the progress of pregnancy that, if dated accurately, can serve as corroborative evidence in determining the duration of gestation.

2. SIGNS OF PREGNANCY

In a healthy woman who previously has experienced spontaneous, cyclic, predictable menstruation, the abrupt **cessation of menses** is highly suggestive of pregnancy. However, it is not until 10 days or more after the expected onset of the next menstrual period that the absence of menses is a reliable indication of pregnancy. When a second menstrual period is missed, the probability of pregnancy is much greater. Cessation or absence of menstruation can be caused by a number of conditions other than pregnancy—most commonly anovulation, which in turn may be due to a number of factors (Chapter 21).

Generally, the anatomic **changes in the breast** that accompany pregnancy are quite characteristic in primiparas but less so in multiparas, whose breasts may contain a small amount of milky material or colostrum for months or even years after the birth of the last child. Occasionally, changes in the breasts similar to those caused by pregnancy are found in women with prolactin-secreting pituitary tumors and in women taking drugs that induce hyperprolactinemia.

During pregnancy, the vaginal mucosa frequently appears dark bluish or purplish-red and congested, the so-called **Chadwick's sign.**

Increased **skin pigmentation** and the appearance of **abdominal striae** are common. However, these signs may be absent during pregnancy or may be associated with the use of estrogen-progestin contraceptives.

The patient's own statements about the presence of a pregnancy must be taken seriously by the physician. If the patient believes she is pregnant, the physician should consider that to be the case until pregnancy is excluded as a possibility.

PROBABLE SIGNS OF PREGNANCY

The probable signs of pregnancy include (1) enlargement of the abdomen; (2) changes in the shape, size, and consistency of the uterus; (3) anatomic changes in the cervix; (4) Braxton Hicks contractions; (5) ballottement; (6) physical outlining of the fetus; and (7) the results of endocrine tests.

1. ENLARGEMENT OF THE ABDOMEN

By 12 weeks of gestation, the uterus usually can be felt through the abdominal wall just above the symphysis pubis, as a tumor; thereafter, the uterus gradually increases in size to the end of pregnancy (Figure 34–1). The abdominal enlargement usually is less pronounced in primiparous than in multiparous women, in whom some of the tone of the abdominal musculature has been lost; indeed, in some multiparous women, the abdominal wall is so flaccid that the uterus sags forward and downward, producing a pendulous abdomen. This results from a physiologic diastasis recti, or widely separated rectus abdominal muscles.

2. CHANGES IN SIZE, SHAPE, & CONSISTENCY OF THE UTERUS

During the first few weeks of pregnancy, the increase in size of the uterus is limited principally to the anteroposterior diameter, but later the body of the uterus is almost globular. On bimanual examination, the body of the uterus during pregnancy feels doughy or elastic and sometimes becomes exceedingly soft.

At about 6–8 weeks after the onset of the last menstrual period, **Hegar's sign** becomes manifest: With one hand on the abdomen and two fingers of the other hand in the vagina, the still-firm cervix is felt, with the elastic body of the uterus above the compressible soft isthmus, which is between the two. Occasionally, softening at the isthmus is so marked that the cervix and the body of the uterus seem to be separate organs.

3. CHANGES IN THE CERVIX

By 6–8 weeks, the cervix often becomes considerably softened. In primigravidas, the consistency of the cervical tissue that surrounds the external os is more like that of the lips than the nasal cartilage, as in nonpregnant women. Other conditions, however, may bring about softening of the cervix. Estrogen-progestin contraceptives, for exam-

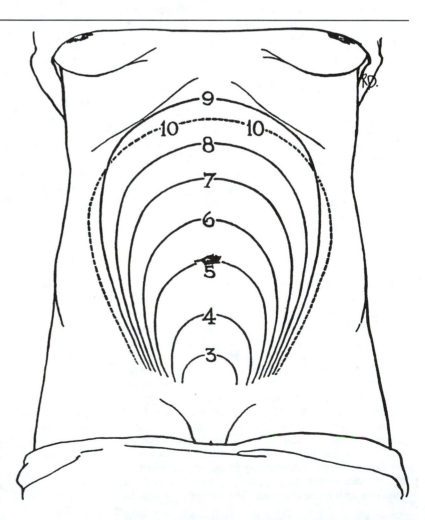

Figure 34–1. Relative height of the fundus at the various lunar months of pregnancy. (Reproduced, with permission, from Eastman NJ, Hellman LM [editors]: *William's Obstetrics*, 13th ed. Appleton-Century-Crofts, 1966.)

ple, commonly act to cause some softening and congestion of the uterine cervix.

As pregnancy advances, the cervical canal may become sufficiently patulous to admit the tip of the examiner's finger.

4. BRAXTON HICKS CONTRACTIONS

During pregnancy, the uterus undergoes palpable but ordinarily painless contractions at irregular intervals from early stages of gestation. These Braxton Hicks contractions may increase in number and amplitude when the uterus is massaged.

5. BALLOTTEMENT

Near mid pregnancy, the volume of the fetus is small compared with the volume of amnionic fluid; and consequently, sudden pressure exerted on the uterus may cause the fetus to sink in the amnionic fluid and then rebound to its original position; the tapping (ballottement) thus produced can be felt by the examining fingers.

6. OUTLINING THE FETUS

In the second half of pregnancy, the outlines of the fetal body may be palpated through the maternal abdominal wall, and outlining becomes easier as term approaches (Chapter 38).

7. ENDOCRINE TESTS FOR PREGNANCY

The presence of **human chorionic gonadotropin (hCG)** in maternal plasma and its excretion in urine provides the basis for endocrine tests for pregnancy. This hormone may be identified in body fluids by a variety of immunoassay or bioassay techniques.

hCG is important in the maternal recognition of pregnancy by virtue of its action on the ovary to prevent involution of the corpus luteum, the principal site of progesterone formation in the first 6–8 weeks of pregnancy. Moreover hCG is a luteinizing hormone-like agent that acts as an LH surrogate in responsive tissues, eg, the ovary (corpus luteum) and testis. The detection of hCG in biologic fluids (urine or serum) is by far the most common test for pregnancy. The student of obstetrics must therefore be familiar with the chemistry, biologic action, and detection of this unique glycoprotein hormone that is produced by the trophoblasts during human pregnancy.

With a sensitive test—eg, radioimmunoassay employing antibodies directed against the β subunit of hCG—the pregnancy hormone can be demonstrated 8–9 days after ovulation, probably on the day of blastocyst implantation. It is estimated that in early pregnancy, the doubling time of hCG concentrations in plasma is 1.4–2 days. The levels of hCG in blood and urine increase from the day of implantation until about 60–70 days of pregnancy. Thereafter, the concentration of hCG declines until a nadir is reached at about 100–130 days of pregnancy.

Inexpensive kits are available that can with certain precautions be used with great precision for quick testing (3–5 minutes). Almost without exception, chemical detection of pregnancy involves the demonstration of hCG in blood or urine. Many different test systems are available, but each is dependent upon recognition of hCG (or a subunit thereof) by an antibody to the hCG molecule. In 1986, there were 39 commercially available urine pregnancy tests. These included tests involving the principles of agglutination inhibition, radioimmunoassay, and enzyme-linked immunosorbent assay (ELISA) methods (see below).

With the recognition that LH and hCG were composed of α and β subunits, that the two subunits of each molecular species could be separated and purified, and that the β subunits of each were structurally distinct at least at the –COOH terminus, antibodies were developed that would specifically recognize epitopes on the β subunit of hCG. In this way, an antibody would be available that could discriminate between LH and hCG. The development of such an antibody has become useful for elucidation of physiologic processes, for early detection of pregnancy, and for monitoring hCG production in persons with neoplastic trophoblastic disease both before and during treatment.

Therefore, antibodies with high specificity for the β subunit of hCG and little cross-reactivity against LH have been raised by immunization of animals (polyclonal antibodies) or by hybridoma techniques (monoclonal antibodies) against recognition sites on the β subunit of hCG; and antibodies have been raised against the α subunit of hCG and LH (which are identical).

Immunoassays of hCG

A. Agglutination Inhibition: Many immunoassay procedures employ the principle of agglutination inhibition, ie, the prevention of flocculation of hCG-coated particles—eg, latex particles to which hCG is covalently bound. The kits commercially available to offices and laboratories that depend upon failure of agglutination of latex particles to detect hCG in urine contain two reagents. The pregnancy test is positive if no agglutination occurs and negative when agglutination occurs. Recently, commercially available kits have been introduced in which the antibody to hCG is directed specifically to epitopes on the β subunit, thus avoiding cross-reactivity with LH.

B. Radioimmunoassays: In radioimmunoassays, [^{125}I]iodohCG is used as the radiolabeled ligand for antibodies raised against hCG (specifically, the β subunit of hCG) and is dependent upon displacement of—or competition with—the radiolabeled ligand by nonradiolabeled hCG in the biologic sample. In radioimmunoassays, "free" and "bound" [^{125}I]iodohCG are separated, and radioactivity that is unbound is assayed. As a result of construction of standard curves, hCG is quantified with great accuracy and sensitivity by this method.

C. Enzyme-Linked Immunosorbent Assay (ELISA): In this assay for hCG, a monoclonal antibody bound to a solid phase support (usually plastic) binds the hCG in the test sample; a second antibody is added to "sandwich" the hCG. It is the second antibody to which an enzyme, eg, alkaline phosphatase, is linked; when substrate for this enzyme is added, a blue color develops whose intensity is related directly to the amount of enzyme and, thus, the amount of second antibody bound. This, in turn, is determined by the amount of hCG present in the test sample. The sensitivity of ELISA for hCG in serum is 50 mIU/mL.

Accuracy of Pregnancy Tests

In a multicenter collaborative study sponsored by the National Institutes of Health, it was concluded that laboratories conducting routine clinical tests could measure hCG accurately at the time of "missed" menses but not necessarily before that time.

"Do It Yourself" Test Kits

Today there are several over-the-counter pregnancy test kits for use at home. These tests employ the principle of hemagglutination inhibition. There appears to be a relatively low false-positive result rate but a high false-negative rate.

POSITIVE SIGNS OF PREGNANCY

The three positive signs of pregnancy are (1) identification of fetal heart action separately and distinctly from that of the mother, (2) perception of active fetal movements by the examiner, and (3) recognition of the embryo or fetus utilizing imaging techniques such as ultrasound or x-ray.

Identification of Fetal Heart Action

Hearing or observing the pulsations of the fetal heart establishes the diagnosis of pregnancy. Contractions of the fetal heart can be identified by auscultation with a special fetoscope by use of the Doppler principle with ultrasound and by use of sonography (Chapter 13). The fetal heartbeat can be detected by auscultation with a stethoscope by an average of 17 weeks of gestation and by 19 weeks in nearly all pregnancies in normal-sized women.

Perception of Fetal Movements

The second positive sign of pregnancy is the detection by the examiner of movements by the fetus. After about 20 weeks of gestation, active fetal movements can be felt, at indeterminate intervals, by placing the examining hand on the woman's abdomen.

Ultrasonic Recognition

A normal intrauterine pregnancy may be demonstrated by pulse echo sonography after only 4–5 weeks of amenorrhea. After 6 weeks of amenorrhea, the small white gestational ring is so characteristic that failure to identify it raises doubts about the presence of pregnancy. Thus, there may be ultrasonic confirmation of pregnancy by the time some of the common tests for hCG in urine become positive. Distinct echoes from the embryonic poles can be demonstrated within the gestational ring by 7 weeks after commencement of the last normal menstrual period. By 8 weeks, fetal brain is seen, and heart action can be detected using Doppler or real-time sonography. By this time, from the length of the embryo, the gestational age can be estimated quite accurately (Chapter 43).

DIFFERENTIAL DIAGNOSIS OF PREGNANCY

The pregnant uterus is sometimes mistaken for other tumors occupying the pelvis or abdomen; less frequently, the reverse error is made. If uncertainty exists, reexamination in a few weeks usually will establish the correct diagnosis.

IDENTIFICATION OF FETAL LIFE OR DEATH

Failure to detect heart wall motion by real-time ultrasonography after 10–12 weeks of gestation is reliable evidence of fetal death. Ancillary findings of sonography in the case of fetal death include scalp edema and sequelae of maceration.

In the early months of pregnancy, the diagnosis of fetal death may present difficulty. Unless ultrasonic techniques are employed, the diagnosis of fetal death can be made with certainty only after it can be shown by repeated examinations that the uterus has remained constant in size or there actually has been a decrease in size of the uterus over a number of weeks. Because trophoblasts of the placenta may continue to produce hCG for several weeks after death of the embryo or fetus, a positive endocrine test for pregnancy does not necessarily mean that the fetus is alive.

In the latter half of pregnancy, cessation of fetal movements usually alerts the woman to the possibility of fetal death, but if fetal cardiac action distinct from that of the mother can still be identified, the fetus is certainly alive. If, by careful auscultation, the fetal heart tones are not heard, the fetus probably is dead. There is a possibility of error, of course, especially in pregnancies in which the fetal heart is remote from the examiner, eg, if the woman is obese or if hydramnios exists.

Ultrasonic instruments in which the Doppler shift principle is employed are of considerable value in the assessment of pregnancies in which the fetal heart cannot be heard by auscultation with a stethoscope. The use of Doppler ultrasound is especially valuable when fetal death is suspected but fetal heart tones are thought to be heard. If fetal heart action is not demonstrated after careful examination, it can be stated that very likely—but not absolutely—the fetus is dead. When carefully performéd, real-time ultrasonic examination will serve to identify the presence or absence of fetal heart motion.

SUGGESTED READINGS

Cunningham FG, MacDonald PC, Gant NF, Leveno KJ, and Gilstrap LC, III (editors): Human Pregnancy: Overview, Organization, and Diagnosis. Chapter 2 in *Williams Obstetrics,* 19th ed., Appleton & Lange, 1993.

35

Physiology of Pregnancy

DATING OF PREGNANCY

Menstrual age, or **gestational age,** is estimated by counting from the first day of the last menstrual period, a time that precedes conception—or about 2 weeks before ovulation and fertilization and nearly 3 weeks before implantation of the fertilized ovum. About 280 days (40 weeks) elapse between the first day of the last menstrual period and delivery of the infant; 280 days corresponds to 9⅓ calendar months, or 10 units of 28 days each.

Obstetricians customarily calculate gestational age on the basis of menstrual age of a given pregnancy. Embryologists, however, cite events in days or weeks from the time of ovulation **(ovulation age)** or conception **(postconception age),** these two being nearly identical. Occasionally, it is of value to divide the period of gestation into three units of three calendar months each, or three **trimesters,** because some important obstetric milestones may be designated conveniently in this way.

HUMAN EMBRYOLOGY

OVUM, ZYGOTE, & BLASTOCYST

During the 2 weeks following ovulation, successive phases of development are as follows: (1) ovulation, (2) fertilization of the ovum, (3) formation of free blastocyst, and (4) implantation of the blastocyst, a process that begins at the end of the first week after conception. Primitive chorionic villi begin to form after implantation.

CLEAVAGE OF THE ZYGOTE

The mature ovum, after fertilization in the uterine tube (fallopian tube, oviduct), becomes a zygote (a diploid cell with 46 chromosomes), which then undergoes segmentation, or cleavage into blastomeres. The first typical mitotic division of the segmentation nucleus of the zygote results in the formation of two blastomeres.

Definitions

Blastocyst: After the morula reaches the uterus, a fluid-filled cavity is formed, converting the morula (see below) to a blastocyst.

Blastomeres: Mitotic division (cleavage) of the zygote (see below) gives rise to daughter cells called blastomeres.

Conceptus: This term is used to refer to all products of conception, ie, embryo (fetus), fetal membranes, and placenta. In particular, the conceptus includes all tissues that develop from the zygote, both embryonic and extraembryonic.

Embryo: The embryo-forming cells, which are grouped as an inner cell mass, give rise to the embryo, which usually is designated when the bilaminar embryonic disk forms. The embryonic period extends until the end of the seventh week, at which time the major structures are present.

Fetus: After the embryonic period, the developing conceptus is referred to as the fetus.

Morula: The solid ball of cells formed by 16 or so blastomeres.

Zygote: The cell that results from the fertilization of the ovum by a spermatozoon.

Within the uterine tube, the fertilized ovum undergoes slow cleavage for 3 days (Figure 35–1). As the blastomeres continue to divide, a solid mulberry-like ball of cells, the **morula,** is produced. The morula enters the uterine cavity about 3 days after fertilization of the ovum. The gradual accumulation of fluid within the morula between blastomeres results in formation of the blastocyst, at one pole of which there is a compact mass of cells, the **inner cell mass,** which is destined to produce the embryo (Figure 35–2), and an outer mass of cells, destined to be the **trophoblasts.**

IMPLANTATION

Before implantation, the zona pellucida disappears and the blastocyst adheres to the endometrial surface, the time of **apposition.** After erosion of the epithelium of the endometrium, the blastocyst sinks into and becomes totally encased within the endometrium, ie, the blastocyst is completely buried in the endometrium. At this time, there

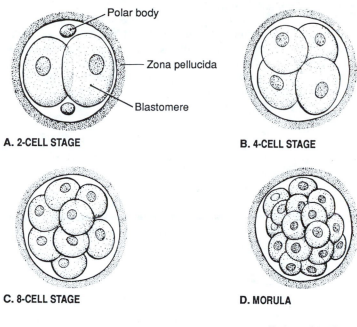

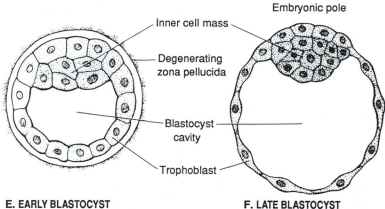

Figure 35–1. Cleavage of the zygote and formation of the blastocyst. **A** to **D** show various stages of cleavage. The period of the morula begins at the 12- to 16-cell stage and ends when the blastocyst forms, which occurs when 50–60 blastomeres are present. **E** and **F** are sections of blastocysts. The zona pellucida has disappeared by the late blastocyst stage (5 days). The polar bodies shown in **A** are small, nonfunctional cells that soon degenerate. (Reproduced, with permission, from Moore KL: *The Developing Human,* 3rd ed. Saunders, 1982.)

clearly are two distinguishable layers of trophoblasts. Thus, the syncytiotrophoblasts are contiguous with maternal decidua (and, later, maternal blood), whereas the cytotrophoblasts are the innermost (embryonic side) layer and ultimately come to be the cell nearest the intravillous space, in which the fetal capillaries course as one conduit of the placental arm of the fetal-maternal communication system.

EARLY TROPHOBLASTS

Human placentation is **hemochorioendothelial,** ie, maternal blood ("hemo-") bathes the syncytiotrophoblasts ("-chorio-"), which in turn are separated from fetal blood by the wall of the capillaries ("-endothelial") of the fetus in the intravillous space. Maternal blood bathes the syn-

cytiotrophoblasts directly, but the fetal blood is separated from the trophoblasts by the endothelium of the fetal capillaries in the intravillous space.

As the lacunae join, a complicated labyrinth is formed that is partitioned by solid trophoblastic columns. The trophoblast-lined labyrinthine channels and the solid cellular columns form the intervillous space and primary villous stalks, respectively.

Maternal blood enters the intervillous space from the spiral arterioles in fountain-like bursts; thus, maternal blood sweeps over and bathes the syncytiotrophoblasts directly (Figure 35–3). The maternal surface of these trophoblasts consists of a complex microvillous structure.

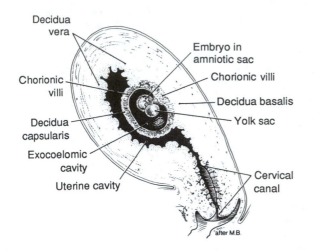

Figure 35–2. Chorion frondosum and chorion laeve of early pregnancy. Three portions of the decidua (basalis, capsularis, and parietalis [vera]) are also illustrated.

THE EMBRYO

The beginning of the embryonic period is taken as the beginning of the third week after ovulation (fertilization)—or the fifth week after the first day of the last menstrual period—and coincides with the expected time of the next menses. Most pregnancy tests in clinical use are positive by this time.

THE FETUS

The end of the embryonic period and the beginning of the fetal period are arbitrarily designated by most embryologists to occur 8 weeks after fertilization, or 10 weeks after the onset of the last menstrual period. At this time, the embryo is nearly 4 cm long. No major new structures are formed thereafter.

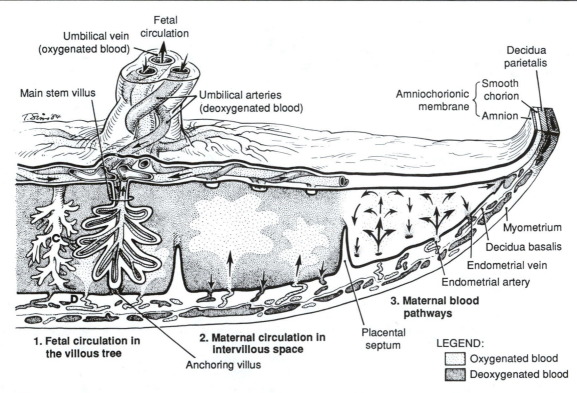

Figure 35–3. Schematic drawing of a section through a full-term placenta: **1.** The relation of the villous chorion (C) to the decidua basalis (D) and the fetal placental circulation. **2.** The maternal placental circulation. Maternal blood flows into the intervillous spaces in funnel-shaped spurts, and exchanges occur with the fetal blood as the maternal blood flows around the villi. **3.** The inflowing arterial blood pushes venous blood into the endometrial veins, which are scattered over the entire surface of the decidua basalis. Note that the umbilical arteries carry deoxygenated fetal blood to the placenta and that the umbilical vein carries oxygenated blood to the fetus. Note that the cotyledons are separated from each other by placental (decidual) septa of the maternal portion of the placenta. Each cotyledon consists of two or more main stem villi and their many branches. (Based on a drawing in Moore KL: *The Developing Human,* 3rd ed. Saunders, 1982.)

ORGANIZATION OF THE PLACENTA

CHORIONIC VILLI

Villi can first be distinguished easily in the human placenta on about the 12th day after fertilization. When the solid trophoblast is invaded by a mesenchymal cord, presumably derived from cytotrophoblast, secondary villi are formed. After angiogenesis occurs in situ from the mesenchymal cord, the resulting villi are termed **tertiary.** Maternal venous sinuses are tapped early, but until the 14th or 15th day after fertilization, maternal arterial blood does not enter the intervillous space. By about the 17th day, both fetal and maternal blood vessels are functional, and a placental circulation is established. The fetal-placental circulation is completed when the blood vessels of the embryo are connected with chorionic blood vessels.

The villi in contact with the decidua basalis proliferate to form the leafy chorion, or **chorion frondosum,** the fetal component of the placenta, whereas those in contact with the decidua capsularis cease to grow and undergo almost complete degeneration, the **chorion laeve.** The greater part of the chorion, thus denuded of villi, is designated the smooth, or bald, chorion or the chorion laeve.

Until near the end of the third month, the chorion laeve remains separated from the amnion by the exocelomic cavity (Figure 35–2). Thereafter, the amnion and chorion are in intimate contact (Figure 35–3). In the human, the chorion laeve and amnion form an avascular amniochorion which is an important site of transfer and metabolic activity.

PLACENTAL COTYLEDONS

Each of the main stem villi and its ramifications constitute a placental cotyledon, the fetal tissue interface of the placental arm of the fetal-maternal communication system (Figure 35–3). The total number of cotyledons remains the same throughout gestation but individual cotyledons continue to grow until term, though less actively in the final weeks.

PLACENTAL SEPTA

These appear to consist of decidual tissue in which trophoblastic elements are encased and thus are probably of dual origin, ie, fetal and maternal.

THE DECIDUA

DECIDUAL REACTION

The decidua is the endometrium of pregnancy and is so named because much of it is shed after parturition. The decidual reaction encompasses the changes that begin in response to progesterone produced after ovulation and prepare the endometrium for implantation and nutrition of the blastocyst.

During pregnancy, the decidua thickens, eventually attaining a depth of 5–10 mm. The portion of the decidua directly beneath the site of implantation forms the **decidua basalis;** that overlying the developing ovum and separating it from the rest of the uterine cavity is the **decidua capsularis** (Figure 35–2). The remainder of the uterus is lined by **decidua parietalis,** or **decidua vera.**

The decidua parietalis and the decidua basalis are composed of three layers each: a surface, or compact zone (**zona compacta**); a middle portion, or spongy zone (**zona spongiosa**), with glands and numerous small blood vessels; and **zona basalis,** or basal zone. The compacta and the spongiosa together form the **zona functionalis** (functional zone). The basal zone remains after delivery and gives rise to new endometrium.

BIOACTIVE SUBSTANCES IN DECIDUA

The concentration of prolactin in amnionic fluid is extraordinarily high compared with the levels in fetal or maternal plasma; this prolactin arises in the decidua.

The factors that regulate prolactin secretion in decidua are not clearly defined, and the physiologic role of prolactin produced in decidua is not known.

CIRCULATION IN THE MATURE PLACENTA

FETAL CIRCULATION

Fetal blood flows to the placenta through the two umbilical arteries, which carry deoxygenated ("venous-like") blood. Blood with a significantly higher oxygen content returns to the fetus from the placenta through the single umbilical vein Figure 35–3.

MATERNAL CIRCULATION

Maternal blood enters the intervillous space in spurts generated by the maternal arterial blood pressure. Continuing influx of arterial blood exerts pressure on the contents of the intervillous space, pushing the blood toward exits in the basal plate, from which it is drained through uterine and other pelvic veins. During uterine contractions, both inflow and outflow are curtailed, though the volume of blood in the intervillous space is maintained, thus providing for continual, though reduced, exchange (Figure 35–3).

THE AMNION

Initially a minute vesicle, it develops into a small sac covering the dorsal surface of the embryo. As it enlarges, it gradually engulfs the growing embryo, which prolapses into its cavity (Figure 35–4). Distention of the amnionic sac eventually brings it into contact with the interior of the chorion; apposition of the mesoblasts of chorion and amnion near the end of the first trimester results in obliteration of the extraembryonic celomic cavity.

There are no blood vessels or nerves in the amnion at any stage of development and, despite the occurrence of suggestive spaces in the fibroblastic and spongy layers, there are no distinct lymphatic channels.

UMBILICAL CORD

The umbilical cord, or funis, extends from the fetal umbilicus to the fetal surface of the placenta. Its exterior is covered by amnion, through which three umbilical vessels may be seen.

PLACENTAL TRANSFER

CHORIONIC VILLUS

Substances that pass from the maternal blood to the fetal blood must traverse (1) the trophoblast, (2) the stroma of the intervillous space, and (3) the fetal capillary wall. Although this histologic "barrier" separates the blood in the maternal and fetal circulations, it does not behave uniformly like a simple physical barrier because throughout pregnancy it actively or passively permits, facilitates, and adjusts the amount and rate of transfer of a wide range of substances to the fetus. After mid pregnancy, the number of Langerhans' cells, or cytotrophoblasts, decreases, and the villous epithelium then consists chiefly of syncytiotrophoblasts. The walls of the villous capillaries likewise become thinner, and the relative number of fetal vessels increases in relation to the villous connective tissue.

TRANSFER BY DIFFUSION

Most substances with a molecular weight less than 500 diffuse readily through the placental tissue interposed between the maternal and fetal circulations. All else equal, the smaller and less ionized the molecule, the more rapid the transfer rate.

Simple diffusion appears to be the mechanism involved in the transfer of oxygen, CO_2, water, and most (not all) electrolytes. Anesthetic gases also pass through the placenta rapidly, apparently by simple diffusion.

Insulin, steroid hormones, and thyroid hormones cross the placenta but at very slow rates. The hormones synthesized in situ in the trophoblasts enter both the maternal and fetal circulations, but not necessarily to the same degree. For example, the concentrations of chorionic gonadotropin and placental lactogen are much lower in fetal plasma than in maternal plasma. Substances of very high molecular weight usually do not traverse the placenta, but there are important exceptions, such as immunoglobulin G (IgG; MW about 160,000), which is transferred by way of a specific trophoblast receptor-mediated mechanism.

The transfer of CO_2 across the placenta is diffusion-limited. Although the transfer of oxygen is blood flow-limited and despite the relatively low Po_2, the fetus normally does not suffer from lack of oxygen. The human fetus has a cardiac output considerably greater per unit of body weight than does the adult. The high cardiac output and, late in pregnancy, the increased oxygen-carrying capacity of fetal blood (attributable to fetal hemoglobin)—and a higher hemoglobin concentration than in adults—compensate effectively for the low oxygen tension.

SELECTIVE TRANSFER & FACILITATED DIFFUSION

The concentrations of a number of substances, which are not synthesized by the fetus, are several times higher in fetal blood than in maternal blood. The concentration of ascorbic acid is 2–4 times higher in fetal plasma than in maternal plasma. The unidirectional transfer of iron across the placenta provides another example of the unique capabilities of the human placenta for transport.

Many viruses, bacteria. and protozoa may cross the placenta and infect the fetus. Malignant cells arising in neoplasias in the pregnant woman can also be transferred to the placenta or fetus.

NUTRITION OF THE FETUS

Because of the small amount of yolk in the human ovum, growth of the fetus from the very early stage of development depends on nutrients obtained from the mother.

GLUCOSE

D-Glucose transfer across the placenta is accomplished by **facilitated diffusion.** Transporter proteins for D-glucose have been isolated from the plasma membrane of the microvilli of human trophoblasts.

LACTATE

Lactate also is transported across the placenta by facilitated diffusion. By way of cotransport with hydrogen ions, lactate is probably transported as lactic acid.

FREE FATTY ACIDS & TRIGLYCERIDES

Neutral fat (triacylglycerols) does not cross the placenta, but glycerol does. The extent of transport of free fatty acids is not known, but active transfer of palmitic acid from the maternal to the fetal side of the human placenta perfused in vitro does occur.

The placental uptake and use of low-density lipoproteins (LDL) by the placenta may account for an additional mechanism for assimilation of essential fatty acids and essential amino acids. The LDL particle of maternal plasma becomes bound to specific LDL receptors in the coated-pit region of the microvilli on the maternal-facing side of the trophoblasts. The LDL particle is taken up by a process of endocytosis. The apoprotein and cholesteryl esters of LDL are hydrolyzed by lysosomal enzymes in trophoblasts to yield (1) cholesterol for progesterone synthesis, (2) free amino acids (including essential amino acids), and (3) an essential fatty acid, linoleic acid, from the hydrolysis of the cholesteryl esters of LDL.

AMINO ACIDS

In addition to the use of LDL, the placenta is known to concentrate a large number of amino acids intracellularly. Neutral amino acids from maternal plasma are taken up by trophoblasts by at least three specific processes. Presumably, the amino acids, concentrated in trophoblasts, are thence transferred to the fetal side by diffusion.

PROTEINS & OTHER LARGE MOLECULES

The transfer of larger proteins across the placenta is generally very limited, but there are important exceptions, especially immunoglobulin G (IgG). In the human, IgG crosses the placenta in large amounts.

Near term, IgG is present in approximately the same concentrations in cord and maternal sera, but the concentrations of IgA and IgM are considerably lower in cord serum.

IONS & TRACE METALS

Iodide transport across the placenta clearly is carrier-mediated by an active process; indeed, the placenta concentrates iodide. Calcium and phosphorus also are actively transported across the placenta from mother to fetus. A calcium-binding protein is present in placenta. Iron is accumulated in placenta by an active, energy-requiring process. The concentrations of zinc in the fetal plasma also are greater than those in maternal plasma.

VITAMINS

Vitamin A (Retinol)
The concentration of vitamin A is greater in fetal than in maternal plasma. Vitamin A in fetal plasma is bound to retinol-binding protein and to prealbumin.

Vitamin C (Ascorbic Acid)
The transport of vitamin C across the placenta from mother to fetus is accomplished by an energy-dependent carrier-mediated process.

Vitamin D (Cholecalciferol)
The levels of the principal vitamin D metabolites, including 25-dihydroxycholecalciferol, are greater in maternal plasma than in fetal plasma.

PHYSIOLOGY OF THE FETUS

FETAL CIRCULATION

The fetal circulation is shown in Figure 35–4. Blood is returned to the placenta through the two **hypogastric arteries,** which distally become the **umbilical arteries.** After birth, the umbilical vessels, the ductus arteriosus, the foramen ovale, and the ductus venosus normally constrict or collapse, and the hemodynamics of the fetal circulation consequently undergo pronounced changes. Clamping of the umbilical cord and expansion of the fetal lungs, either through spontaneous breathing or artificial respira-

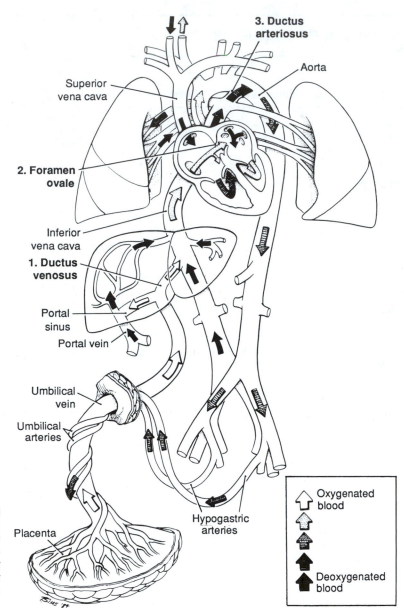

Figure 35–4. The intricate nature of the fetal circulation is evident. The degree of oxygenation of blood in various vessels differs appreciably from that in the postnatal state as a result of oxygenation being provided by the placenta rather than the lungs and the presence of three major vascular shunts: *1.* Ductus venosus. *2.* Foramen ovale. *3.* Ductus arteriosus.

tion, promptly induce a variety of hemodynamic changes in sheep and probably also in humans. The systemic arterial pressure initially falls slightly—apparently the result of the reversal in the direction of blood flow in the ductus arteriosus—but it soon recovers and then rises above the control value.

The ductus is functionally closed 10–96 hours after birth and anatomically closed by 2–3 weeks.

The more distal portions of the hypogastric arteries—which course from the level of the bladder along the abdominal wall to the umbilical ring and into the cord as the umbilical arteries—undergo atrophy and obliteration within 3–4 days after birth to become the **umbilical ligaments;** intra-abdominal remnants of the umbilical vein

form the **ligamentum teres.** The ductus venosus constricts and its lumen closes, resulting in formation of the **ligamentum venosum.**

FETAL BLOOD

Hematopoiesis

Hematopoiesis, in the very early embryo, is demonstrable first in the yolk sac. The next major site of erythropoiesis is the liver and after that the bone marrow. The hemoglobin of fetal blood rises to the adult male level of about 15 g per dL at mid pregnancy, and at term it is somewhat higher—about 18 g per dL. Fetoplacental blood volume appears to be approximately 124 mL per kg of fetus.

Fetal Hemoglobin

In the embryo and fetus, the globin moiety of much of the hemoglobin differs from that of the normal adult. In the embryo, three major forms of hemoglobin may be found. The most primitive forms are Gower-1 and Gower-2. The third form is hemoglobin Portland. Hemoglobin F (so-called fetal hemoglobin or alkaline-resistant hemoglobin) is the next hemoglobin to appear, and hemoglobin A, the final hemoglobin to be formed by the fetus and the major hemoglobin formed after birth in normal adults, is present after the 11th week of gestation in progressively greater amounts as the fetus matures.

At any given oxygen tension and at identical pH, fetal erythrocytes that contain mostly hemoglobin F bind more oxygen than do erythrocytes that contain nearly all hemoglobin A. The major reason for this difference is that hemoglobin A binds 2,3-diphosphoglycerate more avidly than does hemoglobin F, and 2,3-diphosphoglycerate so bound lowers the affinity of the hemoglobin molecule for oxygen. The increased oxygen affinity of the fetal erythrocyte results from a lower concentration of 2,3-diphosphoglycerate compared with that of the maternal erythrocyte, in which the 2,3-diphosphoglycerate level is increased compared with the nonpregnant state. At higher temperatures, the affinity of fetal blood for oxygen decreases. Increases in fetal temperature as a consequence of maternal hyperthermia could significantly compound the effects of fetal hypoxia.

Coagulation Factors in the Fetus

The following factors are low in cord blood: II, VII, IX, X, XI, XII, XIII, and fibrinogen. Without prophylactic vitamin K, vitamin K-dependent coagulation factors usually decrease even further during the first few days after birth, especially in breast-fed infants, and may lead to hemorrhage in the newborn infant.

Fetal Plasma Proteins

The mean total plasma protein and plasma albumin concentrations in maternal and cord blood are similar. Maternal and cord total plasma proteins average 6.5 and 5.9 g/dL, respectively, with maternal and cord plasma albumin levels of 3.6 and 3.7 g per dL, respectively.

IMMUNOCOMPETENCE OF THE FETUS

In the absence of a direct antigenic stimulus in the fetus, such as infection, fetal immunoglobulins consist almost totally of immunoglobulin G (IgG) synthesized by the mother and subsequently transferred across the placenta.

Immunoglobulin G

IgG transport from mother to fetus begins at about 16 weeks of gestation and increases as gestation proceeds.

The bulk of IgG is acquired by the fetus (from the mother) during the last 4 weeks of pregnancy.

Immunoglobulin M

IgM is not transported from mother to fetus; therefore, any IgM in the fetus or newborn was produced in the fetus.

Lymphocytes

B lymphocytes appear in the liver by 9 weeks and are present in the blood and spleen by 12 weeks of gestation. T lymphocytes begin to leave the thymus at about 14 weeks.

Monocytes

Monocytes of newborns are able to process and present antigen when tested with maternal antigen-specific T cells.

Ontogeny of the Immune Response

Morphologic evidence of immunologic competence in the human fetus has been reported as early as 13 weeks of gestational age. Moreover, synthesis of complement late in the first trimester by fetal organs has also been demonstrated.

The human newborn infant does not acquire much in the way of passive immunity from the absorption of humoral antibodies ingested in the colostrum. Nevertheless, IgA ingested in colostrum may provide protection against enteric infections, since the antibody resists digestion and is effective on mucosal surfaces.

In the adult, production of IgM in response to antigen is superseded in a week or so chiefly by production of IgG. In contrast, the IgM response remains the dominant one for weeks to months in the fetus and newborn. Measurement of IgM serum levels in umbilical cord blood and identification of specific antibodies may be of aid in the diagnosis of intrauterine infection.

THE FETAL NERVOUS SYSTEM & SENSORY ORGANS

The earliest proof of synaptic function appears by the eighth week of gestation with flexion of the fetal neck and trunk.

DIGESTIVE SYSTEM

GASTROINTESTINAL TRACT

Development

By the 11th week of gestation, the small intestine undergoes peristalsis and is capable of transporting glucose actively.

Fetal Swallowing

Fetal swallowing appears to have little effect on the amnionic fluid volume early in pregnancy. Late in pregnancy, however, the volume of amnionic fluid appears to be regulated substantially by fetal swallowing, for when swallowing is inhibited, hydramnios is common (see Chapter 53).

Meconium

Meconium consists not only of undigested debris from swallowed amnionic fluid but—to a larger extent—of various products of secretion, excretion, and desquamation by the gastrointestinal tract. Hypoxia has been implicated in evacuation of meconium from the large bowel into the amnionic fluid.

LIVER & PANCREAS

Liver

The liver has a limited capacity for converting free **bilirubin** to bilirubin diglucuronide. The more immature the fetus, the more deficient the system for conjugating bilirubin.

Because the life span of the fetal erythrocyte is shorter than that of normal adult erythrocytes, relatively more bilirubin is produced. Only a small fraction of the bilirubin is conjugated by the fetal liver and excreted through the biliary tract into the intestine and ultimately oxidized to biliverdin.

Most of the cholesterol in the fetus is produced in fetal liver. Indeed, the large demand for LDL cholesterol by the fetal adrenal is met primarily by fetal hepatic synthesis.

Glycogen appears in low concentration in fetal liver during the second trimester, but near term there is a rapid and marked increase in normal fetuses to levels two to three times those in adult liver.

Pancreas

The fetal pancreas responds to hyperglycemia by increasing plasma insulin. The alpha cells of the pancreas, however, do not respond to hypoglycemia and infused alanine by releasing glucagon.

URINARY SYSTEM

By the end of the first trimester, the nephrons have some capacity for excretion through glomerular filtration, though the kidneys are functionally immature throughout fetal life. The ability to concentrate and modify the pH of urine is quite limited even in the mature fetus. Fetal urine is hypotonic with respect to fetal plasma because of low concentrations of electrolytes.

AMNIONIC FLUID

The fluid filling the amnionic sac serves several important functions. It provides a medium in which the fetus can readily move, cushions the fetus against possible injury, helps maintain an even temperature, and provides, when appropriately tested, useful information concerning the health and maturity of the fetus. If the presenting part of the fetus is not closely applied to the lower uterine segment during labor, the hydrostatic action of the amnionic fluid may be important also in dilating the cervix.

The amnionic fluid increases rapidly to an average volume of 400 mL at mid pregnancy; it reaches a maximum of about 1000 mL at 36–38 weeks of gestation. The volume then decreases as term approaches, and if the pregnancy is prolonged, amnionic fluid may become relatively scant.

RESPIRATORY SYSTEM

FETAL LUNG

Surfactant

The principal surface-active component of surfactant is **dipalmitoylphosphatidylcholine,** a unique phosphatidylcholine moiety in which palmitate (a saturated fatty acid) is present in both the *sn*-1 and *sn*-2 positions of this glycerophospholipid. Ordinarily, there is a saturated fatty acid in the *sn*-1 position but a polyunsaturated fatty acid in the *sn*-2 position.

Respiratory distress syndrome is caused by a defect in surfactant biosynthesis in fetal and neonatal lung. Augmented surfactant synthesis normally appears in fetal lungs according to a developmental timetable. Surfactant is formed specifically in the type II pneumocytes that line the alveoli. The type II cells are characterized by multi-vesicular bodies, the cellular progenitors of the lamellar bodies in which surfactant is assembled.

The first indication of maturation of the fetal lung with respect to accelerated surfactant formation is the increased synthesis and secretion of dipalmitoylphosphatidylcholine. At this time, phosphatidylinositol levels in surfactant are high and those of phosphatidylglycerol are low (Figure 35–5). And it is only later in maturation, after a considerable increase in the rate of lecithin synthesis, that there occurs, simultaneously, an increase in phosphatidylglycerol and a decrease in phosphatidylinositol in surfactant.

APOPROTEINS

Surfactant is composed primarily of glycerophospholipids, but in the past 5–10 years the functional importance of the unique apoproteins of surfactant have been investigated. The major apoprotein of surfactant is a glycoprotein (MW about 35,000) referred to as SAP-35. SAP-35 is synthesized in the type II cells, and increased synthesis is related temporally to increased surfactant formation in maturing fetal lungs. The amnionic fluid content of SAP-35 also increases, as does the lecithin:sphingomyelin ratio as a function of gestational age and fetal lung maturity.

FETAL RESPIRATION

Movements of the fetal chest wall have been detected by ultrasonic techniques as early as 11 weeks of gestation. From the beginning of the fourth month, the fetus is capable of respiratory movement sufficiently intense to move amnionic fluid in and out of the respiratory tract.

Fetal breathing movements in the normal human fetus are episodic and irregular, their frequency ranging typically from 30 per min to 70 per min. Asphyxia is followed by cessation of normal breathing movements and the initiation of gasping respiratory efforts. Such cessation of normal respiratory movements may be the consequence of increased levels of fetal β-endorphin.

ENDOCRINE GLANDS

ANTERIOR PITUITARY

The fetal anterior pituitary differentiates into five cell types that secrete six protein hormones: (1) lactotropes, producing prolactin (PRL); (2) somatotropes, producing growth hormone (GH); (3) corticotropes, producing corticotropin (ACTH); (4) thyrotropes, producing thyroid-stimulating hormone (TSH); and (5) gonadotropes, producing luteinizing hormone (LH) and follicle-stimulating hormone (FSH). ACTH is first detected in the fetal pituitary at 7 weeks of gestation, and before the end of the 17th week the fetal pituitary is able to synthesize and store all pituitary hormones. GH, ACTH, and LH have been identified in the pituitary of the human fetus by 13 weeks of gestation. Moreover, the fetal pituitary is responsive to hypophysiotropic hormones and is capable of secreting these hormones from early in gestation.

NEUROHYPOPHYSIS

The fetal neurohypophysis is well developed by 10–12 weeks of gestation, and oxytocin and arginine vasopressin are demonstrable. It is probable that oxytocin as well as arginine vasopressin function in the fetus to conserve water, but these actions may be largely at the level of the lung and placenta rather than the kidney. PGE_2 formation in fetal kidney may serve to attenuate arginine vasopressin action in this organ. The levels of arginine vasopressin in umbilical cord plasma are increased strikingly compared with the levels found in maternal plasma.

FETAL INTERMEDIATE PITUITARY

There is a well-developed intermediate pituitary lobe in the human fetus. The cells of this structure begin to disappear before term and are absent from the pituitary of adults. The principal secretory products of the intermediate lobe cells are α-melanocyte-stimulating hormone (α-MSH) and β-endorphin. The levels of fetal α-MSH decrease progressively with gestation, but the levels of β-endorphin remain unaltered and under fetal control.

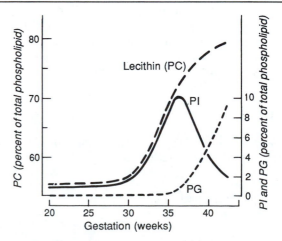

Figure 35–5. Relation between the levels of lecithin (dipalmitoylphosphatidylcholine [PC]), phosphatidylinositol (PI), and phosphatidylglycerol (PG) in amnionic fluid as a function of gestational age.

THYROID

The pituitary-thyroid system is capable of function by the end of the first trimester. Until mid pregnancy, however, secretion of thyroid-stimulating hormone and thyroid hormones is low. There is a considerable increase after this time. Probably very little **thyrotropin** crosses the placenta from mother to fetus, whereas thyroid-stimulating immunoglobulins (formerly called long-acting thyroid stimulators [LATS and LATS protector]) do so when present in high concentrations in the mother.

The human placenta actively concentrates iodide on the fetal side. Therefore, the hazard to the fetus of administering either radioiodide or appreciable amounts of ordinary iodide to the mother is obvious.

Immediately after birth, there are major changes in thyroid function and metabolism. Atmospheric cooling evokes a sudden and marked increase in thyrotropin secretion, which in turn causes a progressive increase in serum thyroxine levels which are maximal 24–36 hours after birth. There are nearly simultaneous elevations of serum triiodothyronine levels.

PARATHYROID GLANDS

There is good evidence that the fetal parathyroids elaborate parathyroid hormone by the end of the first trimester, and the glands appear to respond in utero to regulatory stimuli. Plasma calcium levels in the fetus of 11–12 mg/dL are maintained by active transport from maternal blood. Parathyroid levels in fetal blood are relatively low, and those of calcitonin are high.

ADRENAL GLANDS

The fetal adrenal is much larger in relation to total body size than that of the adult, mainly because of the inner or fetal zone of the cortex. The normally hypertrophied fetal zone involutes rapidly after birth. The fetal zone is scant to absent in rare instances where the fetal pituitary is congenitally absent. (See Placental Hormones, below.)

GONADS

Testosterone is synthesized by the fetal testis from progesterone and pregnenolone by 10 weeks of gestation. The formation of estrogen in fetal ovaries has been demonstrated, but estrogen formation in the ovaries is not required for female phenotypic development.

SEX OF THE FETUS

The sex ratio of human fetuses that reach viability is approximately 106 males to 100 females.

Sex differentiation is discussed in Chapter 21.

THE PLACENTAL HORMONES

PROTEIN HORMONES OF THE PLACENTA

1. CHORIONIC GONADOTROPIN

Chemical Characteristics of hCG

hCG is a glycoprotein (MW about 36,700) with a high carbohydrate content (30%). It is composed of two dissimilar subunits, α and β, which are noncovalently linked. The subunits of hCG have been isolated in pure form, and the primary structure of each has been characterized. There is no intrinsic biologic activity in either separated subunit (neither subunit binds to receptor).

hCG is related structurally to three other glycoprotein hormones: LH, FSH, and TSH. The primary amino acid structure of the α subunits of all four of these human glycoprotein hormones is identical; in contrast, however, although there are certain similarities, there are also clear differences among the amino acid sequences of the β subunits of FSH and TSH as well as those of hCG and LH. The β subunits of hCG and LH, however, are more similar to each other.

Cellular Site of Origin of hCG

The complete hCG molecule is believed to be produced principally in syncytiotrophoblasts rather than in cytotrophoblasts.

Concentrations of hCG in Serum & Urine

The intact (complete) hCG molecule is detectable in the plasma of pregnant women within 8–10 days after the midcycle surge of LH secretion that precedes ovulation. Thus, it is likely that hCG begins to enter maternal blood on the day of blastocyst implantation. Thereafter, the levels of hCG in blood increase rapidly, maximal levels being achieved at about 10 weeks of pregnancy (Figure 35–6).

Assay of hCG

Assays for hCG are of considerable importance because they form the basis for most pregnancy tests (Chapter 34).

Biologic Functions of hCG

The most apparent function of hCG in pregnancy is to

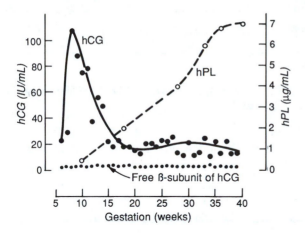

Figure 35–6. Mean concentration of chorionic gonadotropin (hCG) and placental lactogen (hPL) in serum of women throughout normal pregnancy. Free β subunit of hCG is in low concentration or else is undetectable throughout pregnancy. The concentration of free α subunit of hCG in serum increases gradually during pregnancy in a manner similar to that of hPL, albeit in much smaller amounts than hPL. (Data from Ashitaka Y and associates: Production and secretion of hCG and hCG subunits by trophoblastic tissue. Page 51 in: *Chorionic Gonadotropins*. Segal S (editor). Plenum Press, 1980; and Selenkow HA and associates: Patterns of serum immunoreactive human placental lactogen [IR-HPL] and chorionic gonadotropin [IR-HCG] in diabetic pregnancy. Diabetes 1971;20:696.)

maintain the function of the corpus luteum during early gestation.

Fetal testicular testosterone secretion is maximal at the same time in gestation that the rate of placental secretion of hCG is maximal. Thus, at a critical time in male fetal development, hCG serves as an LH surrogate on fetal testes to promote testosterone synthesis and secretion and thereby male sexual differentiation.

2. HUMAN PLACENTAL LACTOGEN

Chemical Characteristics

HPL consists of a single polypeptide chain with a molecular weight of 22,279. HPL contains 191 amino acid residues, compared with 188 in growth hormone; the amino acid sequence in each hormone is strikingly similar (96% homology, including conservative substitutions). HPL also is structurally similar to hPRL, with about 67% sequence homology. For these reasons, it has been suggested that the genes for hPL, hPRL, and hGH evolved from a common ancestral gene by repeated gene duplication.

Secretion & Metabolism

The metabolic clearance rate of hPL is about 175 L per d, considerably greater than that of hCG; and the production rate near term, 1 g or more per day, is the greatest of any known hormone in the human.

Serum Concentration

HPL is demonstrable in syncytiotrophoblasts within 2–3 weeks after conception, and placental lactogen can be detected in the serum of pregnant women as early as the fifth week of gestation (3 weeks after fertilization) (Figure 35–6). Interestingly, hPL is secreted into the maternal but not the fetal compartment.

Metabolic Actions of HPL

These putative actions include (1) lipolysis and an increase in the levels of circulating free fatty acids, thus providing a source of energy for maternal metabolism and fetal nutrition; and (2) inhibition of both the uptake of glucose and of gluconeogenesis in the mother, thus sparing both glucose and protein. The latter proposed anti-insulin action of hPL is believed to lead to an increase in maternal levels of insulin, which favors protein synthesis; this in turn ensures a mobilizable source of amino acids for transport to the fetus.

CHORIONIC ADRENOCORTICOTROPIN & THYROTROPIN

An ACTH-like protein has been isolated from placental tissue, and considerable evidence has accrued to support the proposition that this compound is of placental origin. The physiologic significance of placental ACTH and related compounds is unclear.

The placenta produces chorionic thyrotropin (hCT), but no significant role has been established for this substance in normal human pregnancy.

HYPOTHALAMIC-LIKE-RELEASING HORMONES OF THE PLACENTA

There is an appreciable amount of immunoreactive gonadotropin-releasing hormone (GnRH) and, interestingly, the human placenta can synthesize both GnRH and TRH in vitro.

Indeed, for each known hypothalamic-like releasing or inhibiting hormone described—GnRH, TRH, corticotropin-releasing hormone (CRF), and somatostatin—there are reports of analogous hormones produced in human placenta. The role of these hypothalamic-like releasing or inhibiting hormones in chorionic tissue, however, cannot be resolved at present.

INHIBIN

Inhibin, a glycoprotein hormone that acts preferentially to inhibit FSH release by the pituitary, is known to be produced by human testis and by the granulosa cells of the human ovary. Inhibin is a heterodimer, ie, it is composed of dissimilar α and β subunits. Inhibin also is produced in placenta, and may partially inhibit FSH secretion during pregnancy. In placenta, inhibin is produced in cytotrophoblasts and may act to regulate hCG release or secretion in the placenta.

"PREGNANCY-SPECIFIC" PROTEINS

In the past two decades, a host of proteins referred to as pregnancy-specific or pregnancy-related have been discovered. The precise roles or functions of these proteins produced in placenta or decidua is not defined.

STEROID HORMONES OF THE PLACENTA (Table 35–1)

ESTROGENS

Estrogen Biosynthesis in Placenta

In the placenta but not the ovary, acetate or cholesterol—or even progesterone—cannot serve as precursor for estrogen biosynthesis. Because steroid 17α-hydroxylase activity is not expressed in the human placenta, the conversion of C_{21} steroids to C_{19} steroids—the latter being the immediate precursors of estrogen—is not possible in human placenta.

Plasma-Borne Precursors for Placental Estrogen Biosynthesis

It is now known that plasma-borne dehydroepiandrosterone sulfate (DHEAS), dehydroepiandrosterone (DHEA), androstenedione, and testosterone are converted by the placenta into estrogens. The abundance of DHEAS in the plasma, however, and its much longer half-life uniquely qualify this steroid as the principal circulating precursor of placental estrone and estradiol-17β.

Table 35–1. Steroid production rates in nonpregnant and near-term pregnant women.

Steroid[1]	Production Rate (mg/24 h)	
	Nonpregnant	Pregnant
Estradiol-17β	0.1–0.6	15–20
Estriol	0.02–0.1	50–100
Progesterone	0.1–20	250–600
Aldosterone	0.05–0.1	1–2
Deoxycorticosterone	0.05–0.5	1–12
Cortisol	10–30	10–20

[1]Estrogens and progesterone are produced by placenta. Aldosterone is produced by the maternal adrenal in response to the stimulus of angiotensin II. Deoxycorticosterone is produced in extraglandular tissue sites by way of the 21-hydroxylation of plasma progesterone. Cortisol production during pregnancy is not increased, even through the blood levels are elevated because of decreased clearance caused by increased cortisol-binding globulin (Chapter 36).

FETAL ADRENAL GLANDS

FETAL ADRENAL & ESTROGEN FORMATION IN PLACENTA

Near term, about 50% of estradiol-17β produced in placenta arises from the utilization of maternal plasma DHEAS and 50% from fetal plasma DHEAS.

FETAL ADRENAL CONTRIBUTION TO ESTRIOL FORMATION IN PLACENTA

The disproportionate increase in estriol formation during human pregnancy results from the direct placental formation of estriol from 16α-hydroxylated C_{19} steroids, principally 16α-hydroxydehydroepiandrosterone sulfate. 16α-hydroxydehydroepiandrosterone sulfate arises by synthesis in the fetal adrenal and by 16α-hydroxylation of fetal plasma DHEAS in the fetal liver. A similar mechanism occurs in the maternal compartment (Figure 35–7). However, the fetus is the source of 90% of the precursor of estriol formed in placenta in normal near-term human pregnancy.

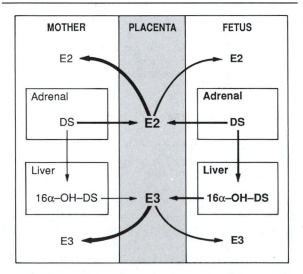

Figure 35–7. Schematic presentation of the biosynthesis of estrogen in human placenta. Near term. 50% of estradiol-17β is derived from fetal adrenal DHEAS (DS) and 50% from maternal DS. On the other hand, 90% of estriol in placenta arises from fetal 16α-hydroxydehydroepiandrosterone sulfate (16α-OH-DS) and only 10% from all other sources. Most (80–90%) of the steroids produced in placenta are secreted into the maternal blood.

FETAL ADRENAL FUNCTION: AN OVERVIEW

It can be estimated that normally, near term, the fetal adrenals must produce 100–200 mg of steroids per day. If one considers that the normal rate of steroid secretion by the adrenals of the nonstressed, resting adult rarely exceeds 20–30 mg per d, it is apparent that the fetal adrenal is a truly remarkable endocrine organ. It is probable that ACTH alone does not give rise to the total physiologic response observed in fetal adrenal growth and steroid secretion; indeed, there is a progressive decrease in the concentration of immunoreactive ACTH in human fetal plasma as pregnancy continues—at a time when the fetal adrenal is growing most rapidly.

The fetal adrenal cortex undergoes rapid involution immediately after birth, and the weight of the adrenals decreases strikingly during the first few weeks of life.

THE SOURCE OF STEROID PRECURSOR IN THE FETAL ADRENAL

It can be calculated that the rate of turnover of the cholesterol pool in the fetus must be six times that of the total cholesterol turnover in the adult just to accommodate the needs of the fetal adrenal for steroidogenesis.

The rate of cholesterol synthesis by fetal adrenal tissue by acetate is insufficient to account for more than a fraction of the steroids produced by the fetal adrenals at term.

Therefore, the fetal adrenal must assimilate cholesterol from the circulation to meet the demands for optimal steroidogenesis. In plasma, cholesterol and cholesteryl esters are present principally in the form of lipoproteins.

Lipoproteins are designated according to density as determined by ultracentrifugation, eg, very low density lipoproteins (VLDL), low-density lipoproteins (LDL), and high-density lipoproteins (HDL). The presence of specific plasma membrane receptors with a high affinity for LDL has been demonstrated in many tissues. After binding of LDL to the plasma membrane receptor, LDL is internalized by an adsorptive endocytotic process. The internalized endocytotic vesicles fuse with lysosomes, and the hydrolytic enzymes of the lysosomes catalyze the hydrolysis of the protein component of LDL, which gives rise to amino acids, and the hydrolysis of the cholesteryl esters of LDL, which gives rise to cholesterol and fatty acids. This same mechanism occurs in the fetal adrenal. Thus, the fetal adrenal is highly dependent upon circulating LDL as a source of cholesterol for steroidogenesis. It appears that three-fourths of the LDL cholesterol is derived from fetal hepatic production; the remainder is of maternal origin.

ESTROGEN PRODUCTION IN PREGNANCY: CLINICAL CORRELATIONS

The pathways of estrogen formation in the placenta are presented schematically in Figure 35–7.

Fetal Anencephaly

In the absence of the fetal zone of the adrenal cortex, as in anencephaly, the rate of formation of placental estrogens (especially estriol) is limited severely because of the lack of precursor formation in the fetus.

Maternal Adrenal Dysfunction

In women with Addison's disease, there is decreased excretion of estrogens in urine during pregnancy, principally resulting from a decrease in maternally derived estrone and estradiol-17β.

Maternal Ovarian Androgen-Producing Tumors

The placenta efficiently converts aromatizable C_{19} steroids (including bioactive testosterone) to estrogens, thereby preventing transplacental passage of bioactive androgen from the mother to the fetus. Indeed, it may be that female fetuses who are virilized in women with androgen-producing tumors are those in whom a nonaromatizable C_{19} steroid androgen is produced by the tumor, eg, 5α-dihydrotestosterone.

Placental Sulfatase Deficiency

Sulfatase deficiency prevents the hydrolysis of C_{19} steroid sulfate precursors of estrogen, the first enzymatic step in the placental use of these circulating prehormones for estrogen biosynthesis. This is an X-linked disorder (all affected fetuses are male) that is associated with the development of ichthyosis later in life.

Glucocorticoid Treatment

Glucocorticoids act to inhibit ACTH secretion by the maternal and fetal pituitary, resulting in decreased maternal and fetal adrenal secretion of placental estrogen precursor and ultimately a decrease in estrogen formation.

Neoplastic Trophoblastic Disease

In hydatidiform mole or choriocarcinoma, there is no fetal adrenal and estrogen formation and is thus limited to the utilization of maternal plasma C_{19} steroids, and the estrogen produced is therefore principally estradiol-17β.

Defect in Fetal LDL Cholesterol Biosynthesis

A successful pregnancy in a woman with abetalipoproteinemia was recently described. The absence of LDL in the maternal plasma led to very low progesterone formation in both the corpus luteum and the placenta; in addition, the levels of estriol were lower than normal. Presumably, the depressed levels of estrogen were the result of decreased LDL formation in the fetus, which was heterozygous for LDL deficiency.

PROGESTERONE

The biosynthesis of progesterone in human pregnancy is accomplished by the placental utilization of maternal plasma LDL cholesterol in syncytiotrophoblast.

Progesterone is formed from cholesterol in all steroidogenic tissues in a two-step enzymatic reaction. First, cholesterol is converted in mitochondria to the steroid intermediate pregnenolone, in a reaction catalyzed by cytochrome P-450, and cholesterol side-chain cleavage enzyme. In turn, pregnenolone is converted to progesterone in microsomes by another P-450 enzyme, 3β-hydroxysteroid dehydrogenase.

The daily production of progesterone in late normal singleton pregnancies is about 250 mg. In some pregnancies with multiple fetuses, however, the daily progesterone production rate may exceed 600 mg per d.

PROGESTERONE METABOLISM DURING PREGNANCY

During pregnancy, there is a disproportionate increase in the concentration of 5α-dihydroprogesterone in plasma, and for that reason the ratio of the concentration of this metabolite to that of progesterone is increased in pregnant women. The mechanisms by which this comes about are not defined, but they may be relevant to the resistance to pressor agents that develops in normal pregnant women. Progesterone is converted also to the potent mineralocorticoid deoxycorticosterone (DOC) in pregnant women and in the fetus. During human pregnancy, the concentration of DOC is increased strikingly in both the maternal and fetal compartments, and the extra-adrenal formation of DOC from circulating progesterone accounts for the vast majority of this mineralocorticosteroid produced in human pregnancy.

SUGGESTED READINGS

Knobil E, Neill JD (editors): *The Physiology of Pregnancy,* 2 vols. Raven Press, 1988.

Cunningham FG, MacDonald PC, Gant NF, Leveno KJ, and Gilstrap LC, III (editors): The Morphological and Functional Development of the Fetus. Chapter 7 in *Williams Obstetrics,* 19th ed., Appleton & Lange, 1993.

Maternal Adaptations to Pregnancy

MATERNAL TISSUES OF THE FETAL-MATERNAL COMMUNICATION SYSTEM

In some ill-defined manner, the implanting blastocyst incites further decidualization of the secretory endometrium. It is likely that this process involves essential elements of the inflammatory process, including blastocyst generation of prostaglandins, platelet-activating factor, and serine proteases (eg, plasminogen activator), which are believed to be important in trophoblast invasion of endometrium. At this time or perhaps earlier, a fetal-maternal communication system is established.

Two maternal tissues are directly involved in the fully developed fetal-maternal communication system: maternal uterine decidua and maternal blood. As the trophoblasts of the blastocyst invade the endometrium, the two distinct arms of the fetal-maternal communication system are established. Trophoblasts invade the endometrial blood vessels. At this time, the **placental arm** of the fetal-maternal communication system is established (Chapter 35). And as the embryo and extraembryonic fetal tissues grow, the fetal membranes develop and ultimately come to lie adjacent to all of the uterine decidua to form the **paracrine arm** of that system (Chapter 35).

THE CARDINAL FUNCTION OF THE DECIDUA IN PREGNANCY MAINTENANCE & PARTURITION

The decidua is the specialized endometrium of pregnancy, being composed largely of decidual cells that develop from the stromal cells (mesenchyme) of the endometrium. Most of the glandular epithelium and glandular structure of endometrium are lost during pregnancy.

A **uterotropin** is an agent that causes uterine preparedness for labor, including cervical effacement and ripening,

the development of gap junctions between myometrial cells, an increase in the number of oxytocin receptors, and increased sensitivity to uterotonins. A **uterotonin** is an agent that brings on the myometrial contractions of labor. There is evidence that the uterine decidua (the endometrium of pregnancy) is one source of the uterotropins and uterotonins that serve to initiate parturition and maintain labor (Chapter 37).

THE DECIDUA

SPECIALIZED FUNCTIONS OF THE ENDOMETRIUM & DECIDUA

The endometrial cavity is patent, ie, anatomically open through the cervical canal, which in turn is open to the vagina, which in turn is open to the external environment. The same is true of the decidua during pregnancy—at least at the lower pole of the interface between the chorion laeve (the innermost of the fetal membranes) and the decidua vera. To be sure, there is functional closure of the cervical canal by way of a "mucous plug," and there are antimicrobial properties ascribed to the cervical mucus. Because the female reproductive tract is "open" to the external environment, it is reasonable to presume that the endometrium and decidua must be able to respond to microbial and immunologic challenges. Decidua probably functions effectively to contain infectious processes at the lower pole of the chorion laeve-decidual interface as a means of preventing the onset of preterm labor (Chapter 37).

UNIQUE DECIDUAL FUNCTIONS

The decidual cells produce prolactin, relaxin, a variety of "pregnancy-specific proteins," prostaglandins, cytokines, and 1,25-dihydroxyvitamin D_3 and are rich in a variety of intriguing enzymes, such as diamine oxidase (see below).

The decidua is the source of prolactin that is found in enormous amounts in the amnionic fluid during human pregnancy. Levels of prolactin of 10,000 ng per mL of amnionic fluid are found during the 20th–24th weeks of pregnancy, compared with levels of 150 ng per mL in plasma of near-term pregnant women. Prolactin produced in decidua preferentially enters amnionic fluid, and little or none enters maternal blood. This is a classic example of the peculiar trafficking of molecules between maternal and fetal tissues of the paracrine arm of the fetal-maternal communication system.

UTERUS

HYPERTROPHY & DILATATION

In the nonpregnant woman, the uterus is an almost solid structure weighing 70 g or so and with a cavity of 10 mL or less. During pregnancy, the uterus is transformed into a relatively thin-walled muscular organ of sufficient capacity to accommodate the fetus, placenta, and amnionic fluid. The total volume of the contents of the uterus at term averages about 5 L. There is a corresponding increase in uterine weight, and the body of the uterus at term weighs approximately 1100 g. During pregnancy, uterine enlargement involves stretching and hypertrophy of existing muscle cells, whereas the appearance of new muscle cells is limited. At the time of parturition, a single myometrial cell is about 500 μm in length, and the nucleus is eccentrically placed in the thickest part of the cell.

During the first few months of pregnancy, hypertrophy of the uterine wall is probably stimulated chiefly by the action of estrogen and perhaps progesterone. But after the third month, the increase in uterine size is in large part related in some manner to the effect of pressure exerted by the expanding products of conception.

Rapid growth of most tissues (perhaps all) is correlated with increased synthesis of **polyamines,** which include **spermidine** and **spermine** and their immediate precursor, **putrescine.** These polyamines are believed to play crucial roles in tissue growth and cell hypertrophy. Polyamine levels in the urine of normally pregnant women are strikingly elevated, and the highest levels are attained at 13–14 weeks of gestation. The increased rate of synthesis of polyamines at this time may be related to the myometrial hypertrophy that occurs during this stage of pregnancy, but it is of interest also that at 13–14 weeks of gestation there is a striking increase in diamine oxidase activity in the blood. This enzyme probably is produced in decidua but is released into blood in large amounts. Indeed, the activity of diamine oxidase in the blood of pregnant women

is 1000 times that found in men or nonpregnant women. This enzyme serves to catalyze the metabolism of polyamines. Thus, it is likely that the rate of polyamine formation is increased strikingly throughout pregnancy, but the rate of metabolism of these growth-promoting agents increases so remarkably, owing to the action of diamine oxidase, that the levels of polyamines decline after 12–14 weeks of gestation.

CHANGES IN UTERINE SIZE, SHAPE, & POSITION

For the first few weeks, the original pear shape of the uterus is maintained, but as pregnancy advances the corpus and fundus assume a more globular form, becoming almost spherical by the third lunar month. Subsequently, the organ increases more rapidly in length than in width and assumes an ovoid shape.

By the end of 12 weeks, the uterus has become too large to remain wholly within the pelvis. As the uterus rises, tension is exerted upon the broad ligaments, which partly unfold their median and lower portions, and upon the round ligaments.

With ascent from the pelvis, the uterus usually undergoes rotation to the right (**dextrorotation),** probably because of the presence of the rectosigmoid on the left side of the pelvis.

CHANGES IN CONTRACTILITY

From the first trimester of pregnancy onward, the uterus undergoes irregular contractions, which normally are painless. Late in pregnancy, these **Braxton Hicks contractions** may cause some discomfort and may account for so-called **false labor.**

UTEROPLACENTAL BLOOD FLOW

Placental perfusion by maternal blood is dependent upon blood flow to the uterus through the uterine and ovarian arteries. There is no question that there is a progressive increase in uteroplacental blood flow during pregnancy. The reported values, which average about 500 mL per min late in pregnancy, are approximations.

CONTROL OF UTEROPLACENTAL BLOOD FLOW

The factors that regulate uteroplacental perfusion remain largely unknown. By the use of animal models and

---

[1]The interested reader should refer to the discussion in Chapter 8 of *Williams Obstetrics,* 19th ed. Appleton & Lange, 1993.

indirect methods of assessing uteroplacental perfusion in the human, however, a partial understanding is evolving.[1]

CHANGES IN THE CERVIX

During pregnancy, pronounced softening and "blush" coloration of the cervix occurs, often demonstrable as early as a month after conception. These changes comprise two of the earliest physical signs of pregnancy (Chapter 35). The factors responsible for these changes are increased vascularity and edema of the entire cervix, together with hypertrophy and hyperplasia of the cervical glands.

Soon after conception, a clot of very thick mucus obstructs the cervical canal. At the onset of labor, if not before, this **mucous plug** is expelled, resulting in a **bloody show.** The glands near the external os proliferate beneath the stratified squamous epithelium of the portio vaginalis, giving the cervix the velvety consistency characteristic of pregnancy.

So-called **erosions of the cervix** during pregnancy probably are not abnormal but rather represent a normal extension or **eversion** of the proliferating endocervical glands and the columnar endocervical epithelium.

OVARIES & FALLOPIAN TUBES

OVARIAN FUNCTION

Ovulation ceases during pregnancy, and the maturation of new follicles is suspended. Ordinarily, the corpus luteum of pregnancy functions maximally during the first 6–7 weeks (4–5 weeks post ovulation) and thereafter contributes little to progesterone production.

RELAXIN

Human relaxin (MW about 6000) is a protein hormone composed of nonidentical A and B chains of similar length. Relaxin has structural features that resemble insulin and insulin-like growth factors I and II. As is the case for insulin, relaxin is synthesized initially as a single-chain preprohormone that includes the signal peptide, ie, the B chain; and the connecting peptide, ie, the A chain.

Human relaxin is secreted by the corpus luteum of pregnancy and possibly by uterine decidua during pregnancy. The pattern of secretion is similar to that of human chorionic gonadotropin. Therefore, appreciable relaxin secretion continues throughout pregnancy.

The decidua has been reported to secrete human relaxin, but significant amounts have not been obtained from decidual tissue. In fact, the amounts of relaxin present in human decidua appear to be quite low compared with the corpus luteum.

The role of relaxin during human pregnancy is not defined. Furthermore, the role of human relaxin in producing softening and effacement of the uterine cervix also is unknown. The topical administration of pharmacologic doses of a highly purified porcine relaxin to the human cervix, however, results in cervical softening and effacement, as well as a higher rate of successful labor inductions in treated versus untreated women.

PREGNANCY LUTEOMA

Clinical observations are consistent with the view that a luteoma of pregnancy represents an exaggeration of the luteinization reaction of the ovary of normal pregnancy and is not a true neoplasm. The luteoma regresses after delivery, and normal ovarian function returns after delivery.

Even though maternal virilization may be prominent, the female fetus usually is not affected, presumably because of the protective role of the placenta through its high capacity to convert androgens and androgen-like steroids to estrogens (Chapter 35).

HYPERREACTIO LUTEINALIS

Hyperreactio luteinalis is a benign lesion of the ovary that causes maternal virilization during pregnancy. While the cellular pattern is similar to that of a luteoma of pregnancy, the two tumors are different grossly. Luteoma is a solid tumor and hyperreactio luteinalis is a cystic tumor. Furthermore, hyperreactio luteinalis commonly is associated with extremely high human chorionic gonadotropin values.

OTHER OVARIAN CHANGES

A **decidual reaction** on and beneath the surface of the ovaries—similar to that found in the endometrial stroma—is common in pregnancy and may be observed at cesarean delivery. These elevated patches of tissue bleed easily and may resemble freshly torn adhesions.

FALLOPIAN TUBES

The musculature of the fallopian tubes undergoes little hypertrophy during pregnancy. The epithelium of the tubal mucosa is flattened compared to that of the nonpregnant state. Decidual cells may develop in the stroma of the endosalpinx, but a continuous decidual membrane is not formed.

VAGINA & PERINEUM

During pregnancy, increased vascularity and hyperemia develop in the skin and muscles of the perineum and vulva, and there is softening of the normally abundant connective tissue of these structures.

The vagina undergoes increased vascularity also. The copious secretion and the characteristic violet color of the vagina during pregnancy (**Chadwick's sign),** similar to the changes that occur in the cervix during pregnancy, probably result chiefly from hyperemia. The vaginal walls undergo a considerable increase in thickness of the mucosa, loosening of the connective tissue, and hypertrophy of the smooth muscle cells to nearly the same extent as in the uterus.

VAGINAL SECRETION

The greatly increased cervical and vaginal secretion during pregnancy consists of a somewhat thick, white discharge. Its pH is acidic, varying from 3.5 to 6.0, the result of increased production of lactic acid from glycogen in the vaginal epithelium by the action of *Lactobacillus acidophilus*. The acidic pH probably acts to control the rate of multiplication of pathogenic bacteria in the vagina.

ABDOMINAL WALL & SKIN

STRIAE GRAVIDARUM

In the later months of pregnancy, reddish, slightly depressed streaks called striae gravidarum commonly develop in the skin of the abdomen and sometimes in the skin over the breasts and thighs. They probably arise as a result of separation of the superficial epidermis, exposing the more vascular dermis underneath.

DIASTASIS RECTI

Occasionally, the muscles of the abdominal walls do not withstand the tension to which they are subjected, and the rectus muscles separate in the midline, creating a diastasis recti of varying extent.

PIGMENTATION

In many women, the midline of the abdominal skin becomes markedly pigmented, assuming a brownish-black color to form the **linea nigra.** Occasionally, irregular brownish patches of varying size appear on the face and neck, giving rise to **chloasma** or **melasma gravidarum** (mask of pregnancy), which usually disappears or at least regresses considerably after delivery.

CUTANEOUS VASCULAR CHANGES

Angiomas, also called **vascular spiders,** develop in about two-thirds of white women and approximately 10% of black women during pregnancy. They appear as tiny red elevations on the skin, especially on the face, neck, upper chest, and arms, with radicles branching outward from a central body. **Palmar erythema** is observed in about two-thirds of white women and one-third of black women. The two conditions frequently occur together but are of no clinical significance and disappear in most women shortly after termination of pregnancy. The high incidence of these disorders in pregnancy is probably related to hyperestrogenemia.

BREASTS

In the early weeks, the pregnant woman often experiences tenderness and tingling of the breasts. After the second month, the breasts increase in size and become nodular as a result of hypertrophy of the mammary alveoli. As the breasts increase in size, delicate veins become visible just beneath the skin. Changes in the nipples and areolae are even more characteristic. The nipples become larger, more deeply pigmented, and more erectile. After the first few months, a thick, yellowish fluid called **colostrum** often can be expressed from the nipples by gentle massage. At that time, the areolae become broader and more deeply pigmented. The depth of pigmentation varies with the woman's complexion. Scattered through the areolae are a number of small elevations, the so-called glands (follicles) of Montgomery, which are hypertrophic sebaceous glands. If the increase in size of the breasts is very extensive, striations similar to those observed in the abdomen may develop. Histologic and functional changes of the breasts induced by pregnancy and lactation are discussed further in Chapter 41.

METABOLIC CHANGES

WEIGHT GAIN

Most of the increase in weight during pregnancy is attributable to the uterus and its contents, the breasts, and increases in blood volume and extravascular extracellular fluid. A smaller fraction of the increased weight is the result of metabolic alterations that result in an increase in cellular water and deposition of new fat and protein, so-called maternal reserves. During the first trimester, the average gain is 1 kg, compared to about 5 kg during each of the last two trimesters.

CALORIC REQUIREMENTS

The excess energy costs of normal pregnancy are approximately 80,000 kcal (335 kJ) or an additional 300 kcal per day.

WATER METABOLISM

Increased water retention is a normal physiologic alteration of pregnancy. It is mediated at least in part by a fall in plasma osmolality of approximately 10 mosm per kg, induced by a resetting of osmotic thresholds for thirst and vasopressin secretion.

At term, the water content of the fetus, placenta, and amnionic fluid amounts to about 3.5 L. About another 3 L accumulate as a result of increases in maternal blood volume and in the size of the uterus and breasts. Thus, the minimum amount of extra water the average woman could be expected to retain during normal pregnancy is about 6.5 L.

PROTEIN METABOLISM

At term, the fetus and placenta together weigh about 4 kg and contain approximately 500 g of protein, or about half of the total increase normally induced by pregnancy. The remaining 500 g of protein is added to the uterus as contractile protein, to the breasts primarily in the glands, and to the maternal blood in the form of hemoglobin and plasma proteins.

The daily requirements for protein intake during pregnancy are increased (Chapter 43), but equally important to an increase in protein in pregnancy is the ingestion of adequate sources of energy foods, eg, carbohydrates and fat. If these are not consumed in adequate amounts, the energy requirements of the mother must be met by catabolism of maternal protein stores. The liberated amino acids used for energy are not available for synthesis of maternal pro-

tein. Therefore, with increasing intake of fat and carbohydrates as energy sources, less dietary protein is required to maintain a positive nitrogen balance. Concentrations of several plasma proteins are altered by pregnancy. The albumin concentration decreases significantly, whereas fibrinogen rises. The concentrations of IgG, IgA, and IgM fall somewhat.

The plasma concentrations of α_1-antitrypsin, α_2-macroglobulin, ceruloplasmin, and transferrin all increase, but complement C3 and haptoglobin apparently are not changed.

CARBOHYDRATE METABOLISM

Pregnancy is potentially diabetogenic. Diabetes mellitus may be aggravated by pregnancy, and clinical diabetes may appear in some women only during pregnancy. Consequently, considerable attention has been focused on the metabolism of carbohydrates and insulin in pregnant women. In healthy women, the fasting plasma glucose concentration falls somewhat during pregnancy, perhaps as a result of increased plasma levels of insulin.

The increased levels of insulin cannot be explained, however, by a change in the metabolism of insulin, because the half-life of insulin during pregnancy is not changed. Although the exact mechanisms responsible for the β cell hypertrophy, hyperplasia, and hypersecretion observed in pregnancy are not understood completely, estrogen, progesterone, and human placental lactogen are probably involved. Finally, the peak in human placental lactogen concentrations corresponds to the greatest insulin responses by the β cell.

The increased basal level of plasma insulin observed in normal pregnancy is associated with several unique responses to the ingestion of glucose. For example, after an oral glucose meal, there is both prolonged hyperglycemia and hyperinsulinemia in pregnant women, with a greater suppression of glucagon. This mechanism probably functions to ensure a sustained postprandial supply of glucose to the fetus. This response is consistent with a pregnancy-induced state of peripheral resistance to insulin.

The existence of tissue resistance to insulin during pregnancy is suggested by three observations: (1) an increased insulin response to glucose (increased plasma level and duration); (2) a reduced peripheral uptake of glucose (increased plasma level and duration); and (3) a suppressed glucagon response. The mechanisms responsible for the tissue resistance to insulin are not fully understood. The plasma levels of human placental lactogen increase with gestation, and this protein hormone is characterized by a growth hormone-like action that may result in increased lipolysis and increased liberation of free fatty acids.

The increased concentration of circulating free fatty acids may also facilitate increased tissue resistance to insulin.

The mechanisms discussed in the preceding paragraphs ensure a continuous supply of glucose for transfer to the fetus. The pregnant woman, however, changes rapidly from a postprandial state characterized by elevated and sustained glucose levels to a fasting state characterized by decreased plasma glucose and amino acids such as alanine. There also are higher plasma concentrations of free fatty acids, triglycerides, and cholesterol in the pregnant woman during fasting (Figure 36–1). When fasting is prolonged in the pregnant woman, these alterations are exaggerated, and ketonemia appears rapidly.

Insulinase activity has been found in the human placenta. It seems unlikely, however, that accelerated degradation of insulin by placental insulinase contributes to the diabetogenic state induced by pregnancy, since the rate of degradation of radiolabeled insulin in vivo does not appear to differ among pregnant and nonpregnant women.

The role of glucagon during pregnancy is not fully defined. The prevailing current view is that β cell sensitivity to a glucose challenge is significantly increased in normal pregnant women but that α cell sensitivity to a glucose stimulus is unaltered.

FAT METABOLISM

The concentrations of lipids, lipoproteins, and apolipoproteins in plasma increase during pregnancy (Figures 36–1 and 36–2). Plasma levels of lipids increase continuously throughout gestation, and there is a positive correlation between the concentrations of lipids (shown in Figure 36–1) with those of estradiol, progesterone, and human placental lactogen.

The concentrations of apolipoproteins A-I, A-II, and B increase until weeks 25, 28, and 30, respectively, and then usually remain unchanged until delivery. The changes in concentration of apolipoprotein B are similar to those of estradiol after a 2-week time shift, and this effect may be causally related.

Plasma lipoprotein cholesterol levels during pregnancy are charted in Figure 36–2.

MINERAL METABOLISM (Other Than Iron)

Plasma copper and ceruloplasmin levels increase considerably early in pregnancy because of the increases in estrogens. Calcium and magnesium levels are reduced very slightly, the reduction probably reflecting for the most part the lowered plasma protein concentration and in turn the decrease in the amount of each electrolyte that is bound to protein. However, there is a small but significant increase in free calcium ion concentration in late pregnancy. Serum phosphorus levels are within the nonpregnant range, and bone turnover is reduced during early pregnancy, returned toward normal during the third trimester, and increased in postpartum lactating women. The status of zinc metabolism in pregnancy is currently somewhat confused.

ACID-BASE EQUILIBRIUM & BLOOD ELECTROLYTES

Normally, the pregnant woman hyperventilates, compared with nonpregnant women, and this causes respiratory alkalosis by lowering the P_{CO_2} of the blood. A moderate reduction in plasma bicarbonate from about 26 mmol/L to about 22 mmol per L partially compensates for the respiratory alkalosis. As a result, there is only a minimal increase in blood pH. The increase in blood pH shifts the oxygen dissociation curve to the left and increases the affinity of maternal hemoglobin for oxygen (**Bohr effect**),

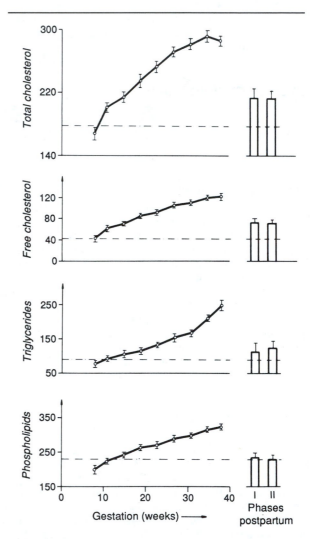

Figure 36–1. Mean (± SEM) plasma lipid concentrations (mg per dL) throughout gestation (N = 42) and during the luteal (I) and follicular (II) phases postpartum (p.p.; N = 23). The dashed lines represent the mean values of the control group (N = 24). TC, total cholesterol; FC, free cholesterol; TG, triglycerides; PL, phospholipids. (Reproduced, with permission, from Desoye G and associates: Correlation of hormones with lipid and lipoprotein levels during normal pregnancy and postpartum. J Clin Endocrinol Metab 1987;64:704.)

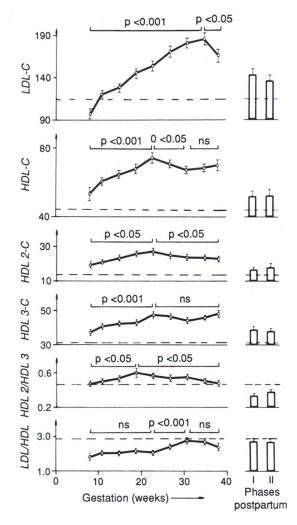

Figure 36–2. Mean (± SEM) plasma lipoprotein cholesterol levels (mg per dL) throughout gestation (N = 42) and during the luteal (I) and follicular (II) phases postpartum (p.p.; N = 23). The dashed lines represent the mean values of the control group (100%). LDL-C, low-density lipoprotein cholesterol; HDL-C, high-density lipoprotein cholesterol; HDL2-C, high-density lipoprotein-2 cholesterol; HDL3-C, high-density lipoprotein-3 cholesterol. (Reproduced, with permission, from Desoye G and associates: Correlation of hormones with lipid and lipoprotein levels during normal pregnancy and postpartum. J Clin Endocrinol Metab 1987;64:704.)

thereby decreasing the oxygen-releasing capacity of maternal blood. Thus, the hyperventilation that results in a reduced maternal P_{CO_2} facilitates transport of CO_2 from the fetus to the mother but appears to impair release of oxygen from the mother's blood to the fetus. The increase in blood pH, however, while minimal, stimulates an increase in 2,3-diphosphoglycerate in maternal erythrocytes that counteracts the Bohr effect by shifting the oxygen dissociation curve back to the right, facilitating oxygen release to the fetus. These subtle but important changes

guarantee that the fetus will have every advantage from blood gas exchange.

Despite large accumulations during pregnancy of sodium and potassium, the serum concentration of these electrolytes decreases. During normal pregnancy, nearly 1000 meq of sodium and 300 meq of potassium are retained.

Sodium and potassium excretion are unchanged during pregnancy even though their filtration by the glomerulus is increased. Obviously, fractional excretion of these electrolytes is decreased, and it has been postulated that progesterone counteracts the natriuretic and kaliuretic effects of aldosterone.

HEMATOLOGIC CHANGES OF NORMAL PREGNANCY

BLOOD VOLUME

The blood volume at or very near term averages about 45% above nonpregnant levels. The degree of expansion varies considerably. In some women there is only a modest increase, and in others, the blood volume nearly doubles.

Maternal blood volume starts to increase during the first trimester, expands most rapidly during the second trimester, and then rises at a much slower rate during the third trimester to reach a plateau during the last several weeks of pregnancy.

The increase in blood volume results from an increase in both plasma and erythrocytes. The usual pattern is an initial rise in plasma volume followed by an increase in the volume of circulating erythrocytes. Although more plasma than erythrocytes is usually added to the maternal circulation, the increase in the volume of circulating erythrocytes is considerable, averaging about 450 mL, or an increase of about one-third.

ATRIAL NATRIURETIC PEPTIDE & PLASMA VOLUME

In the human, increased secretion of atrial natriuretic peptides occurs in response to volume expansion and atrial stretch and in response to a high-sodium diet. Conversely, a low-sodium diet results in a decrease in peptide concentration.

The actual effect of this peptide on plasma volume in the normally pregnant woman remains to be defined. There is no doubt, however, that the peptide has a rapid and effective action on plasma volume during the early puerperium. It seems unlikely that such a potent mediator of volume and sodium homeostasis would not have an effect during pregnancy as well.

CHANGES IN HEMATOCRIT

In spite of augmented erythropoiesis, the concentrations of hemoglobin and erythrocytes, as well as the hematocrit, decrease slightly during normal pregnancy. Consequently, whole blood viscosity decreases. A hemoglobin concentration below 11 g per dL late in pregnancy, however, should be considered abnormal; it is usually due to iron deficiency rather than hypervolemia of pregnancy.

IRON METABOLISM

Iron Stores & Requirements

The total body iron content of normal women is probably in the range of 2–2.5 g, compared to about 4 g in men. The iron requirements of normal pregnancy total about 1 g. About 300 mg are actively transferred to the fetus and placenta, and about 200 mg are lost through various normal routes of excretion. The average increase in the total volume of circulating erythrocytes of about 450 mL during pregnancy uses another 500 mg of iron, since 1 mL of normal erythrocytes contains 1.1 mg of iron.

The amounts of iron absorbed from diet, together with that mobilized from stores, are usually insufficient to meet the demands imposed by pregnancy even though iron absorption from the gastrointestinal tract appears to be moderately increased during pregnancy. Supplemental iron, therefore, is valuable during the latter half of pregnancy, when iron requirements average 6–7 mg per d, and for several weeks after delivery if the infant is to be breastfed.

Without supplemental iron, the maternal **plasma iron concentration** often decreases during pregnancy. Undoubtedly, in most instances, iron deficiency contributes significantly to the fall. The **plasma iron-binding capacity** (transferrin) increases during pregnancy even when iron deficiency has been eliminated by appropriate treatment.

Blood Loss

During normal vaginal delivery and through the next few days, only about half of the erythrocytes added to the maternal circulation during pregnancy are lost. On the average, an amount of maternal erythrocytes corresponding to about 600 mL of predelivery blood is lost during and after vaginal delivery of a single fetus. The average blood loss associated with cesarean or vaginal delivery of twins is about 1 L.

IMMUNOLOGIC & LEUKOCYTE FUNCTIONS

Pregnancy has been assumed to be associated with suppression of a variety of humoral and cell-mediated immunologic functions in order to accommodate the "foreign" semiallogeneic fetal graft. In fact, humoral antibody titers against several viruses are decreased during pregnancy, but only in proportion to the hemodilutional effect of pregnancy.

The prevalence of a variety of autoantibodies is unchanged. Furthermore, α-interferon, which is present in almost all fetal tissues and fluids, most often is absent in normally pregnant women. There is evidence—as yet unexplained—that polymorphonuclear leukocyte chemotaxis and adherence functions are depressed beginning in the second trimester and continuing throughout pregnancy. Thus, both the function and the absolute numbers of leukocytes appear to be important factors when considering the leukocytosis of normal pregnancy.

The blood leukocyte count varies considerably during normal pregnancy. Usually it ranges from 5000/μL to 12,000 per μL, but during labor and the early puerperium it may be markedly elevated. The activity of alkaline phosphatase in the leukocytes is increased from early in pregnancy. Such elevated activity occurs in a wide variety of conditions, including most inflammatory states. During pregnancy, there is neutrophilia consisting predominantly of mature forms; however, an occasional myelocyte is found.

BLOOD COAGULATION

Plasma fibrinogen (factor I) is elevated in normal pregnant women, averaging 300 mg per dL and ranging from 200 mg per dL to 400 mg per dL. The concentration of fibrinogen increases about 50% to average about 450 mg/dL late in pregnancy, with a range of 300–600 mg per dL, resulting in a striking increase in the **erythrocyte sedimentation rate** in normal pregnancy.

Other clotting factors whose activities are increased during normal pregnancy are factor VII (proconvertin), factor VIII (antihemophilic globulin), factor IX (plasma thromboplastin component, Christmas factor), and factor X (Stuart factor). The level of factor II (prothrombin) is usually increased only slightly, whereas the levels of factors XI (plasma thromboplastin antecedent) and XIII (fibrin-stabilizing factor) are decreased somewhat.

The Quick one-stage prothrombin time and the partial thromboplastin time are both shortened slightly as pregnancy progresses. The clotting times of whole blood in either plain glass tubes (wettable surface) or silicone-coated or plastic tubes (nonwettable surface) do not differ significantly in normal pregnant and nonpregnant women.

High-molecular-weight soluble fibrin-fibrinogen complexes circulate in normal pregnancy. An increased capacity for neutralizing heparin has also been described, but plasma antithrombin III does not appear to be reduced. Some of these alterations in coagulation factors during normal pregnancy may be equated with continuing low-grade intravascular coagulation. For example, the number of platelets is reduced slightly, probably because of a shorter half-life in pregnant compared to nonpregnant women. Beta-thromboglobulin, a platelet-specific release protein, also is increased during the second and third trimesters.

During normal pregnancy, the level of maternal plasminogen (profibrinolysin) in plasma increases considerably. Even so, fibrinolytic (plasmin) activity is distinctly prolonged compared with that of the normal nonpregnant state.

CARDIOVASCULAR SYSTEM

HEART

Typically, the resting pulse rate increases about 10–15 beats per min during pregnancy. As the diaphragm is elevated progressively during pregnancy, the heart is displaced to the left and upward, while at the same time it is rotated somewhat on its long axis. As a result, the apex of the heart is moved laterally from its position in the normal nonpregnant state, and an increase in size of the cardiac silhouette is found in radiographs. The extent of these changes is influenced by the size and position of the uterus, the strength of the abdominal muscles, and the configurations of the abdomen and thorax. Variability of these factors makes it difficult to precisely identify moderate degrees of cardiomegaly by physical examination or by simple x-ray studies.

Cardiac volume increases normally by about 75 mL, or a little more than 10%, between early and late pregnancy. Both left ventricular wall mass and end-diastolic dimensions increase during pregnancy, as do heart rate, calculated stroke volume, and cardiac output. The changes in stroke volume are directly proportionate to end-diastolic volume, implying that there is little change in the inotropic state of the myocardium during normal singleton pregnancy and the puerperium. In multifetal pregnancies, however, cardiac output is increased even more than in singleton pregnancies. This occurs predominantly by virtue of an increased inotropic effect as measured by increased fractional shortening of the ventricular diameters. *The increased heart rate and inotropic contractility imply that cardiovascular reserve is reduced.*

The physician must be cautious when interpreting the significance of murmurs during pregnancy—especially systolic murmurs—because some normal cardiac sounds may be enhanced by increases in volume and flow. Normal pregnancy induces no characteristic changes in the electrocardiogram other than slight deviation of the electrical axis to the left as a result of the altered position of the heart.

CARDIAC OUTPUT

Cardiac output at rest, when measured in the lateral recumbent position, increases during the first trimester and remains elevated during the second and third trimesters. Typically, cardiac output in late pregnancy is higher when the woman is in the lateral recumbent position than when she is supine, since in the supine position the large uterus and its contents often impede venous return to the heart. Despite the increase in cardiac output, arterial blood pressure decreases because of a decrease in peripheral vascular resistance.

During the first stage of labor, maternal cardiac output increases moderately, and during the second stage of labor, with vigorous expulsive efforts, cardiac output is greater. Most of the increase in cardiac output induced by pregnancy is lost soon after delivery.

FACTORS CONTROLLING VASCULAR REACTIVITY IN PREGNANCY

Normal pregnant women are refractory to the pressor effects of angiotensin II, while hypertensive women and those destined to become hypertensive are sensitive to the pressor effects of infused angiotensin II (Chapter 57). A variety of physiologic processes probably act to control vascular reactivity to angiotensin II. These factors include alterations in circulating plasma levels of renin, angiotensin II, aldosterone, and possibly prostaglandins.

Renin, Angiotensin II, & Plasma Volume

In normotensive pregnant women, there are marked increases in the concentrations of plasma renin, renin activity, renin substrate, angiotensin II, and aldosterone, as well as a blunted pressor response to infused angiotensin II. Most of these responses to normal pregnancy are reversed in women with pregnancy-induced hypertension (Chapter 57).

Concisely stated, it appears likely that vascular reactivity in human pregnancy is controlled, at least in part, by (1) the action of prostaglandins or prostaglandin-related substances on vascular smooth muscle; (2) the action of progestin, which may modify the prostaglandin effect; (3) alterations in the cyclic nucleotide system of vascular smooth muscle; and (4) changes in intracellular calcium concentration. The control or restitution of these factors may be useful, ultimately, in preventing pregnancy-induced hypertension (Chapter 57). Preliminary clinical trials using low-dose aspirin to block thromboxane formation are encouraging.

CIRCULATION

The posture of the pregnant woman affects **arterial blood pressure.** Typically, blood pressure in the brachial artery is highest when she is sitting, lowest when lying in the lateral recumbent position, and intermediate when supine, except for some women who become quite hypotensive in the supine position. Arterial blood pressure usually decreases to a nadir during the second trimester or early third trimester and rises thereafter. A sustained rise of 30 mm Hg systolic or 15 mm Hg diastolic under basal conditions may be indicative of an abnormality—most likely pregnancy-induced hypertension (see Chapter 57).

OTHER CIRCULATORY EFFECTS RESULTING FROM THE SUPINE POSITION

In the supine position, the large pregnant uterus rather consistently compresses the venous system that returns blood from the lower half of the body to the extent that cardiac filling may be reduced and cardiac output decreased. Infrequently, this causes significant arterial hypotension, sometimes referred to as the **supine hypotensive syndrome.**

When the pregnant woman is supine, uterine arterial pressure is significantly lower than that in the brachial artery. In the presence of systemic hypotension, as occurs with spinal analgesia, the decrease in uterine arterial pressure is even more marked than in arteries above the level of aortic compression. A substantial number of women destined to develop pregnancy-induced hypertension exhibit more than a 20 mm Hg increase in diastolic blood pressure when they are turned from the lateral to the supine position. The exact mechanism responsible for this **supine-pressor response** remains to be defined.

BLOOD FLOW TO SKIN

Increased cutaneous blood flow during pregnancy acts to dissipate excess heat generated by the increased metabolism imposed by pregnancy.

RESPIRATORY TRACT

ANATOMIC CHANGES

The level of the diaphragm rises about 4 cm during pregnancy. The subcostal angle widens as the transverse diameter of the thoracic cage increases about 2 cm. The thoracic circumference increases about 6 cm but not sufficiently to prevent a reduction in the residual volume of air in the lungs created by the elevated diaphragm. Diaphragmatic excursion is greater during pregnancy, and as a result the tidal volume increases.

PULMONARY FUNCTION

At any stage of normal pregnancy, the amount of oxygen delivered by the increase in tidal volume clearly exceeds the oxygen need imposed by the pregnancy. Moreover, the amount of hemoglobin in the circulation and, in turn, the total oxygen-carrying capacity increases during normal pregnancy, as does cardiac output. As a consequence, maternal **arteriovenous oxygen difference** is decreased.

The respiratory rate is little changed during pregnancy, but the **tidal volume, minute ventilatory volume,** and **minute oxygen uptake** increase as pregnancy advances.

The **maximum breathing capacity** and **forced or timed vital capacity** are not altered appreciably. The **functional residual capacity** and the **residual volume** of air are decreased as a consequence of the elevated diaphragm. **Lung compliance** is unaffected by pregnancy, whereas **airway conductance** is increased and **total pulmonary resistance** is reduced (Figure 36–3).

The **closing volume,** or the lung volume at which airways in the dependent parts of the lung begin to close during expiration, is higher in pregnancy.

The increased respiratory effort characteristic of pregnancy and, in turn, the reduction in PCO_2, most likely is induced by progesterone and to a lesser degree by estrogen. The site of action of the hormones appears to be central, through a direct stimulatory effect on the respiratory center.

URINARY SYSTEM

KIDNEY

The kidney increases slightly in size during pregnancy and has been found to be 1.5 cm longer during the early puerperium than when measured 6 months later.

The glomerular filtration rate (GFR) and renal plasma flow (RPF) increase early in pregnancy, the former as much as 50% by the beginning of the second trimester and the latter not quite so much. The elevated glomerular filtration has been found by most investigators to persist to term, whereas renal plasma flow decreases during late pregnancy.

LOSS OF NUTRIENTS

As a result of augmented renal function, amino acids and water-soluble vitamins are lost in the urine of pregnant women in much greater amounts than in the urine of nonpregnant women. These losses, however, are not clinically significant in the healthy gravida.

TESTS OF RENAL FUNCTION

During pregnancy, the concentrations in plasma creatinine and urea normally decrease as a consequence of increased glomerular filtration. **Creatinine clearance** is a useful test to estimate renal function in pregnancy provided complete urine collection is made over an accurately timed period—several hours at least. **Urine concentration tests** may give results that are misleading. The failure of a pregnant woman to excrete a concentrated urine after fluids have been withheld for approximately 18 hours does not necessarily imply renal damage.

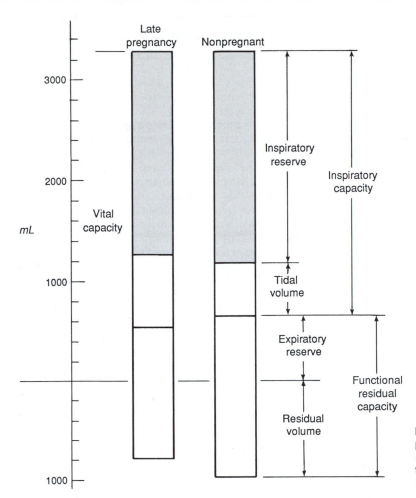

Figure 36–3. Lung volume and capacities in pregnancy. (From Hytten F.E., Leitch I.: *The Physiology of Human Pregnancy* (ed. 2). Oxford: Blackwell Scientific Publications, Ltd., 1971, p. 120. Used with permission.)

URINALYSIS

Glycosuria during pregnancy is not necessarily abnormal. The increase in glomerular filtration, together with an impaired tubular reabsorptive capacity for filtered glucose, accounts for most cases. Even though glycosuria is common during pregnancy, the possibility of diabetes mellitus cannot be ignored. **Proteinuria** and **hematuria** do not occur normally during pregnancy except occasionally to a slight extent during or soon after vigorous labor.

HYDRONEPHROSIS & HYDROURETER

In pregnant women, after the uterus rises completely out of the pelvis, it rests upon the ureters, compressing them at the pelvic brim. Typically, ureteral dilatation above the pelvic brim is more marked on the right side, probably due to a cushioning effect on the left ureter provided by the sigmoid colon and perhaps as a result of greater compression of the right ureter from dextrorotation of the uterus. The right ovarian vein complex lies obliquely over the right ureter and may contribute significantly to right ureteral dilatation. Another possible mechanism causing hydronephrosis and hydroureter is hormonal, presumably an effect of progesterone.

After delivery there is resolution, so that by 6–8 weeks the urinary tract has returned to prepregnancy dimensions. Stretching and dilatation do not continue long enough to impair permanently the elasticity of the ureter unless infection supervenes.

URINARY BLADDER

From the fourth month of pregnancy onward, the increased size of the uterus, together with the hyperemia that affects all pelvic organs and the hyperplasia of the muscle and connective tissues, elevates the bladder trigone and causes thickening of its posterior (intraureteric) margin. Continuation of this process to the end of pregnancy produces marked deepening and widening of the trigone. The bladder mucosa undergoes no change other than an increase in size and tortuosity of its blood vessels.

Toward the end of pregnancy—particularly in nulliparas, in whom the presenting part often engages before the onset of labor—the entire base of the bladder is pushed forward and upward, converting the normal convex surface into a concavity. As a result, the pressure of the presenting part impairs the drainage of blood and lymph from the base of the bladder, often rendering the area edematous, easily traumatized, and probably more susceptible to infection. Both urethral pressure and length have been shown to be decreased in women following vaginal but not abdominal delivery, suggesting that pregnancy or delivery may play a role in the pathogenesis of urinary stress incontinence (Chapter 15).

GASTROINTESTINAL TRACT

As pregnancy progresses, the stomach and intestines are displaced by the enlarging uterus. As a result of the positional changes in these viscera, the physical findings in certain diseases are altered. The appendix, for instance, is usually displaced upward and somewhat laterally as the uterus enlarges, and at times it may reach the right flank (Chapter 60).

Tone and motility of the gastrointestinal tract are usually decreased, leading to prolongation of gastric emptying times and intestinal transit. This may be due to progesterone, which is present in large amounts during pregnancy; to decreased levels of **motilin,** a hormonal peptide known to have smooth muscle stimulating effects; or to both causes. During labor, especially after administration of analgesic agents, **gastric emptying time** typically is prolonged. A major hazard of general anesthesia for delivery is regurgitation and aspiration of either food-laden or highly acidic gastric contents (Chapter 44).

Pyrosis (heartburn), common during pregnancy, is most likely caused by reflux of acidic secretions into the lower esophagus, the altered position of the stomach probably contributing to its frequent occurrence.

The gums may become hyperemic and softened during pregnancy and may bleed when mildly traumatized, as with a toothbrush. A focal, highly vascular swelling of the gums, the so-called **epulis of pregnancy,** develops occasionally but typically regresses after delivery. There is no credible evidence that pregnancy per se incites tooth decay.

Hemorrhoids are fairly common during pregnancy. They are caused in large measure by constipation and the elevated pressure in veins below the level of the enlarged uterus.

LIVER & GALLBLADDER

LIVER

There is no change in liver size or morphology during normal pregnancy. There may be a slight increase in hepatic blood flow, however.

The normal changes induced by pregnancy often change liver function tests in the same direction as those found in patients with hepatic disease. Total **alkaline phosphatase** activity in serum almost doubles during normal pregnancy. Much of the increase is attributable to alkaline phosphatase isozymes from the placenta, which are heat-stable up to 65 °C. There is a decrease in **plasma albumin** concentration to an average 3 g per dL late in pregnancy, compared with 4.3 g per dL in nonpregnant women. The reduction in serum albumin, combined with a slight increase in globulins in plasma that occurs normally during pregnancy, results in a decrease in the albumin-globulin ratio similar to that seen in certain hepatic diseases. Plasma **cholinesterase** activity is reduced during normal pregnancy about the same as the decrease in the concentration of albumin.

Leucine aminopeptidase activity is markedly elevated during pregnancy, and at term it reaches approximately three times the nonpregnant value. This probably results from the appearance of a pregnancy-specific enzyme (or enzymes) with distinct substrate specificities. Interestingly, aminopeptidase has oxytocinase activity.

Sulfobromophthalein excretion is somewhat decreased during normal pregnancy, while at the same time the ability of the liver to extract and store sulfobromophthalein is increased. **Spider nevi** and **palmar erythema,** both of which occur in patients with liver disease, are commonly found in normal pregnant women, most likely as a result of the increased circulating estrogens during pregnancy, but they disappear soon after delivery.

GALLBLADDER

Gallbladder function is altered during pregnancy, and it is commonly accepted that pregnancy predisposes to formation of gallstones (see Chapter 60).

ENDOCRINE GLANDS

Some of the most important endocrine changes of pregnancy have been discussed elsewhere, especially in Chapter 35.

PITUITARY

The pituitary enlarges during pregnancy by approximately 136% compared to nonpregnant controls, and striking enlargement of microadenomas of the pituitary can occur during pregnancy (see Chapter 60).

PITUITARY GROWTH HORMONE

Although placental lactogen (hPL) is abundant in the blood of pregnant women, the level of pituitary growth hormone is increased only slightly. After delivery, hPL rapidly disappears, but growth hormone is elevated for some time—though at levels lower than late pregnancy values. The relative lack of these hormones, with loss of their diabetogenic effect, may account in part for the usually abrupt and marked reduction in insulin requirements of women with diabetes mellitus during the early puerperium.

PROLACTIN

During the course of human pregnancy, there is a marked increase in the levels of prolactin in the maternal plasma. In fact, the levels increase to such an extent that the mean concentration of prolactin at term is 150 ng per mL, a value ten times greater than normal. Paradoxically, these levels decrease even in women who are breast feeding.

The physiologic cause of the marked increase in prolactin prior to parturition is not certainly known; however, estrogen stimulation increases the number of anterior pituitary lactotrophs (prolactin-producing cells) and may stimulate the release of prolactin from these cells. Thyroid-releasing hormone acts to cause an increased level of prolactin in pregnant compared to nonpregnant women, but the response decreases in each trimester as pregnancy advances. Serotonin also is believed to increase prolactin, but prolactin-inhibiting factor (probably identical to dopamine) is believed to inhibit its secretion.

The principal function of maternal serum prolactin is believed to be to ensure lactation.

Prolactin also is found throughout the course of gestation in high concentration in the fetal plasma, attaining highest concentrations during the last 5 weeks of pregnancy. Prolactin also is present in amnionic fluid in high concentrations—indeed, levels of 10,000 ng per mL can be measured in the amnionic fluid at 20–26 weeks of gestation. The site of synthesis for amnionic fluid prolactin appears to be the uterine decidua.

The function of amnionic fluid prolactin is not known.

β-LIPOTROPIN

The major precursor for a number of pituitary and probably chorionic peptide hormones is proopiomelanocortin, a large peptide chain that is processed at a variety of sites by specific proteolytic enzymes. One of the major fragments from this process is a 91-amino-acid chain, β-lipotropin. This compound may then be cleaved again to give two additional fragments, one a 58-amino-acid peptide called γ-lipotropin and the other a 31-amino-acid chain called β-endorphin. β-Endorphin is a potent endogenous opioid that is elevated in a variety of stressful situations, including labor, in parallel with pituitary ACTH.

Maternal plasma concentrations of β-lipotropin, β-endorphin, and γ-lipotropin increase steadily throughout pregnancy. Their levels are lower in women delivering vaginally who have epidural analgesia than in women receiving either a narcotic or no analgesia. The specific physiologic function of these opioid agents in maternal plasma during pregnancy and labor has not been established. However, such agents obviously could serve to blunt the pain of childbirth.

THYROID

During pregnancy, there is moderate enlargement of the thyroid caused by hyperplasia of the glandular tissue and increased vascularity. However, normal pregnancy does not cause significant thyromegaly, and any goiter in pregnancy should be considered pathologic. The basal metabolic rate increases progressively during normal pregnancy by as much as 25%. Most of this increase in oxygen consumption is the result of the metabolic activity of the products of conception. If the body surface of the fetus is considered along with that of the mother, the predicted and the measured basal metabolic rates are quite similar.

Thyroxine

Beginning as early as the second month of pregnancy, the concentration of **thyroxine** (T_4) rises sharply in the maternal plasma to a plateau, which is maintained until after delivery. The plateau is reached at levels of 9–16 µg/dL, as compared with 5–12 µg per dL in nonpregnant euthyroid women.

This elevation of circulating thyroid hormone is not indicative of hyperthyroidism. During pregnancy, the **thyroxine-binding proteins** of plasma, principally an α-globulin, are increased considerably. Thyroid-binding globulin levels in plasma are 7.1 mg per dL in the first trimester, 9 mg per dL in the second trimester, and 8.9 mg per dL in the third trimester, compared to values of 3.6 mg per dL for normal nonpregnant women. Even though the total concentrations of thyroxine and triiodothyronine (T_3) are elevated, the amounts of unbound, or effective, hormone are not appreciably higher. The increase in circulating estrogens during pregnancy presumably is the major cause of these changes in hormone levels and binding capacity.

Reverse Triiodothyronine (rT_3)

Reverse T_3 is formed from the inner ring (5-deiodinase) monodeiodination of thyroxine. The level of reverse triiodothyronine in maternal blood is 3–5 times less than in fetal blood and amnionic fluid, probably because the conversion of thyroxine to reverse triiodothyronine occurs in fetal membranes and in the placenta.

There is almost no transfer of thyroxine, triiodothyronine, or reverse triiodothyronine from the maternal into the fetal compartment. Therefore, fetal thyroid function appears to be independent of maternal thyroid status. This protection of the fetus probably is the consequence of the previously mentioned placental inner ring deiodination of thyroxine.

Thyroid-Stimulating Immunoglobulin (TSI)

The usually protected status of the fetal thyroid is overcome in some cases of Graves' disease. Thyroid-stimulating immunoglobulin (TSI)—formerly known as long-acting thyroid stimulator (LATS)—may cross the placenta in women with Graves' disease and stimulate the fetal thyroid to produce neonatal thyrotoxicosis.

Thyroid-Releasing Hormone (TRH)

Thyroid-releasing hormone is a neurotransmitter present throughout the brain but in highest concentrations in the hypothalamus. This compound stimulates the synthesis and release of TSH from the anterior pituitary. It is not increased during normal pregnancy, but it does cross the placenta and may stimulate the fetal pituitary to increase TSH. The role, if any, of maternal TRH in fetal homeostasis is not clear at this time.

Thyroid-Stimulating Hormone (TSH)

TSH is not bound by a carrier protein in the blood but circulates in the free form. Its concentration is not elevated by pregnancy, and it does not cross the placenta. Thus, there is no correlation between maternal and fetal TSH.

A thyrotropic substance obtained from human placenta has been identified as **chorionic thyrotropin,** but its role (if any) in stimulating the thyroid is unclear. In women with hydatidiform moles, increased thyroid activity is probably due chiefly to the action of chorionic gonadotropin, which is known to have intrinsic thyroid-stimulating activity.

PARATHYROID & CALCIUM METABOLISM

The regulation of calcium concentration is closely related to magnesium, phosphate, parathyroid hormone, vitamin D, and calcitonin physiology. Any alteration of one of these factors is likely to change the others.

Parathyroid Hormone & Calcium Interrelationships

Acute or chronic decreases in plasma calcium or acute decreases in magnesium stimulate the release of parathyroid hormone, whereas increases in calcium and magnesium suppress parathyroid hormone levels. The known actions of parathyroid hormone are presented in Table 36–1. The net effect of the action of this hormone on bone resorption, intestinal absorption, and kidney reabsorption is to increase extracellular fluid calcium and decrease phosphate.

Parathyroid hormone concentrations in plasma decrease during the first trimester, then increase progressively throughout the remainder of pregnancy. Increased parathyroid hormone levels probably result from increased plasma volume, increased glomerular filtration rate, and increased fetal transfer of calcium, all resulting in chronic suppression of calcium concentration in the pregnant woman. Despite the observed decrease in total calcium concentration during pregnancy, ionized calcium, which is the major feedback mechanism regulating secretion of parathyroid hormone, is decreased only slightly during pregnancy. Estrogens appear to block the action of parathyroid hormone on bone resorption, resulting in another mechanism to increase parathyroid hormone during pregnancy. The net result of these actions is a "physiologic hyperparathyroidism" of pregnancy, probably in order to supply the fetus with adequate calcium.

Calcitonin & Calcium Interrelationships

The calcitonin-secreting C cells are derived embryologically from the neural crest and are located predominantly in the parafollicular areas of the thyroid gland. Calcium and magnesium increase the biosynthesis and secretion of calcitonin. Various gastric hormones (gastrin, pentagastrin, glucagon, and pancreozymin) and food ingestion also increase calcitonin plasma levels.

The known actions of calcitonin are shown in Table 36–1 and can generally be considered to oppose those of parathyroid hormone and vitamin D to protect the calcification of the skeleton during times of calcium stress. Pregnancy and lactation are two examples of profound calcium stress, and calcitonin levels during these times are higher than in nonpregnant women.

Table 36–1. Relationship between parathyroid hormone (PTH), vitamin D, and calcitonin to calcium (Ca), phosphate (P), and magnesium (Mg).[1]

	Bone Resorption			Intestinal Absorption		Kidney Resorption			Extracellular Fluid	
	Ca	P	Mg	Ca	Mg	Ca	P	Mg	Ca	P
PTH	↑	↑	↑	↑	↑	↑	↓	↑	↑	↓
Vitamin D	↑	↑↑	—	↑	↑	—	—	—	↑	↑
Calcitonin	↓	↓	↓	—	↓	↓	↓	↓	↓	↓

[1]Modified from Tsang RC, Donovan EF, Steichen JJ: Calcium physiology and pathology in the neonate. Pediatr Clin North Am 1976;23:611.

Vitamin D & Calcium Interrelationships

Vitamin D is produced in the skin or ingested and is converted into 25-hydroxyvitamin D_3 in the liver. This product then is converted in the kidney, decidua, and placenta to 1,25-dihydroxyvitamin D_3, which is most likely the biologically active compound, whose known actions are listed in Table 36–1.

The actual mechanism of control of 1,25-dihydroxyvitamin D_3 production and release is unknown, but the conversion of 25-hydroxyvitamin D_3 to 1,25-dihydroxyvitamin D_3 is facilitated by parathyroid hormone and by low calcium and phosphate plasma levels and opposed by calcitonin.

ADRENAL GLANDS

In normal pregnancy, there is probably little morphologic change in the maternal adrenal glands.

Cortisol

There is a considerable increase in the concentration of circulating cortisol during pregnancy, but much of it is bound by cortisol-binding globulin, or **transcortin.** The rate of cortisol secretion by the maternal adrenal is not increased—and is probably decreased compared to the nonpregnant state. The metabolic clearance rate of cortisol, however, is lower during pregnancy.

In early pregnancy, the levels of circulating corticotropin (ACTH) are strikingly reduced. As pregnancy progresses, the levels of ACTH and free cortisol rise. This apparent paradox is not fully understood.

Aldosterone

As early as the 15th week of normal pregnancy, the maternal adrenal secretes greatly increased amounts of aldosterone. By the third trimester, about 1 mg per d is secreted. If sodium intake is restricted, aldosterone secretion is elevated even further. At the same time, levels of renin and angiotensin II substrate are normally increased, especially during the latter half of pregnancy. This gives rise to increased plasma levels of angiotensin II, which, by acting on the zona glomerulosa of the maternal adrenal glands, probably accounts for the markedly elevated secretion of aldosterone. It has been suggested that the increased secretion of aldosterone during normal pregnancy affords protection against the natriuretic effect of progesterone.

Deoxycorticosterone

There is a striking increase in the maternal plasma levels of deoxycorticosterone (DOC) during pregnancy. In nonpregnant women and during the first two trimesters of pregnancy, the levels of plasma DOC are less than 100 pg per mL. During the last few weeks of pregnancy, DOC levels rise to 1500 pg per mL or more.

DOC in maternal plasma arises primarily by way of the 21-hydroxylation of plasma progesterone, and this transformation occurs in tissue sites of mineralocorticoid action, ie, kidney, skin, and blood vessels. Great person-to-person variability in this peripheral conversion is known to exist. Finally, DOC sulfate in maternal plasma arises at least in part by way of placental formation of DOC sulfate from the utilization of fetal plasma pregnenolone-3,21-disulfate.

DEHYDROEPIANDROSTERONE SULFATE

As discussed in Chapter 35, the levels of dehydroepiandrosterone sulfate circulating in maternal blood and excreted in the urine are not increased during normal pregnancy. On the contrary, they are decreased as a consequence of an increased rate of removal through extensive 16α-hydroxylation in the maternal liver and through estrogen formation in the placenta.

ANDROSTENEDIONE & TESTOSTERONE

Maternal plasma levels of androstenedione and testosterone are increased during pregnancy. The source of this increased C_{19} steroid production is unknown, but it is probably the ovary.

MUSCULOSKELETAL SYSTEM

Progressive **lordosis** is a characteristic feature of normal pregnancy. Compensating for the anterior position of the enlarging uterus, the lordosis shifts the center of gravity back over the lower extremities. There is increased mobility of the sacroiliac, sacrococcygeal, and pubic joints during pregnancy, presumably as a result of hormonal changes. Their mobility may contribute to the alteration of maternal posture and, in turn, cause discomfort in the lower back, especially late in pregnancy.

SUGGESTED READINGS

Cunningham FG, MacDonald PC, Gant NF, Leveno KJ, and Gilstrap LC, III (editors): Maternal Adaptations to Pregnancy.

Chapter 8 in *Williams Obstetrics*, 19th ed., Appleton & Lange, 1993.

37

Parturition: Biomolecular & Physiologic Processes

Physiologically and clinically, parturition is divisible into three distinct but overlapping phases: (1) uterine preparation for labor, (2) forceful contractions of active labor and delivery, and (3) puerperal contraction and involution of the uterus. The first phase is commonly identifiable by distinctive signs of the preparatory process, including ripening of the cervix, increasing frequency of painless uterine contractions, and uterine irritability. The second phase begins with the **onset of labor**—the regular, forceful, painful uterine contractions that bring about cervical dilatation and descent of the fetus—and ends with delivery. The second phase is divided further into the **three stages of labor** (see below). The third phase begins after delivery, with persistent contractions of the uterus that ensure puerperal hemostasis, and proceeds through complete involution of the uterus, a process that returns this organ to the nonpregnant state.

UTERINE CHANGES OF PREGNANCY

Stretching, cell replication, inflammation, trauma, and foreign tissue grafts all are known stimulators of prostaglandin formation, and each of these processes is fundamental to pregnancy. During human pregnancy, the uterus increases in size from an organ of about 50 g to one that at term weighs more than 1 kg. This comes about by way of a tenfold increase in myometrial cell size as a consequence of cellullar hypertrophy. And during this same time, the volume capacity of the uterus increases by several orders of magnitude. It is no wonder, therefore, that one of the great mysteries of human pregnancy is the quiescence of the uterus during more than 99% of pregnancy. It has been stated that "the uterus is remarkably tolerant of its burden during this time."

PROGESTERONE & HUMAN PARTURITION

Immediately after ovulation in women, the granulosa cells of the follicle (from which the ovum was extruded) are luteinized to form the corpus luteum. This temporary organ within an organ secretes progesterone in prodigious amounts, but only for a brief time. The life span of the corpus luteum of the nonfertile ovarian cycle of women is about 12–14 days, but by 10 days the secretion of progesterone begins to decline abruptly (Chapter 35). With implantation of the blastocyst, however, hCG is produced in the trophoblasts and enters maternal blood by way of the placental arm of the fetal-maternal communication system. Compared with the amount of LH produced by the pituitary, hCG is produced in massive quantities, and this LH surrogate acts to rescue the corpus luteum and to prolong the functional life span of this progesterone-producing organ. This important function of the blastocyst is probably crucial for optimizing conditions for the success of early pregnancy.

Progesterone acts to effect secretory changes in the endometrium, which are believed to be optimal for implantation of the blastocyst. Progesterone, the "progestational steroid," is important—perhaps essential—to the maintenance of mammalian pregnancy. Nonetheless, the corpus luteum of human pregnancy functions for only a short time, even though the plasma levels of hCG are massive. In fact, corpus luteum function begins to decline by about 6 weeks of gestation (menstrual age), and by 8 weeks little or no progesterone is being produced by the ovary. Thus, the life span of the corpus luteum during pregnancy is only 4–6 weeks—but this is longer than that of the corpus luteum of the menstrual cycle, which is only 10–14 days (Chapter 20).

If progesterone withdrawal is artificially achieved during human pregnancy by whatever means, abortion or labor does ensue. Removal of the corpus luteum in early human pregnancy (before 8 weeks of gestation) results in abortion. And in other abnormal circumstances—eg, ectopic pregnancies and fetal demise—a decrease in progesterone formation may precede the onset of uterine contractions and delivery of a decidual cast (ectopic pregnancy; see Chapter 35) or a dead fetus. Progesterone withdrawal, however, is not an immediate accompaniment or result of fetal demise; rather, it may occur many weeks after fetal death. Pharmacologically induced inhibition of progesterone action or progesterone formation in human pregnancy also causes abortion or increased sensitivity of myometrium to uterotonic agents (Chapter 9). On the other hand, the administration of progesterone to women does not prevent or arrest preterm labor.

OXYTOCIN & HUMAN PARTURITION

Oxytocin means "quick birth" or "hastening birth." In 1906, uterotonic bioactivity was discovered in extracts of the posterior pituitary. By 1909, the uterotonic property of these extracts was demonstrated after administration to women, and by 1911 these crude preparations were in use in clinical obstetrics. In 1950, DuVigneaud determined the structure of oxytocin, the uterotonic agent of the posterior pituitary; he was later awarded the Nobel Prize for his pioneering work. Oxytocin is a nonapeptide synthesized in the cell bodies of the supraoptic and paraventricular neurons and transported along the axons to the neural lobe of the posterior pituitary in membrane-bound vesicles for storage and later release.

The increase in oxytocin receptors in the uterus before (or during) the onset of labor is an important marker of the preparatory events preceding parturition. Oxytocin may act to maximize the myometrial forces involved in the expulsive phase (second stage) of labor; it may act to ensure uterine contraction and thereby decrease blood loss after delivery; it may act synergistically with other uterotonins produced within the uterus to maintain labor; and it is important in milk let-down during lactation. But there is scant or no evidence that oxytocin is the initiator of human parturition or that oxytocin is the primary uterotonin of human labor.

PHYSIOLOGY OF UTERINE CONTRACTIONS

The final event in initiating a uterine contraction is an increase in the intracellular concentration of ionic calcium (Ca^{2+}) in myometrial smooth muscle cells in response to the action of a uterotonin. The ATP-energy-dependent translocation of calcium to a stored form in the sarcoplasmic reticulum is associated with uterine relaxation.

The body of the uterus and the cervix, though they are parts of the same organ, must respond to parturition in quite different ways. On the one hand, during most of pregnancy, it is essential that the myometrium be distensible but remain quiescent. On the other hand, the cervix must remain rigid and unyielding. Synchronously with the events involved in parturition, however, the cervix must soften, yield, and then dilate. The fundus must be transformed from the relaxed, quiescent organ characteristic of most of pregnancy to one of violent contractions of sufficient force and efficiency to drive the fetus through the cervix and on through the birth canal. Failure of timely interaction between the functions of the cervix and the fundus portends an unfavorable pregnancy outcome. But despite the apparent reversal of roles between cervix and fundus before and during labor, there is evidence that both

processes are regulated by common agents, the uterotropins-uterotonins of parturition.

There are three principal structural components in the cervix: smooth muscle, collagen, and connective tissue, ie, the ground substance. In the ground substance are formed important constituents of the cervix, the glycosaminoglycans: dermatan sulfate and hyaluronic acid. The smooth muscle content of the cervix varies from upward to downward—from 25% to only 6%. There is in the human, however, no apparent role for smooth muscle in the cervical "ripening" process; rather, this process seemingly involves changes that occur in collagen and connective tissue; thus, with "ripening," cervical flexibility increases as collagen and protein concentrations decrease.

THREE STAGES OF LABOR

Customarily and for good clinical reasons, labor—the second phase of parturition—is divided into three separate stages.

The **first stage of labor** commences when uterine contractions (myometrial forces) of sufficient **frequency, intensity,** and **duration** to bring about readily demonstrable effacement and dilatation of the cervix are attained. The first stage ends when the cervix is fully dilated, ie, when the cervix is sufficiently dilated (about 10 cm) to allow passage of the fetal head. The first stage of labor, therefore, is that stage in which **cervical effacement and dilatation** occur.

The **second stage of labor** begins when dilatation of the cervix is complete and ends with delivery of the infant. The second stage of labor is the stage of **expulsion of the fetus.**

The **third stage of labor** begins with delivery of the infant and ends with delivery of the placenta and fetal membranes. The third stage of labor is the stage of **separation and expulsion of the placenta.**

In addition to these classic three stages of labor, some obstetricians categorize a period of prelabor and a latent phase of labor (phase 1 of parturition) that precede active labor (stages 1, 2, and 3), which is the second phase of parturition. **Prelabor** has been identified as the period of increased uterine activity that occurs for a few weeks before active labor. During this time, the increased uterine activity is believed to facilitate softening of the cervix, some cervical effacement, slight to modest cervical dilatation, and expansion of the lower uterine segment, ie, the time of uterine preparedness for labor. A **latent phase of labor** has been described that precedes active labor by several hours (Chapter 46). During the latent phase, uterine contractions typically are infrequent, produce some discomfort, and may be irregular; nonetheless, these contractions apparently can generate sufficient force to facilitate slow effacement and dilatation if biochemical changes have occurred that lead to ripening and softening of the cervix.

"LIGHTENING"

A few weeks before the onset of labor, the abdomen of the pregnant woman commonly undergoes a change in shape. The fundal height decreases somewhat; at times this event is reported by the mother with the words, "the baby dropped." This phenomenon is the consequence of the development of a well-formed lower uterine segment, the descent of the fetal head to or even through the pelvic inlet, and to some degree a reduction in the volume of amnionic fluid.

FALSE LABOR

For a variable time before the establishment of true or effective labor, women may experience so-called false labor. The uterine contractions of false labor are characterized by irregularity in occurrence and brevity of duration; most often, the discomfort produced is confined to the lower abdomen and groin. In contrast, the discomfort produced by the uterine contractions characteristic of true labor begins first in the fundal region and then radiates over the uterus and through to the lower back.

Uterine irritability that causes discomfort but does not represent true labor (in that cervical dilatation does not occur) may develop at any time during pregnancy. False labor is observed most commonly late in pregnancy and in parous women. It often stops spontaneously but may proceed rapidly to the effective contractions of true labor. Therefore, the report of relatively infrequent and short-lived (but uncomfortable) uterine contractions cannot be dismissed summarily. All too frequently when this is done, delivery takes place without benefit of the assistance of professional personnel or facilities essential for optimal care of mother and offspring.

"SHOW"

A fairly dependable sign of the impending onset of labor (provided no rectal or vaginal examination has been performed in the preceding 48 hours) is "show" or "bloody show," which consists of the discharge from the vagina of a small amount of blood-tinged mucus, representing extrusion of the plug of mucus that was filling the cervical canal during pregnancy. "Show" is a late sign, for labor usually ensues during the next several hours to a few days. Normally, only a few drops of blood escape with the mucous plug; more substantial bleeding is suggestive of an abnormal condition.

CHARACTERISTICS OF UTERINE CONTRACTIONS IN LABOR

Unique among physiologic muscular contractions, those of labor are painful. Therefore, the common designation in many languages for such contractions is "pain." The cause of the pain is not definitely known.

Uterine contractions are involuntary and for the most part independent of extrauterine control. Neural blockade from caudal or epidural analgesia, if initiated quite early in labor, is sometimes associated with a reduction in the frequency and intensity of uterine contractions, but not after labor is well established. Moreover, in paraplegic women and in women who have undergone bilateral lumbar sympathectomy, there are normal, though painless, contractions.

The interval between contractions diminishes gradually from about 10 minutes at the onset of the first stage of labor to as little as 1 minute or less in the second stage. Periods of relaxation between contractions, however, are essential to the welfare of the fetus, because unremitting contraction of the uterus may interfere with uteroplacental blood flow of sufficient magnitude to produce fetal hypoxia. In the active phase of labor, the duration of each contraction ranges from 30 to 90 seconds, averaging about 1 minute. There is appreciable variability in the intensity of uterine contractions during apparently normal labor, and pressures range normally from 20 mm Hg to 60 mm Hg.

With labor, the uterus differentiates into two distinct parts. The actively contracting upper segment becomes thicker as labor advances; the lower portion, comprising the lower segment of the uterus and the cervix, is relatively passive compared with the upper segment, and it develops into a much thinner-walled passage for the fetus. The lower uterine segment is analogous to a greatly expanded and thinned-out isthmus of the uterus of nonpregnant women, the formation of which is not solely a phenomenon of labor. The lower segment develops gradually as pregnancy progresses and then thins remarkably during labor (Figures 37–1 and 37–2).

If the entire sac of uterine musculature, including the lower uterine segment and cervix, were to contract simultaneously and with equal intensity, the net expulsive force would be decreased markedly. Therein lies the importance of the division of the uterus into an actively contracting upper segment and a more passive lower segment that differ not only anatomically but also physiologically. The upper segment contracts, retracts, and expels the fetus; in response to the force of the contractions of the upper segment, the ripened lower uterine segment and cervix dilate and thereby form a greatly expanded, thinned-out muscular and fibromuscular tube through which the fetus can pass.

The myometrium of the upper uterine segment does not relax to its original length after contractions; rather, it becomes relatively fixed at a shorter length—the tension, however, remaining the same as before the contraction. The function of the ability of the upper portion of the uterus, or active segment, to contract down on its diminishing contents, with myometrial tension remaining constant, is to take up slack, ie, to maintain the advantage gained with respect to expulsion of the fetus and to maintain the uterine musculature in firm contact with the intrauterine contents. As a consequence of retraction, each suc-

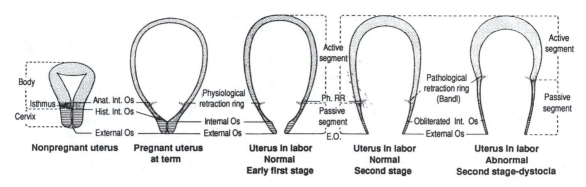

Figure 37–1. Sequence of development of the segments and rings in the uterus in pregnant women at term and in labor. Note comparison between the uterus of a nonpregnant woman, the uterus at term, and the uterus during labor. The passive lower segment of the uterine body is derived from the isthmus; the physiologic retraction ring develops at the junction of the upper and lower uterine segments. The pathologic retraction ring develops from the physiologic ring. Anat.Int.Os, anatomic internal os; Hist.Int.Os, histologic internal os; Ph.R.R., physiologic retraction ring; E.O., external os.

cessive contraction commences where the preceding one left off, so that the upper part of the uterine cavity becomes slightly smaller with each successive contraction. Because of the shortening of its muscular fibers with each contraction, the upper uterine segment (active segment, Figure 37–1) becomes progressively thickened throughout the first and second stages of labor and tremendously thickened immediately after birth of the baby. The phenomenon of retraction of the upper uterine segment is contingent upon a decrease in the volume of its contents. For its contents to be diminished—particularly early in labor, when the entire uterus is virtually a closed sac with only a minute opening at the cervix—there is a requirement that the musculature of the lower segment must stretch, per-

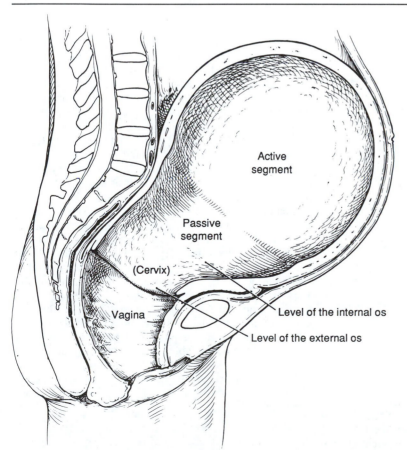

Figure 37–2. The uterus at the time of vaginal delivery. The active upper segment of the uterus retracts about the fetus as the fetus descends through the birth canal. In the passive lower segment, there is considerably less myometrial tone.

mitting more and more of the intrauterine contents to occupy the lower segment. Indeed, the upper segment retracts only to the extent that the lower segment distends and the cervix dilates.

The relaxation of the lower uterine segment is by no means complete relaxation but rather the opposite of retraction. The fibers of the lower segment become stretched with each contraction of the upper segment, after which these are not returned to the previous length but remain relatively fixed at the greater length; the tension, however, remains essentially the same as before. The musculature still manifests tone, still resists stretch, and still contracts somewhat on stimulation.

INTRA-ABDOMINAL PRESSURE

After the cervix is dilated fully, the most important force in expulsion of the fetus is increased intra-abdominal pressure from contraction of the abdominal muscles synchronously with forced respiratory efforts with the glottis closed. In obstetric jargon, this usually is referred to as "pushing." The nature of the force produced is similar to that involved in defecation, but the intensity is usually much greater. The important role served by intra-abdominal pressure in fetal expulsion is most clearly attested to by the labors of women who are paraplegic.

CERVICAL EFFACEMENT

Effacement ("obliteration," or "taking up") of the cervix is shortening of the cervical canal from approximately 2 cm in length to a mere circular orifice with almost paper-thin edges. This process takes place from above downward; it occurs as the muscle fibers in the vicinity of the internal os are pulled upward, or "taken up," into the lower segment, while the condition of the external os remains temporarily unchanged. As illustrated in Figure 37–3, the edges of the internal os are drawn upward several centimeters to become, functionally, part of the lower uterine segment. Effacement may be compared with a funneling process in which the whole length of a narrow cylinder is converted into a very obtuse, flaring funnel with only a small circular orifice for an outlet. As a result of increased myometrial activity during phase 1 of parturition, appreciable effacement of the ripened cervix is sometimes attained before true labor begins. Such effacement usually facilitates expulsion of the mucous plug from the cervical canal as the canal shortens.

CERVICAL DILATATION

In order for the head of the average fetus at term to pass through the cervix, the canal must dilate to a diameter of about 10 cm. When sufficient dilatation is attained for the fetal head to pass through, the cervix is said to be fully dilated. There may be no fetal descent during cervical ef

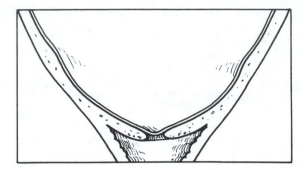

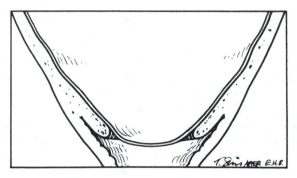

Figure 37–3. Cervical canal obliterated; ie, the cervix is completely effaced. ***Top,*** primigravida. ***Bottom,*** multipara.

facement, but as a rule the station of the presenting part descends somewhat as the cervix dilates. During the second stage, descent of the fetal presenting part typically occurs rather slowly but steadily in nulliparas. In multiparas, however—particularly those of high parity—descent may be very rapid.

The pattern of cervical dilatation that takes place during the course of normal labor takes on the shape of a sigmoid curve. As depicted in Figure 37–4, two phases of cervical dilatation can be defined: the latent phase and the active phase. The active phase has been subdivided further as the acceleration phase, the phase of maximum slope, and the deceleration phase. The duration of the latent phase is more variable and subject to sensitive changes by extraneous factors and by sedation (prolongation of latent phase) and myometrial stimulation (shortening of latent phase). The duration of the latent phase has little bearing on the subsequent course of labor, whereas the characteristics of the accelerated phase usually are predictive of the outcome of a particular labor. The completion of cervical dilatation during the active phase of labor is accomplished by cervical retraction about the presenting part of the fetus. After complete cervical dilatation, the second stage of labor commences; thereafter, only progressive descent of the presenting fetal part is available to assess the progress of labor.

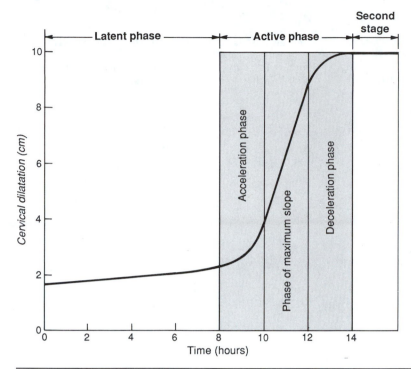

Figure 37–4. Composite of the average dilatation curve for nulliparous labor based on analysis of the data derived from the patterns traced by a large, nearly consecutive series of gravidas. The first stage is divided into a relatively flat latent phase and a rapidly progressive active phase. In the active phase, there are three identifiable component parts: an acceleration phase, a linear phase of maximum slope, and a deceleration phase. (Courtesy of L Casey; redrawn from Friedman EA: *Labor: Clinical Evaluation and Management,* 2nd ed. Appleton, 1978.)

DESCENT

In many nulliparas, engagement of the fetal head is accomplished prior to the onset of labor, and further descent does not occur until late in labor. In others in whom engagement of the fetal head initially is not so extensive, further descent occurs during the first stage of labor. In the descent pattern of normal labor, a typical hyperbolic curve is formed when the station of the fetal head is plotted as a function of the duration of labor. Active descent usually takes place after cervical dilatation has progressed for some time. In nulliparas, increased rates of descent are observed ordinarily during the phase of maximum slope of cervical dilatation. At this time, the speed of descent increases to a maximum, and this maximal rate of descent is maintained until the presenting fetal part reaches the perineal floor.

THIRD STAGE OF LABOR

The third stage of labor, which begins immediately after delivery of the fetus, involves separation and expulsion of the placenta. As the baby is born, the uterus spontaneously contracts down on its diminishing contents. Normally, by the time the infant is completely delivered, the uterine cavity is nearly obliterated and the organ consists of an almost solid mass of muscle whose walls are several centimeters thick above the lower segment, with the fundus lying just below the level of the umbilicus. This sudden diminution in uterine size inevitably is accompanied by a decrease in the area of the placental implantation site. In order for the placenta to accommodate itself to this reduced area, it increases in thickness; but because of limited placental elasticity, it is forced to buckle. The resulting tension causes the weakest layer of the decidua—the spongy layer, or decidua spongiosa—to give way, and cleavage takes place at that site. Therefore, separation of the placenta results primarily from a disproportion created between the unchanged size of the placenta and the reduced size of the underlying implantation site. During cesarean section, this phenomenon may be observed directly when the placenta is implanted posteriorly.

After the placenta has separated from its implantation site, the pressure exerted upon it by the uterine walls causes it to slide downward into the flaccid lower uterine segment or the upper part of the vagina. In some cases, the placenta may be expelled from those locations by an increase in abdominal pressure, but women in the recumbent position frequently cannot expel the placenta spontaneously. An artificial means of completing the third stage is therefore generally required. The usual method employed is alternately to compress and elevate the fundus, while exerting minimal traction on the umbilical cord.

SUGGESTED READINGS

Challis JRG, Olson DM: Parturition. Page 2177 in: *The Physiology of Reproduction.* Vol 2. Knobil E, Neill JD (editors). Raven Press, 1988.

Cunningham FG, MacDonald PC, Gant NF, Leveno KJ, and Gilstrap LC, III (editors): Parturition: Biomolecular and Physiologic Processes. Chapter 10 in *Williams Obstetrics,* 19th ed., Appleton & Lange, 1993.

Friedman EA: *Labor: Clinical Evaluation and Management,* 2nd ed. Appleton, 1978.

The Pelvis; Fetal Attitude, Lie, Presentation, & Position

I. THE PELVIS

The mechanisms of labor are essentially processes of accommodation of the fetus to the bony passage through which it must pass. Accordingly, the size and shape of the pelvis are extremely important in obstetrics.

The adult pelvis is composed of four bones: the sacrum, the coccyx, and two innominate bones. Each innominate bone is formed by the fusion of the ilium, the ischium, and the pubis. The innominate bones are joined firmly to the sacrum at the sacroiliac synchondroses and to one another at the symphysis pubis. Consideration of the pelvis will be limited to those features of importance in childbearing.

PELVIC ANATOMY: OBSTETRIC CONSIDERATIONS

The true pelvis lies beneath the linea terminalis and is the portion that is important in childbearing. The true pelvis is bounded above by the promontory and alae of the sacrum, the linea terminalis, and the upper margins of the pubic bones and below by the pelvic outlet. The cavity of the true pelvis can be described as an obliquely truncated, bent cylinder with its greatest height posteriorly.

The walls of the true pelvis are partly bony and partly ligamentous. The posterior boundary is the anterior surface of the sacrum, and the lateral limits are formed by the inner surface of the ischial bones and the sacrosciatic notches and ligaments. In front, the true pelvis is bounded by the pubic bones, the ascending superior rami of the is-

chial bones, and the obturator foramina, which they partially enclose.

Extending from the middle of the posterior margin of each ischium are the ischial spines, which are of great obstetric importance since the distance between them usually represents the shortest lateral diameter of the pelvic cavity (Figure 38–1). Moreover, since the ischial spines can be felt readily by vaginal or rectal examination, they serve as landmarks in determining the level to which the presenting part of the fetus has descended into the true pelvis.

The sacrum forms the posterior wall of the pelvic cavity. Its upper anterior margin, corresponding to the body of the first sacral vertebra and designated the promontory, may be felt on vaginal examination and can provide a landmark for clinical pelvimetry.

The appearance of the pubic arch is characteristic. The descending inferior rami of the pubic bones unite at an angle of 90–100 degrees to form a rounded arch under which the fetal head may readily pass.

PELVIC JOINTS

Symphysis Pubis

Anteriorly, the pelvic bones are joined together by the symphysis pubis. The symphysis has a certain degree of mobility that increases during pregnancy, particularly in multiparas.

Sacroiliac Joints

Posteriorly, the pelvic bones are joined by the articulations between the sacrum and innominate bones (sacroiliac joints). These joints also have a certain degree of mobility.

Relaxation of the Pelvic Joints

During pregnancy, relaxation of these joints is probably the result of hormonal changes. The symphysis pubis also

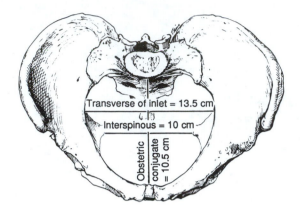

Figure 38–1. Adult female pelvis demonstrating anteroposterior and transverse diameters of the pelvic inlet and transverse (interspinous) diameter of the mid pelvis. The obstetric conjugate normally is greater than 10 cm.

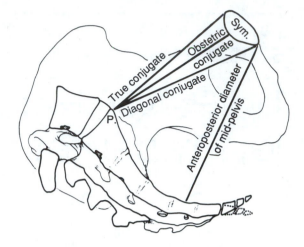

Figure 38–2. Three anteroposterior diameters of the pelvic inlet are illustrated: the true conjugate, the more important obstetric conjugate, and the clinically measurable diagonal conjugate. The anteroposterior diameter of the mid pelvis is also shown. P, sacral promontory; Sym, symphysis pubis.

increases in width during pregnancy (more in multiparas than in primigravidas) and returns to normal soon after delivery.

PLANES & DIAMETERS OF THE PELVIS

It is difficult to describe the exact location of an object within the pelvis. For convenience, therefore, the pelvis is described as having four imaginary planes: (1) the plane of the pelvic inlet (superior strait), (2) the plane of the pelvic outlet (inferior strait), (3) the plane of the mid pelvis (least pelvic dimensions), and (4) the plane of greatest pelvic dimensions.

PELVIC INLET

Four diameters of the pelvic inlet are usually measured: anteroposterior, transverse, and two obliques. The obstetrically important anteroposterior diameter is the shortest distance between the promontory of the sacrum and the symphysis pubis and is designated the **obstetric conjugate** (Figure 38–2). Normally, the obstetric conjugate measures 10 cm or more.

The transverse diameter is at right angles to the obstetric conjugate and represents the greatest distance between the linea terminalis on either side (Figure 38–1). The segment of the obstetric conjugate from the intersection of these two lines to the promontory is designated the **posterior sagittal diameter** of the plane of the inlet. The oblique diameters have no obstetric significance.

The anteroposterior diameter of the pelvic inlet, which

has been identified as the **true conjugate,** does not represent the shortest distance between the promontory of the sacrum and the symphysis pubis (Figure 38–2). The shortest distance is the **obstetric conjugate,** which is the shortest anteroposterior diameter through which the head must pass in descending through the pelvic inlet.

The obstetric conjugate cannot be measured directly with the examining fingers. For clinical purposes, however, it is sufficient to estimate the length of the obstetric conjugate indirectly by measuring the distance from the lower margin of the symphysis to the promontory of the sacrum, ie, the **diagonal conjugate** (Figure 38–2), and subtracting 1.5–2 cm from the result (see Pelvic Size and Its Clinical Estimation, below).

MID PELVIS

The interspinous diameter—10 cm or somewhat more—is usually the smallest diameter of the pelvis (Figure 38–1). The anteroposterior diameter, through the level of the ischial spines, normally measures at least 11.5 cm. The posterior component (posterior sagittal diameter) between the sacrum and the intersection with the interspinous diameter is usually at least 4.5 cm.

PELVIC OUTLET

The outlet of the pelvis consists of two approximately triangular areas not in the same plane but having a common base, which is a line drawn between the two ischial tuberosities (Figure 38–3). The apex of the posterior triangle is at the tip of the sacrum, and the lateral boundaries

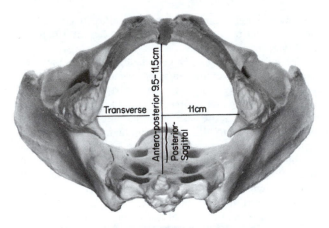

Figure 38–3. Pelvic outlet with diameters marked. Note that the anterior-posterior diameter may be divided into anterior and posterior sagittal diameters.

are the sacrosciatic ligaments and the ischial tuberosities. The anterior triangle is formed by the area under the pubic arch. Three diameters of the pelvic outlet are usually described: anteroposterior, transverse, and posterior sagittal. The anteroposterior diameter (9.5–11.5 cm) extends from the lower margin of the symphysis pubis to the tip of the sacrum (Figure 38–3). The transverse diameter (11 cm) is the distance between the inner edges of the ischial tuberosities. The posterior sagittal diameter extends from the tip of the sacrum to a right-angled intersection with a line drawn between the ischial tuberosities. The normal **posterior sagittal diameter** of the outlet usually exceeds 7.5 cm (Figure 38–3).

In obstructed labors caused by a narrowing of the mid pelvis or pelvic outlet, the prognosis for vaginal delivery often depends on the length of the posterior sagittal diameter of the pelvic outlet.

CALDWELL–MOLOY CLASSIFICATION

In 1933, two American obstetricians developed a classification of the pelvis that is still used. The classification is based upon the shape of the pelvis, and familiarity with the classification helps the physician to understand the mechanisms of labor in normally and abnormally shaped pelves.

A line drawn through the greatest transverse diameter of the inlet divides it into anterior and posterior segments. The shapes of these segments are important determinants in this method of classification (Figure 38–4). The character of the posterior segment determines the type of pelvis, and the character of the anterior segment determines the tendency. Many pelves are not pure but mixed types, eg, a gynecoid pelvis with android "tendency," meaning that the posterior pelvis is gynecoid and the anterior pelvis is android in shape.

Gynecoid Pelvis

This type of pelvis has anatomic characteristics ordinarily associated with the female pelvis. The prognosis for vaginal delivery is best with this type of pelvis.

Android Pelvis

The posterior sagittal diameter at the inlet is much shorter than the anterior sagittal diameter, limiting the use of the posterior space by the fetal head. The extreme android pelvis presages a very poor prognosis for vaginal delivery. The frequency of difficult forceps operations and stillbirths increases substantively when there is a small android pelvis.

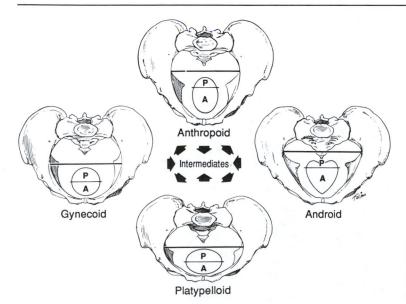

Figure 38–4. The four parent pelvic types of the Caldwell-Moloy classification. A line passing through the widest transverse diameter divides the inlet into posterior (P) and anterior (A) segments.

Anthropoid Pelvis

This type of pelvis is characterized by an anteroposterior diameter of the inlet greater than the transverse, forming more or less an oval anteroposteriorly, with the anterior segment somewhat narrow and pointed.

Platypelloid Pelvis

This type of pelvis has a flattened gynecoid shape, with a short anteroposterior and a wide transverse diameter.

Intermediate Type Pelves

Intermediate or mixed types of pelves are much more frequent than pure types.

PELVIC SIZE & ITS CLINICAL ESTIMATION

PELVIC INLET MEASUREMENTS

Diagonal Conjugate

The diagonal conjugate measurement is of the greatest importance—and every practitioner of obstetrics should be familiar with the technique of its measurement and the interpretation of the result.

The examiner first introduces two fingers into the vagina to evaluate the mobility of the coccyx by attempting to move it to and fro. The anterior surface of the sacrum is then palpated methodically from below upward, and its vertical and lateral curvatures are noted. In normal pelves, only the last three sacral vertebrae can be felt without in-

denting the perineum, whereas in markedly contracted pelves the entire anterior surface of the sacrum usually is readily accessible.

The index and second fingers, held firmly together, are carried up and over the anterior surface of the sacrum, where, by sharply depressing the wrist, one can discern the promontory with the tip of the third finger as a projecting bony margin at the base of the sacrum. With the finger closely apposed to the most prominent portion of the upper sacrum, the vaginal hand is elevated until it reaches the pubic arch, and the immediately adjacent point on the index finger is marked as shown in Figure 38–5. The hand is withdrawn, and the distance between the mark and the tip of the third finger is measured.

Transverse contraction of the inlet can be measured only by x-ray or CT scan. Such a contraction may exist even in the presence of an adequate anteroposterior diameter.

Engagement

By engagement it is meant descent of the biparietal plane of the fetal head to a level below that of the pelvic inlet (Figure 38–6). When the biparietal (widest) diameter of the normally flexed fetal head has passed through the inlet, the head is engaged. Although engagement of the fetal head is usually regarded as a phenomenon of labor, in nulliparas it commonly occurs during the last few weeks of pregnancy. With engagement, the fetal head serves as an internal pelvimeter to demonstrate that the pelvic inlet is ample for that fetus.

Whether the head is engaged may be ascertained either by rectal or vaginal examination or by abdominal palpation. If the lowest part of the occiput is at or below the level of the spines, the head is usually engaged, since the distance from the plane of the pelvic inlet to the level of

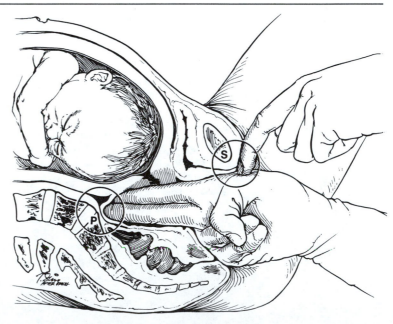

Figure 38–5. Vaginal examination to determine the diagonal conjugate. P, sacral promontory; S, symphysis pubis.

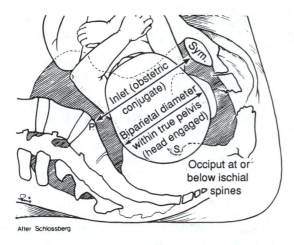

Figure 38–6. When the lowermost portion of the fetal head is at or below the ischial spines, it is usually engaged. Exceptions occur when there is considerable molding or caput formation, or both. P, sacral promontory; Sym, symphysis pubis; S, ischial spine.

the ischial spines is approximately 5 cm in most pelves, and the distance from the biparietal plane of the unmolded fetal head to the vertex is about 3–4 cm. Engagement may be ascertained less accurately by abdominal examination. (See Leopold's maneuvers, below.)

Fixation of the fetal head is its descent through the pelvic inlet to a depth that prevents its free movement in any direction when bimanual pressure is exerted over the lower abdomen. Fixation is not necessarily synonymous with engagement.

PELVIC OUTLET MEASUREMENTS

An important dimension of the pelvic outlet that is accessible for clinical measurement is the diameter between the ischial tuberosities, variously called the **biischial diameter,** the **intertuberous diameter,** and the **transverse diameter of the outlet** (Figure 38–3). A measurement of over 8 cm is considered normal. Measurement of the transverse diameter of the outlet can be estimated by placing a closed fist of known width against the perineum between the ischial tuberosities. Usually the closed fist is wider than 8 cm. The shape of the subpubic arch can be evaluated at the same time by palpating the pubic rami from the subpubic region toward the ischial tuberosities.

MID-PELVIS ESTIMATION

Clinical estimation of mid pelvis capacity by any direct form of measurement is not possible. If the ischial spines are prominent, the sidewalls are felt to converge, the concavity of the sacrum is very shallow, and the biischial diameter of the outlet is less than 8 cm, one should suspect a

contraction in this region. However, the mid pelvis can be precisely measured only by imaging studies.

IMAGING PELVIMETRY: X-RAY & COMPUTED TOMOGRAPHY

X-RAY PELVIMETRY

Status of X-Ray Pelvimetry

There are at least five anatomic and mechanical factors of importance in successful vaginal delivery: (1) the size and shape of the bony pelvis, (2) the size of the fetal head, (3) the force of the uterine contractions, (4) the moldability of the fetal head, and (5) the presentation and position of the fetus. Only the first of these factors is susceptible to reasonably precise radiographic measurement, which means that it is possible to retrieve only this one factor from the realm of the unknown.

X-ray pelvimetry has the following advantages over manual estimation of pelvic size: (1) It can provide precise mensuration to a degree unobtainable clinically, and (2) it can provide exact mensuration of two important diameters not otherwise obtainable, ie, the transverse diameter of the inlet and the interischial spinous diameter (transverse diameter of the mid pelvis). This information may prove critical during breech delivery.

Indications for X-Ray Pelvimetry

Because of the expense involved as well as potential radiation hazards, radiographic pelvic measurement is not necessary in the great majority of cases. There are, however, clinical circumstances in which x-ray pelvimetry is part of good obstetric practice. Examples are the patient with a history of injury or disease likely to affect the bony pelvis and the fetus presenting as a breech when vaginal delivery is anticipated.

Hazards of Diagnostic Radiation

The recognized dangers to the fetus from diagnostic radiation are chromosomal mutations and an increased risk of cancer in later life. Many geneticists and radiobiologists believe, on the basis of animal experimentation, that the only entirely safe dose of irradiation is no radiation. *The slight risk from x-ray pelvimetry, however, seems justifiable whenever information critical to the welfare of the fetus or mother is likely to be obtained.*

The concept that the use of x-ray pelvimetry should be limited has been endorsed by the American College of Radiology and the American College of Obstetricians and Gynecologists.

COMPUTED TOMOGRAPHY (CT Scanning)

Because of the slight risk of childhood cancer associated with x-ray exposure, digital radiographs obtained with computed tomographic scanners have been used to measure pelvic diameters. The obvious advantage of this technique is a reduction in radiation exposure a range of 44–425 millirads. Furthermore, the accuracy is greater than that of conventional x-ray pelvimetry, and the procedure is easier to perform. The cost is comparable to that of conventional x-ray pelvimetry.

II. FETAL ATTITUDE OR POSTURE

In the later months of pregnancy, the fetus assumes a characteristic **posture** sometimes called also its **attitude** or **habitus** (Figure 38–7). This characteristic posture results partly from the natural growth of the fetus and partly from a process of accommodation to the uterine cavity.

LIE OF THE FETUS

The lie of the fetus is the relation of its long axis to that of the mother and is either **longitudinal** or **transverse.** Occasionally, the fetal and maternal axes may cross at a 45-degree angle, forming an **oblique lie,** which is unstable and always becomes longitudinal or transverse during the course of labor. Longitudinal lies are present in over 99% of labors at term.

PRESENTATION

The presenting part determines the presentation. Accordingly, in longitudinal lies, the presenting part is either the fetal head or the breech, creating cephalic and breech presentations, respectively. When the fetus lies with its long axis transverse to that of the mother, the shoulder is the presenting part.

Cephalic presentations are classified according to the relation of the head to the body of the fetus (Figure 38–7). Ordinarily, the head is flexed sharply so that the chin is in contact with the thorax. Such a presentation is usually referred to as a **vertex** or **occipital presentation.** Much less commonly, the fetal neck may be sharply extended so that the occiput and back come in contact and the face is foremost in the birth canal **(face presentation).** The fetal head may assume a position between these extremes—partially flexed in some cases, with the anterior (large) fontanelle, presenting **(sincipital presentation);** or partially extended in other cases, with the brow presenting **(brow presentation).** As labor progresses, sincipital and brow presentations are almost always converted into vertex or face presentations by flexion or extension, respectively.

When the fetus presents as a breech, the thighs may be flexed and the legs extended over the anterior surfaces of the body **(frank breech presentation).** A complete breech presentation occurs when the thighs are flexed on the abdomen and the legs upon the thighs. An incomplete breech presentation occurs when one or both feet, or one or both knees, are lowermost.

POSITION

The position of the fetus is the relation of an arbitrarily chosen portion of the presenting part to the right or left side of the birth canal. Accordingly, with each presentation there may be two positions, right or left. The occiput, chin, and sacrum are the determining points in vertex, face, and breech presentations, respectively (Figure 38–8).

Variety

For still more accurate orientation, the relation of a given portion of the presenting part to the anterior, transverse, or posterior portion of the mother's pelvis is considered. Since there are two positions, it follows that there must be six varieties for each presentation (Figure 38–8).

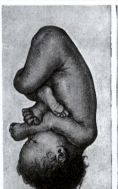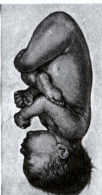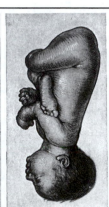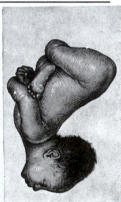

Figure 38–7. Differences in attitude of the fetus in vertex, sinciput, brow, and face presentations.

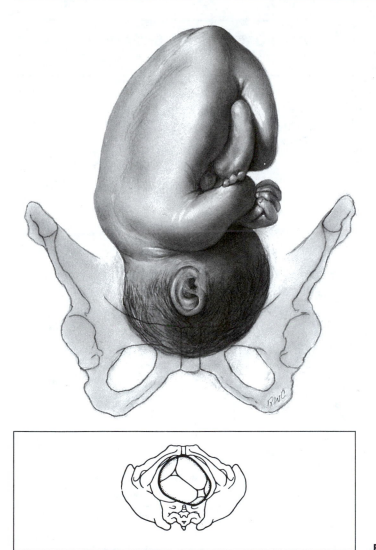

Figure 38–8. Vertex presentation.

The presenting part in any presentation may be in either the left or right position, which means that there are left and right occipital (LO, RO), left and right mental (LM, RM), and left and right sacral (LS, RS) presentations. Since the presenting part in each of the two positions may be directed anteriorly (A), transversely (T), or posteriorly (P), there are thus six varieties of each of these three presentations.

In shoulder presentations, the acromion (or the scapula) is the portion of the fetus arbitrarily chosen to orient it with the maternal pelvis. Since it is impossible to differentiate precisely the several varieties of shoulder presentation by clinical examination and since such differentiation serves no practical purpose, it is customary to refer to all transverse lies of the fetus simply as shoulder presentations.

Frequency of the Various Presentations & Positions

At or near term the incidence of the various presentations is approximately as follows: vertex, 96%; breech, 3.5%; face, 0.3%; and shoulder, 0.4%. About two-thirds of all vertex presentations are in the left occipital position and one-third in the right.

Reasons for the Predominance of Cephalic Presentations

The most logical explanation for the predominance of cephalic presentations seems to be that the uterus is piriform in shape. Although the fetal head at term is slightly larger than the breech, the entire podalic pole of the fetus—ie, the breech and its flexed extremities—is bulkier than the cephalic pole and more movable. The cephalic pole is composed of the fetal head only, because the upper extremities are some distance away, are small, and are less protruding than the buttocks and lower extremities combined. The high incidence of breech presentations in hydrocephalic fetuses accords with this theory, since in this circumstance the cephalic pole of the fetus is definitely larger than the podalic pole.

The cause of breech presentation may be some circumstance that prevents normal version from taking place, eg, a septum that protrudes into the uterine cavity. A peculiarity of fetal attitude—particularly extension of the vertebral column, as occurs in frank breeches—may also prevent the fetus from turning.

DIAGNOSIS OF PRESENTATION & POSITION OF THE FETUS

ABDOMINAL PALPATION: LEOPOLD'S MANEUVERS
(Figure 38–9)

In order to obtain satisfactory results, the examination of the abdomen should be conducted systematically, employing four maneuvers suggested by Leopold and Sporlin in 1894.

During the first three maneuvers, the examiner stands at

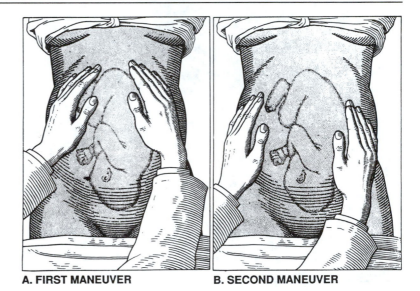
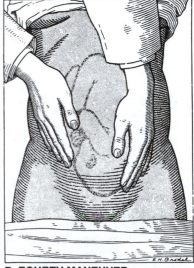

A. FIRST MANEUVER

B. SECOND MANEUVER

C. THIRD MANEUVER

D. FOURTH MANEUVER

Figure 38–9. Palpation in left occiput anterior position (maneuvers of Leopold). See text for explanation.

the side of the bed and faces the patient; for the last maneuver, the examiner turns and faces toward the patient's feet.

First Maneuver

The examiner gently palpates the fundus with the tips of the fingers of both hands in order to determine which fetal pole is present in the fundus.

Second Maneuver

The palms of the examiner's hands are placed on either side of the abdomen, and gentle but deep pressure is exerted. On one side, a hard, resistant structure is felt (the back); and on the other, numerous nodulations (the small parts).

Third Maneuver

Employing the thumb and fingers of one hand, the examiner grasps the lower portion of the patient's abdomen just above the symphysis pubis. If the presenting part is not engaged, a movable body will be felt, usually the fetal head. If by careful palpation it can be shown that the cephalic prominence is on the same side as the small parts, the head must be flexed, and therefore the vertex is the presenting part. When the cephalic prominence of the fetus is on the same side as the back, the head must be extended.

Fourth Maneuver

The examiner faces the mother's feet and—using the tips of the first three fingers of each hand—exerts deep pressure in the direction of the axis of the pelvic inlet. If the head presents, one hand is arrested sooner than the other by a rounded body, the cephalic prominence, while the other hand descends more deeply into the pelvis. In vertex presentations, the prominence is on the same side as the small parts, and in face presentations it is on the same side as the back. The ease with which the prominence is felt is indicative of the extent to which descent has occurred. So long as the cephalic prominence is readily palpable, the vertex has not descended to the level of the ischial spines.

VAGINAL EXAMINATION

Before labor begins, the diagnosis of fetal presentation and position by vaginal examination may be somewhat inconclusive, because the presenting part must be palpated through the closed cervix and lower uterine segment. During labor, however, after dilatation of the cervix, important information may be obtained.

In attempting to determine presentation and position by vaginal examination, it is advisable to pursue a definite routine that consists of three maneuvers as follows:

(1) Two gloved fingers are introduced into the vagina and carried up to the presenting part. Differentiation of vertex, face, and breech is then readily accomplished.

(2) If the vertex is presenting, the examiner's fingers are introduced into the posterior aspect of the vagina. The fingers are then swept forward over the fetal head toward the maternal symphysis. The examiner's fingers must cross the sagittal suture, and its course is outlined, with small and large fontanelles at the opposite ends.

(3) The positions of the two fontanelles then are ascertained, ie, anterior and posterior.

AUSCULTATION

In cephalic presentations, the point of maximal intensity of fetal heart sounds is usually midway between the maternal umbilicus and the anterior-superior spine of her ilium, whereas in breech presentations it is usually about level with the umbilicus.

SONOGRAPHY

Employing ultrasonography, the fetal head and body can be located usually without difficulty.

SUGGESTED READINGS

Caldwell WE, Moloy HC: Anatomical variations in the female pelvis and their effect in labor with a suggested classification. Am J Obstet Gynecol 1933;26:479.

Mechanism of Normal Labor in Occipital Presentation

The fetus is in the occipital (vertex) presentation in approximately 96% of all labors.

CARDINAL MOVEMENTS OF A LABOR IN OCCIPITAL PRESENTATION

The cardinal movements of labor are (1) engagement (2) descent, (3) flexion, (4) internal rotation, (5) extension, (6) external rotation, and (7) expulsion. These movements are illustrated in Figure 39–1. The mechanisms of labor consist of a combination of all these movements going on at the same time. For example, as part of the process of engagement, there is both flexion and descent of the head. Concomitantly, the uterine contractions bring about important modifications in the attitude, or habitus, of the fetus, especially after the head has descended into the pelvis. These changes consist principally of straightening of the fetus, with loss of its dorsal convexity and closer application of the extremities and small parts to the body. As a result, the fetal ovoid is transformed into a cylinder—with, normally, the smallest possible cross section passing through the birth canal.

ENGAGEMENT

Engagement of the fetal head occurs when the biparietal diameter passes through the pelvic inlet. The fetal head usually enters the pelvic inlet either in the transverse diameter or in one of the oblique diameters.

Asynclitism

Although the fetal head tends to accommodate to the transverse axis of the pelvic inlet, the sagittal suture, while remaining parallel to that axis, may not lie exactly midway between the symphysis and the sacral promontory. The sagittal suture is frequently deflected either posteriorly toward the promontory or anteriorly toward the symphysis, as shown in Figure 39–2.

DESCENT

Descent is brought about by one or more of four forces: (1) pressure of the amnionic fluid, (2) direct pressure of the fundus upon the breech, (3) contraction of the abdominal muscles, and (4) extension and straightening of the fetal body.

FLEXION

As soon as the descending head meets resistance, flexion occurs, and the appreciably shorter suboccipitobregmatic diameter is substituted for the longer occipitofrontal diameter.

INTERNAL ROTATION

This movement is a turning of the head in such a manner that the occiput gradually moves from its original position anteriorly toward the symphysis pubis or, less commonly, posteriorly toward the hollow of the sacrum.

EXTENSION

When, after internal rotation, the sharply flexed head reaches the vulva, it undergoes extension, which brings the base of the occiput into direct contact with the inferior margin of the symphysis pubis. With increasing distention of the perineum and vaginal opening, an increasingly

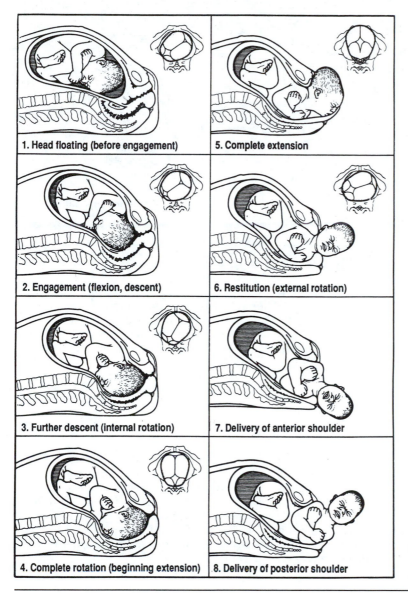

1. Head floating (before engagement)

2. Engagement (flexion, descent)

3. Further descent (internal rotation)

4. Complete rotation (beginning extension)

5. Complete extension

6. Restitution (external rotation)

7. Delivery of anterior shoulder

8. Delivery of posterior shoulder

Figure 39–1. Cardinal movements in the mechanism of labor and delivery, left occiput anterior position.

large portion of the occiput gradually appears. The head is delivered by further extension as the occiput, bregma, forehead, nose, mouth, and finally the chin pass successively over the anterior margin of the perineum.

EXTERNAL ROTATION

The delivered head next undergoes restitution. If the occiput was originally directed toward the left, it rotates toward the left ischial tuberosity; if it was originally directed toward the right, the occiput rotates to the right. The return of the head to the oblique position (restitution) is followed by completion of external rotation to the transverse position, a movement that corresponds to rotation of the fetal body, serving to bring its bisacromial diameter into relation with the anteroposterior diameter of the pelvic outlet. Thus, one shoulder is anterior, behind the symphysis, and the other is posterior. This movement is apparently brought about by the same pelvic factors that cause internal rotation of the head.

LABOR IN OCCIPUT POSTERIOR POSITIONS

In the great majority of labors with the fetus presenting in occiput posterior positions, the mechanism of labor is identical to what occurs in the transverse and anterior varieties, except that the occiput must rotate to the symphysis pubis through 135 degrees instead of 90 degrees and 45 degrees, respectively.

If rotation is incomplete, **transverse arrest** results. If

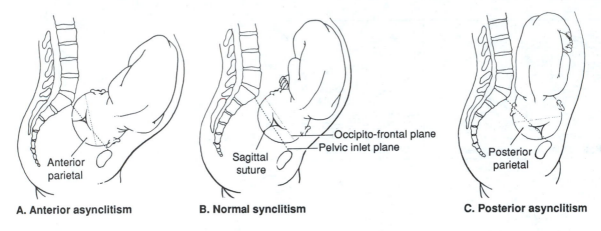

A. Anterior asynclitism   B. Normal synclitism   C. Posterior asynclitism

Anterior parietal

Sagittal suture

Occipito-frontal plane
Pelvic inlet plane

Posterior parietal

Figure 39–2. Synclitism and asynclitism.

rotation toward the symphysis does not take place, the occiput usually rotates to the direct occiput posterior position, a condition known as **persistent occiput posterior.** Both transverse arrest and persistent occiput posterior positioning represent deviations from the normal mechanisms of labor and are considered further in Chapter 46.

CHANGES IN SHAPE OF THE FETAL HEAD

CAPUT SUCCEDANEUM

In prolonged labors before complete dilatation of the cervix, the portion of the fetal scalp immediately over the cervical os becomes edematous, forming a swelling known as caput succedaneum. The swelling usually attains a thickness of only a few millimeters, but in prolonged labors it may be severe enough to prevent differentiation of the various sutures and fontanelles. More commonly, the caput is formed when the head is in the lower portion of the birth canal and frequently only after the resistance of a rigid vaginal outlet is encountered. It occurs over the most dependent portion of the head.

MOLDING

Of considerable importance is the degree of molding that the head undergoes. Because the various bones of the skull are not firmly united, movement may occur at the sutures. These changes are of greatest importance in contracted pelves, when the degree to which the head is capable of molding may make the difference between successful vaginal delivery and a difficult forceps application or caesarean delivery.

SUGGESTED READINGS

Mechanisms of Normal Labor in Occiput Presentation. Chapter 13 in *Williams Obstetrics,* 19th ed., Cunningham FG, MacDonald PC, Gant NF, Leveno KJ, and Gilstrap LC, III (editors). Appleton & Lange, 1993.

40

The Newborn Infant

ADAPTATION OF THE NEWBORN TO AIR BREATHING

INITIATION OF AIR BREATHING

Conclusive evidence of episodic respiratory movements in utero during normal human pregnancy has been obtained by use of ultrasound. Very soon after birth, the breathing pattern shifts from one of shallow episodic inspirations to one characterized by regular deep inhalations. It is now apparent that aeration of the newborn lung is not inflation of a collapsed structure but the rapid replacement of bronchial and alveolar fluid by air. Delay in removal of fluid from the alveoli probably contributes to the syndrome of **transient tachypnea of the newborn.**

As the fluid is replaced by air, there is considerable reduction in pulmonary vascular compression and, in turn, lowered resistance to blood flow. With the fall in pulmonary arterial blood pressure, the ductus arteriosus normally closes. Closure of the foramen ovale is more variable.

Normally, from the first breath after birth, progressively more residual air accumulates in the lung, and with each successive breath, a lower pulmonary opening pressure is required. In the mature normal infant, by about the fifth breath of air, the pressure-volume changes achieved with each respiration are very similar to those of the normal adult. This requires the presence of surface-active materials (surfactants) that prevent collapse of the lung with each respiration (Chapter 35). Lack of sufficient surfactant leads to the prompt development of respiratory distress syndrome (Chapter 55).

The Stimuli to Breathe Air

Some explanations of this phenomenon are as follows:

A. Physical Stimulation: The handling of the infant may provoke respiration through stimuli reaching the respiratory center reflexly from the skin.

B. Compression of Fetal Thorax at Delivery: Compression of the fetal thorax incidental to vaginal delivery and the expansion that follows delivery may help initiate respiration.

C. Deprivation of Oxygen and Accumulation of Carbon Dioxide: Lack of oxygen may stimulate respiration after birth. Observations on both animals and humans, however, have shown that profound lack of oxygen produces apnea.

MANAGEMENT OF DELIVERY

Immediate Care

As the head of the infant is delivered, either vaginally or by cesarean delivery, the face is immediately wiped and the mouth and nares suctioned. A soft rubber ear syringe or its equivalent inserted with care is quite suitable for the purpose.

Once the cord has been severed, the infant is immediately placed supine with the head lowered and turned to the side in a heated unit that has appropriate thermal regulation and is equipped for immediate intensive care. To minimize heat loss, the baby is wiped dry.

Evaluation of the Infant

Before and during delivery, careful consideration must be given to the following determinants of infant well-being: (1) health status of the mother; (2) fetal (gestational) age; (3) duration of labor; (4) duration of rupture of the membranes; (5) kinds, amounts, times, and routes of administration of analgesics; (6) kind and duration of anesthesia; and (7) degree of difficulty encountered in effecting delivery. The obstetrician inspects the infant for any visible abnormalities during delivery and until the cord is severed, and the infant is then handed over to a trained associate for further care.

A readily discernible heartbeat of 100 per min or more is acceptable. Persistent bradycardia requires prompt resuscitation. Next, the mouth, nares, and pharynx are carefully suctioned.

Most normal infants take a breath within a few seconds

after delivery and cry within half a minute. If respirations are infrequent, suction of the mouth and pharynx followed by light slapping of the soles of the feet and rubbing of the back usually serve to stimulate breathing. Prolongation of these intervals beyond 1 and 2 minutes, respectively, indicates an abnormality. Continued lack of breathing indicates either marked central depression or mechanical obstruction and demands active resuscitation.

Lack of Effective Respirations

Important causes of failure to establish effective respirations include the following: (1) fetal hypoxemia from any cause; (2) drugs administered to the mother; (3) gross immaturity of the fetus; (4) upper airway obstruction; (5) pneumothorax; (6) other lung abnormalities, either intrinsic (eg, hypoplasia) or extrinsic (eg, diaphragmatic hernia); (7) aspiration of amnionic fluid grossly contaminated with meconium; (8) central nervous system injury; and (9) septicemia.

METHODS USED TO EVALUATE THE NEWBORN'S CONDITION

APGAR SCORE

A useful aid in the evaluation of the infant is the Apgar scoring system applied at 1 minute and again at 5 minutes after birth (Table 40–1). In general, the higher the score (up to a maximum of 10), the better the condition of the infant. The 1-minute Apgar score determines the need for immediate resuscitation. Most infants at birth are in excellent condition, as indicated by Apgar scores of 7–10, and require no aid other than perhaps simple nasopharyngeal suction. **Mildly to moderately depressed infants** score 4–7 at 1 minute, demonstrating depressed respirations, flaccidity, and pale to blue color. Heart rate and reflex irritability, however, are good. **Severely depressed infants** score 0–4, with heart rate slow to inaudible and reflex responses depressed or absent. Resuscitation, including artificial ventilation, should be started immediately.

Note: A baby who is flaccid, apneic, covered with meconium, and with a heart rate below 100 per min obviously needs active intervention, and in such cases there is no need for considering further the 1-minute Apgar score. Pharyngeal suction, endotracheal intubation, endotracheal suction, and positive pressure oxygenation should be instituted as soon as possible.

The Apgar score is a clinical tool useful only to help identify those neonates who might require resuscitation and to monitor the effectiveness of resuscitative measures. Unfortunately, attempts have been made to relate the Apgar score to long-term outcome. What is more, for reasons that are not entirely clear, erroneous definitions of asphyxia have been established on the basis of the Apgar score alone. Because of these misconceptions, the Committee on Maternal and Fetal Medicine of the American College of Obstetricians and Gynecologists and the Committee on Fetus and Newborn of the American Academy of Pediatrics have issued a joint statement on the use and misuse of the Apgar score.

UMBILICAL CORD BLOOD ACID-BASE & BLOOD GAS MEASUREMENTS

An objective method of diagnosing hypoxia in the newborn has been the identification of umbilical arterial metabolic acidemia at birth. Normal values for acid-base and blood gas measurements are listed in Table 40–2. Acidemia has been defined as an umbilical arterial pH of less than 7.20. However, a pH between 7.10 and 7.19 is associated with a vigorous neonate in OVER 80% of cases.

An umbilical cord arterial pH above 7.20 is convincing evidence that obstetric management of labor did not result in fetal asphyxia. Detection of an umbilical cord pH of less than 7.20, however, may be the result of respiratory, metabolic, or mixed acidosis. Most often, these low pH levels are not due to metabolic acidemia, and it is only a metabolic acidosis of severe magnitude and long duration that results in serious fetal damage. Gilstrap and colleagues (1989) suggest that a diagnosis of asphyxia should be based on an arterial pH less than 7.00, a 1-minute Apgar less than 3, and evidence of organ dysfunction.

Table 40–1. Apgar scoring system.

Sign	0	1	2
Heart rate	Absent	Slow (< 100)	> 100
Respiratory effort	Absent	Slow, irregular	Good, crying
Muscle tone	Flaccid	Some flexion of extremities	Active motion
Reflex irritability	No response	Grimace	Vigorous cry
Color	Blue, pale	Body pink, extremities blue	Completely pink

Table 40–2. Umbilical arterial and venous pH and blood gas determinations at birth in 146 normal neonates.[1]

	Arterial				Venous			
	Mean	SD[2]	Range	SEM[3]	Mean	SD[2]	Range	SEM[3]
pH	7.28	0.05	7.15–7.43	0.004	7.35	0.05	7.24–7.49	0.0004
P_{CO_2} (mm Hg)	49.2	8.4	31.1–74.3	0.68	38.2	5.6	23.2–49.2	0.46
P_{O_2} (mm Hg)	18.0	6.2	3.8–33.8	0.50	29.2	5.9	15.4–48.2	0.48
Bicarbonate (meq/L)	22.3	2.5	13.3–27.5	0.20	20.4	2.1	15.9–24.7	0.17

[1]Modified from Yeomans ER and associates: Umbilical cord pH pCO_2 and bicarbonate following uncomplicated term vaginal deliveries. Am J Obstet Gynecol 1985;151:798.

ACTIVE RESUSCITATION

Successful active resuscitation requires (1) skilled personnel who are immediately available; (2) a suitably heated, well-lighted, appropriately large work area; (3) equipment to deliver oxygen by intermittent positive pressure through a face mask and to carry out endotracheal intubation with endotracheal suction and positive-pressure oxygenation; and (4) drugs, syringes, needles, and catheters for possible intravenous administration of naloxone (Narcan), sodium bicarbonate, and, rarely, administration of sublingual epinephrine. The site of every delivery, vaginal or abdominal, must be so equipped for resuscitation, and the equipment should be thoroughly checked before each delivery.

VENTILATION BY MASK

Inadequate respirations that persist much beyond 1 minute lead to a falling heart rate and decreased muscle tone and call for a quick but careful physical examination—especially of the mouth, nose, pharynx, neck, and chest—and the administration of oxygen. If the mouth and pharynx are free of liquid and foreign material and no physical obstruction to breathing is identified, oxygen may be delivered through a well-fitting mask at a pressure of about 20 cm H_2O in 1- to 2-second bursts to deliver oxygen into the bronchi. If this maneuver does not *promptly* stimulate breathing and correct the evidence of hypoxia, tracheal intubation is necessary under direct visualization with an appropriate laryngoscope.

TRACHEAL INTUBATION

After clearing the airway, endotracheal intubation is followed by intermittent positive-pressure ventilation with oxygen delivered from a bag connected to the tracheal tube. If the stomach expands, the tube is almost certainly in the esophagus rather than in the trachea. Once adequate spontaneous respirations have been established, the tube can usually be removed safely.

CAUSES OF PERSISTENT DEPRESSION OF THE NEWBORN

Acidosis

Sodium bicarbonate, 1 meq per kg, is injected through the umbilical vein of the severely depressed, hypoxic newborn who does not respond promptly to establishment of an airway and positive-pressure oxygen administration. This dose may be repeated if a favorable clinical response is not achieved.

Opioid Drugs

Meperidine (Demerol) and similar drugs given to the mother an hour or less before delivery may cause respiratory depression in the newborn infant. In such cases, naloxone (Narcan) may be given in a dose of 10 μg per kg.

Hypovolemia

Some severely depressed newborn infants are hypovolemic. Hypovolemia may occur without fetal hemorrhage having been detected, eg, with sepsis, fetal-to-maternal hemorrhage, trauma to the placenta, cord compression with obstruction of the umbilical vein and pooling of blood in the placenta, and twin-to-twin transfusion. At least partial restoration of intravascular volume and correction of severe anemia are essential for improvement in the volume-depleted infant.

CARDIAC MASSAGE

If fetal heart action was present just before delivery but cannot be demonstrated after birth—or if the heart stops after birth—external cardiac massage may be initiated. *Immediately,* the airway must be cleared, the trachea intubated, and adequate pulmonary ventilation established. External cardiac massage is effected with two fingers applied to the anterior chest wall in the lower midline at a rate of about 120 per min. Four compressions of the chest are alternated with inflation of the lung. A delay of several minutes in cardiac massage most likely will result in an unfortunate outcome—either death or permanent marked impairment of central nervous system function.

COMMON ERRORS IN RESUSCITATION OF THE NEWBORN

If resuscitation efforts are not promptly successful, the failure may be due to some easily correctable technical error. Common errors include the following:

1. Failure to check resuscitation equipment beforehand
   a. Damaged resuscitation bag
   b. Laryngoscope with weak or flickering light
   c. Nonsterile umbilical catheter
2. Use of a cold resuscitation table
3. Unsuccessful intubation
   a. Hyperextension of neck
   b. Inadequate suctioning
   c. Excessive force
4. Inadequate ventilation
   a. Improper head position
   b. Improper application of mask
   c. Placement of tracheal tube into esophagus or right main stem bronchus
   d. Failure to secure tracheal tube
5. Failure to detect and determine the cause of poor chest movements or persistent bradycardia
6. Failure to detect and treat hypovolemia
7. Failure to perform cardiac massage

ROUTINE NEWBORN CARE

ESTIMATION OF GESTATIONAL AGE

A rapid yet rather precise estimate of gestational age of the newborn infant may be made soon after delivery by examining (1) sole creases, (2) breast nodules, (3) scalp hair, (4) ear lobes, and, in the case of males, (5) testes and scrotum—as outlined in Table 40–3. A more definitive estimate can be made in a few days with the help of neurologic examination (Chapter 59). Unfortunately, estimates of gestational age based upon physical and neurologic examination of the neonate are often unacceptably inaccurate in preterm and growth-retarded infants. It is unwise to rely on these evaluations alone in such neonates.

CARE OF THE EYES

Because of the possibility of infection of the eyes of the newborn during passage through the vagina of a mother with gonorrhea, prophylactic measures have been devel-

Table 40–3. Rapid estimation of gestational age of the newborn.

| | Gestational Age | | |
Sites	36 Weeks or Less	37–38 Weeks	39 Weeks or More
Sole creases	Anterior transverse crease only	Occasional creases anterior two-thirds	Sole covered with creases
Breast nodule diameter	2 mm	4 mm	7 mm
Scalp hair	Fine and fuzzy	Fine and fuzzy	Coarse and silky
Ear lobe	Pliable, no cartilage	Some cartilage	Stiffened by thick cartilage
Testes and scrotum	Testes in lower canal, scrotum small, few rugae	Intermediate	Testes pendulous, scrotum full, extensive rugae

oped to prevent **gonococcal ophthalmia neonatorum** and the resulting blindness.

Technique of Silver Nitrate Prophylaxis

The region about each eye should be irrigated with sterile water applied to the nasal side of the eye and allowed to run off the opposite side. The lower lid should then be drawn down and 1% silver nitrate solution dropped into the lower cul-de-sac. In over half of cases, silver nitrate produces chemical conjunctivitis manifested by redness, edema, or discharge which develops in 24 hours and lasts 2–3 days.

Antibiotic Prophylaxis

Penicillin serves as an alternative to silver nitrate in prophylaxis of gonococcal ophthalmia neonatorum. Penicillin ointment, 100,000 units per g, is placed in the eyes of the newborn baby, or penicillin is injected intramuscularly.

Tetracycline ointment, 1%, or **erythromycin ointment,** 0.5%, afford effective prophylaxis against gonorrhea. Both should serve also to prevent chlamydial conjunctivitis or at least reduce its incidence. Laga and colleagues (1988) reported that tetracycline ointment is as effective as silver nitrate solution in preventing gonococcal ophthalmia. While both tetracycline and silver nitrate afforded substantive protection against *Chlamydia trachomatis* infection, approximately 10% of exposed infants developed chlamydial conjunctivitis despite prophylaxis. Newer techniques are described in the 19th edition of *Williams Obstetrics.*

PERMANENT INFANT IDENTIFICATION

A foolproof system for proper identification of every infant must be in operation at all hours and should prevent separation of the infant from its mother until identification bands are placed on both the mother and the neonate. A second identification system consists of taking footprints rather than fingerprints or palmprints. This is done because the ridges in the feet are more pronounced and because it is easier to obtain footprints from newborn infants.

SUBSEQUENT CARE

Temperature

The temperature of the infant drops rapidly immediately after birth. Chilling incites shivering and increases oxygen requirements. Consequently, the infant must be cared for in a warm crib in which temperature control is regulated closely. During the first few days of life, the infant's temperature is unstable, responding to slight stimuli with considerable fluctuations above or below normal.

Vitamin K

Administration of vitamin K should be done routinely, as described in Chapter 55.

Umbilical Cord

Loss of water from Wharton's jelly leads to mummification of the cord shortly after birth. Within 24 hours, it loses its characteristic bluish-white, moist appearance and soon becomes dry and black. Gradually, the line of demarcation appears just beyond the skin of the abdomen, and in a few days the stump sloughs, leaving a small granulating wound that after healing forms the umbilicus. Separation usually takes place within the first 2 weeks (range, 3–45 days). Because the umbilical cord dries more quickly and separates more readily when exposed to the air, a dressing is not recommended. Strict aseptic precautions should therefore be observed in the immediate care of the cord. Some obstetricians apply bacitracin ointment to the stump (American College of Obstetricians and Gynecologists).

Care of the Skin

Infants should be promptly patted dry to minimize heat loss caused by evaporation. Not all the vernix caseosa is removed, but the excess, as well as blood and meconium, is gently wiped off. It is unwise to wash a newborn until its temperature has stabilized. Handling of the baby should be minimized.

Stools & Urine

For the first 2 or 3 days after birth, the contents of the colon are composed of soft, brownish-green **meconium,** which is composed of desquamated epithelial cells from the intestinal tract, mucus, and epidermal cells and lanugo (fetal hair) that have been swallowed with the amnionic fluid. The characteristic color results from bile pigments. The passage of meconium and urine in the minutes immediately after birth or during the next few hours verifies patency of the gastrointestinal and urinary tracts.

After the third or fourth day, as a consequence of ingesting milk, meconium is replaced by light yellow homogeneous feces with a characteristic odor.

Icterus Neonatorum

About one-third of all babies develop so-called **physiologic jaundice of the newborn** between the second and fifth days of life. At birth there is hyperbilirubinemia of 1.8–2.8 mg per dL, increasing during the next few days but with wide individual variations. Between the third and fourth days, the bilirubin in mature infants commonly reaches somewhat more than 5 mg per dL, the concentration at which jaundice usually becomes noticeable. Most of the bilirubin is free, or unconjugated. One cause—but not the sole cause—of hyperbilirubinemia is immaturity of the hepatic cells, resulting in slight conjugation of bilirubin with glucuronic acid and reduced excretion in bile (Chapter 55). Reabsorption of free bilirubin as a result of enzymatic splitting of bilirubin glucuronide by intestinal conjugase activity in the newborn intestine also appears to contribute significantly to the transient hyperbilirubinemia. Jaundice is more common and usually more severe and prolonged in preterm infants than in term infants because of greater hepatic enzymatic immaturity. Infants who are term but small for gestational age, however, metabolize bilirubin in a manner similar to term infants. Increased erythrocyte destruction from any cause contributes to hyperbilirubinemia.

Table 40–4. Criteria for early discharge.[1]

1. Delivery is vertex, single, sterile, and vaginal.
2. Apgar scores of > 7 at 1 and 5 minutes.
3. Gestational age of 38–42 weeks and weight of 2700–4000 g.
4. Minimum length of stay of 24 hours; a transition to normal thermoregulation in an open crib, completion of 2 successful feedings, evidence of stool and void, completion of neonatal screening for metabolic disease and blood type and Coombs' test (Rh-negative and O mothers) prior to discharge.
5. Vital signs within normal ranges at discharge:
   Axillary temperature   36.1–37.2 °C
   Heart rate   110–150/min
   Respiratory rate   30–60/min
6. A normal neonatal hospital course with no signs or symptoms that require continuous observation:
   Blood dextrose maintained > 45 mg/dL
   Hematocrit 45–65%
   ABO-incompatible infants must be held until 48 hours and released only if they do not require therapy for hemolysis.
7. Physical examination completed by the physician or a trained assistant.
8. Demonstration of mother's understanding and ability to provide adequate care for her newborn; infant care education provided on a one-to-one or classroom basis by the nursing staff prior to discharge. Finally the mother must agree to return the baby for screening tests for a variety of diseases due to inborn error in metabolism (see text).
9. Signed documentation by mother that states her obligation to participate in follow-up care.

[1]Reproduced, with permission, from Conrad PD, Wilkening RB, Rosenberg AA: Safety of newborn discharge in less than 36 hours in an indigent population. *Am J Dis Child* 1989;**143**:98. Copyright 1989, American Medical Association.

Initial Weight Loss

Because the infant may receive little nutrition for the first 3 or 4 days of life and at the same time produces a considerable amount of urine, feces, and sweat, it progressively loses weight until the mother's flow of milk or other feeding has been established. Preterm infants lose relatively more weight and regain their birth weight more slowly than do term infants. Infants who are small for gestational age but otherwise healthy regain their initial weight more quickly when fed than do preterm infants.

If the normal infant is nourished properly, the birth weight is usually regained by the end of the tenth day. Subsequently, weight typically increases steadily at the rate of about 25 g daily for the first few months, to double the birth weight by 5 months of age and to triple it by the end of the first year.

Feeding

Because of the stimulating effect of nursing on mother and baby, it is advisable to commence regular nursing within the first 12 hours postpartum. Most term infants thrive best when fed at intervals of about 4 hours. Preterm or growth-retarded infants require feedings at shorter intervals. In most instances, a 3-hour interval is satisfactory.

Circumcision

There is no absolute medical indication for routine circumcision of the newborn.

Screening for Disease

The following laboratory tests should be performed upon cord blood samples obtained at delivery from all newborns: (1) hematocrit, (2) blood type and Rh status, (3) direct Coombs test, and (4) a serologic test for syphilis. Phenylalanine screening on whole blood (after feeding) is required throughout the United States. A variety of other screening tests are required by law in some states. These tests include (1) screening tests for a variety of aminoacidurias, including leucine, isoleucine, homocysteine, and valine; (2) thyroid function tests; (3) hemoglobinopathies; and (4) galactosemia. Other similar screening tests probably will be added to this list in the future (Table 40–4).

Abnormalities of the Newborn Infant

These are considered in Chapters 55 and 59.

SUGGESTED READINGS

American Academy of Pediatrics Committee on Fetus and Newborn: Use and abuse of the Apgar score. Pediatrics 1986;78:1148.

American College of Obstetricians and Gynecologists Committee on Maternal and Fetal Medicine: Use and misuse of the Apgar Score. November, 1986.

American College of Obstetricians and Gynecologists: Control of Infections in Obstetric and Nursing Areas. Chap 6, p 128, in: *Guidelines for Perinatal Care,* 2nd ed. Washington, 1988.

Cunningham FG, MacDonald PC, Gant NF, Leveno KJ, and Gilstrap LC, III (editors): The Newborn Infant. Chapter 17 in *Williams Obstetrics,* 19th ed., Appleton & Lange, 1993.

Gilstrap LC, Leveno KJ, Burris J, Williams ML, Little BB: Diagnosis of birth asphyxia based on fetal pH, Apgar score, and newborn cerebral dysfunction. Am J Obstet Gynecol 1988;161:825.

Laga M et al: Prophylaxis of gonococcal and chlamydial ophthalmia neonatorum: A comparison of silver nitrate and tetracycline. N Engl J Med 1988;318:653.

Yeomans ER et al: Umbilical cord pH, PCO_2, and bicarbonate following uncomplicated term vaginal deliveries. Am J Obstet Gynecol 1985;151:798.

41

The Puerperium

The puerperium is the period of confinement just after birth, and the term has been extended to include the subsequent weeks during which the reproductive tract returns to its normal nonpregnant state. The plan for follow-up care generally practiced by most obstetricians—at least until recently—covers the 6 weeks following delivery. The "normal nonpregnant state" then includes those permanent structural changes in the cervix, vagina, and perineum that were acquired during labor and delivery. By 6 weeks after delivery or not much longer than that in women who are not breast feeding, pituitary-ovarian synchrony appropriate for resumption of ovulation is usually reestablished.

INVOLUTION OF THE UTERUS

Immediately after expulsion of the placenta, the fundus of the contracted uterus is about midway between the umbilicus and symphysis or slightly higher. The body of the uterus now consists mostly of myometrium covered by serosa and lined by basal decidua. The anterior and posterior walls are in close apposition, and each measures 4–5 cm in thickness. Because its vessels are compressed by the contracted myometrium, the puerperal uterus appears ischemic on section when compared with the reddish-purple hyperemic pregnant organ. During the next 2 days, the uterus remains approximately the same size and then shrinks, so that within 2 weeks it has descended into the cavity of the true pelvis and can no longer be felt above the symphysis. It normally regains its previous nonpregnant size within about 4 weeks.

Within 2 or 3 days after delivery, the decidua remaining in the uterus becomes differentiated into two layers. The superficial layer becomes necrotic and is sloughed in the lochia. The basal layer adjacent to the myometrium, which contains the fundi of endometrial glands, remains intact and is the source of new endometrium.

The process of endometrial regeneration is rapid except at the placental site. Elsewhere, the free surface becomes covered by epithelium within a week or 10 days, and the entire endometrium is restored during the third week.

Complete extrusion of the placental site takes up to 6 weeks. This process is of great clinical importance, since late puerperal hemorrhage may occur if it is defective. Immediately after delivery, the placental site is about the size of the palm of the hand, but it rapidly decreases in size until by the end of the second week it is 3–4 cm in diameter.

The vagina and vaginal outlet in the first part of the puerperium form a capacious, smooth-walled passage that gradually diminishes in size but rarely returns to its nulliparous dimensions. The rugae reappear by the third week. The hymen is represented by several small tags of tissue, which during cicatrization are converted into the myrtiform caruncles characteristic of parous women.

CHANGES IN THE ABDOMINAL WALL

As a result of rupture of the elastic fibers of the skin and the prolonged distention caused by the enlarged pregnant uterus, the abdominal walls remain soft and flabby for a while. The return to normal of these structures requires several weeks. Recovery is aided by exercise. Except for silvery striae, the abdominal wall usually resumes its prepregnancy appearance, but when the muscles are atonic, it may remain lax. There may be marked separation (diastasis) of the rectus muscles.

CHANGES IN THE URINARY TRACT

Cystoscopic examination soon after delivery shows not only edema and hyperemia of the bladder wall but, frequently, submucous extravasation of blood. In addition, the puerperal bladder has an increased capacity and a relative insensitivity to intravesical fluid pressure. Therefore, overdistention, incomplete emptying, and excessive residual urine must be watched for closely. The paralyzing effect of anesthesia—especially conduction analgesia—and the temporarily disturbed neural function of the bladder are undoubtedly contributory factors. Residual urine and bacteriuria in a traumatized bladder, coupled with the dilated renal pelves and ureters, create optimal conditions for the development of urinary tract infection. The dilated ureters and renal pelves return to the prepregnant state 2–8 weeks after delivery.

LACTATION

Colostrum

By the second postpartum day, a modest amount of colostrum—the liquid secreted by the breasts for the first 5 days after delivery—can be expressed from the nipples. Colostrum contains a higher percentage of protein—much of it globulin—than is present in milk and more minerals but less sugar and fat. Even so, colostrum contains rather large fat globules ("colostrum corpuscles") thought by some to be epithelial cells that have undergone fatty degeneration and by others to be mononuclear phagocytes containing fat. Colostrum undergoes gradual conversion to mature milk in about 5 days.

Antibodies are readily demonstrable in colostrum. Its content of immunoglobulin A may offer protection to the fetus against enteric infection.

Milk

The major components of milk are proteins, lactose, water, and fat. Milk is isotonic with plasma, with lactose accounting for half of the osmotic pressure. The major proteins in milk—α-lactalbumin, β-lactoglobulin, and casein—are synthesized in the rough endoplasmic reticulum of the alveolar secretory cell. The essential amino acids are derived from the blood, and nonessential amino acids are derived from the blood or synthesized in the mammary gland. Most of the proteins of milk are unique proteins not found elsewhere.

In normal circumstances, the quantity of flow and duration of lactation are controlled in large part by the repeated stimulus of nursing. Prolactin is essential for lactation; women with extensive pituitary necrosis, as in Sheehan syndrome, do not lactate (Chapter 50). Although plasma prolactin falls after delivery to lower levels than during pregnancy, each act of suckling triggers a rise in the prolactin level. Presumably, a stimulus from the breast curtails the release of prolactin-inhibiting factor from the hypothalamus, which in turn induces a transient increase in secretion of prolactin by the pituitary.

IMMUNOLOGIC CONSEQUENCES OF BREAST FEEDING

Antibodies are present in human colostrum and milk but are poorly absorbed—if at all—from the infant's gut. The predominant immunoglobulin in milk is secretory IgA, a macromolecule that is important in antimicrobial processes in the mucous membranes across which it is secreted. It is believed that secretory IgA in mother's milk may act locally within the infant's gastrointestinal tract. For example, milk contains secretory IgA antibodies against **Escherichia coli,** and it is known that breast-fed babies are less prone to enteric infections than bottle-fed babies. It has been suggested that IgA exerts its action by preventing bacterial adherence to epithelial cell surfaces, thus preventing tissue invasion.

Recent attention is being directed to a possible role of maternal lymphocytes in breast milk in fetal immunologic processes. It has been reported that human milk contains both T and B lymphocytes.

CLINICAL ASPECTS OF THE PUERPERIUM

IMMEDIATELY AFTER LABOR

After delivery of the placenta, the uterus should be firm, with its upper margin just below the umbilicus. As long as it remains in this condition, there is no danger of postpartum hemorrhage from uterine atony. To guard against such an occurrence, the uterus should be palpated through the abdominal wall at frequent intervals after completion of the third stage of labor (ie, delivery of the placenta). If relaxation is detected, the uterus should be massaged through the abdominal wall until it remains contracted. Blood may accumulate within the uterus without external evidence of bleeding. This condition may be detected early by identifying uterine enlargement through frequent palpation of the fundus during the first few hours postpartum. Since the likelihood of significant hemorrhage is greatest immediately postpartum, an attendant should remain with the mother for at least 1 hour after completion of the third stage of labor.

SUBSEQUENT DISCOMFORT

The discomfort from cesarean delivery and its causes and management are discussed in Chapter 52. During the first few days after vaginal delivery, the mother may be uncomfortable for a variety of reasons, including afterpains, episiotomy incisions, birth canal lacerations, breast engorgement, and, at times, postspinal headache. It is prudent to provide codeine, 60 mg, or aspirin, 600 mg, at intervals as frequent as every 3 hours when awake during the first few days after delivery. Uterine contractions are commonly accentuated during nursing, giving rise at times to troublesome afterpains (see below).

The repaired episiotomy or lacerations may be uncomfortable. Early application of an icebag to the perineum may minimize swelling. Most women also appear to obtain relief from periodic application of a local anesthetic spray at the site of episiotomy or laceration. Severe discomfort may mean that a sizable hematoma has formed in the genital tract. Therefore, careful examination is warranted, especially whenever oral analgesics do not provide sufficient relief. The episiotomy incision is normally firmly healed and nearly asymptomatic by the third week after delivery.

FEVER

Breast engorgement, which is common on the third or fourth day of the puerperium, may cause a rise in temperature. This so-called **milk fever** is caused by extreme vascular and lymphatic engorgement, but it does not last more than 24 hours. Any rise of body temperature in the puerperium implies infection, most likely somewhere in the genitourinary tract.

AFTERPAINS

In primiparas, the puerperal uterus tends to remain tonically contracted unless blood clots, fragments of placenta, or other foreign bodies are retained in its cavity, causing hypertonic contractions. In multiparas especially, the uterus often contracts vigorously at intervals, the contractions giving rise to painful sensations that occasionally are severe enough to require an analgesic. In some women, they may last for days. Afterpains are particularly noticeable when the infant suckles, presumably because of the release of oxytocin. They usually decrease in intensity and become quite mild by the third day after delivery.

LOCHIA

Beginning early in the puerperium, there is continued sloughing of decidual tissue that results in vaginal discharge of variable quantities of lochia. Microscopically lochia consists of erythrocytes, shreds of decidua, epithelial cells, and bacteria. Microorganisms are found in lochia pooled in the vagina and are present in most cases even in discharge from the uterine cavity.

For the first few days after delivery, the content of blood in the lochia is sufficient to color it red (lochia rubra). After 3 or 4 days, the lochia becomes progressively paler (lochia serosa). After the tenth day, because of a marked admixture with leukocytes and a reduced fluid content, the lochia assumes a white or yellowish-white color (lochia alba). Foul-smelling lochia may signal infection and should be investigated.

MICTURITION

Diuresis regularly occurs between the second and fifth days even when intravenous fluids were not massively infused during labor and delivery. Normal pregnancy is associated with an increase in extracellular water. Puerperal diuresis represents a reversal of this process as the fluid-retaining stimuli of pregnancy-induced hyperestrogenism and elevated venous pressure in the lower half of the body are removed and as residual hypervolemia is dissipated. In preeclampsia, both retention of fluid antepartum and diuresis postpartum may be greatly increased (Chapter 57).

The rate of accumulation of urine in the bladder after delivery may be quite variable. In most hospitals, intravenous fluids are nearly always infused during labor and for an hour or so after delivery. Oxytocin in antidiuretic doses is commonly infused in the intravenous fluid after the third stage of labor. As a consequence of the volume of fluid infused and the sudden withdrawal of the antidiuretic effect of oxytocin, rapid filling of the bladder is common. Moreover, both bladder sensation and the capability of the bladder to empty spontaneously may be diminished by anesthesia—especially conduction analgesia—and by painful lesions in the genital tract, such as extensive episiotomy, lacerations, or hematomas. It is not surprising, therefore, that urinary retention with overdistension of the bladder is a common complication of the early puerperium. Once overdistension occurs, bladder function becomes further impaired, and ascending infection of the urinary tract is a likely consequence.

BLOOD STUDIES

Leukocytosis occurs during and after labor, with counts sometimes as high as $30,000/\mu L$. The increase reflects chiefly granulocytes. There is relative lymphopenia and an absolute eosinopenia. Normally, during the first few days after delivery, the hemoglobin, hematocrit, and erythrocyte count fluctuate moderately. In general, however, if they fall much below the levels present just before or during early labor, the patient has lost a considerable amount of blood (Chapter 58). By 1 week after delivery, blood volume has returned to almost the usual nonpregnant level.

LOSS OF WEIGHT

In addition to the loss of an average of about 12 lb as a consequence of evacuation of the contents of the uterus and normal blood loss, there is generally further loss of body weight during the puerperium of about 5 lb. This weight loss is accounted for by fluid lost chiefly through urination, as described above.

MILD DEPRESSION

The mother may show some degree of depression a few days after delivery ("baby blues," "postpartum blues"), probably the result of a number of factors: (1) the emotional letdown following pregnancy and delivery, (2) the discomforts of the early puerperium, (3) fatigue from loss of sleep, (4) anxiety about her ability to care for the infant, and (5) fears that she has become less attractive. Anticipation, recognition, and reassurance are usually the only treatment required. If the problem persists or worsens, symptoms of psychotic depression are sought and psychiatric consultation is considered.

AMBULATION

Women are now out of bed well within the first 24 hours after vaginal delivery. The advantages of early ambulation are confirmed by well-controlled studies. Women feel better and stronger after early ambulation, and bladder complications and constipation are less frequent. Early ambulation has also reduced the incidence of thrombosis and pulmonary embolism during the puerperium. For the first ambulation at least, an attendant should be present in case of dizziness or fainting.

CARE OF THE BREASTS & NIPPLES

The nipples require little attention during the puerperium other than cleanliness and attention to fissures. Since dried milk is likely to accumulate and irritate the nipples, cleansing of the areolae with water and mild soap is helpful before and after nursing. Occasionally it is necessary to use a nipple shield for 24 hours or longer. A nursing brassiere that provides support without constriction is desirable. Suppression of lactation in the woman who does not nurse her infant is considered in Chapter 50.

IMMUNIZATIONS

The D-negative woman who is not isoimmunized and whose baby is D-positive is given 300 μg of anti-D immune globulin shortly after delivery (Chapter 55). Women who are not already immune to rubella or rubeola are candidates for vaccination before discharge. The mother should also receive a tetanus toxoid booster injection unless contraindicated.

TIME OF DISCHARGE

If there are no puerperal complications, hospitalization is seldom warranted for more than 3 days for primiparas and 2 days for multiparas. Indeed, because of hospitalization costs, many women request discharge after a 1-day stay. This is certainly acceptable as long as physician access is readily available and appropriate neonatal screening is performed for hypothyroidism, phenylketonuria, and other congenital disorders. Following uncomplicated postoperative cesarean delivery, the patient is usually ready for discharge on the fourth day, and in some hospitals earlier.

RETURN OF MENSTRUATION & OVULATION

If the woman does not nurse, menstrual flow will probably return within 6–8 weeks after delivery. At times, however, it is difficult clinically to predict a specific date for the first menstrual period after delivery. A minority of women bleed small to moderate amounts intermittently starting soon after delivery. Menses may not appear as long as nursing continues, but great variations are observed, since in lactating women the first period may occur as early as the second or as late as the 18th month after delivery. It has long been recognized that ovulation is much less frequent in women who breast feed than in those who do not. Nonetheless, pregnancy can occur during the period of lactation.

FOLLOW-UP CARE

By the time of discharge from the hospital after vaginal delivery and a normal in-hospital puerperium, the mother can resume most activities, including bathing, driving, and household functions. Although some obstetricians recommend that she not go back to work or school for several weeks, there is no evidence that doing so earlier causes any physical harm.

There is little scientific evidence on which to base recommendations about resumption of sexual activity. It is most unlikely that there are increased risks from intercourse after 2 weeks from the date of delivery except perhaps the risk of dyspareunia, which can be minimized by careful repair of the episiotomy.

Delay of examination of the mother until 6 weeks postpartum has become the standard practice of some obstetricians, but the reasons for waiting until that time are not altogether clear. It seems more reasonable to schedule appointments for follow-up examination during the third week following delivery. The third week is quite satisfactory both to identify any abnormalities of the later puerperium and to initiate contraceptive practices.

Family planning techniques and follow-up care are discussed further in Chapter 27.

SUGGESTED READINGS

The puerperium. Chapter 13 in: *Williams Obstetrics,* 19th ed. Cunningham FG, MacDonald PC, Gant NF, Leveno KJ, Gilstrap LC (editors). Appleton & Lange, 1993.

Management of Normal Pregnancy

42

Prenatal Care

The objective of prenatal care is to ensure that every wanted pregnancy culminates in the delivery of a healthy baby without impairing the health of the mother. It is self-evident that pregnancy should be considered a normal physiologic state. *It is essential for the physician who assumes responsibility for prenatal care to be familiar with the normal physiologic changes of pregnancy as well as the pathologic changes that may develop during pregnancy.*

NORMAL DURATION OF PREGNANCY

The mean duration of pregnancy calculated from the first day of the last normal menstrual period for a large number of healthy women has been identified to be very close to 280 days, or 40 weeks. It is customary to estimate the expected date of delivery by adding 7 days to the date of the first day of the last normal menstrual period and counting back 3 months (**Naegele's rule**). For example, if the woman's last menstrual period began on September 10, the expected date of delivery would be June 17. It is apparent that pregnancy is erroneously considered to have begun about 2 weeks before ovulation if the duration of pregnancy is so calculated from the first day of the last menstrual period. Nonetheless, clinicians persist in using **gestational age** or **menstrual age,** calculated from the first day of the last menstrual period, to identify temporal events in pregnancy; embryologists and other reproductive biologists more often employ **ovulatory age** or **fertilization age,** both of which are typically 2 weeks shorter.

It has become customary to divide pregnancy into three equal parts, or **trimesters,** of slightly more than 13 weeks (3 calendar months) each. There are certain major obstetric problems that cluster in each of these time periods. For example, most spontaneous abortions occur during the first trimester, whereas almost all cases of pregnancy-induced hypertension become clinically evident during the third trimester.

GENERAL PRINCIPLES OF PRENATAL CARE

Every word and every act by all health professionals who come in contact with the pregnant woman should im-

---

Definitions

Nulligravida: A woman who is not now and never has been pregnant.

Gravida: A woman who is or has been pregnant, irrespective of the pregnancy outcome. With the establishment of the first pregnancy, she becomes a primigravida and with successive pregnancies a multigravida.

Nullipara: A woman who has never completed a pregnancy beyond an abortion. She may or may not have had one or more spontaneous or elective abortions.

Primipara: A woman who has been delivered once of a fetus or fetuses that reached the stage of viability. Therefore, the completion of any pregnancy beyond the stage of abortion bestows parity upon the mother.

Multipara: A woman who has completed two or more pregnancies to the stage of viability. It is the number of pregnancies reaching viability and not the number of fetuses delivered that determines parity. Parity is not greater if a single fetus, twins, or quintuplets were delivered, nor lower If the fetus or fetuses were stillborn.

Parturient: A woman in labor.

Puerpera: A woman who has just given birth.

---

press upon her both the importance and the availability of prenatal care for her fetus and herself. Prenatal care should be initiated as soon as there is a reasonable likelihood of pregnancy. This may be as early as a few days after a missed menstrual period—especially for the woman who desires an abortion—but it should be no later than the second missed period for anyone.

At the initial visit, personnel familiar with obstetric care should attempt to identify and assess the following: (1) the probability of pregnancy (including urine testing for human chorionic gonadotropin when indicated); (2) the woman's desire for the pregnancy to continue; (3) any current health problems; (4) any previous major illnesses, including those in previous pregnancies; (5) the outcomes of previous pregnancies; and (6) all medications being taken. The woman is instructed to bring with her at the next visit a few days later all drugs she is currently taking.

Physical evaluation at the initial screening visit includes determination of blood pressure, height, and weight.

The following laboratory tests are initiated at the first visit:

(1) Hemoglobin concentration, hematocrit, platelet count, sickle cell screening for black women, glucose and creatinine concentration, serologic test for syphilis, identification of blood types and of antibodies to red cell antigens, and presence of antibody to rubella. The Centers for Disease Control as well as the American College of Obstetrics and Gynecology recommend routine screening for hepatitis B antigen.

(2) Urine glucose, protein, and screening of a clean-catch midstream urine specimen to identify significant bacteriuria.

A physician should be consulted whenever a problem is suspected that might require immediate attention. Any woman who is considering abortion should be offered counseling at this time.

Finally, the patient is given explicit instructions about how to get help promptly in case a problem develops. Either at the initial visit or at a subsequent visit within 2 weeks, a comprehensive general health examination should be done as described below. Previous health records and laboratory data are reviewed at that time.

INITIAL COMPREHENSIVE EVALUATION

The major goals of the initial health examination are (1) to define the health status of the mother and fetus, (2) to determine the gestational age of the fetus, and (3) to initiate a plan for continuing obstetric care. Once the health status of the mother and fetus has been defined, the initial plan for subsequent care may range from relatively infrequent routine visits to prompt hospitalization because of serious maternal or fetal disease.

History

In general, history taking from the pregnant woman proceeds as for any medical patient. It is mandatory that all data important to the care of the mother and fetus be clearly recorded so that all members of the health care team who use the record can interpret them correctly.

The menstrual history is extremely important. The woman who spontaneously menstruates regularly every 28 days or so is most likely to ovulate at midcycle. Thus, the gestational age (menstrual age) becomes simply the number of weeks since the onset of the last menstrual period. Without regular, predictable, cyclic, spontaneous menses that suggest ovulatory cycles, accurate dating of pregnancy by physical examination is difficult. Thus, it is important to ascertain whether or not steroidal contraceptives were used before the pregnancy and, if so, when.

Obstetric Examination

The cervix is inspected with a speculum lightly lubricated with water. Next, in order to identify cytologic abnormalities, specimens are obtained by gentle swabbing from the lower half of the cervical canal and a scraping from the squamocolumnar junction, spread on slides, and

fixed immediately in ether-alcohol or with an appropriate aerosol spray. The outer half of the cervical canal is again swabbed slowly to obtain material for culture to identify **Neisseria gonorrhoeae.**

The character of vaginal secretions is noted. A moderate amount of white mucoid discharge is normal.

The speculum is then removed and the digital pelvic examination is completed by palpation, with special attention paid to the consistency, length, and dilatation of the cervix; to the fetal presenting part, especially if late in pregnancy; to the bony architecture of the pelvis; and to any anomalies of the vagina and perineum, including cystocele, rectocele, and relaxed or torn perineum. The vulva and contiguous structures are also carefully inspected. (The pelvic examination is described in more detail in Chapter 44.)

Physical Examination

The general physical examination should be thorough as for any complete medical examination.

Further Instructions

After the history and physical examination have been completed, the expectant mother is instructed about diet, relaxation and sleep, bowel habits, exercise, bathing, clothing, recreation, smoking, drug and alcohol ingestion, and follow-up visits, including steps to take if an appointment is missed. Usually it is possible to assure her that she may anticipate an uneventful pregnancy followed by an uncomplicated delivery. At the same time, she is tactfully instructed about the following danger signals, which must be reported immediately, day or night:

1. Any vaginal bleeding
2. Swelling of the face or fingers
3. Severe or continuous headache
4. Dimness or blurring of vision
5. Abdominal pain
6. Persistent vomiting
7. Chills or fever
8. Dysuria
9. Escape of fluid from the vagina
10. Marked change in frequency or intensity of fetal movements

SUBSEQUENT PRENATAL CARE

RETURN VISITS

Subsequent prenatal examinations have traditionally been scheduled at intervals of 4 weeks until 28 weeks, then every 2 weeks until 36 weeks, and then weekly thereafter. Often, however, important information can be gained from a more flexible appointment schedule.

In essentially all pregnancies, the fetal heart may be first heard between 16 and 19 weeks of gestation when carefully listened for with a DeLee fetal stethoscope (Chapter 45). Obviously, the ability of the examiner to hear unamplified fetal heart sounds will depend upon several factors, including the patient size and the examiner's hearing acuity.

Measurement of the height of the uterine fundus above the symphysis can provide useful information. Between 20 and 31 weeks of gestation, the fundal height in centimeters usually equals the gestational age in weeks. The bladder must be emptied before making the measurement.

GESTATIONAL AGE

For the great majority of pregnancies, the most important question to be answered through prenatal examination is, "How old is the fetus?" Fortunately, it is possible to identify the gestational age of the fetus with considerable precision through an appropriately timed, carefully performed clinical examination coupled with information about the date of onset of the last menstrual period. When the date of onset of the last menstrual period and the fundal height are repeatedly in temporal agreement, the duration of gestation can be firmly established. When gestational age cannot be clearly identified, sonography is likely to be of considerable value (Chapter 43).

PRENATAL SURVEILLANCE

History & Physical Examination

At each return visit, steps are taken to identify the wellbeing of both the patient and her fetus. Certain information—obtained by interrogation and by examination—is especially important in this regard:

A. Fetal:
  1. Fetal heart rate(s)
  2. Size of fetus(es), actual and rate of change
  3. Amount of amnionic fluid
  4. Presenting part and station (late in pregnancy)
  5. Fetal activity
B. Maternal:
  1. Blood pressure, actual and extent of change
  2. Weight, actual and amount of change
  3. Symptoms, including headache, altered vision, abdominal pain, nausea and vomiting, vaginal bleeding, discharge of fluid from the vagina, and dysuria
  4. Distance to the uterine fundus from the symphysis
  5. A carefully performed vaginal examination late in pregnancy often provides valuable information concerning the presenting part and its station as well as cervical consistency, dilatation, and effacement.

Subsequent Laboratory Tests

If the initial results were normal, most of the procedures need not be repeated. Hematocrit determination and the serologic test for syphilis, if syphilis is prevalent in the population cared for, should be repeated at about 28–32 weeks of gestation.

Determination of maternal serum α-fetoprotein concentration at 16–18 weeks is recommended to screen for open neural tube defects and some chromosomal anomalies. Precise knowledge of gestational age is paramount for accuracy of this screening test (see Chapter 54).

For women at risk for gestational diabetes, screening for glucose intolerance is recommended between 24 and 28 weeks by the American College of Obstetricians and Gynecologists. Following a 50-g oral glucose challenge, if plasma glucose at 1 hour exceeds 140 mg/dL, then a 3-hour 100-g test is recommended (see Chapter 60). Some recommend that all women be given a 1-hour 50-g glucose challenge. For women without risk factors for gestational diabetes, a random plasma glucose determination can be used to rule out overt diabetes.

Other screening tests may be applied selectively to populations at high risk for the condition sought. For example, serologic testing for human immunodeficiency virus should be performed for women who take illicit intravenous drugs or who may be at risk for other reasons (see Chapter 60). Any woman who desires testing for HIV should be screened.

Women at high risk for sexually transmitted diseases may benefit from cultures to identify *Chlamydia trachomatis* infections.

WEIGHT GAIN & NUTRITION DURING PREGNANCY

It generally is recommended that pregnant women gain around 10–12 kg (22–27 lb) during pregnancy. Of the recommended additional weight, normal physiologic events account cumulatively for about 9 kg as fetus, placenta, amnionic fluid, uterine hypertrophy, increase in maternal blood volume, breast enlargement, and dependent edema as a result of mechanical factors. The remainder appears to be mostly maternal fat. In most pregnant women, this result may be achieved by eating, according to appetite, a diet adequate in calories, protein, essential fatty acids, minerals, and vitamins. Seldom, if ever, should maternal weight gain be restricted below this level. Indeed, failure of a small or normal-sized pregnant woman to gain weight is an ominous sign.

The Food and Nutrition Board of the National Research Council periodically recommends dietary allowances for women, including those who are pregnant or lactating. In addition to 300 kcal and 30 g/d of protein, all of the recommended increases, with the exception of iron, can be supplied by eating a normal diet.

Of the approximately 300 mg of iron transferred to the fetus and placenta and the 500 mg incorporated, if available, into the expanding maternal hemoglobin mass, nearly all is utilized during the latter half of pregnancy. During that time, the average iron requirements imposed by the pregnancy itself are about 6 mg/d, and there is in addition a need for nearly 1 mg to compensate for maternal excretion—a total of about 7 mg of iron daily. Few women have sufficient iron stores to supply this amount of iron. Moreover, the diet seldom contains enough iron to meet this demand.

Therefore, every pregnant woman should be given at least 30 mg of elemental iron supplied as the simple iron salt, such as ferrous gluconate, sulfate, or fumarate. This amount should be taken once daily throughout the latter half of pregnancy and while lactating.

The practice of supplying vitamin supplements prenatally is a deeply ingrained habit of many obstetricians even though scientific evidence to show that the usual vitamin supplements are of benefit to either the mother or her fetus is quite meager. The Committee on Maternal Nutrition of the National Research Council has pointed out that in most cases routine pharmaceutical supplementation of vitamin and mineral preparations to pregnant women is of doubtful value, except for iron and perhaps folic acid.

Such vitamin and mineral preparations should of course not be regarded as substitutes for food.

GENERAL HYGIENE

EXERCISE

In general, it is not necessary for the pregnant woman to limit exercise provided she does not become excessively fatigued or risk injury to herself or her fetus. The American College of Obstetricians and Gynecologists recommends that women who are accustomed to aerobic exercise before pregnancy should be allowed to continue this activity during pregnancy. It cautions, however, against starting new aerobic exercise programs or intensifying training efforts. For example, in women who previously were sedentary, aerobic activity more strenuous than walking is not recommended because of possible injury.

With some pregnancy complications, the mother and her fetus may benefit from a very sedentary existence; for example, women with pregnancy-induced hypertension appear to do so (see Chapter 57).

EMPLOYMENT

Nearly half of all women of childbearing age in the United States are now in the labor force, and even larger proportions of socioeconomically less fortunate women are working. Common sense dictates that any occupation that subjects the pregnant woman to severe physical strain should be avoided. Ideally, no work or play associated with undue fatigue should be continued. Adequate periods of rest should be provided during the working day. Women with a history of complications of pregnancy that are likely to occur again (eg, low-birth-weight infants) probably should minimize physical work.

TRAVEL

Travel is not contraindicated for the pregnant woman who has no complications. Travel in pressurized aircraft offers no unusual risk. At least every 2 hours, the pregnant woman should walk about. Perhaps the greatest risk with travel—especially international travel—is the development of a complication in a region remote from facilities adequate for treatment.

COITUS

Whenever abortion or preterm labor is a threat, coitus should be avoided. Otherwise, it has been generally accepted that in healthy pregnant women sexual intercourse usually does no harm before the last 4 weeks or so of pregnancy. It has long been the custom of many obstetricians to recommend abstinence from intercourse during the last 4 weeks of pregnancy—a recommendation undoubtedly not followed in many instances.

IMMUNIZATION

There has been some concern over the safety of various immunization techniques during pregnancy. The recommendations of the American College of Obstetricians and Gynecologists with appropriate updating for specific immunizations during pregnancy are summarized in Table 42–1.

SMOKING

Mothers who smoke during pregnancy frequently bear smaller infants than do nonsmokers. There is also evidence that smoking mothers have a significantly greater number of unsuccessful pregnancies because of an increase in perinatal deaths. In view of the obvious dangers to people who smoke, cigarettes should be avoided completely by women irrespective of any deleterious effects on pregnancy.

ALCOHOL

Excessive ingestion of alcohol by the expectant mother is likely to produce abnormalities in the fetus. Chronic alcoholism can lead to fetal maldevelopment, commonly referred to as **fetal alcohol syndrome,** the features of which

Table 42–1. Summary of recommendations for immunization during pregnancy.

Live virus vaccines
    Measles—contraindicated
    Mumps—contraindicated
    Poliomyelitis—not routine; increased risk exposure
    Rubella—contraindicated
    Yellow fever—travel to endemic areas
Inactivated virus vaccines
    Influenza—serious underlying disease
    Rabies—same as nonpregnant
Inactivated bacterial vaccines
    Cholera—to meet international travel requirements
    Meningococcal meningitis—same as nonpregnant
    Plague—selective vaccination of exposed persons
    Typhoid fever—travel to endemic areas
Toxoids
    Tenanus-diphtheria—same as nonpregnant
Hyperimmune globulins
    Hepatitis B—postexposure prophylaxis: give along with hepatitis B vaccine initially, then vaccine alone at 1 and 6 months.
    Rabies—postexposure prophylaxis
    Tetanus—postexposure prophylaxis
    Varicella—same as nonpregnant
Pooled immune globulins
    Hepatitis A—postexposure prophylaxis
    Measles—postexposure prophylaxis

are discussed in Chapter 55. Women with chronic and severe drinking problems must be discouraged from becoming pregnant until these problems are brought under control. Serious consideration should be given to early pregnancy termination in alcoholic women.

Differences of opinion persist in regard to the possible adverse effects on the fetus from social drinking. Evidence has been presented, however, that a linear relationship between alcohol consumption and fetal damage exists. From the evidence available, the best advice to the woman who is pregnant or contemplating pregnancy would seem to be not to drink alcohol during pregnancy.

CAFFEINE

In 1980, the Food and Drug Administration advised pregnant women to limit caffeine intake. The Fourth International Caffeine Workshop concluded shortly thereafter that there was no evidence that caffeine increased teratogenic or reproductive risk. Most studies of human pregnancy report no association between caffeine consumption and birth defects or low birth weight.

RECREATIONAL DRUGS

Any patient suspected of using "street drugs" should be considered to be using not one drug but a variety. Cocaine and "crack cocaine" have been associated with an increased incidence of fetal growth retardation, placental abruption, and more disturbingly, an abnormal neurologic development in the infant following birth. Depending upon state laws, any patient suspected of drug abuse in pregnancy may be screened, and if the drug test is positive, active attempts at withdrawal from the drug should be instituted.

MEDICATIONS

With rare exceptions, any drug that exerts a systemic effect in the mother will cross the placenta to reach the embryo and fetus. Some drugs commonly ingested during pregnancy and their possible adverse fetal effects are considered in Chapter 54.

COMMON COMPLAINTS

NAUSEA & VOMITING

Nausea and vomiting are common complaints during the first half of pregnancy. Typically, nausea and vomiting commence between the first and second missed menstrual period and continue until about the time of the fourth missed period. Nausea and vomiting are usually worse in the morning but may continue throughout the day.

The genesis of pregnancy-induced nausea and vomiting is not clear. It may be that the hormonal changes of pregnancy are responsible. Chorionic gonadotropin, for instance, has been implicated on the basis that its levels are rather high at the same time that nausea and vomiting are most common. Moreover, in women with hydatidiform mole, in whom levels of chorionic gonadotropin typically are much higher than in normal pregnancy, nausea and vomiting are often prominent clinical features. Emotional factors undoubtedly contribute to the severity of the nausea and vomiting of pregnancy. Very infrequently, vomiting may be so severe that dehydration, electrolyte and acid-base disturbances, and starvation become serious problems.

Seldom is the treatment of nausea and vomiting of pregnancy so successful that the affected expectant mother is afforded complete relief. However, the unpleasantness and discomfort can usually be minimized. Eating small feedings at more frequent intervals but stopping short of satiation is of value. A combination of doxylamine succinate plus pyridoxine (Bendectin) was given for many years for pregnancy-induced nausea and vomiting, but the preparation is no longer available because of legal concerns. Promethazine or prochlorperazine suppositories can be prescribed for severe nausea and vomiting.

The syndrome of severe nausea and vomiting requiring hospitalization for successful management is referred to as **hyperemesis gravidarum.** Prompt correction of fluid and electrolyte imbalances usually relieves the symptoms.

Therapeutic abortion for management of this problem is rarely required.

VARICOSITIES

Varicosities, generally resulting from congenital predisposition, are exaggerated by prolonged standing, pregnancy, and advancing age. Varicosities usually become more prominent as pregnancy advances, as weight increases, and as the length of time spent upright is increased. As shown in Figure 42–1, these may be severe. The symptoms produced by varicosities vary from cosmetic blemishes on the lower extremities and mild discomfort at the end of the day to severe discomfort that requires prolonged rest with the feet elevated.

The treatment of varicosities of the lower extremities during pregnancy is generally limited to periodic rest with elevation of the legs, or use of elastic stockings, or both. Surgical correction during pregnancy generally is not advised, though the symptoms rarely may be so severe that injection, ligation, or even stripping of the veins is necessary to keep the patient ambulatory.

Occasionally, **superficial thrombophlebitis** complicates preexisting varicose veins. Treatment is discussed in Chapter 50.

HEMORRHOIDS

Varicosities of rectal veins occasionally first appear during pregnancy. More often, pregnancy causes exacerbation or recurrence of previous symptoms. Aggravation of hemorrhoids during pregnancy is undoubtedly related to increased pressure in the rectal veins caused by obstruction of venous return by the large pregnant uterus and to the tendency toward constipation during pregnancy. Pain and swelling are usually relieved by topically applied anesthetics, warm soaks, and agents that soften the stool.

HEARTBURN

Heartburn—one of the most common complaints of pregnant women—usually is caused by reflux of gastric or duodenal contents into the lower esophagus. The in-

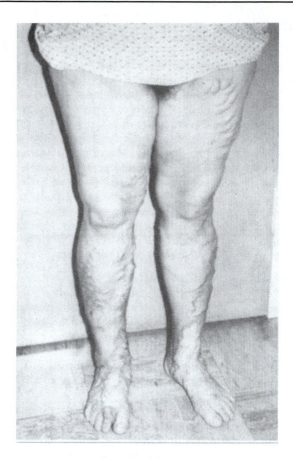

Figure 42–1. Massive varices during pregnancy in a multiparous woman. Well-fitting support hose provided considerable relief until surgical correction was performed late in the puerperium.

creased frequency of regurgitation during pregnancy most likely results from upward displacement and compression of the stomach by the uterus combined with decreased gastrointestinal motility. In some pregnant women, the cardia actually herniates through the diaphragm. In most case, symptoms are mild and relieved by a regimen of more frequent but smaller meals and avoidance of bending over or lying flat. Antacid preparations may provide relief.

SUGGESTED READINGS

American College of Obstetricians and Gynecologists: Immunization during pregnancy. Tech Bull No. 160, October 1991.

American College of Obstetricians and Gynecologists: Management of diabetes mellitus in pregnancy. Tech Bull No. 92, March 1986.

American College of Obstetricians and Gynecologists: Women and exercise. Tech Bull No. 87, September 1986.

Centers for Disease Control: Prevention of perinatal transmission of hepatitis B virus: Prenatal screening of all pregnant women for hepatitis B surface antigen. MMWR 1988;37:341.

43

Evaluation of Fetal Health

A number of social factors, including overall better nutrition and improved economic status, have contributed to a remarkable decrease in neonatal mortality and morbidity rates in the past 30 years. Broader availability of prenatal care and advances in medical technology have also contributed to this desirable result. The technologic advances useful in fetal monitoring are the subject of this chapter.

AMNIOCENTESIS

The ability to enter the amnionic sac without undue risk to the mother or fetus has influenced obstetric care remarkably.

Risks

The three major risks from amniocentesis are (1) trauma to the fetus, to the placenta, or, less often, to the umbilical cord or maternal structures; (2) infection; and (3) abortion or preterm labor. Surgical asepsis is mandatory.

Anti-D globulin (Rh_o D immune globulin) is commonly administered to nonsensitized Rh(D)-negative women at the time of amniocentesis (see Chapter 55).

Several attempts have been made to identify the overall risk of amniocentesis performed near mid pregnancy. In one study, however, no significant differences were found in fetal loss rate, birth weights, birth defects, neonatal complications, or growth and development at 1 year of age. The overall fetal loss was 3.5% for the amniocentesis group and 3.2% for the control group. The overall accuracy of prenatal diagnosis was 99.4%.

Bloody Tap

Blood contaminating the amnionic fluid may complicate the techniques for study and the interpretation of the results. Erythrocytes may inhibit the replication in culture of fetal cells from amnionic fluid. Moreover, blood may change the apparent level of various constituents of amnionic fluid under study, especially α-fetoprotein from fetal blood.

ASSESSMENT OF AMNIONIC FLUID SURFACTANT (Fetal Lung Maturity)

Amniocentesis was initially employed chiefly to estimate the concentration of bilirubin or bilirubin-like pigment in amnionic fluid and in that way to identify hemolytic disease in the fetus (see Chapter 55). Currently, it probably is used most often to determine the relative concentration of surfactant-active phospholipids as a means of determining whether the fetus has or has not developed lung maturity.

Several tests have been developed to predict mature or immature fetal lungs.

Lecithin-Sphingomyelin (L/S) Ratio

Before 34 weeks of gestation, lecithin and sphingomyelin are present in amnionic fluid in similar concentrations. At about 34 weeks, the concentration of lecithin relative to sphingomyelin begins to rise. With an L/S ratio greater than 2, the risk of respiratory distress is slight unless the mother has diabetes.

Obviously, there are times when the risk to the fetus from a hostile intrauterine environment will be greater than the risk of death from respiratory distress, even though the L/S ratio is less than 2.

Phosphatidylglycerol

Surfactant action insufficient to prevent respiratory distress, even though the L/S ratio is 2, is thought to be due in part to lack of phosphatidylglycerol and thus absence of its enhancement of surface-active properties. The identification of phosphatidylglycerol in amnionic fluid provides substantial assurance—but not a guarantee—that respiratory distress will not develop.

Phosphatidylglycerol has not been detected in blood, meconium, and vaginal secretions; consequently, these contaminants do not confuse the interpretation.

Foam Stability (Shake) Test

To reduce the time and effort inherent in precise measurement of the L/S ratio, the foam stability test, or so-called shake test, is recommended. The test depends upon the ability of surfactant in amnionic fluid, when mixed appropriately with ethanol, to generate stable foam at the air-liquid interface. The technique takes no more than 30 minutes to complete. If the ring of foam persists for 15 minutes, the risk of respiratory distress is very low. There are, however, two problems with the test: (1) slight contamination of amnionic fluid, reagents, or glassware—or errors in measurement—may alter the test results markedly; and (2) false-negative tests are rather common—ie, failure of the ring of foam to persist intact for 15 minutes in the tube containing diluted amnionic fluid is not necessarily predictive of respiratory distress.

AMNIOCENTESIS TO IDENTIFY INHERITED DISORDERS

These disorders are discussed in Chapter 54.

FETAL BLOOD SAMPLING[1]

PERCUTANEOUS UMBILICAL BLOOD SAMPLING (Cordocentesis)

Percutaneous umbilical blood sampling has revolutionized the diagnosis and therapy of fetal disorders. Although the technique is not simple (Figure 43–1), the indications for the procedure are increasing rapidly, and any list provided here would be outdated by the time of its publication. While genetic indications are expanding most rapidly, the procedure is also being used for diagnosis and treatment of fetal hypoxia and isoimmunization.[1]

REAL-TIME SONOGRAPHY

Real-time sonography has proved valuable for monitoring the products of conception in a variety of ways that include the following:

(1) Very early identification of intrauterine pregnancy.
(2) Demonstration of the size and rate of growth of the amnionic sac and the embryo.
(3) Identification of multiple fetuses, including conjoined twins.
(4) Measurements of the fetal head, abdominal circumference, femur, and other anatomic landmarks.
(5) Detection of fetal anomalies.
(6) Demonstration of hydramnios or oligohydramnios.

(7) Identification of the location, size, and "maturity" of the placenta.
(8) Demonstration of placental abnormalities such as hydatidiform mole.
(9) Identification of uterine tumors or anomalous development.
(10) Detection of a foreign body such as an intrauterine device.

FETAL SURVEILLANCE USING REAL-TIME SONOGRAPHY

Using real-time sonography, fetal breathing can be seen and the fetal heartbeat demonstrated as early as 7 weeks of gestation, trunk movement as early as 8 weeks, and limb movement as early as 9 weeks. Filling and intermittent emptying of the fetal urinary bladder are especially obvious with real-time sonography. Sonographic confirmation of fetal movements, fetal tone, fetal breathing, and the presence of normal amounts of amnionic fluid provides evidence of fetal well-being (see Biophysical Profile, below).

DOPPLER ULTRASOUND

Doppler ultrasound is used most commonly as an office procedure to detect fetal heart tones as early as 10–12 weeks of gestation. It is also used to detect the movement of red blood cells in vessels, and this principle is used to assess—directly or indirectly—a variety of altered measurements of blood flow within maternal and fetal vessels. For example, using the Doppler effect, the velocity of blood in a vessel can be measured.

DETERMINATION OF INDEXED FLOW FROM WAVEFORM ANALYSIS

Doppler waveforms of vessels have been described in a variety of ways, but all are based upon the relationship between systole and diastole. The most common measurements are some variation of the systolic/diastolic ratio. Ratios have been used to reduce the same potential error factors in the numerator and denominator. The use of a ratio obviates most problems of measuring the angle of insonation. Thus, indirectly determined indices are not measurements of actual flow; however, they may provide useful information about flow.

Systolic/Diastolic Ratio

The systolic/diastolic ratio—also known as the S/D ratio, the A/B ratio, or the Stuart index—is the simplest index to calculate. It is arrived at by dividing the maximal

---

[1]Fetal scalp blood sampling is discussed on p 338; fetoscopically directed blood sampling has been replaced by cordocentesis.

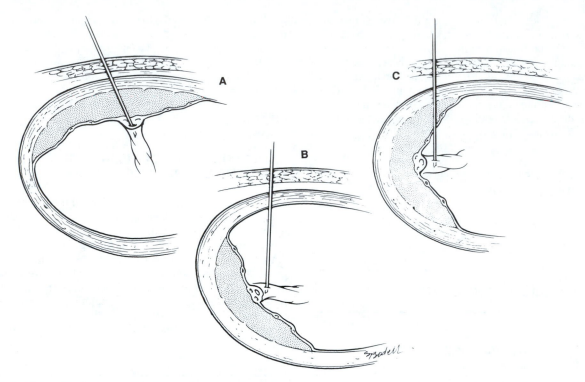

Figure 43–1. Umbilical cord blood sampling. Access to the umbilical artery or vein varies, depending upon both the placental location and the position of cord insertion into the placenta. *A:* With an anterior placenta, the needle may traverse the placenta. *B:* With a posterior implantation, the needle usually passes through the amnionic fluid before penetrating an umbilical vessel. *C:* With a lateral or fundal placenta, the needle may pass through the placenta and amnionic cavity to enter the umbilical vessel. (Redrawn after Queenan JT, King JC: Intrauterine transfusion for severe Rh-EBF: Past and future. Contemp Ob/Gyn 1987;30:51.)

systolic Doppler shift by the end-diastolic shift and is most often determined from measurements of the maternal uterine or fetal umbilical artery, using either pulsed or continuous-wave Doppler (Figure 43–2). In both vessels, the index gradually decreases as gestation progresses. Since larger fetal vessels have low or absent diastolic flow, the systolic/diastolic ratio is not useful for assessing fetal aortic blood flow.

Pourcelot or Resistance Index

The Pourcelot index is the difference in systolic and diastolic shifts divided by the systolic value ($[S-D])/S$. The index is best used in studies of umbilical and uterine arteries, since low diastolic values limit or prevent its use in the fetal aorta or other vessels without significant continuous diastolic flows.

Pulsatility Index

This index usually is calculated as the difference in systolic and diastolic shifts divided by the mean of the systolic and diastolic shifts ($[S-D]$/mean), which requires digitized waveform analysis for calculating the mean of the frequencies represented. Because of the mean value in the denominator, this index can be used for low- or no-diastolic-flow vessels such as the fetal descending aorta.

CLINICAL APPLICATIONS OF DOPPLER ULTRASOUND

Applications of this technology are discussed throughout this book in relation to its use in the diagnosis and management of a variety of pregnancy complications.

ASSESSMENT OF FETAL CARDIAC FUNCTION

The measurement of fetal cardiac function with Doppler ultrasound has immediate clinical importance. For example, the mean right ventricular output has been determined to be 307 mL per kg per minute and the left ventricular output 232 mL per kg per minute (right- to left-ventricular output ratio 55:45). Reversible ductal constriction has been observed in three fetuses whose mothers received indomethacin for treatment of preterm labor, whereas such changes were not observed in 25 normal pregnancies. Using a variety of techniques, several groups have reported convincing evidence that fetal cardiac arrhythmias can be diagnosed and appropriately treated in utero.

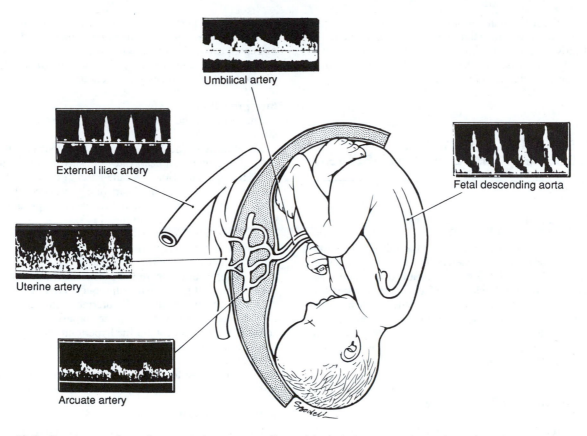

Figure 43–2. Doppler waveforms from normal pregnancy. Shown (clockwise) are normal waveforms from the maternal arcuate, uterine, and external iliac arteries and from the fetal umbilical artery and descending aorta. Reversed end-diastolic flow velocity is apparent in the external iliac artery, whereas continuous diastolic flow characterizes the uterine and arcuate vessels. Continuous "negative" flow in the umbilical waveform segment is from the umbilical vein, whose direction of flow is opposite that of the artery. Finally, note the greatly diminished end-diastolic flow in the fetal descending aorta. (Modified from Copel J and colleagues: Williams Supplement No. 16. Appleton & Lange, January/February, 1988.)

ASSESSMENT OF FETAL WELL-BEING

The use of Doppler measurements of blood flow is considered in the discussion of specific clinical conditions elsewhere in this book, eg, fetal growth retardation (Chapter 59), postterm pregnancy (Chapter 59), and pregnancy-induced hypertension (Chapter 57).

IMAGING STUDIES

RADIOGRAPHY, AMNIOGRAPHY, & FETOGRAPHY

These techniques have been almost completely abandoned since the advent of sonography.

MAGNETIC RESONANCE IMAGING

Use of MRI during pregnancy appears to be safe for the fetus and mother. However, the conclusion of the National Institutes of Health Consensus Development Conference was that "pregnant women, especially early in pregnancy, not undergo the procedure unless they have a clear medical need that cannot be resolved by other means."

ASSESSMENT OF FETAL MOVEMENTS & WELL-BEING

The fetus that is felt by the mother late in pregnancy to move consistently, is most often healthy. Conversely, a sudden decrease in fetal movements is a sign of fetal distress. The absolute number of movements per day appears to be less important than a marked change in frequency of fetal movements. In the case of cessation of fetal movements, fetal heart sounds have been observed commonly to disappear within the next 24 hours.

ANTEPARTUM BIOPHYSICAL ASSESSMENT OF FETAL WELL-BEING

Changes in the fetal heart rate can be used in two ways to evaluate fetal well-being. One is commonly referred to as the **contraction stress test** and the other as the **nonstress test,** or fetal heart acceleration test. A third antepartum test of fetal well-being that has gained widespread acceptance is the **biophysical profile.** The profile consists of a nonstress test plus three to five other assessments of fetal well-being, which include amnionic fluid volume, fetal respiratory motions, fetal tone, fetal movement, and placental grading. Four of the latter five parameters can be obtained only with real-time ultrasound equipment.

CONTRACTION STRESS TEST

The fetal heart rate is recorded from an externally placed ultrasound transducer. Uterine activity is identified with an external tocographic transducer. Although actual intrauterine pressure is not recorded, the onset, the time of maximum intensity, and the cessation of the contraction can be identified with reasonable precision. The maternal blood pressure is recorded initially and at least every 10 minutes during the procedure.

Baseline uterine activity and fetal heart rate are recorded for 15–20 minutes. If, by chance, spontaneous uterine contractions that last 40–60 seconds and recur approximately three times in 10 minutes are detected, the response of the fetal heart rate to the contractions is evaluated as described below. In the absence of demonstrable spontaneous uterine activity, oxytocin is usually administered intravenously. The initial rate of infusion of 0.5 mU per min through a constant-speed infusion pump is doubled every 15–20 minutes until uterine contractions lasting 40–60 seconds with a frequency of three every 10 minutes are established.

To avoid the difficulties associated with the intravenous infusion of oxytocin and yet stimulate the uterus to contract somewhat, the breast stimulation or, more correctly, the **nipple stimulation test,** has been employed. The basis for the test presumably was that tactile stimulation of the nipple would stimulate the release of exogenous oxytocin from the neurohypophysis.

Indications & Contraindications

The following conditions may contraindicate the use of oxytocin—and perhaps nipple stimulation—to perform a contraction stress test: (1) threatened preterm labor, (2) placenta previa, (3) hydramnios, (4) multiple fetuses, (5) rupture of the membranes, (6) previous preterm labor, and (7) previous classical cesarean section.

Interpretation

The results of the contraction stress test have been classified as follows:

A. Positive: There is consistent and persistent late deceleration of the fetal heart rate—ie, slowing of the heart rate develops some time after the onset of the uterine contraction, the nadir for the heart rate is reached after the peak of uterine contraction, and recovery occurs after the contraction is completed (Figure 43–3).

B. Negative: At least three contractions in 10 minutes, each lasting at least 40 seconds, are identified without late deceleration of the fetal heart rate.

C. Suspicious: There are inconsistent late decelerations that do not persist with subsequent contractions.

D. Hyperstimulation: If uterine contractions are more frequent than every 2 minutes or last longer than 90 seconds, or if persistent uterine hypertonus is suspected, a late deceleration does not necessarily indicate uteroplacental disease.

E. Unsatisfactory: The frequency of contractions is less than three per 10 minutes, or the tracing is poor.

False-Negative Tests

It is now apparent that a negative contraction stress test is usually (not always) compatible with uteroplacental function sufficient to maintain the fetus alive in utero for at least another week.

False-Positive Tests

The high false-positive rate with the contraction stress test is troublesome. Therefore, most advocates of the test recommend use of other tests, including assessment of fetal heart rate accelerations in response to fetal movement (see Nonstress Test, below). Most often, the fetus is not in serious jeopardy if the fetal heart rate accelerates with fetal movement and the contraction stress test is usually repeated within 24 hours.

Others recommend a biophysical profile (see below) or at least an ultrasonic evaluation of amnionic fluid volume before deciding that the contraction stress test is falsely positive. The presence of a positive contraction stress test along with a nonreactive fetal heart rate pattern is associated with serious fetal malformations often enough that real-time ultrasound screening for fetal anomalies is recommended by some.

NONSTRESS TEST

Fetal movement typically is accompanied by transient acceleration of the fetal heart rate. This phenomenon serves as the basis for the "nonstress test," or fetal heart acceleration test.

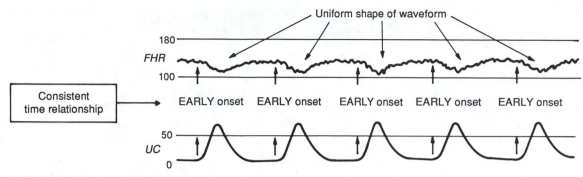

A. Early deceleration (HC) Uniform shape – early timing

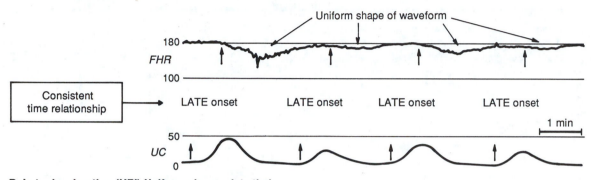

B. Late deceleration (UPI) Uniform shape – late timing

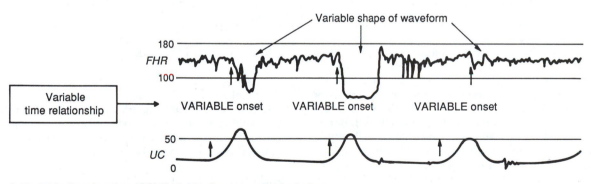

C. Variable deceleration (CC) Variable shape – variable timing

Figure 43–3. Fetal heart rate decelerations in relation to the time of onset of uterine contractions. HC, head compression; UPI, uteroplacental insufficiency; CC, cord compression. (Reproduced, with permission, from Hon EH: *An Atlas of Fetal Heart Rate Patterns.* Harty, 1968.)

An ultrasonic transducer to detect the fetal heartbeat is placed as described for the oxytocin test. Each time fetal movement is felt by the mother, she presses a button to record the instant of movement on the same moving paper strip the heart rate is being recorded on.

Interpretation

The nonstress test is generally considered normal when two or more fetal movements are accompanied by acceleration of the fetal heart rate of 15 beats per min for at least 15 seconds' duration within a 20-minute period (Figure 43–4). A nonreactive tracing is one without acceptable fetal heart rate accelerations over a 40-minute period. These are the most widely accepted criteria for a normal test, but many variations have been offered. Absence of fetal movements is considered unsatisfactory for testing, but prolonged absence of movements is an ominous sign unless it occurs during a period of fetal sleep. Smith and associates (1988) described the **fetal acoustic stimulation test,** in which they used an artificial larynx placed against

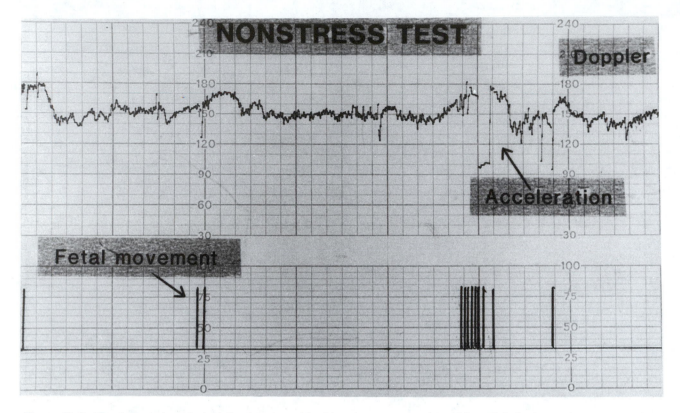

Figure 43–4. Reactive nonstress test. Notice increase of fetal heart rate to more than 15 beats/min for longer than 15 seconds following fetal movements, indicated by the vertical marks on the lower part of the recording. (Photo courtesy of K Leveno.)

the maternal abdomen to "awaken the fetus" and reduce the number of falsely nonreactive tests.

A heart rate tracing with a spontaneous variable deceleration of at least 15 beats per min for 15 seconds or longer, usually associated with oligohydramnios, is suggestive of umbilical cord jeopardy and should be followed by an assessment of amnionic fluid volume or delivery. A prolonged > 1 minute) and severe (< 90 beats per min or 40 beats below baseline) deceleration, regardless of type, has been reported to be associated with a high incidence of intrapartum fetal distress. Many obstetricians recommend delivery when such a deceleration is detected. This pattern of deceleration apparently may occur with either a contraction stress test or with a nonstress test.

The fetus whose heart rate does not accelerate over a longer period is likely to be quite sick. Leveno and colleagues (1983) reported 27 pregnancies from a High Risk Pregnancy Unit in which heart rate acceleration was absent or less than 10 beats per min over 80 minutes. All were associated with features of uteroplacental insufficiency. In this series, four fetuses were stillborn and, despite delivery by cesarean section before labor, seven of the other 16 neonates died.

Observations reported to date imply that acceleration of the fetal heart with fetal movement most often—but certainly not always—indicates that the fetus will survive in utero for at least 1 more week.

BIOPHYSICAL PROFILE

Manning and associates (1980) were the first to report the use of a biophysical profile to assess fetal well-being. The test they originally described consists of a nonstress test with an additional four observations made with the use of real-time ultrasound. The five components of their biophysical profile are as follows:

(1) A reactive nonstress test.
(2) Fetal breathing movements consisting of one or more episodes within 30 minutes and lasting 30 seconds or more.
(3) Fetal movements consisting of three or more discrete body or limb movements within 30 minutes.
(4) Adequate fetal tone, defined as one or more episodes of limb extension with return to flexion within 30 minutes.
(5) Adequate amnionic fluid volume, defined as one or more 1-cm or larger pockets of fluid in two perpendicular planes.

For each of the five components, a normal observation is given a score of 2 and an abnormal observation a score of 0. In the absence of oligohydramnios, a score of 8–10 is normal, 6 is equivocal, and 4 or less is abnormal. Baskett

(1988) emphasized that falsely abnormal tests are more common in preterm fetus.

Oligohydramnios

Although the identification of diminished amnionic fluid alone is not at present considered a single test of fetal well-being, it may assume such a role in the future. Because of its association with postterm pregnancy and fetal growth retardation, oligohydramnios is discussed in detail in Chapter 59.

"Modified" Biophysical Profile

Manning and associates (1987) have modified their original biophysical profile by selective use of the nonstress test. Specifically, they now assess the fetus ultrasonically, and if all four parameters are normal, they do not perform the nonstress test. A normal test score is then 8 out of 8.

Other Biophysical Profile Tests

Other variations of the original biophysical profile have been reported by Shime and associates (1984), who omit fetal tone from their biophysical profile; and by Vintzileos and associates (1983), who add a sixth factor for placental grading.

Eden et al (1988) begin with the nonstress test and, if it is reactive, assess only amnionic fluid volume, which they consider to be normal if a 2-cm pocket is identified.

VALUE OF ANTEPARTUM TESTS USING FETAL HEART RATE & OTHER BIOPHYSICAL PARAMETERS

These tests are now widely in use at least in the United States. However, dispute continues about the relative merits of each in identifying the fetus in jeopardy. The nonstress test appears to be favored by many because it is easier to perform; however, opinion differs about which is the best test to evaluate fetal well-being. Each test evaluates different end points.

The contraction stress test apparently is a more sensitive—certainly an earlier—indicator of fetal jeopardy.

In a large prospective but nonrandomized trial comparing the contraction stress and nonstress tests, there were eightfold fewer stillbirths when the contraction stress test was the primary fetal surveillance method. Finally, once a nonreactive nonstress test was present, serious fetal compromise already was present.

False-Positive Tests

Thacker and Berkelman (1986) reported that the false-positive rates for all three tests were excessively high for fetal mortality and morbidity, with generally poor sensitivities and specificities for the stress tests.

False-Negative Tests

The likelihood of a fetus dying within 1 week of a nor-

mal or reassuring test is less than 1:1000. Unfortunately, such good results are not always obtained.

Summary

In summary, the following statements seem appropriate:

(1) A week can prove to be a dangerously long time in the life of a fetus!

(2) Anything that focuses attention on the fetus is likely to improve care.

(3) No test of fetal well-being, including cardiotocographic and biophysical profile tests, provides complete reassurance no matter how meticulously performed and interpreted.

(4) Finally, the false-positive rates of all these tests are excessively high, and their specificity and sensitivity are extremely variable among medical centers.

ANTEPARTUM BIOPHYSICAL ASSESSMENT OF FETAL WELL-BEING AT PARKLAND HOSPITAL

At our institution, antepartum fetal heart rate testing is based upon the following rationale established by Leveno and colleagues (1983): (1) the **presence of fetal heart rate accelerations** following fetal movement does not reliably predict fetal health, and (2) the **absence of fetal heart accelerations** for 80–90 minutes or the presence of significant decelerations is associated with a high incidence of fetal jeopardy, especially if this pattern has evolved from a previously normal picture. *Therefore, antepartum electronic fetal heart rate monitoring is not done to predict continuing fetal health but rather to determine when there may be fetal jeopardy.*

This distinction is extremely important. Specifically, fetal heart rate accelerations probably do not predict fetal well-being for a definable time period, and this renders outpatient monitoring impractical since the fetus may deteriorate rapidly in women not evaluated clinically on a daily basis.

On an antepartum unit, fetal heart rate monitoring is done every 7 days in selected high-risk women. Daily fetal heart rate monitoring is done for pregnancies associated with (1) oligohydramnios, (2) prematurely ruptured membranes, and (3) maternally perceived decreased fetal activity (Leveno and Cunningham, 1988).

The method consists of placing the woman in a semi-Fowler position and recording blood pressure at the beginning of the session. A 20-minute fetal heart rate recording is performed, with the woman noting spontaneous fetal movements by pressing an event marker. The interpretation of the fetal heart rate recording is as follows:

(1) A heart rate acceleration of more than 10 beats per min is considered normal. Neither the number of accelerations nor their duration is considered.

(2) The heart rate tracing must be of good technical quality.

(3) If the recording quality is technically unsatisfactory in the first 20 minutes or if accelerations are not seen, the recording is continued after 20 minutes for a total of 40 minutes.

(4) If, after 40 minutes, the tracing is still technically unsatisfactory, the test should be repeated later the same day.

(5) If, after the first 40 minutes, accelerations are not seen in a good-quality record, a *physician* should personally repeat the tracing by sitting at the bedside and recording the fetal heart rate for an *additional* 40 minutes.

(6) The lack of fetal heart rate accelerations for 80–90 minutes in a good-quality record is considered an ominous finding.

(7) Significant decelerations of any type require clinical reevaluation.

(8) A sinusoidal fetal heart rate pattern should be considered indicative of fetal anemia, often associated with hydrops due to various causes.

(9) A transient late deceleration may be the result of supine hypotension; therefore, the blood pressure should be checked and the patient's position changed if there is hypotension.

Delivery should be considered if there are significant spontaneous decelerations or if no fetal heart rate accelerations are observed for 90 minutes. This antepartum fetal heart rate assessment does not replace obstetric judgment.

INTRAPARTUM SURVEILLANCE OF THE FETUS

A goal to be constantly pursued during labor is the preservation of fetal well-being by early detection and correction of fetal distress.

ELECTRONIC MONITORING OF FETAL HEART RATE & UTERINE CONTRACTIONS

With each uterine contraction, there is a temporary variable reduction in the flow of oxygenated maternal blood through the placental intracotyledonary spaces. Hon (1974) aptly pointed out that labor is a stress test for the fetus that may be handicapped by (1) intrinsic fetal disease, (2) placental disease, (3) cord compression, (4) maternal disease, (5) drugs administered for analgesia and anesthesia, or (6) maternal hypotension resulting from the supine position, conduction analgesia, or both. To detect fetal distress during labor, he and others urged that continuous beat-to-beat recording of the fetal heart rate be made

concomitant with the pressure changes generated by the uterine contractions.

INTERNAL MONITORING OF FETAL HEART RATE

The fetal heart rate may be identified as beat to beat by attaching a unipolar electrode directly to the fetus and another electrode to the mother and, after appropriate filtration and amplification, recording each contraction of the fetal heart on a time-calibrated moving-strip recorder.

To be able to attach an electrode to the fetus, the cervix must be dilated at least 1 cm, and, of course, the membranes above the cervix must be ruptured. It is important that the electrode be attached to the fetus at a benign site, usually on the vertex or buttock. Care must be taken to avoid the face, eyes, and genitalia.

INTRAUTERINE PRESSURE MEASUREMENTS

Measurements of intrauterine pressure are made by directly coupling the fluid to some sort of recording device. In clinical practice, a fluid-filled plastic catheter is positioned in utero so that the distal tip is located in amnionic fluid above the presenting fetal part.

EXTERNAL (INDIRECT) ELECTRONIC MONITORING

The necessity for rupture of the membranes and invasion of the uterus may be avoided by use of external detectors to identify fetal heart action and characterize uterine activity. External monitoring does not provide the precision of measurement of fetal heart rate afforded by internal monitoring or any quantification of uterine pressure.

The fetal heart rate may be detected in a number of ways through the maternal abdominal wall overlying the uterus. The easiest technique to use during the antepartum and early intrapartum periods employs the ultrasound Doppler principle.

TERMINOLOGY TO DESCRIBE FETAL HEART RATE

Since the fetal heart rate is rarely fixed but instead shows frequent periodic variations, standardized terminology has been proposed to try to describe more precisely both baseline activity and periodic variations from the baseline.

The **baseline fetal heart rate** is the modal rate that prevails apart from any periodic accelerations or decelerations associated with uterine contractions. A baseline rate between 120 and 160 beats per min is considered **normal,** a rate of 100–119 **mild bradycardia,** and a rate of less than 100 **marked bradycardia.** A baseline rate between

161 and 180 beats per min is considered **mild tachycardia and a rate of 181 or more is marked tachycardia.**

The **periodic fetal heart rate** represents deviations from baseline that are related to uterine contractions. **Acceleration** and **deceleration** are variations in fetal heart rate above or below the baseline rate. Three major patterns of deceleration are described:

(1) **Uniform patterns of deceleration** reflect the shape of the simultaneously recorded uterine contractions. With the uniform pattern of **early deceleration,** the onset, nadir, and recovery of the fetal heart rate to baseline coincide with the onset, peak, and end of the uterine contraction (Figure 43–3). Early decelerations are usually attributed to compression of the fetal head, though the stimulus to early deceleration may be more ominous. With **late deceleration,** the onset of slowing occurs as the contraction intensity peaks, the nadir in heart rate is reached well after the peak, and recovery is not achieved until after the uterine contraction has subsided (Figure 43–3). Late decelerations are likely to be the consequence of uteroplacental insufficiency.

(2) **Variable patterns of deceleration, or nonuniform decelerations,** are characterized by a decrease in heart rate beginning at no fixed time in relation to uterine contractions and by waveforms that differ in shape from those of the uterine contractions and from each other, and may be nonrepetitive (Figure 43–3). Variable decelerations are most often the consequence of cord compression.

(3) **Combined (mixed) patterns of deceleration** have features of both of the patterns described above.

CONSEQUENCES OF DECELERATION PATTERNS

The pattern of early deceleration (Figure 43–3) is apt to result from a transient increase in intracranial pressure from head compression, which stimulates the vagus nerve, thereby slowing the heart. Early decelerations may, however, have a more ominous origin, eg, compression of the umbilical cord. Prompt sterile vaginal examination is indicated to identify the status of the cervix and presenting part and to rule out a prolapsed cord. Treatment includes ascertaining that the mother is reclining comfortably on her side and checking the monitor, especially if external, to make certain it is functioning properly. Early decelerations that are severe and prolonged or persistent—and certainly if accompanied by gross meconium staining of the amnionic fluid—must not be ignored.

The **pattern of late deceleration** (Figure 43–3) is likely to result from hypoxia and associated metabolic derangement and acidosis from uteroplacental insufficiency. After termination of the uterine contractions, the heart rate may return to or rise transiently above normal baseline in the less severely affected fetus or remain low in the severely affected fetus. The fetus stressed to an intermediate degree may demonstrate tachycardia between contractions. Delivery can be safely delayed only if the uteroplacental insufficiency is promptly corrected, as, for

example, the relief of uterine overactivity by immediately stopping oxytocin stimulation or by correcting maternal hypotension and thereby improving uteroplacental perfusion. Otherwise, prompt delivery is most often indicated.

The **pattern of variable deceleration (nonuniform deceleration)** (Figure 43–3) is apt to result from compression of the umbilical cord. Vaginal examination should be done promptly to search for cord prolapse and determine the degree of cervical dilatation and the station and position of the presenting part. The position of the mother should be changed so that she is lying on her side or turned to the opposite side. If decelerations persist or worsen, either immediate measurement of fetal scalp blood pH or prompt delivery is indicated. Since this heart rate pattern signifies umbilical cord compression, it usually recurs. In such women, there is anticipation of an increased likelihood of abdominal delivery. Therefore, if serious umbilical cord compression recurs and persists, emergency cesarean delivery is done immediately.

Various deceleration patterns do not always reflect the causes ascribed to them. Although the classification presented above has served as a guide to the interpretation of various patterns of fetal heart rate responses during labor, its rigid application may lead to erroneous diagnosis and treatment.

Beat-to-Beat Variability

Later in pregnancy, there is normally a beat-to-beat variation in the fetal heart rate; ie, the time interval between the same locus (eg, the R wave) in consecutive electrical systoles is not fixed. The variation was attributed by Hon (1974) to the continuous interaction of sympathetic and parasympathetic nerve action on the heart.

Absence of beat-to-beat variability in some circumstances late in pregnancy may be indicative of fetal compromise. In fact, fetal heart rate variability may be the most important aspect of the overall clinical evaluation of the fetus in utero. Gilstrap and associates (1987) reported that fetal acidosis, defined as a blood pH of less than 7.20, was unlikely as long as fetal beat-to-beat variability was present. However, an otherwise normal preterm fetus or the fetus who is "asleep" may not demonstrate beat-to-beat variability. Moreover, medications in doses commonly used during labor and in preparation for delivery may ablate beat-to-beat variability. These drugs include meperidine, morphine, alphaprodine, barbiturates, agents used for conduction or general anesthesia, diazepam, phenothiazines, atropine, scopolamine, and perhaps magnesium sulfate in large doses. Unfortunately, recordings made with externally applied detecting devices are unreliable for identifying the presence or absence of beat-to-beat variation.

Sinusoidal Fetal Heart Rate Pattern

A sinusoidal fetal heart rate pattern—especially when marked—can prove to be an ominous sign of fetal deterioration. For example, Katz and colleagues (1983) observed that with sinusoidal oscillations of more than 25 beats per min, death of the fetus or newborn infant was very common. A marked sinusoidal fetal heart rate pattern has often been identified in fetuses who were severely anemic.

Several drugs have been reported to produce a sinusoidal fetal heart rate pattern, including alphaprodine, meperidine, and butorphanol.

Persistent Fetal Tachycardia or Bradycardia

Tachycardia without deceleration may be the consequence of febrile illness, a response to hypoxia, or, rarely, a reaction to fetal thyrotoxicosis. Gilstrap and colleagues (1987) identified umbilical arterial blood acidemia (pH < 7.20) in seven of 32 neonates (22%) with tachycardia during the second stage of labor. They defined tachycardia as 160 beats per min or greater. Pure metabolic acidemia or respiratory acidemia were noted in two neonates, and the remaining five had mixed metabolic-respiratory acidemia. None of these acidemic neonates needed resuscitation.

Mild bradycardia without deceleration or acceleration is not necessarily evidence for fetal distress. Young and colleagues (1979) found no evidence of acidosis during labor and delivery in several fetuses who demonstrated persistent bradycardia in the range of 100–119 beats per min, and the neonatal outcomes were good. Interestingly, an occiput posterior or transverse position was identified in each instance. The authors ascribed the mild bradycardia to a vagal response induced by persistent head compression in the occiput posterior position. Umbilical arterial blood acidemia (pH < 7.20) was identified by Gilstrap and colleagues (1987) in 16 of 53 neonates (30%), with mild bradycardia defined as 90–119 beats per min and detected during second-stage labor. Two each of the acidemic neonates had pure metabolic or respiratory acidemia, and the remaining 12 had mixed metabolic-respiratory acidemia. None of these acidemic neonates required resuscitation.

These workers also noted umbilical arterial blood acidemia in 25 of 63 neonates (40%), with moderate to severe bradycardia defined as less than 90 beats per min. Eight neonates had metabolic acidemia and four had respiratory acidemia. The remaining 13 neonates had mixed metabolic-respiratory acidemia. Only one of the neonates with pure metabolic acidemia required resuscitation.

An important cause of presumed fetal bradycardia is fetal death, with the *maternal* heart rate being recorded by the monitor but erroneously considered to be the fetal heart rate. Especially before performing any heroic treatment on the basis of electronic monitoring data, it is always wise to listen carefully to the fetal heart with an appropriate stethoscope while simultaneously checking the maternal pulse rate. Another approach is to look for fetal heart motion with real-time ultrasound.

Fetal Cardiac Arrhythmias

Intermittently recurring cardiac arrhythmias of ectopic origin may cause concern. The generally favorable neonatal outcome usually is not improved by pregnancy intervention or attempts at pharmacologic treatment in utero unless evidence of fetal heart failure (hydrops) is present.

Normal Fetal Heart Rate Pattern

The absence of an ominous fetal heart rate pattern is generally predictive of a good fetal outcome. However, there have been documented instances of cardiac arrest and death of a fetus without detection of such a pattern.

FETAL SCALP BLOOD SAMPLING

Internal electronic fetal monitoring has superseded the need for fetal scalp blood sampling. Today, fetal scalp blood sampling is not used widely at major teaching hospitals.

COMPLICATIONS FROM INTERNAL ELECTRONIC & PHYSICOCHEMICAL MONITORING

Routine use of internal monitoring techniques is liable to predispose to early amniotomy and its potential dangers, including cord prolapse, infection, and perhaps more stress for the fetus not cushioned by amnionic fluid during labor.

ASSESSMENT OF RESULTS OF ELECTRONIC MONITORING

Not all clinical studies can be interpreted as showing a reduced fetal mortality rate associated with continuous electronic monitoring, and good outcomes have also been reported using systematic clinical monitoring. Continuous recording of fetal heart rates and uterine pressures per se does not provide continuous surveillance of the fetus. Trained personnel must be immediately available to activate the electronic techniques, to inspect and analyze almost continuously the data being recorded, and to act promptly on the findings.

CLINICAL MONITORING

The status of the fetus can often be satisfactorily monitored clinically by trained individuals who closely adhere to the guidelines listed below, which are emphasized in Chapter 43. In summary, the fetal heart rate is carefully monitored at brief intervals during and immediately after a uterine contraction until the infant is actually delivered; the frequency and intensity of uterine contractions are carefully estimated; and the rates of cervical dilatation and descent of the presenting part are determined periodically.

INTRAPARTUM SURVEILLANCE OF THE FETUS

In about 60% of labors, the fetus is monitored clinically as described above and in Chapter 43. Continuous electronic monitoring currently is reserved for the following circumstances:

(1) Variations in the fetal heart rate detected by auscultation *and for which immediate delivery is not considered necessary.*
(2) Meconium in amnionic fluid.
(3) Induction or augmentation of labor with oxytocin.
(4) Previous cesarean delivery.
(5) Increased likelihood of uteroplacental insufficiency or compromised fetus:

(a) Hypertension.
(b) Bleeding.
(c) Preterm and postterm pregnancies.
(d) Small fetus, probably growth-retarded.
(e) Abnormal presentations.
(f) Previous unexplained stillbirth.
(g) Sickle cell hemoglobinopathies.
(h) Hemolytic disease of the fetus.
(i) Diabetes.

SUGGESTED READINGS

Baskett TF: Gestational age and fetal biophysical assessment. Am J Obstet Gynecol 1988;158:332.

Eden RD et al: A modified biophysical profile for antenatal fetal surveillance. Obstet Gynecol 1988;71:365.

Freeman RK: The use of the oxytocin challenge test for antepartum clinical evaluation of utero-placental respiratory function. Am J Obstet Gynecol 1975;121:481.

Freeman RK, Anderson G, Dorchester W: A prospective multi-institutional study of antepartum fetal heart rate monitoring: II. Contraction stress test versus nonstress test for primary surveillance. Am J Obstet Gynecol 1982;143:778.

Gilstrap LC III et al: Second-stage fetal heart rate abnormalities and type of neonatal acidemia. Obstet Gynecol 1987;70:191.

Goldaber K et al: Pathologic fetal acidemia. Obstet Gynecol 1991;78:1103.

Hon EH: Fetal heart rate monitoring. In: *Modern Perinatal Medicine.* Gluck L (editor). Year Book, 1974.

Katz M et al: Clinical significance of sinusoidal fetal heart rate pattern. Br J Obstet Gynaecol 1983;90:832.

Leveno KJ, Cunningham FG: Forecasting fetal health. Williams Supplement No. 19. Appleton & Lange, August-September, 1988.

Leveno KJ et al: Perinatal outcome in absence of antepartum fetal heart rate acceleration. Obstet Gynecol 1983;61:347.

Manning FA, Platt LD, Sipos L: Antepartum fetal evaluation: Development of a fetal biophysical profile. Am J Obstet Gynecol 1980;136:787.

Manning FA et al: Fetal biophysical profile scoring: Selective use of the nonstress test. Am J Obstet Gynecol 1987;156:709.

Reed KL et al: Cardiac Doppler flow velocities in human fetuses. Circulation 1956;73:41.

Shime J et al: Prolonged pregnancy: Surveillance of the fetus and the neonate and the course of labor and delivery. Am J Obstet Gynecol 1984;148:547.

Smith CV et al: Fetal acoustic stimulation testing: II. Predictive value of a reactive test. J Reprod Med 1988;33:217.

Thacker SB, Berkelman RL: Assessing the diagnostic accuracy and efficacy of selected antepartum fetal surveillance techniques. Obstet Gynecol Surv 1986;41:121.

Vintzileos AM et al: The fetal biophysical profile and its predictive value. Obstet Gynecol 1983;62:271.

Young BK et al: Fetal blood and tissue pH with moderate bradycardia. Am J Obstet Gynecol 1979;135:45.

Zalar RW, Quilligan EJ: The influence of scalp sampling on the cesarean section rate for fetal distress. Am J Obstet Gynecol 1979;135:239.

44

Conduct of Normal Labor & Delivery; Analgesia & Anesthesia

NORMAL LABOR & DELIVERY

ADMISSION PROCEDURES

Early admission to the labor and delivery unit is especially important if, during antepartum care, the gravida, her fetus, or both have been identified as being at risk.

1. DIAGNOSIS OF LABOR

Differentiation of false and true labor can be based on the following features:

(1) **True labor:**
　　Contractions occur at regular intervals
　　Intervals gradually shorten
　　Intensity gradually increases
　　Discomfort noted in back and abdomen
　　Cervix dilates
　　Not stopped by sedation
(2) **False labor:**
　　Contractions occur at irregular intervals
　　Intervals remain long
　　Intensity remains unchanged
　　Discomfort noted chiefly in lower abdomen
　　Cervix does not dilate
　　Usually relieved by sedation

Inquiries are made about the status of the fetal membranes and whether there has been any vaginal bleeding, fluid leakage from the vagina, and, if so, how much and when it started. The frequency and intensity of uterine contractions and when they first became uncomfortable should also be ascertained.

The physician should obtain a history and do a physical examination that includes assessment of the heart rate, fetal presentation, and size of the fetus. The fetal heart rate should be checked, especially at the end of a contraction and immediately thereafter, to identify any pathologic slowing of the fetal heart rate.

2. ADMISSION VAGINAL EXAMINATION

Careful attention to the following is essential in order to obtain needed information and minimize bacterial contamination from multiple examinations:

(1) **Amnionic fluid:** If there is a question about whether rupture of the membranes has occurred, the vulva and the vaginal introitus are cleansed, a sterile speculum is inserted, and fluid is sought in the posterior vaginal fornix.
(2) **Cervix:** Softness, degree of effacement (length), extent of dilatation, and location of the cervix with respect to the presenting part and vagina are ascertained as described below.
(3) **Presenting part:** The nature of the presenting part should be positively determined and, ideally, its position as well.
(4) **Station:** The degree of descent of the presenting part into the birth canal is identified.
(5) **Pelvic architecture:** The diagonal conjugate, ischial spines, pelvic sidewalls, and sacrum are reevaluated for adequacy.
(6) **Vagina and perineum:** The distensibility of the vagina and the firmness of the perineum are assessed.

The Cervix
The degree of effacement of the cervix usually is expressed in terms of percentage of the length of the cervix (see Chapter 38). The amount of cervical dilatation is ascertained and expressed in centimeters. The position of

the cervical os in relation to the fetal head is categorized as posterior, mid, or anterior.

Station

When the lowermost portion of the presenting fetal part is at the level of the ischial spines, it is said to be at zero station (Chapter 38).

Detection of Ruptured Membranes

Rupture of the fetal membranes is significant for three reasons: (1) If the presenting part is not fixed in the pelvis, the possibility of prolapse of the cord and cord compression is greatly increased; (2) labor is likely to occur soon if the pregnancy is at or near term; and (3) if the fetus remains in utero 24 hours or more after rupture of the membranes, there is a likelihood of serious intrauterine infection.

Several diagnostic tests for the detection of ruptured membranes have been recommended, but none are completely reliable. One commonly used test is performed with **nitrazine test papers.** The pH of the vaginal secretion is estimated by inserting a sterile cotton-tipped applicator deeply into the vagina and then touching it to a strip of nitrazine paper and comparing the color reaction with a standard chart. The pH of vaginal secretions ranges between 4.5 and 5.5, while that of amnionic fluid is 7.0–7.5. A false reading may be obtained with intact membranes in women who have an unusually large amount of bloody show, since blood, like amnionic fluid, is not acidic.

3. OTHER ADMISSION PROCEDURES

Vital Signs & Review of Pregnancy Record

The maternal blood pressure, temperature, pulse, and respiratory rate are recorded. The pregnancy record is promptly reviewed to identify complications. Any problems identified during the antepartum period as well as any that were anticipated should be prominently displayed in the pregnancy record along with the plan of management.

Preparation of Vulva & Perineum

The patient is placed in the dorsal lithotomy position on a bedpan. The attendant holds a sponge to the introitus to prevent wash water from running into the vagina. Scrubbing is from anterior toward posterior on the introitus.

In many hospitals, the hair on the lower half of the vulva and on the perineum is removed either by shaving or by clipping.

Vaginal Examinations

After the vulvar and perineal regions have been prepared properly and the examiner has donned sterile gloves, the labia are spread widely with thumb and forefinger to expose the vaginal opening and to keep the examining fingers from coming in contact with the inner surfaces of the labia. The index and third fingers of the examining hand are then introduced into the vagina.

Enema

Early in labor, a cleansing enema is generally given to minimize subsequent contamination by feces.

Laboratory Studies

A hematocrit should be obtained, and a labeled clotted tube should be kept on hand for blood grouping and screening if needed or for routine serologic testing.

MANAGEMENT OF THE FIRST STAGE OF LABOR

As soon as possible after admission, the remainder of the general physical examination is completed. The physician must then draw upon these results and other information compiled during the antepartum period. A rational plan for monitoring labor can then be formulated based on the needs of the fetus and the mother.

1. MONITORING FETAL WELL-BEING DURING LABOR

It is mandatory for a good pregnancy outcome that a program be established to provide careful surveillance of the well-being of both the mother and the fetus. All observations must be properly recorded.

Fetal Heart Rate

The heart rate of the fetus may be identified with a suitable stethoscope or Doppler ultrasonic device.

Changes in the fetal heart rate that are most likely to be ominous are almost always detectable immediately after a uterine contraction. Therefore, it is imperative that the fetal heart be monitored by auscultation immediately after a contraction. To avoid confusing maternal and fetal heart actions, the maternal pulse should be counted as the fetal heart rate is counted. Otherwise, maternal tachycardia may be misinterpreted as a normal fetal heart rate.

Fetal distress, ie, loss of fetal well-being, is suspected if the fetal heart rate immediately after a contraction is repeatedly below 120 per min. Fetal distress is probable if the rate is less than 100 per min, even though there is recovery to a rate in the 120–160 range before the next contraction. When decelerations of this magnitude are found after a contraction, the fetus may be in jeopardy and further labor, if allowed, is often best monitored electronically as described in Chapter 43.

The appropriate frequency of fetal heart rate auscultation is not known. During the first stage of labor, in the absence of any abnormalities, the fetal heart is best checked immediately after a contraction at least every 30 minutes. For women with pregnancies at high risk, most obstetricians recommend continuous electronic monitoring; however, intermittent auscultation every 15 minutes during the first stage is an acceptable alternative.

Uterine Contractions

With the palm of one hand lightly on the abdomen over the uterus, the examiner determines the time of onset of the contraction. The intensity of the contraction is gauged from the degree of firmness the uterus achieves.

Attendance in Labor

Given a choice, most women probably would prefer the nearly continuous presence of the obstetrician or of a compassionate, well-trained obstetric associate to that of a metal cabinet and its wires and tubes that invade her and her fetus. However, because of the ease of the procedure, the pervasive threat of legal liability for mishaps, and simply because the trend to continuous electronic fetal monitoring has become almost an accepted reality, it seems unlikely that continuous electronic fetal monitoring will be used less often in the future. It is important to note, however, that the monitor itself is not a mystical talisman. Electronic monitors are merely extensions of doctors' and nurses' eyes and hands. Simply stated, the physician or nurse must be present to interpret the information gathered from electronic monitors.

2. MATERNAL MONITORING & MANAGEMENT DURING LABOR

Maternal Position During Labor

The normal gravida need not be confined to bed early in labor prior to the use of analgesia. In bed, however, the mother should be allowed to assume the position she finds most comfortable. She must not be restricted to lying supine.

Subsequent Vaginal Examinations

During the first stage of labor, the need for subsequent vaginal examinations will vary considerably. When the membranes rupture, the examination should be repeated immediately if the fetal head was not definitely engaged at the previous vaginal examination. The fetal heart rate should be checked immediately and during the next uterine contraction to help detect cord compression.

Analgesia

Analgesia and anesthesia are discussed later in this chapter; however, the timing, the method of administration, and the size of initial and subsequent doses of systemically acting analgesic agents are based to a great extent on the anticipated time of delivery. A repeat vaginal examination is often appropriate, therefore, before more analgesia is administered.

Maternal Vital Signs

Temperature, blood pressure, and pulse are taken every 1–2 hours. The blood pressure is taken between contractions.

If membranes have been ruptured or if there is a borderline elevation, the temperature should be checked hourly during labor.

Amniotomy

Amniotomy may shorten the length of labor slightly, but there is no evidence that shorter labor is beneficial to the fetus or to the mother. Indeed, the reverse may be true. If amniotomy is performed, aseptic technique should be attempted.

Oral Intake

In essentially all circumstances, food and oral fluids should be withheld during active labor and delivery. Gastric emptying time is remarkably prolonged once labor is established and analgesics are administered. As a consequence, ingested food and most medications remain in the stomach and are not absorbed, but they can be vomited and aspirated.

Intravenous Fluids

Once active labor is established, an intravenous infusion should be started. An infusion system is advantageous during the immediate puerperium in order to administer oxytocin prophylactically and at times therapeutically when uterine atony persists. Moreover, with longer labors, the administration of glucose, some salt, and water to the otherwise fasting woman at the rate of 60–120 mL per h is efficacious to combat dehydration and acidosis.

Urinary Bladder Function

Bladder distention must be avoided, since it can lead to subsequent bladder hypotonia and infection. In the course of each abdominal examination, the suprapubic region should be palpated in order to detect a filling bladder. If the bladder is distended and the patient cannot void, catheterization is indicated.

MANAGEMENT OF THE SECOND STAGE OF LABOR

1. IDENTIFICATION

With full dilatation of the cervix, which signifies the onset of the second stage of labor, the patient typically begins to bear down, and with descent of the presenting part she develops the urge to defecate. Uterine contractions and the accompanying expulsive forces may last 1½ minutes and recur at times after a myometrial resting phase of no more than a minute.

2. DURATION

The median duration of the second stage is 50 minutes in nulliparas and 20 minutes in multiparas, but it can be highly variable.

Fetal Heart Rate

For the low-risk fetus, the heart rate should be auscultated at least every 15 minutes, whereas in those at high risk 5-minute intervals are recommended. Slowing of the fetal heart rate induced by head compression is common during contractions and the accompanying maternal expulsive efforts. If recovery of the fetal heart rate is prompt after the contraction and expulsive efforts cease, labor is allowed to continue.

Not all instances of slowing of the fetal heart during the second stage of labor are the consequence of head compression, however. The vigorous force generated within the uterus by its contraction and by the mother's expulsive efforts may reduce placental perfusion considerably. Descent of the fetus through the birth canal and the consequent reduction in uterine volume may trigger some degree of premature separation of the placenta, with further compromise of fetal well-being. Descent of the fetus is more likely to tighten a loop of umbilical cord around the fetus—especially the neck—sufficiently to obstruct umbilical blood flow. Prolonged, uninterrupted expulsive efforts by the mother can be dangerous to the fetus in this circumstance. Maternal tachycardia, which is common during the second stage, must not be mistaken for a normal fetal heart rate.

Maternal Expulsive Efforts

In most cases, bearing down is reflex and spontaneous in the second stage of labor, but occasionally the patient does not employ her expulsive forces to good advantage and coaching is desirable. She should not be encouraged to "push" beyond the time of completion of each uterine contraction. Instead, she and the fetus should be allowed to rest and recover from the combined effects of the uterine contraction, breath holding, and physical effort. During this period of active bearing down, the fetal heart rate auscultated immediately after the contraction is apt to be slow, but it should recover to normal range before the next expulsive effort.

Preparation for Delivery

Actual delivery of the fetus can be accomplished with the mother in a variety of positions. The most widely used and often the most satisfactory is the dorsal lithotomy position on a delivery table with leg supports and appropriate draping in such a way that only the immediate area about the vulva is exposed.

In the past, the major reason for care in scrubbing, gowning, and gloving was to protect against the introduction of infectious agents. Although this reason remains valid, concern today must also be extended to the health care providers because of the threat of exposure to human immunodeficiency virus. Recommendations for protection of those who care for women during labor and delivery are summarized in Chapter 60.

SPONTANEOUS DELIVERY

1. DELIVERY OF THE HEAD

As the head becomes increasingly visible, the vaginal outlet and vulva are stretched further until they ultimately encircle the largest diameter of the baby's head. This encirclement of the largest diameter of the fetal head by the vulvar ring is known as **crowning.**

Unless an episiotomy has been made, the perineum by now is extremely thin and—in the case of the nulliparous woman especially—almost at the point of rupture with each contraction. At the same time, the anus becomes greatly stretched and protuberant, and the anterior wall of the rectum may be easily seen through it. Failure to perform an episiotomy by this time invites perineal lacerations and some degree of permanent relaxation of the pelvic floor with its possible sequelae of cystocele, rectocele, and uterine prolapse (see Chapter 15).

Ritgen Maneuver

By the time the head distends the vulva and perineum during a contraction sufficiently to open the vaginal introitus to a diameter of 5 cm or so, it is desirable to drape a towel over one gloved hand to protect it from the anus and then exert forward pressure on the chin of the fetus through the perineum just in front of the coccyx, while the other hand exerts pressure superiorly against the occiput (Figure 44–1). This maneuver allows the physician to control delivery of the head.

Clearing the Nasopharynx

To minimize the likelihood of aspiration of amnionic fluid debris and blood that might occur once the thorax is delivered and the infant can inspire, the face is quickly wiped and the nares and mouth are aspirated.

Nuchal Cord

Next, the index finger should be passed to the neck of the fetus to ascertain whether it is encircled by one or more coils of the umbilical cord. Coils occur in about 25% of cases and ordinarily do no harm. If a coil is felt, it should be drawn down between the fingers and, if loose enough, slipped over the infant's head. If it is applied too tightly to the neck to be slipped over the head, it should be cut between two clamps and the infant delivered promptly.

2. DELIVERY OF THE SHOULDERS

In most cases, the shoulders appear at the vulva just after external rotation and are born spontaneously. Occasionally a delay occurs, and immediate extraction may appear advisable. In that event, the sides of the head are

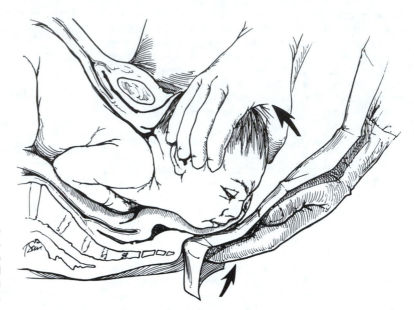

Figure 44–1. Near completion of the delivery of the fetal head by the modified Ritgen maneuver. Moderate upward pressure is applied to the fetal chin by the posterior hand covered with a sterile towel while the suboccipital region of the fetal head is held against the symphysis.

grasped with the two hands and *gentle* downward traction is exerted until the anterior shoulder appears under the pubic arch. Then, by an upward movement, the posterior shoulder is delivered and the anterior shoulder usually drops down from beneath the symphysis. An equally effective method entails completion of delivery of the anterior shoulder before the posterior shoulder (Figure 44–2).

The rest of the body almost always follows the shoulders without difficulty, but in case of prolonged delay its birth may be hastened by *moderate* traction on the head and moderate pressure on the uterine fundus. Hooking the fingers in the axillae should be avoided, however, since doing so may injure the nerves of the upper extremity.

3. CLAMPING THE CORD

The umbilical cord is cut between clamps placed 4 or 5 cm from the fetal abdomen, and later an umbilical cord clamp is applied 2 or 3 cm from the fetal abdomen.

If after delivery the infant is placed at the level of the vaginal introitus or below and the fetoplacental circulation is not immediately occluded by clamping the cord, as much as 100 mL of blood may be shifted from the placenta to the infant.

MANAGEMENT OF THE THIRD STAGE OF LABOR

Immediately after delivery of the infant, the height of the uterine fundus and its consistency are ascertained. As long as the uterus remains firm and there is no unusual bleeding, watchful waiting until the placenta is separated is the usual practice. Uterine massage is not performed.

1. SIGNS OF PLACENTAL SEPARATION

Since attempts to express the placenta prior to its separation are futile and dangerous, it is most important that the following signs of placental separation be recognized:

(1) The uterus becomes globular and, as a rule, firmer. This sign is the earliest to appear.
(2) There is often a sudden gush of blood.
(3) The uterus rises in the abdomen because the placenta, having separated, passes down into the lower uterine segment and the vagina, where its bulk pushes the uterus upward.
(4) The umbilical cord protrudes farther out of the vagina, indicating that the placenta has descended.

When the placenta has separated, the physician first ascertains that the uterus is firmly contracted. The mother, if she is not anesthetized, may be asked to bear down, and the intra-abdominal pressure so produced may be adequate to expel the placenta. If these efforts fail or if spontaneous expulsion is not possible because of anesthesia, the physician—again having made certain that the uterus is contracted firmly—exerts pressure with a hand on the fundus to expel the detached placenta into the vagina.

2. DELIVERY OF THE PLACENTA

Placental expression should never be forced before placental separation lest the uterus be turned inside out. **Inversion of the uterus** is one of the grave mishaps associated with delivery (see Chapter 49). As pressure is applied to the body of the uterus, the umbilical cord is kept slightly taut. The uterus is lifted cephalad with the abdom-

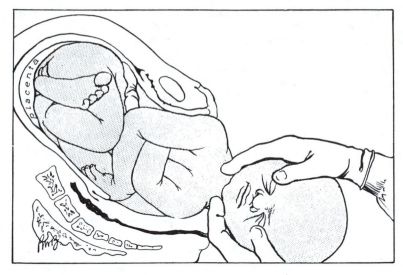

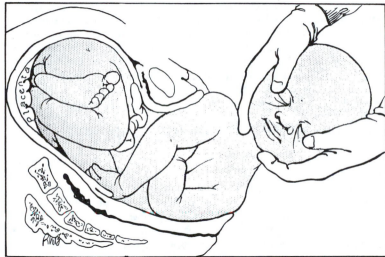

Figure 44–2. ***Top:*** Gentle downward traction to bring about descent of anterior shoulder. ***Bottom:*** Delivery of anterior shoulder completed; gentle upward traction to deliver the posterior shoulder.

inal hand. This maneuver is repeated until the placenta reaches the introitus.

Traction on the cord, however, must not be used to pull the placenta out of the uterus. As the placenta passes through the introitus, pressure on the uterus is discontinued. The placenta is then gently lifted away from the introitus. Care is taken to prevent the membranes from being torn off and left behind. If the membranes start to tear, they are grasped with a clamp and removed by gentle traction. *The placenta should be examined carefully to ascertain whether it has been delivered in its entirety from the uterine cavity.*

Manual Removal of Placenta

If at any time there is brisk bleeding and the placenta cannot be delivered, manual removal is indicated, with safeguards described in Chapter 49.

THE "FOURTH STAGE" OF LABOR

The hour immediately following delivery of the placenta is a critical period referred to by some obstetricians as the "fourth stage of labor." It is mandatory that the uterus be evaluated frequently throughout this period by an attendant who places a hand frequently on the fundus and massages it at the slightest sign of relaxation. At the same time, the vaginal and perineal region is inspected frequently to guarantee prompt identification of any excessive bleeding.

OXYTOCIC AGENTS

After the uterus has been emptied and the placenta has been delivered, the primary mechanism by which hemostasis is achieved at the placental site is vasoconstriction produced by a well-contracted myometrium. Oxytocin, ergonovine maleate (Ergotrate), and methylergonovine maleate (Methergine) are employed in various ways in the conduct of the third stage of labor, principally to stimulate myometrial contractions and thereby reduce the blood loss.

1. OXYTOCIN

The synthetic form of the octapeptide oxytocin is commercially available in the United States as Syntocinon and Pitocin; 1 mg of oxytocin is equal to about 500 USP units. Each milliliter of injectable oxytocin contains 10 USP units of oxytocin, which is not effective by mouth. The half-life of intravenously infused oxytocin is very short, perhaps 3 minutes.

Cardiovascular Effects

Because of the danger of maternal hypotension, oxytocin should not be given intravenously as a large bolus but rather as a dilute solution by continuous intravenous infusion.

Antidiuresis

Another important adverse effect of oxytocin is antidiuresis, caused primarily by reabsorption of free water. In women who are undergoing diuresis in response to the administration of water, the continuous intravenous infusion of 20 mU of oxytocin per minute usually produces a demonstrable decrease in urine flow. When the rate of infusion is raised to 40 mU per min, urinary flow is strikingly reduced.

If an intravenous infusion is in place, one should add 20 units (2 mL) of oxytocin per liter, which is administered after delivery of the placenta at a rate of 10 mL per min for a few minutes until the uterus remains firmly contracted and bleeding is controlled. The infusion rate is then reduced to 1–2 mL per min until the mother is ready for transfer from the recovery suite to the postpartum unit, when the infusion is usually discontinued.

2. ERGONOVINE & METHYLERGONOVINE

Ergonovine is an alkaloid obtained either from ergot, a fungus that grows on rye and some other grains, or synthesized in part from lysergic acid. Methylergonovine is a similar alkaloid made from lysergic acid. The alkaloids are dispensed as the maleate (Ergotrate and Methergine, respectively), either in solution for parenteral use or in tablets for oral use.

Effects

Whether given intravenously, intramuscularly, or orally, ergonovine and methylergonovine are powerful stimulants of myometrial contraction, exerting an effect that may persist for hours. The sensitivity of the pregnant uterus to ergonovine and methylergonovine is very great.

An intravenous dose of as little as 0.1 mg—or an oral dose of only 0.25 mg—results in the tetanic contraction that occurs almost immediately after intravenous injection of the drug and within a few minutes after intramuscular or oral administration. Moreover, the response is sustained with little tendency toward relaxation.

The parenteral administration of these alkaloids, especially by the intravenous route, sometimes initiates transient but severe hypertension. Such a reaction is most likely to occur when conduction analgesia is used for delivery and in women who are prone to develop hypertension.

Oxytocics During & After Delivery

Oxytocin, ergonovine, and methylergonovine are all employed widely in the conduct of the normal third stage of labor. Oxytocin and ergonovine—especially the latter—given before delivery of the placenta will decrease blood loss somewhat; however, oxytocin, ergonovine, or methylergonovine—especially the latter two—given before delivery of the placenta may entrap an undiagnosed and therefore undelivered second twin. This may prove injurious, if not fatal, to the entrapped fetus. In most cases following uncomplicated vaginal delivery, the third stage of labor can be conducted with acceptable blood loss without using alkaloids of ergot.

LACERATIONS OF THE BIRTH CANAL

Lacerations of the vagina and perineum are classified as first, second, or third degree. Such lacerations most often are preventable with an appropriate episiotomy and avoidance of midforceps delivery. A **first-degree laceration** involves the fourchette, the perineal skin, and vaginal mucous membrane but not the underlying fascia and muscle; a **second-degree laceration** involves, in addition to skin and mucous membrane, the fascia and muscles of the perineal body but not the rectal sphincter; and a **third-degree laceration** extends through the skin, mucous membrane, and perineal body and involves the anal sphincter. Some obstetricians apply the term **fourth-degree lacerations** to third-degree tears that extend through the rectal mucosa to expose the lumen of the rectum.

Since the repair of perineal tears is virtually the same as that of episiotomy incisions—albeit often less satisfactory because of irregular lines of tissue cleavage—the technique of repairing lacerations is discussed in the next section.

EPISIOTOMY & REPAIR

The incision may be made in the midline (median or midline episiotomy), or it may begin in the midline but be directed laterally and downward away from the rectum (mediolateral episiotomy).

An episiotomy substitutes a straight, neat surgical incision for the ragged laceration that otherwise frequently results. An episiotomy is easier to repair and heals better than a tear. With mediolateral episiotomy, the likelihood of lacerations into the rectum is reduced.

Timing of Episiotomy

It is common practice to perform an episiotomy when the head is visible during a contraction to a diameter of 3–4 cm. Although it is slightly more awkward to perform an episiotomy with forceps in place, blood loss from the episiotomy is somewhat less with this technique, and the resultant tamponade of the perineal floor by the fetal head is effected earlier than is otherwise the case.

Midline Versus Mediolateral Episiotomy

The advantages and disadvantages of the two types of episiotomies may be listed as follows:

(1) **Median episiotomy:**
Easy to repair
Faulty healing rare
Less painful in puerperium
Dyspareunia rarely follows
Anatomic end results almost always excellent
Blood loss less
Extension through the anal sphincter and into rectum rather common
(2) **Mediolateral episiotomy:**
More difficult to repair
Faulty healing more common
Pain for a few days in one-third of cases
Dyspareunia occasionally follows
Anatomic end results more or less faulty in about 10% of cases (depending on operator)
Blood loss greater
Extension through sphincter uncommon

The possibility of extension of a median episiotomy into the rectal sphincter is much greater when the perineal body is short, when the fetus is large, when the occiput is posterior, in midforceps deliveries, and in breech deliveries. It is good practice, in general, to use mediolateral episiotomy in the circumstances mentioned but to employ the median incision otherwise.

Repair of Episiotomy

The most common practice is to defer repair of the episiotomy until after the placenta has been delivered.

There are many ways to close the episiotomy incision, but hemostasis and anatomic restoration without excessive suturing are essential for success with any method. A technique commonly employed is shown in Figure 44–3. The suture material ordinarily used is 000 chromic catgut. The technique of repairing a third-degree laceration with extension into the wall of the rectum is shown in Figure 44–4.

If the rectal mucosa was involved, stool softeners should be prescribed for a week. Enemas, of course, should be avoided.

Pain After Episiotomy

An ice collar applied early tends to reduce swelling and allay discomfort. Aerosol sprays containing a local anesthetic are helpful at times. Analgesics such as codeine give considerable relief. Since pain may be a signal of a large vulvar, paravaginal, or ischiorectal hematoma or perineal cellulitis, it is essential to examine these sites carefully if pain is severe or persistent.

ANESTHESIA & ANALGESIA

For obstetrics, there is no completely safe and satisfactory method of pain relief. Therefore, the advantages of pain relief in labor must offset its disadvantages. In fact, analgesia and anesthesia, when employed by skilled personnel, actually may be beneficial rather than detrimental to both fetus and mother.

During labor, there are two patients the obstetrician and anesthesiologist must care for: the mother and the fetus. In one sense the two parties have a conflict of interest in that the respiratory center of the fetus is highly vulnerable to sedative and anesthetic drugs, so that when these agents are given to the mother they rapidly traverse the placenta and may cause respiratory depression in the newborn infant.

Analgesia

While analgesia is not absolutely necessary for all spontaneous vaginal deliveries, it may spare the mother unnecessary suffering. Analgesia is essential to the safe and humane conduct of many abnormal deliveries. Obstetric analgesia may be required for 12 hours or even longer. Analgesic agents should exert little or no deleterious effect on uterine contractions and voluntary expulsive efforts. If they do, labor may be prolonged and postpartum hemorrhage may be an added risk.

Anesthesia

Labor begins without warning, and obstetric anesthesia may be required within a few hours after a full meal. Moreover, gastric emptying is delayed during pregnancy and prolonged even more during labor, especially after analgesics are given. Vomiting with aspiration of gastric contents is a constant threat and often a major cause of serious maternal morbidity and even death.

PRINCIPLES OF PAIN RELIEF

The three essentials of obstetric pain relief are simplicity, safety, and the preservation of fetal homeostasis. With respect to the latter, the most important factor is the transfer of oxygen, which is dependent on the concentration of inhaled oxygen, uterine blood flow, the oxygen gradient

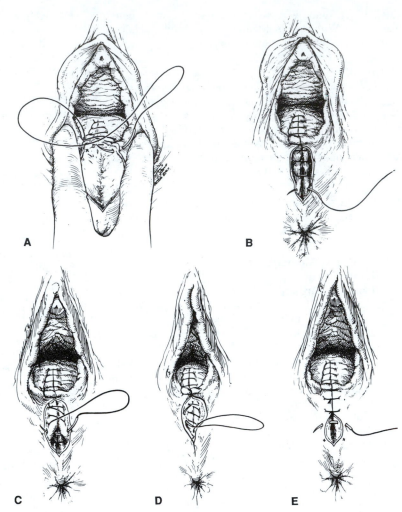

Figure 44–3. Repair of median episiotomy. **A:** Chromic catgut, preferably 000, is used as a continuous suture to close the vaginal mucosa and submucosa. **B:** After closure of the vaginal incision and reapproximation of the cut margins of the hymenal ring, the suture is tied and cut. Next, three or four interrupted sutures of 00 or 000 catgut are placed in the fascia and muscle of the incised perineum. **C:** A continuous suture is now carried downward to unite the superficial fascia. **D:** Completion of repair. The continuous suture is carried upward as a subcuticular stitch. (An alternative method of closure of skin and subcutaneous fascia is illustrated in E.) **E:** Completion of repair of median episiotomy. A few interrupted sutures of 000 chromic catgut are placed through the skin and subcutaneous fascia and loosely tied. This closure avoids burying two layers of catgut in the more superficial layers of the perineum.

across the placenta and umbilical blood flow. Impaired fetal oxygenation most often is the consequence of either compression of the umbilical cord or prolonged or repeated decreases in placental perfusion. Prominent causes of reduced placental perfusion include hypertonic uterine contractions, severe pregnancy-induced hypertension, hemorrhage, premature separation of the placenta, and hypotension from spinal or epidural analgesia.

With any form of analgesia, there should be close supervision to avoid falls from bed and vomiting with aspiration. Similarly, assiduous attention to blood pressure and anesthetic levels should follow administration of spinal and epidural analgesia in all cases.

The obstetrician should master an effective method of parenteral analgesia such as provided by meperidine plus promethazine and become expert in local, pudendal, and low spinal (saddle block) analgesia. Continuous lumbar epidural analgesia may also be administered by the obstetrician in appropriate circumstances. General anesthesia should be immediately available for laparotomy.

Proper psychologic management of the pregnant woman throughout pregnancy and labor is a useful tranquilizer. Fear potentiates pain. Great benefits can be obtained by couples who attend childbirth preparation classes. Women who are taught what kind and degree of pain to expect with labor generally have less fear and therefore less pain. Conversely, women who attempt natural childbirth but who eventually request intrapartum analgesia should never be allowed to feel they have "failed."

ANALGESIA & SEDATION DURING LABOR

A narcotic such as meperidine plus one of the tranquilizer drugs such as promethazine usually are indicated for pain relief during labor. With a successful program of analgesia and sedation, the mother should be able to rest quietly between contractions. Discomfort usually is felt at the peak of an effective uterine contraction, but the pain is not unbearable.

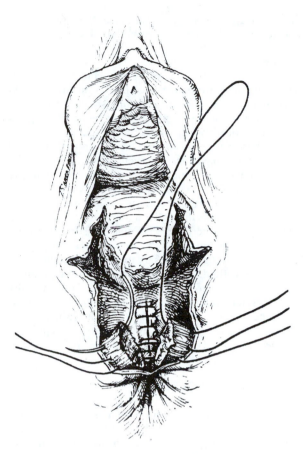

Figure 44–4. Repair of complete perineal tear. The rectal mucosa has been repaired with interrupted, fine chromic catgut sutures. The torn ends of the sphincter ani are next approximated with two or three interrupted chromic catgut sutures. The wound is then repaired, as in a second-degree laceration or an episiotomy.

Meperidine, 50–100 mg, with promethazine, 25 mg, may be administered intramuscularly at intervals of 3–4 hours. In general, a small dose given more frequently is preferable to a large one administered less often. Then, if delivery follows rapidly after the injection, the neonate is less likely to be depressed by the medication. The size of the mother must be taken into account in determining the size of the dose.

A more rapid effect is achieved by giving these drugs intravenously, but in general not more than 50 mg of meperidine or more than 25 mg of promethazine should be given at one time by this route. Whereas analgesia is maximal about 45 minutes after an intramuscular injection, it develops in about 5 minutes following intravenous administration. The depressant effect on the fetus follows closely behind the peak analgesic effect in the mother.

NARCOTIC ANTAGONISTS

Narcotics used during labor may impair respiratory function in the newborn. Prompt ventilation is mandatory in such cases. Naloxone hydrochloride (Narcan) is a narcotic antagonist capable of reversing respiratory depression induced by opioid narcotics by displacing the narcotic from specific receptors in the central nervous system. Unfortunately, it concomitantly blocks the analgesic and euphoriant effects of the narcotic.

GENERAL ANESTHESIA

Without exception, all anesthetic agents that depress the maternal central nervous system cross the placenta and depress the fetal central nervous system. Aspiration of acid gastric contents and obstruction of the airway with particulate matter are constant hazards with any general anesthetic. Fasting before anesthesia is not always an effective safeguard, since fasting gastric juice, even though free of particulate matter, is likely to be strongly acidic and thus can produce fatal aspiration pneumonitis. Tracheal intubation remains the most effective means of minimizing this risk.

1. INHALATION ANESTHESIA

Nitrous oxide (N_2O) is the only anesthetic gas in current use for obstetric analgesia and anesthesia in the United States. It may be used to provide pain relief during labor as well as at delivery. This agent produces analgesia and altered consciousness but by itself does not provide true anesthesia. Nitrous oxide does not prolong labor or interfere with uterine contractions. Satisfactory analgesia often is obtained with a concentration of 50% nitrous oxide and 50% oxygen, but its use requires that personnel be in close attendance. During the second stage of labor, when a uterine contraction begins, a well-fitting clear mask is placed on the patient's face and she is encouraged to take three deep breaths and then to bear down.

Nitrous oxide is commonly used as part of a balanced general anesthesia that is popular for cesarean delivery and some forceps deliveries. It is given along with oxygen in a 50:50 mixture, and a short-acting barbiturate (usually thiopental) is given intravenously along with a muscle relaxant (usually succinylcholine) just prior to tracheal intubation. With this technique, high concentrations of potent inhalational anesthetics are avoided.

Halothane, enflurane, and isoflurane are used to supplement nitrous oxide during maintenance of general anesthesia. These halogenated hydrocarbons cross the placenta readily and are capable of producing narcosis in the fetus.

2. ASPIRATION DURING GENERAL ANESTHESIA

Pneumonitis from inhalation of gastric contents has been the most common cause of anesthetic deaths in obstetrics. Aspirated particulate matter may cause airway obstruction that, unless promptly relieved, can prove rapidly fatal. Gastric juice is likely to be free of particulate matter during fasting, but it is extremely acidic and capable of inducing a lethal chemical pneumonitis. The aspiration of strongly acidic gastric juice is probably more common and perhaps even more dangerous than aspiration of gastric contents that contain particulate matter buffered somewhat by food.

Important to effective prophylaxis are (1) fasting for at least 6 and preferably 12 hours before anesthesia; (2) use of agents to reduce gastric acidity during the induction and maintenance of general anesthesia; (3) skillful tracheal intubation accompanied by pressure on the cricoid cartilage to occlude the esophagus; and (4) at completion of the operation, extubation with the patient awake and lying on her side with head lowered.

Clinical Findings

The woman who aspirates stomach contents may develop evidence of respiratory distress immediately or as long as several hours after aspiration, depending in part upon the material aspirated, the severity of the process, and the acuity of her attendants. Aspiration of a large amount of solid material causes obvious signs of airway obstruction. Smaller particles without acidic liquid may lead to patchy atelectasis and later to bronchopneumonia.

When highly acidic liquid is inspired, tachypnea, bronchospasm, rhonchi, rales, atelectasis, cyanosis, tachycardia, and hypotension are likely to develop. At sites of injury, protein-rich fluid containing numerous erythrocytes exudes from capillaries into the lung interstitium and alveoli to cause decreased pulmonary compliance, shunting of blood, and severe hypoxemia. Radiographic changes may not appear immediately and may be quite variable in any case. Therefore, a clear chest x-ray alone should not rule out aspiration of a significant amount of strongly acidic gastric contents.

Prevention

A. Fasting: Gastric emptying in labor is even more retarded, and women in early labor should be advised to fast before coming to the hospital and certainly thereafter. Despite these precautions, it should be assumed that any woman in labor has both gastric particulate matter as well as acidic contents in her stomach. If general anesthesia is used soon after eating, a nasogastric tube should be inserted during surgery. With irrigation, the likelihood of vomiting and aspiration during extubation is lessened.

B. Antacids: The practice of administering antacids shortly before induction of anesthesia probably has done more to reduce the mortality rate associated with obstetric anesthesia than any other single practice. It is essential that the antacid disperse promptly throughout all of the gastric contents to neutralize the hydrogen ion effectively;

but it is equally important that the antacid, if aspirated, not incite comparably serious pulmonary problems.

Treatment

Suspicion of aspiration of gastric contents demands close monitoring for evidence of pulmonary damage. As much as possible of the inhaled fluid should be immediately wiped out of the mouth and removed from the pharynx and trachea by suction. Saline lavage is not recommended because it probably further disseminates the acid throughout the lung. If large particulate matter is inspired, prompt bronchoscopy may be indicated to relieve airway obstruction. Otherwise, bronchoscopy not only is unnecessary but may contribute to morbidity and mortality.

Oxygen delivered through a tracheal tube in increased concentration by intermittent positive pressure often is required to raise and maintain the arterial P_{O_2} at 60 mm Hg. Frequent suctioning is necessary to remove secretions, including edema fluid. Mechanical ventilation that produces positive end-expiratory pressure may prove lifesaving by preventing the complete collapse of the now surfactant-poor lung on expiration and, partially at least, the outpouring of protein-rich fluid from pulmonary capillaries into the interstitium and alveoli.

REGIONAL ANALGESIA

A variety of nerve blocks have been developed over the years to provide pain relief for the woman in labor and at delivery. Since they are designed to be implemented without loss of consciousness (anesthesia), they are correctly referred to as regional analgesics.

Pain in the first stage of labor originates mostly in the uterus. Visceral sensory fibers from the uterus, cervix, cardinal ligaments, and upper vagina pass through Frankenhäuser's ganglion, which lies just lateral to the cervix, into the pelvic plexus and then to the middle and superior hypogastric plexuses. From there, the fibers travel in the lumbar and lower thoracic sympathetic chains to enter the spinal cord through the white rami communicantes associated with the tenth, 11th, and 12th thoracic and first lumbar nerves. Early in the first stage of labor, the pain of uterine contractions is transmitted chiefly through the 11th and 12th thoracic nerves.

The motor pathways to the uterus leave the spinal cord at the level of the seventh and eighth thoracic vertebrae. Theoretically, any method of sensory block that does not also block the motor pathways to the uterus can be used for analgesia during labor.

Although painful contractions of the uterus continue during the second stage of labor, much of the pain of vaginal delivery arises in the lower genital tract. Painful stimuli from the lower genital tract are transmitted primarily through the pudendal nerve, the peripheral branches of which provide sensory innervation to the perineum, anus, and the more medial and inferior parts of the vulva and clitoris. The pudendal nerve passes across the posterior surface of the sacrospinous ligament just as the ligament attaches to the ischial spine (Figure 44–5). The sensory nerve fibers of the pudendal nerve are derived from the ventral branches of the second, third, and fourth sacral nerves.

1. ANESTHETIC AGENTS

Some of the more commonly used local anesthetics include chloroprocaine, tetracaine, lidocaine, and bupivacaine. Administration of small-volume boluses allows careful monitoring for early signs of toxicity.

Although appropriate use of these anesthetics almost always proves to be safe for the mother and fetus, the potential exists for toxic reactions that may prove life-threatening to both. Administration of these agents must be followed by monitoring for adverse reactions, and equipment and personnel to manage these reactions must be immediately available.

Serious toxicity usually follows injection of an anesthetic into a vessel, but it may be induced by administration of excessive amounts because of miscalculation of the dose. Since many of these agents are manufactured in more than one concentration and ampule size to be used for specific local or regional blocks, a thorough knowledge of the ones selected for use is essential for safety. Life-threatening systemic toxicity from local anesthetics may involve the central nervous system or cardiovascular system.

2. LOCAL INFILTRATION

Local infiltration of anesthetic is useful only for delivery. It is of particular value in the following circumstances: (1) before episiotomy and delivery; (2) after delivery, into the site of lacerations to be repaired; and (3) around the episiotomy wound if adequate analgesia is lacking. Local infiltration analgesia is the "safest" technique. Sufficient time, however, must be allowed to establish analgesia.

3. PUDENDAL BLOCK

Pudendal block usually works well and is an extremely safe and relatively simple means of providing analgesia for spontaneous delivery.

A tubular director that allows 1–1.5 cm of a 15-cm-long 22-gauge needle to protrude beyond its tip is used to guide the needle into position over the pudendal nerve (Figure 44–5). The end of the director is placed against the vaginal mucosa just beneath the tip of the ischial spine. The needle is pushed beyond the tip of the director into the mucosa, and a mucosal wheal is made with 1 mL of 1% lidocaine solution or an equivalent dose of another local anesthetic with similar high tissue penetration and rapid action. Aspiration is attempted before this and all subsequent injections to guard against intravascular infusion. The needle is then advanced until it touches the sacrospinous ligament, which is infiltrated with 3 mL of lidocaine. The needle is advanced farther through the ligament, and as it pierces the loose areolar tissue behind the ligament, the resistance of the plunger decreases. Another 3 mL of

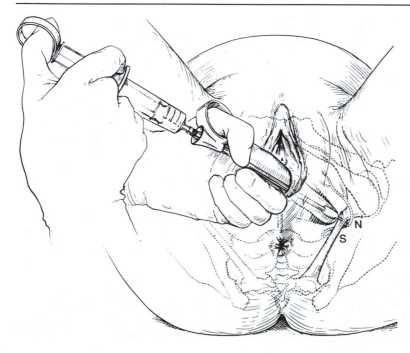

Figure 44–5. Local infiltration of the pudendal nerve. Transvaginal technique showing the needle extended beyond the needle guard and passing through the sacrospinous ligament (S) to reach the pudendal nerve (N).

the anesthetic solution is injected into this region. Next, the needle is withdrawn into the guide, the tip of the guide is moved to just above the ischial spine, and the needle is inserted through the mucosa. After aspiration again to avoid intravascular injection, the remainder of the 10 mL vial of solution is deposited. Most obstetricians elect to perform pudendal block bilaterally so that discomfort of perineal distention with delivery is minimized.

Within 3–4 minutes after injection, the successful pudendal block will allow pinching of the lower vagina and posterior vulva bilaterally without pain. It is often of benefit before pudendal block to infiltrate the fourchette, perineum, and adjacent vagina directly at the site where the episiotomy is to be made with 5–10 mL of 1% lidocaine solution. Then, if delivery occurs before pudendal block becomes effective, an episiotomy can be made without pain. By the time of the repair, the pudendal block usually has become effective.

4. SPINAL (SUBARACHNOID) BLOCK

Introduction of a local anesthetic into the subarachnoid space to effect spinal block has long been used for uncomplicated cesarean and vaginal delivery of normal women of low parity. *Because of the smaller subarachnoid space during pregnancy, the same amount of anesthetic agent in the same volume of solution produces much higher blockade in parturients than in nonpregnant women.* The smaller space is probably the consequence of engorgement of the internal vertebral venous plexus, which in turn is the consequence of compression by the uterus of the inferior vena cava and adjacent large veins.

Vaginal Delivery

Low spinal block is a popular form of analgesia for delivery. The level of analgesia extends to the tenth thoracic dermatome, which corresponds to the level of the umbilicus. Blockade to this level provides excellent relief from the pain of uterine contractions. The term **saddle block** has been incorrectly applied to this level of analgesia, since the area of skin anesthetized is greater than what would be in contact with a saddle.

Cesarean Delivery

For cesarean delivery, a higher level of spinal sensory blockade is essential to at least the level of the eighth thoracic dermatome, which is just below the xiphoid process. Since a larger area is to be anesthetized, a somewhat larger dose of anesthetic is necessary, and this increases the frequency and severity of toxic reactions. Depending upon the mother' size, 8–10 mg of tetracaine or 50–75 mg of lidocaine is administered. Undue delay between intrathecal injection of anesthetic agent and delivery of the infant should be avoided in order to ensure a safe dose level and adequate operative time. Therefore, catheterization of the bladder and shaving of the operative field should be done before the anesthetic is administered. Preanalgesic intra-

venous volume expansion usually prevents dangerous hypotension.

Complications with Spinal Analgesia

A number of complications may follow induction of spinal analgesia, and it is imperative that close clinical monitoring of vital signs be performed. This includes assessment of the level of analgesia, which should stabilize by 10–20 minutes.

Maternal hypotension may develop soon after injection of the analgesic agent. This is the consequence of vasodilatation from sympathetic blockade compounded by obstructed venous return caused by uterine compression of the vena cava and adjacent large veins. Importantly, in the supine position, even in the absence of maternal hypotension—at least as measured in the brachial artery—placental blood flow may be reduced significantly. Important to prophylaxis and to treatment of spinal hypotension are (1) uterine elevation and displacement to the left of the abdomen; (2) acute hydration with a balanced salt solution; and (3) at the first sign of a decrease in blood pressure after hydration, the intravenous injection of 10–15 mg of ephedrine.

Complete spinal blockade with respiratory paralysis may complicate spinal analgesia. Most often, total spinal blockade is the consequence of administration of a dose of analgesic agent far in excess of that tolerated by pregnant women. Hypotension and apnea develop promptly and must be immediately treated to prevent cardiac arrest. In the undelivered woman, the uterus is displaced laterally to minimize aortic and vena caval compression. Effective ventilation is established—through a tracheal tube when possible—to protect against aspiration. When the patient is hypotensive, intravenous fluids are given, and ephedrine may be helpful to increase cardiac output. Elevation of the legs will increase venous return and help reverse hypotension. Preparation should be made for cardiac resuscitation in the event of cardiac arrest.

Any puncture of the dura may on occasion result in a "spinal headache." Such headaches are believed to be the consequence of continued leakage of cerebrospinal fluid through the punctured dura. Headache is absent in the supine position but severe in the upright position. Most such headaches respond to bed rest, hydration, and analgesics. Occasionally, however, the patient's own blood may have to be injected into the epidural space in this region to seal the "leak." This so-called "blood patch" is virtually always successful in rapidly correcting such headaches.

5. EPIDURAL (PERIDURAL) ANALGESIA

Relief from the pain of uterine contractions and delivery—vaginal or abdominal—can be accomplished by injecting a suitable local anesthetic agent into the epidural or peridural space. The epidural space, in effect, is a potential area that contains areolar tissue, fat, lymphatics, and the internal venous plexus, which becomes engorged during pregnancy so that it reduces the volume of the space. It is limited peripherally by the ligamentum flavum and centrally by the dura matter, and it extends from the base of the skull to almost the end of the sacrum. The portal of entry into the epidural space for obstetric analgesia is either through a lumbar intervertebral space (**lumbar epidural analgesia**) or through the sacral hiatus and sacral canal (**caudal epidural analgesia**). Although one injection may be used, more often the injections are repeated through an indwelling plastic catheter or the agent is given by continuous infusion using a volumetric pump.

Continuous Lumbar Epidural Block

Complete analgesia for the pain of labor and vaginal delivery necessitates a block from the tenth thoracic to fifth sacral dermatomes. For abdominal delivery, block is essential beginning at the eighth thoracic level and extending to the first sacral dermatome. The spread of the epidurally injected anesthetic agent will depend upon the location of the catheter tip as well as the dose, concentration, and volume of anesthetic agent used and whether the patient is placed in the head-down, horizontal, or head-up position. It is important that the meninges not be perforated, since if this happens the anesthetic enters the subarachnoid space and, in the much larger dose used to achieve epidural analgesia, rapidly produces total spinal blockade.

Before injection of any local anesthetic agent, a test dose is given and the woman observed for features of toxicity from intravascular injection and signs of spinal blockade from subarachnoid injection. If there is no evidence of these mishaps, a full dose is given carefully and analgesia is maintained by intermittent boluses of similar volume, or small volumes of the drug are delivered continuously by infusion pump.

When vaginal delivery is anticipated in 10–15 minutes, a rapidly acting agent is given through the epidural catheter to effect perineal analgesia.

Complications

Both lumbar and caudal epidural analgesia for labor and delivery may provide welcome relief from the pain of labor. It is imperative that close observation, including monitoring of the level of analgesia, be maintained.

Puncture of the dura, along with inadvertent subarachnoid injection, is always a potential complication, so personnel and facilities must be immediately available to manage the complications of high spinal block.

By blocking sympathetic tracts, epidurally injected analgesic agents may cause hypotension. In nonhypertensive and normally hypervolemic pregnant women, hypotension induced by epidural analgesia usually can be prevented by rapid infusion of a balanced salt solution or treated successfully as described for spinal analgesia. Despite these precautions, hypotension is the most common side effect and develops in about one-third of patients.

Convulsions are an uncommon but serious complication that require anticonvulsants and frequently tracheal intubation and control of respiration.

Epidural block induced prior to well-established labor may be followed by desultory labor. The precise role played by epidural analgesia in this phenomenon is not clear, since this sequence of events also is seen in its absence. During the second stage of labor, epidural analgesia that provides effective pain relief is likely to reduce maternal expulsive efforts. As a consequence, epidural block may lead to delay or, less frequently, failure of descent of the presenting part and spontaneous rotation to the occiput anterior position. Therefore, with epidural analgesia there is likely to be an increased necessity for forceps deliveries and forceps rotations.

SUGGESTED READINGS

Cox SM, Bost JE, Faro S, Carpenter RJ: Epidural anesthesia during labor and the incidence of forceps delivery. Tex Med 1987;83:45.

Crawford JS: Some maternal complications of epidural analgesia for labour. Anesthesia 1985;40:1219.

Gibbs CP, Banner TC: Effectiveness of Bicitra as a preoperative antacid. Anesthesiology 1984;61:97.

Abnormalities of Labor, Delivery, & the Puerperium

45

Dystocia Due to Abnormalities of the Expulsive Forces & Precipitate Labor

Dystocia ("difficult labor") is characterized by abnormally slow progress of labor. It is the consequence of four distinct abnormalities that may exist singly or in combination:

(1) Abnormalities of the expulsive forces (Chapter 45).

(2) Abnormalities of presentation, position, or development of the fetus (see Chapter 46).

(3) Abnormalities of the maternal bony pelvis—ie, pelvic contraction (see Chapter 47).

(4) Abnormalities of the birth canal other than those of the bony pelvis that form an obstacle to fetal descent (see Chapter 48).

Pelvic contraction is often accompanied by uterine dysfunction, and the two together constitute the most common cause of dystocia. Similarly, faulty presentation or unusual fetal size or shape may be accompanied by uterine dysfunction. *As a generalization, uterine dysfunction is common whenever there is disproportion between the presenting part of the fetus and the birth canal.*

UTERINE DYSFUNCTION

As described in Chapter 37, the **first stage of labor** has commonly but somewhat artificially been divided into two distinct phases: a latent phase and an active phase. Typically, the **latent phase** will be of several hours' duration, during which time the cervix undergoes softening and effacement but only slight dilatation. This phase of cervical change is characterized by uterine contractions of mild intensity, short duration, and variable frequency.

During the **active phase** that follows, the cervix dilates more rapidly at 1–2 cm per h, and there is descent of the presenting part through the birth canal (Figure 45–1).

The active phase of labor has been subdivided further into three additional divisions or phases: the acceleration phase, the phase of maximum slope, and the deceleration phase. The acceleration and deceleration phases may never be identified during rapid labor. In fact, to anticipate a deceleration phase in labor can result in the delivery of many babies under less than optimal circumstances.

The descent of the presenting part normally begins well before the cervix reaches full dilatation and proceeds until the presenting part reaches the perineum. It should be noted that this pattern is highly variable. The fetal presenting part in nulliparous women may be at the +1 or even +2 station before the onset of labor, whereas in parous women, descent of the presenting part may not begin until the cervix is almost fully dilated.

The sigmoid curve for cervical dilatation and the slope of fetal descent should be considered at best as idealized visual aids to understanding the temporal relationships of cervical dilatation and the descent of the presenting part (Figure 45–1).

Failure of the cervix to dilate or of the presenting part to descend is cause for concern. Prolongation of either the **first or second stage of labor** may result in increased perinatal and maternal morbidity. Any delay in cervical dilatation during the first stage or prolongation of the second stage of labor should alert the obstetrician to possible danger.

Uterine dysfunction in any phase of cervical dilatation is characterized by lack of progress, since one of the prime characteristics of normal labor is its progression. Prolongation of the latent phase has been defined as 20 hours in nulliparas and 14 hours in multiparas and a protracted active phase as cervical dilatation of less than 1.2 cm per h in nulliparas and less than 1.5 cm in multiparas (Figure 45–1, Table 45–1). The diagnosis of uterine dysfunction in the latent phase is difficult and sometimes can be made

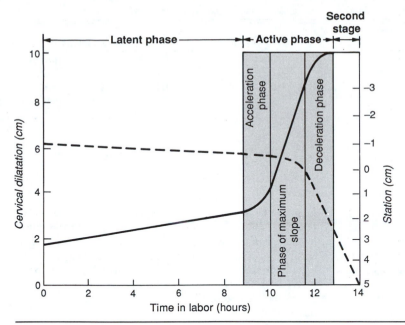

Figure 45–1. Composite of cervical dilatation and fetal descent curves, illustrating their interrelationship and their component phases. (Courtesy of Cohen W, Friedman EA [editors]: *Management of Labor*. University Park Press, 1983.)

only in retrospect. One of the most common errors is to treat women for uterine dysfunction who are not yet in active labor.

There have been three significant advances in the treatment of uterine dysfunction: (1) the realization that undue prolongation of labor may contribute to perinatal morbidity and mortality; (2) the use of very dilute intravenous infusions of oxytocin in the treatment of certain types of uterine dysfunction; and (3) the more frequent use of cesarean delivery rather than difficult midforceps delivery to effect delivery when oxytocin fails or its use is inappropriate (Table 45–2).

Types of Dysfunction

Uterine contractions of labor are normally characterized by a gradient of myometrial activity, being greatest and lasting longest at the fundus (fundal dominance) and diminishing toward the cervix. In addition to a gradient of activity, there is a time differential in the onset of the contractions in the fundus, midzone, and lower segments of the uterus.

The lower limit of pressure of contractions required to dilate the cervix is 15 mm Hg. Actually, a normal spontaneous uterine contraction often exerts a pressure of about 60 mm Hg.

It is possible, therefore, to define two types of uterine dysfunction: (1) In **hypotonic uterine dysfunction,** there

Table 45–1. Abnormal labor patterns, diagnostic criteria, and methods of treatment.[1]

Labor Pattern	Diagnostic Criterion		Preferred Treatment	Exceptional Treatment
	Nulliparas	Multiparas		
Prolongation disorder (Prolonged latent phase)	> 20 h	> 14 h	Therapeutic rest	Oxytocin or cesarean deliveries for urgent problems
Protraction disorders 1. Protracted active phase dilatation 2. Protracted descent	< 1.2 cm/h < 1.0 cm/h	< 1.5 cm/h < 2 cm/h	Expectant and supportive	Cesarean delivery for CPD[2]
Arrest disorders 1. Prolonged deceleration rate 2. Secondary arrest of dilatation 3. Arrest of descent 4. Failure of descent	> 3 h > 2 h > 1 h No descent in deceleration phase or second stage of labor	> 1 h > 2 h > 1 h	Without CPD: oxytocin With CPD: cesarean delivery	Rest if exhausted Cesarean delivery

[1]Modified from Cohen W, Friedman EA (editors): *Management of Labor*. University Park Press, 1983.

Table 45–2. Neonatal apgar scores by labor pattern in nulliparas and perinatal mortality by delivery method.

Labor Pattern	Percent of Apgar Scores Less than 5		Perinatal Mortality per 1,000 by Delivery Method		
	At 1 min	*At 5 min*	*Spontaneous*	*Low Forceps*	*Midforceps*
Normal	12.7	3.2	1.5	2.8	10.8[a]
Prolongation disorder	12.9	4.6	0.0	0.0	10.8[a]
Protraction disorders	23.7[a]	3.1	0.0	12.0[a]	28.5[a]
Arrest disorders	25.2[a]	8.0[a]	16.1[a]	24.4[a]	38.3[a]

[a]Statistically significant, p < 0.01.
Modified from Cohen and Friedman, 1983.

is no basal hypertonus, and uterine contractions have a normal (synchronous) gradient pattern, but the slight rise in pressure during a contraction is insufficient to dilate the cervix at a satisfactory rate. This type of uterine dysfunction usually occurs during the active phase of labor, after the cervix has dilated to more than 4 cm. (2) In **hypertonic (incoordinate) uterine dysfunction,** either basal tone is elevated or the pressure gradient is distorted, perhaps by contraction of the fundus of the uterus with more force than the midsegment or by complete asynchronism of the impulses originating in each cornu—or a combination of the two mechanisms. This type of dysfunction is typically encountered in the latent phase of labor.

In hypotonic uterine dysfunction, contractions become less frequent and the uterus is easily indentable even at the acme of a contraction. Contractions of the hypertonic or incoordinate variety are typically much more painful yet ineffective.

Hypotonic dysfunction often responds to treatment with oxytocin. The opposite is most often true of hypertonic dysfunction, in which the abnormal pattern of uterine contractions is more likely to become accentuated and the tone of the uterine muscle increased.

Etiology

Moderate degrees of pelvic contraction and fetal malposition may cause hypotonic uterine dysfunction. Overdistention of the uterus, as with twins and with hydramnios, may contribute to the condition. In many—perhaps half—of instances, however, the cause of uterine dysfunction is unknown.

Complications

Procrastination often leads to an unfortunate outcome, whereas intervention too early results in needless cesarean deliveries. Fetal and neonatal deaths are accompaniments of intrauterine infection that commonly develops in prolonged dysfunctional labor. Maternal exhaustion may occur if labor is greatly prolonged; however, supportive therapy with intravenous fluids should be initiated and delivery effected before these complications appear.

Treatment of Hypotonic Uterine Dysfunction

Two questions must be answered before a plan for treat-

ment can be formulated: (1) Has the woman actually been in active labor? If the cervix has been observed to undergo distinct changes in effacement and in dilatation to 4 cm at least, it is correct to conclude that there has been real, albeit abnormal, labor. (2) Is there cephalopelvic disproportion? Uterine dysfunction often serves as protection against pelvic contraction or abnormalities of fetal size or presentation.

A. Amniotomy: Most often, once the diagnosis of active labor followed by hypotonic uterine dysfunction has been made and the head is well fixed in the pelvis, the membranes, if intact, should be ruptured and (ideally) an intrauterine pressure catheter and fetal scalp electrode placed. Close observation may be employed for 30–60 minutes to see if the amniotomy will improve the quality of contractions. Next, a decision must be made about whether to stimulate labor with oxytocin or to effect cesarean delivery. The presence of meconium in the amnionic fluid may be an ominous sign, and this observation makes close monitoring of the fetal heart rate and uterine contraction pattern even more critical.

The choice of whether to augment labor with hypotonic uterine dysfunction has been for many years an empirical decision based largely upon clinical judgments about fetal size, presentation, and position as well as clinical assessment of pelvic size.

B. Oxytocin Augmentation: It should be established that the birth canal is probably adequate for the size of the fetal head and that the fetal head is well flexed so as to utilize its smallest diameters to negotiate the birth canal. A contracted pelvis is most unlikely when all of the following criteria are met:

(1) The diagonal conjugate is normal.
(2) The pelvic sidewalls are nearly parallel.
(3) The ischial spines are not prominent.
(4) The sacrum is not flat.
(5) The subpubic angle is not narrow.
(6) The occiput is known to be the presenting part.
(7) The fetal head is engaged or descends through the pelvic inlet with fundal pressure.

If these criteria are not met, the alternatives are cesarean delivery or perhaps oxytocin stimulation. If oxytocin is used, it is mandatory that the fetal heart rate and the contraction pattern frequency, intensity, duration, and timing in relation to the fetal heart rate be observed closely. If fetal heart action is monitored discontinuously, it is imperative that it be checked *immediately following contractions* rather than a minute or more afterward.

C. Technique for Intravenous Oxytocin Administration: Ten units of oxytocin are thoroughly mixed with 1 L of aqueous solution, usually 5% glucose in water.

Since the oxytocin solution contains 10 mU per mL, its rate of flow is easily calculated. Use of a constant infusion pump enhances the precision of the dosage delivered, especially in the lower range. *With the flow shut off,* a needle is inserted into an arm vein—or, preferably, into an already well-functioning intravenous infusion line—and the flow started to deliver no more than 1 mU per min.

For **augmentation of labor** in true hypotonic dysfunction, 1 mU of oxytocin should not initiate tetanic uterine contractions, though one should be prepared to stop the flow if the uterus is overly sensitive to the drug. The flow can be increased gradually at intervals not greater than 30 minutes to yield no more than 10 mU per min. The American College of Obstetricians and Gynecologists (1987) recommends increasing the dose at 30- to 60-minute intervals by 1–2 mU per min. It is rarely necessary to exceed this rate in the treatment of uterine dysfunction. For the **induction of labor,** if a flow rate of 30–40 mU per min fails to initiate satisfactory uterine contractions, faster rates are not likely to do so.

The mother should never be left alone while the oxytocin infusion is running. Uterine contractions must be evaluated continually and oxytocin shut off immediately if contractions exceed 1 minute in duration or if the fetal heart rate decelerates significantly. When either occurs, immediate discontinuation of the oxytocin nearly always corrects the disturbances, preventing harm to mother and fetus. The oxytocin concentration in plasma rapidly falls, since the mean half-life of oxytocin is approximately 5 minutes.

Caution: Oxytocin has potent antidiuretic action. Whenever 20 mU per min or more of oxytocin is infused, water intoxication may lead to convulsions, coma, and even death.

The following precautions should be observed when using oxytocin to treat hypotonic dysfunction:

(1) The patient must be in true labor, not false or prodromal labor. Labor must have progressed to 3–4 cm of dilatation. One of the most common mistakes in obstetrics is to try to stimulate labor in women who have not been in active labor.

(2) There must be no other discernible evidence of mechanical obstruction to safe delivery.

(3) Do not use oxytocin in cases involving abnormal presentations of the fetus and marked uterine overdistention such as gross hydramnios, a large singleton fetus, or multiple fetuses.

(4) In general, women of high parity (more than five deliveries) should not be given oxytocin because their uteri rupture more readily than those of women of lower parity.

(5) The condition of the fetus must be good, as evidenced by a normal heart rate and lack of heavy contamination of the amnionic fluid with meconium. A dead fetus is, of course, no contraindication to the use of oxytocin unless there is overt fetopelvic disproportion or a transverse lie.

(6) The obstetrician must note the time of the first contraction after administration of the drug and be prepared to discontinue its use if a tetanic contraction occurs. The frequency, intensity, and duration of contractions—and uterine tone *between* contractions, must not exceed those of normal spontaneous labor.

(7) Continuous electronic monitoring of the fetal heart and uterine activity should be maintained. Internal scalp electrode and pressure monitoring devices are used as soon as it is prudent to insert them.

One characteristic of intravenous oxytocin is that when successful, it acts promptly, leading to noticeable progress with little delay. Therefore, the drug need not be used for an indefinite period of time to stimulate labor. It should be employed for no more than a few hours; if by then the cervix has not changed appreciably and if predictably easy vaginal delivery is not imminent, cesarean delivery should be performed. Oxytocin administration by any route other than in a dilute intravenous solution as described above is not recommended.

Treatment of Hypertonic Uterine Dysfunction

Hypertonic uterine dysfunction is characterized by uterine pain that appears to be out of proportion to the intensity of contractions and certainly out of proportion to their effectiveness in effacing and dilating the cervix. This type of uterine dysfunction characteristically occurs prior to the cervix reaching a dilatation of 4 cm or more. This is a relatively uncommon cause of dysfunctional labor, and placental abruption must always be considered as a possible cause of uterine hypertonus.

Oxytocin is rarely, if ever, indicated in the presence of uterine hypertonus with a living fetus. Cesarean delivery should be employed if fetal distress is suspected. If the membranes are intact and there is no other evidence of fetopelvic disproportion, administration of morphine or meperidine will relieve pain and rest the mother as well as arrest the abnormal uterine activity. When she awakes, it is hoped that more effective labor will be evident. Such management must not lead to undue procrastination and unrecognized fetal distress, including the defecation of copious amounts of meconium into the amnionic fluid—and, in turn, serious meconium aspiration by the fetus.

CLASSIFICATION & MANAGEMENT OF LABOR DISORDERS

Labor disorders have been divided into three types: prolonged latent phase disorders, protraction disorders, and arrest disorders. Their diagnostic criteria and treatment approaches are summarized in Table 45–1.

The diagnosis of a **prolonged latent phase** is based on the passage of time with failure of the cervix to dilate past 3–4 cm. Unfortunately, this diagnosis is most often made in retrospect. The most frequent causes are early uses of narcotic or sedative analgesics in excessive doses and the use of regional epidural analgesia. Thus, treatment usually consists of allowing these drugs to be metabolized and cleared from the maternal circulation if sufficient time is available—ie, if the membranes have not been ruptured for too long a time and the fetus and mother are in no imminent danger. If waiting does not achieve the desired result, 85% of such patients will respond to an oxytocin infusion.

As simple as these diagnoses and management options may seem, the problem remains that a prolonged latent phase may be due (1) injudicious use of analgesics, (2) false labor, (3) hypertonic uterine dysfunction, or (4) "unknown" reasons. Thus, if analgesic causes are not present and if delivery is not mandated for fetal or maternal reasons, heavy sedation with narcotics should be tried. When the patient awakens in 6–7 hours, she usually will be in progressive labor if the disorder was due to hypertonic uterine dysfunction or will not be in labor if she had been in false labor. In the 2–3% of patients who revert to the same pattern as before the sedation, a diagnosis of hypertonic uterine dysfunction is most likely.

The two **protraction disorders** are closely related and should be considered together. The diagnosis is established when the cervix fails to dilate at the rates listed in Table 45–1 or when the presenting part fails to descend at the rates listed in the table but progress continues. The most frequent causes of these disorders are unknown, but approximately one third of cases are due to varying degrees of cephalopelvic disproportion.

Treatment of the protraction disorders is not clearly established except when cephalopelvic disproportion can be documented, in which case cesarean delivery is indicated. In other circumstances, supportive measures such as hydration and psychologic support can be instituted, bearing in mind that even with oxytocin stimulation the rate of dilatation of the cervix and the rate of descent of the presenting part cannot be accelerated.

The **arrest disorders** are considered to be present (Table 45–1) when there is no cervical dilatation for 2 hours, when the deceleration phase is prolonged, or when the presenting part fails to descend for 1 hour or longer. Friedman (1978) maintains that approximately one-half of these patients have "insurmountable obstruction" and recommends the judicious use of intravenous oxytocin but cautions that such efforts, while effective in dilating the cervix and ultimately resulting in vaginal delivery, may subject the fetus to substantial risks of hypoxic injury as well as birth trauma.

The author's approach has been to assess the quality of uterine contractions with an internal pressure catheter. An adequate contraction pattern is considered to be at least three contractions per 10 minutes lasting at least 45 seconds with an amplitude of 50 mm Hg or more. An arrest pattern in the face of such contractions is unlikely to respond to an oxytocin augmentation, and cesarean delivery is performed instead. If, however, the contraction pattern is inadequate, oxytocin augmentation is performed as previously discussed under treatment of hypotonic dysfunction and techniques of intravenous oxytocin.

INADEQUATE VOLUNTARY EXPULSIVE FORCE

With full cervical dilatation, women usually feel the urge to "bear down" or "push" each time the uterus contracts. Typically, the laboring woman inhales deeply, closes her glottis, and contracts her abdominal musculature repetitively to increase intra-abdominal pressure throughout the time of uterine contraction. The combined contractions of the uterus and the abdominal musculature propel the fetus down the vagina and through the vaginal outlet.

Causes of Inadequate Expulsive Forces

Conduction analgesia is likely to reduce the reflex urge for the woman to "push" and at the same time may impair her ability to contract the abdominal muscles sufficiently to increase intra-abdominal pressure. Loss of consciousness associated with general anesthesia certainly imposes these adverse effects, as does heavy sedation.

Management

Careful selection of analgesic agents and the timing of their administration are important to prevent compromise of voluntary expulsive efforts. With rare exceptions, intrathecal analgesia or general anesthesia should not be administered until all conditions for a safe forceps delivery have been met (Chapter 51). With continuous epidural analgesia, it may be necessary to allow the paralytic effects to wear off so that the mother in response to coaching can generate intra-abdominal pressure sufficient to move the fetal head into a position appropriate for low forceps delivery. The alternatives—a possibly difficult forceps vaginal delivery or cesarean delivery—are unsatisfactory options in the absence of evidence of fetal distress.

LOCALIZED ABNORMALITIES OF UTERINE ACTION

Very rarely, localized **rings or constrictions of the uterus** develop in association with prolonged rupture of the membranes and protracted labors. The most common type is the so-called **pathologic retraction ring of Bandl.**

In rare instances, uterine contractions disappear without leading to the birth of the child. The fetus then dies and may be retained in utero for months or years, undergoing mummification. This condition is known as **missed labor.**

PRECIPITATE LABOR & DELIVERY

Precipitate—ie, extremely rapid—labor and delivery may result from abnormally low resistance of the soft parts of the birth canal, from abnormally strong uterine and abdominal contractions, or, very rarely, from the absence of painful sensations and thus a lack of awareness of vigorous labor.

Clinical Findings

A. Maternal Effects: Precipitate labor combined with a long, firm cervix and a vagina, vulva, or perineum that resists stretch may lead to rupture of the uterus or extensive lacerations of the cervix, vagina, vulva, or perineum. The uterus that contracts with unusual vigor before delivery is likely to be hypotonic after delivery, with hemorrhage from the placental implantation site as the consequence.

B. Effects on Fetus and Neonate: Perinatal mortality and morbidity from precipitate labor may be increased considerably for several reasons. First, the tumultuous uterine contractions often prevent appropriate uterine blood flow and oxygenation of the fetal blood. Second, resistance of the birth canal to expulsion of the head may cause intracranial trauma. Moreover, Erb-Duchenne palsy is associated with such labors in a third of cases. Third, during an unattended birth, the infant may fall to the floor and be injured or may need resuscitation that is not immediately available.

Treatment

Any oxytocic agents being administered should be stopped immediately. Tocolytic agents such as ritodrine and parenteral magnesium sulfate may prove effective.

SUGGESTED READINGS

American College of Obstetricians and Gynecologists: Induction and augmentation of labor. Tech Bull No. 110, November 1987.

Caldeyro-Barcia R, Alvarez H, Reynolds SRM: A better understanding of uterine contractility through simultaneous recording with an internal and a seven channel external method. Surg Obstet Gynecol 1950;91:641.

Cohen W, Friedman EA (editors): *Management of Labor.* University Park Press, 1983.

Friedman EA: *Labor: Clinical Evaluation and Management,* 2nd ed. Appleton, 1978.

46

Dystocia Due to Abnormalities in Presentation, Position, or Development of the Fetus

BREECH PRESENTATION

Breech presentation is common remote from term. Most often, however, at some time before the onset of labor, the fetus turns spontaneously to a vertex presentation, so that breech presentation persists in only about 3–4% of singleton deliveries.

The fundamental difference between labor and delivery in cephalic and breech presentations is that with cephalic presentation, once the head is delivered, the rest of the body usually follows without difficulty, whereas with breech presentation, successively larger and much less compressible parts of the fetus are born. With breech presentation, an increased frequency of the following complications can be anticipated: (1) perinatal morbidity and mortality from difficult delivery; (2) low birth weight from prematurity, growth retardation, or both; (3) prolapsed cord; (4) placenta previa; (5) fetal anomalies and developmental abnormalities that appear after the newborn period; (6) maternal uterine anomalies and tumors; (7) multiple fetuses; and (8) operative delivery, especially cesarean delivery.

Etiology

Factors other than gestational age that appear to predispose to breech presentation include uterine relaxation associated with high parity, multiple fetuses, hydramnios, oligohydramnios, hydrocephalus, anencephalus, previous breech delivery, uterine anomalies, and tumors in the pelvis and perhaps implantation of the placenta in either cornual-fundal region of the uterus.

Diagnosis

A. Types of Breech Presentation: With a **frank breech** presentation, the lower extremities are flexed at the hips and extended at the knees; thus, the feet lie in close proximity to the head. A **complete breech** presentation differs in that one or both knees are flexed rather than both extended. With **incomplete breech** presentation, one or both hips are not flexed and one or both feet or one or both knees lie below the breech, ie, a foot or knee is lowermost in the birth canal (see Chapter 38).

B. Physical Examination: A breech presentation may be diagnosed by physical examination using Leopold's maneuvers or by vaginal examination (see Chapter 38). The presentation can be confirmed with imaging techniques.

C. Imaging Studies: Sonography ideally should be used to confirm a clinically suspected breech presentation and to identify, if possible, any fetal anomalies. Unfortunately, sonography cannot be used in most cases to identify the relationship of the lower extremities to the fetal pelvis. This information often is essential in planning the route of delivery (see below).

If the woman is in labor and vaginal delivery is being considered, the type of breech presentation is of considerable importance. In such cases, radiation exposure may be reduced considerably by using CT pelvimetry.

Imaging techniques can be used to provide information about the type of breech presentation, the presence or absence of a flexed fetal head, and accurate measurements of the pelvis (see Chapter 38).

Prevention

Whenever a breech presentation is recognized during the third trimester, an attempt may be made to substitute a vertex presentation by **external version.** External version is more readily accomplished in multiparous women with lax abdominal walls than in nulliparous women. Because of possible trauma, anesthesia should never be used.

If properly and gently performed, external version is a benign procedure. However, fetal and maternal injury and hemorrhage may occur. Immunoprophylaxis with anti-D globulin before external version is attempted has been recommended for Rh negative women.

Management

A. External Cephalic Version: Version substitutes one pole of a longitudinal presentation for the other or converts an oblique or transverse lie into a longitudinal presentation. According to whether the head or breech is made the presenting part, the operation is designated cephalic or podalic version, respectively. In **external versions,** the manipulations are performed exclusively through the abdominal wall; in **internal versions,** the entire hand is introduced into the uterine cavity.

External cephalic version is more likely to be successful (1) if the presenting part has not descended into the pelvis; (2) if there is a normal amount of amnionic fluid; (3) if the fetal back is not positioned posteriorly; and (4) if the patient is not obese. The fetal heart action must be continuously monitored, usually with a Doppler sound instrument, so that the obstetrician can continuously hear the fetal heart rate during the procedure. Sonography, when immediately available, often proves helpful. Anesthesia should never be used lest undue force be applied.

In the early stages of labor, before the membranes have ruptured, the same indications apply. They may then be extended to oblique presentations as well, though these unstable lies usually convert spontaneously to longitudinal lies as labor progresses.

B. Recommendations for Delivery: To try to minimize infant mortality and morbidity rates, cesarean delivery is now commonly used in the following circumstances in all but the extremely immature fetus whose potential for survival is negligible.

1. Breech presentation and a large fetus.
2. Breech presentation and any degree of contraction or unfavorable shape of the pelvis (Chapter 38).
3. Breech presentation and a hyperextended head.
4. Breech presentation not in labor, with maternal or fetal indications for delivery such as pregnancy-induced hypertension or rupture of the membranes for 12 hours or more.
5. Breech presentation and uterine dysfunction.
6. Complete or footling breech presentation.
7. Breech presentation, active labor, and an apparently healthy but preterm fetus of 26 weeks' gestation or longer.
8. Breech presentation and severe fetal growth retardation.
9. Breech presentation and previous perinatal death or previous offspring suffering from birth trauma.
10. Breech presentation and a request by the mother for sterilization.

C. Vaginal Delivery: Vaginal delivery should be relatively safe for a frank breech presentation (1) if the pelvis is in no way contracted when examined by imaging pelvimetry (a previous cephalic delivery by itself is not proof that the pelvis may not be "contracted" for a breech delivery); (2) if the fetus is judged to be less than 8 lb by two or more examiners or when weight is estimated ultrasonically; (3) if labor is established; and (4) if individuals skilled in breech delivery, in providing appropriate anesthesia, and in infant resuscitation are in immediate attendance. Even when every attempt is made to fulfill these criteria, the outcome for the infant is not always as good as when delivery is by cesarean.

There are three general methods of breech delivery through the vagina:

1. Spontaneous breech delivery–The infant is expelled entirely spontaneously without any traction or manipulation other than support of the infant. This form of delivery of mature infants is rare.

2. Partial breech extraction–The infant is delivered spontaneously as far as the umbilicus, but the remainder of the body is extracted.

3. Total breech extraction–The entire body of the infant is extracted by the obstetrician.

D. Management of Labor: A woman admitted in labor with a breech presentation requires the immediate attention of nursing and medical personnel.

1. Stage of labor–If labor is too far advanced, insufficient time may be available to obtain imaging pelvimetry, and this alone may force the decision for abdominal rather than vaginal delivery. *Regardless, the time available to accomplish all necessary nursing and medical procedures is the first priority to be established in the laboring woman with a breech presentation.*

2. Fetal condition–The presence or absence of gross fetal abnormalities such as hydrocephaly or anencephaly can be ascertained rapidly with the use of sonography or x-ray examination. CT pelvimetry will usually document flexion of the fetal head; if it does not, a plain film of the abdomen will suffice.

3. Intravenous fluids and laboratory values–Possible emergency induction of anesthesia or hemorrhage from lacerations or uterine atony from halogenated anesthetics are but two of many reasons for immediate placing of an indwelling intravenous catheter that can be used to administer medications or fluids, including blood. The same site can be used prior to administering fluids to obtain blood for hematocrit, typing, and cross-matching.

4. Electronic fetal monitoring–Continuous electronic monitoring of fetal heart rate and uterine contractions is started immediately. When membranes are ruptured, the risk of umbilical cord prolapse is increased. Therefore, vaginal examination should be done after rupture of the membranes to check for umbilical cord prolapse. Special attention should be directed to the fetal heart rate for the first 5–10 minutes following rupture to make certain there has not been an occult cord prolapse. After rupture, internal electronic monitoring of the fetal heart rate and uterine contractions is preferable because of the more reliable information provided by these techniques.

5. Recruitment of nursing and medical personnel–For labor, one-on-one nursing should be maintained because of the risk of umbilical cord prolapse or occlusion, and the obstetrician must be readily available in case of emergency.

6. Route of delivery–The obstetrician should decide the route of delivery as soon as possible after admission.

E. Timing Of Delivery: In general, preparations for breech extraction should be in place by the time the buttocks or the feet appear at the vulva. It is essential that the delivery team include (1) an obstetrician skilled in the art of breech extraction; (2) an associate scrubbed and gowned to assist with the delivery; (3) an anesthesiologist who can quickly induce general anesthesia when needed; (4) an individual trained to resuscitate the infant effectively, including tracheal intubation; and (5) someone to provide general assistance.

Delivery is easier and perinatal morbidity and mortality rates are thus lower when the fetus is allowed to deliver spontaneously to the umbilicus. If fetal distress develops before this time, a decision must be made about whether to perform total breech extraction or, what is more likely, cesarean delivery. At the minimum, the birth canal must be capacious enough to allow passage of the fetus without trauma, and the cervix must be effaced and fully dilated. If these conditions are not met, cesarean delivery is almost always preferable.

F. Extraction of Complete or Incomplete Breech and Frank Breech: The technique of breech extraction differs in complete and incomplete breech versus frank breech extraction. Specific techniques for vaginal deliveries of breech presentations are discussed and illustrated in Chapter 25, "Techniques for Breech Delivery," in Cunningham FG, MacDonald PC, Gant NF, Leveno KJ, Gilstrap LC (editors): *Williams Obstetrics,* 19th ed. Appleton & Lange, 1993.

G. Anesthesia: The fetus should be allowed to deliver spontaneously to the umbilicus. Analgesia for episiotomy and intravaginal manipulations needed for breech extraction can usually be accomplished with pudendal block and local infiltration of the perineum (Chapter 44). Nitrous oxide plus oxygen by inhalation provides further relief from pain. If for any reason general anesthesia is desired, it can be quickly induced with thiopental plus a muscle relaxant and maintained with nitrous oxide. Continuous epidural analgesia cannot be confidently recommended.

H. Internal Podalic Version: There are few (or no) indications for internal podalic version other than for delivery of the second twin (Chapter 56). The maneuver consists of inserting a hand into the uterine cavity, grasping one or both feet, and drawing them through the cervix while exerting pressure transabdominally in the opposite direction on the upper portion of the body. The maneuver is followed by breech extraction.

I. Cesarean Delivery: There is little question that perinatal mortality and morbidity from trauma and hypoxia can be reduced by liberal use of cesarean delivery. Certainly, the fetus in the breech position is likely to benefit from cesarean delivery performed early in labor but at the expense of a substantial increase in maternal morbidity and a slight increase in maternal mortality rates.

Prognosis

With breech presentation, both the mother and the fetus are at greater risk.

A. Maternal Risk: Labor is usually not prolonged, but because of the greater frequency of operative delivery, including cesarean delivery, there is a higher maternal morbidity rate and a slightly higher mortality rate for pregnancies complicated by persistent breech presentation. This risk is probably even greater if an emergency rather than an elective cesarean delivery is performed.

B. Risk to Fetus or Infant: The prognosis for the fetus in a breech presentation is considerably worse than in a vertex presentation. The major contributors to this perinatal loss are preterm delivery, congenital anomalies, and birth trauma. However, it has been suggested that the breech presentation might be a factor identifying an already abnormal fetus. In one report, one-third of children with cerebral palsy who were in breech presentation at birth had major noncerebral malformations.

FACE PRESENTATION

In face presentation, the head is hyperextended so that the occiput is in contact with the fetal back and the chin (mentum) is the presenting part. The incidence is approximately 1:1200 deliveries.

Etiology

Extended positions of the head occur more frequently when the pelvis is contracted or the fetus is very large. In multiparous women, the pendulous abdomen is another factor that predisposes to face presentation.

In exceptional instances, marked enlargement of the neck or coils of cord about the neck may cause extension. Anencephalic fetuses naturally present by the face because of faulty development of the cranium.

Diagnosis

The error of mistaking a breech for a face presentation on vaginal palpation can be avoided by remembering that the fetal anus is always on a line with the ischial tuberosities whereas the fetal mouth and malar prominences form the corners of a triangle.

Mechanism of Labor

The mechanism of labor in these cases consists of the cardinal movements of labor. Descent is brought about by the same factors as in vertex presentations. Extension results from the relation of the fetal body to the deflected head, which is converted into a two-armed lever, the longer arm of which extends from the occipital condyles to the occiput. When resistance is then encountered, the occiput must be pushed toward the back of the fetus while the chin descends (Figure 46–1).

The object of internal rotation of the face is to bring the

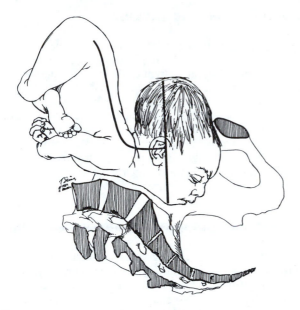

Figure 46–1. Face presentation. The occiput is on the longer end of the head lever. The chin is directly posterior. Vaginal delivery is impossible unless the chin rotates anteriorly. (Reproduced, with permission, from Cunningham FG, MacDonald PC, Gant NF, Leveno KJ, Gilstrap LG [editors]: *Williams Obstetrics*, 19th ed. Appleton & Lange, 1993.)

chin under the symphysis pubis. Unless the head is unusually small, natural delivery cannot otherwise be accomplished. Only with rotation of the chin to the anterior position can vaginal delivery occur.

Management

In the absence of a contracted pelvis and with effective spontaneous labor and no evidence of fetal distress, successful vaginal delivery will usually follow. If labor is allowed, careful monitoring of the fetal heart is probably better done with external devices so as to avoid damage to the face and eyes. Face presentations among term-size fetuses occur more commonly when there is some degree of contraction of the pelvic inlet. Therefore, cesarean section often proves to be the best method for delivery.

BROW PRESENTATION

Brow presentation is rare, occurring in approximately 1:4600 deliveries. The causes are essentially the same as those of face presentation. With brow presentation, that portion of the fetal head between the orbital ridge and the anterior fontanelle presents at the pelvic inlet. The fetal head thus occupies a position midway between full flexion (occiput) and full extension (mentum, or face). Except when the fetal head is small or the pelvis is unusually large, engagement of the fetal head and subsequent delivery cannot take place as long as the presentation persists.

Diagnosis

The presentation may be recognized by abdominal palpation when both the occiput and chin can be easily palpated, but vaginal examination is usually necessary (Figure 46–2).

Mechanism of Labor

The mechanism of labor varies greatly with the size of the fetus. With a very small fetus and a large pelvis, labor is generally easy. With larger fetuses, however, labor is usually very difficult, since engagement is impossible until after marked molding develops that shortens the occipitomental diameter. More commonly, either flexion to an occiput presentation or extension to a face presentation occurs.

Management

The principles underlying the management of brow presentations are much the same as those for face presentation. If, by chance, spontaneous labor is progressing without any evidence of distress in the closely monitored fetus and without unduly vigorous uterine contractions, no interference is necessary. If labor becomes either unduly vigorous or, more likely, ineffective—or if fetal distress is suspected—prompt cesarean delivery is indicated.

Prognosis

In the transient varieties of brow presentation, the prognosis depends upon the ultimate presentation. When brow presentation persists, the prognosis is poor for vaginal delivery of an uncompromised infant unless the fetus is small or the birth canal is huge.

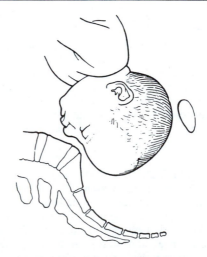

Figure 46–2. Brow posterior presentation. (Reproduced, with permission, from Cunningham FG, MacDonald PC, Gant NF, Leveno KJ, Gilstrap LG [editors]: *Williams Obstetrics*, 19th ed. Appleton & Lange, 1993.)

TRANSVERSE LIE

Transverse lie occurs in approximately 1:420 deliveries. The shoulder is usually over the pelvic inlet, with the head lying in one iliac fossa and the breech in the other. This condition is referred to as a **shoulder** or **acromion presentation.** The side of the mother toward which the acromion is directed determines the designation of the lie as right or left acromial. Moreover, since in either position the back may be directed anteriorly or posteriorly and superiorly or inferiorly, it is customary to distinguish varieties as dorsoanterior and dorsoposterior.

Etiology

The common causes of transverse lie are (1) unusual relaxation of the abdominal wall, resulting from grand multiparity; (2) preterm fetus; (3) placenta previa; (4) abnormal uterus; and (5) contracted pelvis.

Diagnosis

The abdomen is unusually wide from side to side, whereas the fundus of the uterus extends scarcely above the umbilicus. On palpation, with the first Leopold maneuver no fetal pole is detected in the fundus. On the second maneuver, a ballottable head is found in one iliac fossa and the breech in the other. The third and fourth maneuvers are negative.

On vaginal examination in the early stages of labor, the side of the thorax, if it can be reached, may be recognized by the "gridiron" feel of the ribs above the pelvic inlet. When dilatation is further advanced, the scapula and the clavicle are distinguished on opposite sides of the thorax. The position of the axilla indicates the side of the mother toward which the shoulder is directed. Later in labor, the shoulder becomes tightly wedged in the pelvic canal, and a hand and arm frequently prolapse into the vagina and through the vulva.

Management

The spontaneous birth of a fully developed infant is manifestly impossible in a persistent transverse lie. At term, both the fetus and the mother will die unless appropriate measures are taken. Before the onset of labor, with the membranes intact, external version may be attempted. The onset of active labor in a woman with a transverse lie is an absolute indication for cesarean delivery.

Prognosis

A. Maternal Risks: Even with the best of care, the chance of maternal death will be increased slightly for four reasons: (1) the frequent association of transverse lie with placenta previa, (2) the increased likelihood of cord accidents, (3) the almost inevitable necessity for major operative interferences, and (4) the likelihood of sepsis after rupture of the membranes and extrusion of the arm through the vagina.

B. Risk to Fetus or Infant: The risks to the fetus-infant include prematurity, cord prolapse, and trauma.

COMPOUND PRESENTATION

Any condition that prevents complete occlusion of the pelvic inlet by the fetal head may cause a compound presentation, in which an extremity prolapses alongside the presenting part with both presenting in the pelvis simultaneously. In most cases, the prolapsed part should be left alone, since most often it will not interfere with labor. Electronic fetal heart rate monitoring and intrauterine pressure monitoring are preferable. Cesarean delivery can be done for fetal distress or uterine dysfunction.

Perinatal loss is due to preterm delivery, prolapsed cord, and traumatic obstetrical procedures.

PERSISTENT OCCIPUT POSTERIOR POSITIONS

In 10% of cases or less, spontaneous rotation of the occiput to the anterior position does not occur. Transverse narrowing of the mid pelvis undoubtedly is one cause.

The conduct of labor and delivery need not differ remarkably from occiput anterior presentation. Fetal status is best monitored by continuous electronic techniques. In most instances, delivery can be accomplished without great difficulty once the head reaches the perineum.

The possibilities for vaginal delivery are (1) to await spontaneous delivery, (2) to proceed with forceps delivery, (3) to accomplish forceps rotation of the occiput to the anterior position and delivery, or (4) to attempt manual rotation to the anterior position. Cesarean delivery is indicated if forceps or manual intervention is tried without prompt success.

PERSISTENT OCCIPUT TRANSVERSE POSITION

In the absence of an abnormality of the pelvic architecture, the occiput transverse position is probably a transitory one as the occiput rotates to the anterior position. If hypotonic uterine dysfunction—either spontaneous or the consequence of conduction analgesia—does not develop, spontaneous rotation is usually soon completed.

If rotation ceases because of lack of uterine action and in the absence of pelvic contraction, the occiput may be manually rotated anteriorly or posteriorly and forceps delivery accomplished from either the anterior or the posterior position. Another approach is to rotate the occiput to the anterior position with Kielland forceps (Chapter 51). If failure of spontaneous rotation is caused by hypotonic uterine dysfunction *without cephalopelvic disproportion,* dilute oxytocin may be infused while the fetal heart rate and the uterine contractions are closely monitored.

The genesis of the occiput transverse position is not always so simple, nor is management so benign. With platypelloid or android pelves, there may not be adequate room for rotation of the occiput to either the anterior or the posterior position. With an android pelvis, the head may not even be engaged yet the scalp may be visible through the vaginal introitus as a consequence of considerable molding and caput formation. This situation is fraught with danger to both the fetus and the mother. If forceps are tried, undue force must not be applied; if forceps intervention is not promptly successful, a cesarean delivery should be accomplished.

FETAL MACROSOMIA

Several factors—alone or in combination—may be operative in the genesis of macrosomia: (1) large size of the parents, especially the mother; (2) grand multiparity; (3) maternal diabetes; (4) maternal obesity; (5) prolonged gestation; and (6) previous delivery of an infant weighing more than 4000 g.

With large fetuses, dystocia may arise because the head becomes not only larger but harder and less moldable with increasing weight. Moreover, dystocia may be caused by the arrest of even larger shoulders at either the pelvic brim or the outlet. About 5.3% of neonates are macrosomic (4000 g or more), and only 0.4% weigh 4500 g or more.

Diagnosis

The diagnosis of macrosomia is often not made until after fruitless attempts at delivery. Nevertheless, clinical examination should enable experienced examiners to arrive at a fairly accurate estimate of fetal size. Sonographic evaluation of the dimensions of the head, thorax, and abdomen often enhances the accuracy of the estimate.

Prognosis

Since macrosomic infants are more often born to multiparous mothers and to women with diabetes, both the maternal and fetal risks are increased.

SHOULDER DYSTOCIA

With shoulder dystocia, the head is delivered, causing the cord to be drawn into the pelvis and compressed before the delivery of the shoulders.

Incidence, Etiology, & Contributing Factors

The cause of shoulder dystocia is fetal macrosomia and not simply an increase in fetal weight to above an arbitrarily defined weight of 4000 g. Thus, fetal macrosomia is an increase in body size in relation to head size, the result often being a larger shoulder girdle than a fetal head. A predictable diagnosis of fetal macrosomia is extremely difficult, and a reliable prediction of shoulder dystocia is impossible.

Contributing Factors

A. Antepartum Factors: Any maternal or fetal factor that contributes to an increased incidence of fetal macrosomia also naturally increases the incidence of shoulder dystocia.

1. Maternal obesity–Maternal obesity alone is diffi-

cult to distinguish from gestational diabetes or overt diabetes. Women weighing over 250 lb have an estimated eightfold greater incidence of shoulder dystocia in labor than women weighing less than 200 lb.

2. Diabetes mellitus–The association of macrosomia with mild diabetes mellitus is well established and is a significantly important contributing factor to shoulder dystocia.

3. Postterm pregnancy–Many fetuses continue to grow after 42 weeks. The association of an increased incidence of shoulder dystocia and postterm pregnancy is now an accepted fact.

B. Intrapartum Factors:

1. Prolonged second stage of labor–The incidence of shoulder dystocia is increased in infants weighing 4000 g or more if the second stage of labor is arrested or prolonged.

2. Oxytocin induction–Large infants often are associated with dysfunctional labors, and oxytocin frequently is indicated in dysfunctional labor. Furthermore, the management of postterm pregnancy consists of induced labor and delivery, and a postterm gestation often is associated with an increased incidence of macrosomia and shoulder dystocia.

3. Midforceps and vacuum extraction–For many of the same reasons discussed under oxytocin induction or augmentation, there is a significant increase in the incidence of shoulder dystocia with midforceps or vacuum extractions.

Management

Because shoulder dystocia cannot be predicted, there always will be the unexpected case. Therefore, the practitioner of obstetrics must be well versed in the management principles of this occasionally devastating complication.

Reduction of the time between delivery of the head and delivery of the body is of great importance to survival, but overly vigorous traction on the head or neck, or excessive rotation of the body may cause serious damage to the infant.

A large mediolateral episiotomy and adequate anesthesia are necessary. The next step is to clear the infant's mouth and nose. Having completed the above steps, a variety of methods or techniques have been described to free the anterior shoulder from its impacted position beneath the maternal symphysis pubis. These techniques are described and illustrated in Chapter 20, "Dystocia Due to Abnormalities in Presentation, Position, or Development of the Fetus," in Cunningham FG, MacDonald PC, Gant NF, Leveno KJ, Gilstrap LG (editors): *Williams Obstetrics,* 19th ed. Appleton & Lange, 1993.

One should first attempt to free the impacted shoulder by simple abdominal pressure applied over the symphysis. If this is not successful, the McRoberts maneuver (sharply flexing the maternal thighs onto her abdomen) is added. If still unsuccessful, the posterior fetal arm and shoulder are delivered or the shoulder girdle is rotated into the oblique position. In the exceptional case when none of the above are possible, the cephalic replacement technique may be tried (flexing the fetal head and pushing it back and upward into the uterus). As a last resort, it may be necessary to deliberately fracture the clavicle.

Prognosis

A. Fetal Consequences: Shoulder dystocia, if not appropriately managed, may be associated with fractured humeri or clavicles, Erb's palsy, asphyxia, and death. Prompt physiotherapy may improve brachial nerve damage in some cases of Erb's palsy (Chapter 55).

B. Maternal Consequences: Uterine atony and vaginal and cervical lacerations are the major maternal risks. Puerperal infection is a problem, but significant infection can usually be prevented with the use of perioperative broad-spectrum antimicrobials (Chapter 50).

HYDROCEPHALUS AS A CAUSE OF DYSTOCIA

Internal hydrocephalus is present in about 1:2000 fetuses and accounts for about 12% of all severe malformations present at birth. Associated defects are common, with spina bifida occurring in about one-third of cases. Breech presentation is found in about one-third of these spina bifida cases. Whatever the presentation, gross cephalopelvic disproportion is the rule, with serious dystocia the usual consequence.

Diagnosis

The thickness of the abdominal wall usually prevents detection of the thin, elastic hydrocephalic cranium. The high head forces the body of the infant upward, with the result that the fetal heart is often loudest above the umbilicus, a circumstance leading to a suspicion of breech presentation. Vaginally, the broader dome of the head feels tense, but more careful palpation may disclose very large fontanelles, wide suture lines, and an indentable, thin cranium characteristic of hydrocephalus. Radiography or sonography provides confirmation by demonstration of a large, globular head. Sonography is recommended in all cases, however, to compare the diameter of the lateral ventricles to the biparietal diameter of the head and to evaluate the thickness of the cerebral cortex as well as to compare the size of the head with that of the thorax and abdomen.

Management

The size of the hydrocephalic head must usually be reduced if the head is to pass through the birth canal. Needle aspirations of the fetal cerebral ventricles can be accomplished transabdominally or vaginally to drain the ventricles and allow vaginal delivery.

The antepartum identification of fetal hydrocephaly has resulted in successful "shunt" of the ventricles. However, not all such attempts have been successful—not only because of mechanical problems but also because many of these fetuses have multiple abnormalities, some of them lethal.

Prognosis

Rupture of the uterus is a danger and may occur before complete dilatation of the cervix. Hydrocephalus predisposes to rupture not only because of the obvious disproportion but also because the great transverse diameter of the cranium overdistends the lower uterine segment. When fetal hydrocephalus is overlooked, the maternal mortality rate is high.

LARGE FETAL ABDOMEN AS A CAUSE OF DYSTOCIA

Enlargement of the fetal abdomen sufficient to cause grave dystocia is usually the result of a greatly distended bladder, ascites, or enlargement of the kidneys or liver. Occasionally, the abdomen of a fetus affected with edema may attain such proportions that spontaneous delivery is impossible. An enlarged abdomen and intra-abdominal accumulation of fluid can be diagnosed in utero by careful sonographic examination.

Management

If the abdominal enlargement is not discovered until the fetal head has been delivered, decompression of the fetal abdomen may be accomplished using a large-gauge long needle which is inserted through the midline of the maternal abdomen into the fetal abdomen. Fluid in the fetal bladder or peritoneal cavity promptly escapes.

If the diagnosis of gross enlargement of the fetal abdomen is made before delivery, the decision must be made whether or not to perform a cesarean delivery. In general, irrespective of the route of delivery, the prognosis is very poor for the fetus with abdominal enlargement severe enough to cause dystocia.

CONJOINED TWINS

The embryologic basis of incomplete twinning is considered in Chapter 56. Generally, cesarean delivery is preferred if the diagnosis is known, but vaginal delivery can occur. This is possible because such pregnancies seldom go to term; because conjoined twins may not greatly exceed the size of a normal fetus; and because the connection between the halves is sometimes flexible.

SUGGESTED READINGS

Acker DB et al: Risk factors for Erb-Duchenne palsy. Obstet Gynecol 1988;71:389.

Dystocia due to abnormalities in presentation, position, or development of the fetus. Chapter 20 in: Cunningham FG, MacDonald PC, Gant NF, Leveno KJ, Gilstrap LG (editors): *Williams Obstetrics,* 19th ed. Appleton & Lange, 1993.

Fortunato SJ, Mercer LJ, Guzick DS: External cephalic version with tocolysis: Factors associated with success. Obstet Gynecol 1988;72:59.

Johnson SR, Kolberg BH, Varner MW: Maternal obesity and pregnancy. Surg Gynecol Obstet 1987;164:431.

Nelson KB, Ellenberg JH: Antecedents of cerebral palsy: Multivariate analysis of risk. N Engl J Med 1986;315:81.

47

Dystocia Due to Pelvic Contraction

Any contraction of the pelvic diameters that diminishes the capacity of the pelvis can create dystocia during labor. Pelvic contractions may be classified as follows:

(1) Contraction of the pelvic inlet
(2) Contraction of the mid pelvis
(3) Contraction of the pelvic outlet
(4) Generally contracted pelvis (combinations of the above)

CONTRACTED PELVIC INLET

The pelvic inlet is usually considered to be contracted if its shortest anteroposterior diameter is less than 10 cm or if the greatest transverse diameter is less than 12 cm. The anteroposterior diameter of the pelvic inlet is commonly approximated by measuring manually the diagonal conjugate, which is about 1.5 cm greater. Therefore, inlet contraction usually is defined as **a diagonal conjugate of less than 11.5 cm.** The configuration of the pelvic inlet (Caldwell-Moloy classification; see Chapter 38) also is an important determinant of the adequacy of any pelvis, independent of actual measurements.

Size of Fetal Head

Inability to push the head into the pelvis, however, does not necessarily mean that vaginal delivery is impossible. A clear demonstration of a flexed fetal head that overrides the symphysis pubis is presumptive evidence of disproportion, however.

Measurement of the fetal biparietal diameter and head circumference by ultrasonic means allows precise measurement. A cephalic circumference measurement usually is preferable, however, since the head of the fetus in the breech presentation may be elongated in the occipitofrontal diameter (dolichocephaly). This dolichocephalic head may also be observed in multifetal gestations and in cases of oligohydramnios.

Presentation & Position of the Fetus

A contracted pelvic inlet plays an important part in the production of abnormal presentations. Face and shoulder presentations occur three times more frequently in women with contracted pelves, and prolapse of the cord and of the extremities occurs four to six times more frequently. In normal nulliparous women, the presenting part commonly descends into the pelvic cavity before the onset of labor at term. When the pelvic inlet is greatly contracted, however, descent usually does not occur until after the onset of labor if it occurs at all.

Course of Labor

When the pelvic deformity is sufficiently pronounced to prevent the head from readily entering the inlet, the course of labor is prolonged, and in many cases spontaneous labor is never achieved. The effects on the mother and fetus when this happens are severe.

A. Maternal Effects: While maternal and fetal effects resulting from inlet contraction are arbitrarily divided in the subsequent discussion, it must be remembered that bony dystocia may result in serious consequences to either or both patients.

1. Abnormalities in cervical dilatation–Normally, dilatation of the cervix is facilitated by the hydrostatic action of the unruptured membranes or, after their rupture, by direct application of the presenting part against the cervix. In contracted pelves, however, when the head is arrested in the pelvic inlet, the entire force exerted by the uterus acts directly upon the portion of membranes that overlie the dilating cervix.

After rupture of the membranes, the absence of pressure exerted by the fetal head against the cervix and lower uterine segment predisposes to less effective uterine contractions. With degrees of pelvic contractions incompatible with vaginal delivery, the cervix seldom dilates satisfactorily. Thus, the behavior of the cervix has prognostic value.

2. Danger of uterine rupture–When the disproportion between the head and the pelvis is so pronounced that engagement and descent do not occur, the lower uterine segment becomes increasingly stretched, and the danger of its rupture becomes imminent. In such cases, a **pathologic retraction ring** may develop and can be felt as a transverse or oblique ridge extending across the uterus somewhere between the symphysis and the umbilicus. Whenever this condition is noted, prompt cesarean delivery must be employed to terminate labor and prevent rupture of the uterus.

3. Production of fistulas—When the presenting part is firmly wedged into the pelvic inlet but does not advance for a considerable time, portions of the birth canal lying between it and the pelvic wall may be subjected to excessive pressure. As the circulation is impaired, the resulting necrosis may become manifest several days after delivery by the appearance of vesicovaginal, vesicocervical, or rectovaginal fistulas.

4. Intrapartum infection—Infection is another serious danger to which the mother and the fetus are exposed in labors complicated by prolonged rupture of the membranes. The danger of infection is increased by repeated vaginal examinations and other intravaginal and intrauterine manipulations.

B. Fetal Effects: Prolonged labor in itself is deleterious to the fetus. In women in labor for more than 20 hours or with a second stage of labor of more than 3 hours, there is a significant increase in perinatal mortality rates. If the pelvis is contracted and there is associated early rupture of the membranes, intrapartum infection is a serious complication for the mother and an important cause of fetal and neonatal death.

1. Caput succedaneum formation—A large caput succedaneum frequently develops on the most dependent part of the head during labor if the pelvis is contracted. The caput may reach almost to the pelvic floor while the head is still not engaged, and without recognizing this, an inexperienced physician may make premature and unwise attempts at forceps delivery. Typically, the large caput disappears within a few days after birth.

2. Molding of the fetal head—Under the pressure of strong uterine contractions, the bones of the skull overlap one another at the major sutures, a process referred to as molding. This process may reduce the biparietal diameter by 0.5 cm or so without causing cerebral injury; with greater degrees of molding, the likelihood of intracranial injury increases.

Fractures of the skull are occasionally encountered, usually following forcible attempts at delivery, though sometimes they may occur with spontaneous delivery.

3. Prolapse of the cord—A serious fetal complication is prolapse of the cord, which is facilitated by imperfect adaptation between the presenting part and the pelvic inlet.

Treatment

Management of inlet contraction is determined principally by the prognosis for safe vaginal delivery. If, on the basis of the criteria reviewed, a spontaneous delivery that is safe for both mother and child cannot be anticipated, cesarean delivery should be accomplished.

Prognosis

The prognosis for successful vaginal delivery of a term-sized fetus in cases of severe inlet contraction with an an-

teroposterior diameter of less than 9 cm is nearly hopeless. For the borderline group in which the anteroposterior diameter is slightly below 10 cm, the prognosis for vaginal delivery is influenced significantly by a number of variables, including the following:

(1) All presentations but the occiput are unfavorable.

(2) The size of the fetus is of obvious importance.

(3) The shape of the pelvic inlet plays an important role.

(4) Uterine dysfunction is common with significant disproportion.

(5) In general, orderly spontaneous cervical dilatation indicates that vaginal delivery most likely will be successful.

(6) Extreme asynclitism and marked molding of the head without engagement are unfavorable prognostic signs.

(7) Knowledge of the outcomes of previous labors and deliveries at term is helpful, as well as previous infant weights.

(8) Successful vaginal delivery is hindered by coincidental conditions that impair uteroplacental perfusion.

CONTRACTED MID PELVIS

Although the definition of midpelvic contractions has not been established with the precision possible for inlet contractions, the mid pelvis is probably contracted when the sum of the interischial spinous and posterior sagittal diameters (normally, 10.5 plus 5 cm, or 15.5 cm) falls to 13.5 or less. There is reason to suspect that midpelvic contraction exists whenever the **interischial spinous diameter is less than 10 cm.** When it is smaller than 9 cm, the mid pelvis is definitely contracted. The preceding definitions of midpelvic contraction do not, of course, imply that dystocia will necessarily occur but simply that it may occur, depending also upon the size and shape of the fore pelvis and the size of the fetal head as well as the degree of midpelvis contraction.

Diagnosis

Midpelvis contraction should be suspected when on vaginal examination the spines are prominent, the pelvic side walls converge, or the sacrosciatic notch is narrow. The relationship between the intertuberous and interspinous diameters of the ischium is sufficiently constant that narrowing of the interspinous diameter can be anticipated when the intertuberous diameter is narrow.

Treatment

In the management of labor complicated by midpelvis contraction, the main injunction is to allow the natural forces of labor to push the biparietal diameter beyond the potential interspinous obstruction.

Only when the head has been allowed to descend to such an extent that the perineum is bulging and the vertex is actually visible is it reasonably certain that the head has passed the obstruction. It is then usually safe to apply forceps. Strong suprafundal pressure should not be used to try to force the head past the obstruction.

The use of forceps or a vacuum extractor to effect delivery in a midpelvis contraction—usually undiagnosed—has been responsible to a great extent for the stigma attached to these operations.

Prognosis

Midpelvis contraction probably is more common than inlet contraction and frequently is a cause of transverse arrest of the fetal head and of potentially difficult mid-forceps operations.

CONTRACTED PELVIC OUTLET

Contraction of the pelvic outlet is usually defined as diminution of the interischial tuberous diameter to 8 cm or less. Outlet contractions occur in approximately 0.9% of primigravidas.

It is apparent in Figure 47–1 that a short intertuberous diameter with consequent narrowing of the anterior triangle must inevitably force the fetal head posteriorly. Whether delivery can take place, therefore, depends partly on the size of the posterior triangle or, more specifically, the interischial tuberous diameter and the posterior sagittal diameter of the outlet.

A contracted outlet may cause dystocia not so much by itself as through the often associated midpelvis contraction. Outlet contraction without concomitant midplane contraction is rare.

Even when the disproportion between the size of the fetal head and the pelvic outlet is not sufficiently great to give rise to severe dystocia, it may play an important part in the production of perineal tears. With increasing narrowing of the pubic arch, the occiput cannot emerge directly beneath the symphysis pubis but is forced increasingly farther down upon the ischiopubic rami.

GENERALLY CONTRACTED PELVIS

Since the contraction involves all portions of the pelvic canal, labor is not rapidly completed after the fetal head has passed the pelvic inlet. The prolongation of labor is caused not only by the resistance offered by the pelvis but also in many instances by the faulty spontaneous uterine contractions that frequently accompany diminution in the size of the pelvis.

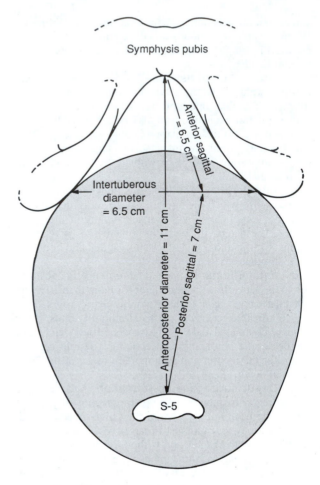

Figure 47–1. Diagram of pelvic outlet in which the intertuberous diameter is narrow (6.5 cm) and the posterior sagittal diameter is quite short (7 cm), precluding vaginal delivery of most term-sized fetuses. Int. tub. diam, intertuberous diameter; Sym., symphysis pubis; S-5, fifth sacral vertebra.

PELVIC FRACTURES & PREGNANCY

Trauma from automobile collisions is the most common cause of pelvic fracture in pregnant women. Bilateral fractures of the pubic rami often compromise the capacity of the birth canal by callus formation or malunion.

SUGGESTED READINGS

Dystocia due to pelvic contraction. Chapter 21 in: Cunningham FG, MacDonald PC, Gant NF, Leveno KJ, Gilstrap LG (editors): *Williams Obstetrics,* 19th ed. Appleton & Lange, 1993.

48

Dystocia Due to Soft Tissue Abnormalities of the Reproductive Tract

VULVAR ABNORMALITIES

Incomplete vulvar atresia usually results from adhesions or scars following injury or infection. For example, extensive perineal inflammation and scarring from hidradenitis suppurativa, lymphogranuloma venereum, or Crohn's disease may create difficulties with vaginal delivery as well as with episiotomy or laceration repair. Rarely, **condylomata acuminata** may be so extensive as to make vaginal delivery undesirable.

VAGINAL ABNORMALITIES

Occasionally, the vagina is divided by a **longitudinal septum,** which may be complete, extending from the vulva to the cervix, or (more often) incomplete, limited to either the upper or lower portion of the canal. Such conditions are frequently associated with other abnormalities in development of the genital tract, and their detection should always prompt careful examination to ascertain whether there is a coexistent uterine or renal deformity (Chapter 5). A complete longitudinal septum usually does not cause dystocia, since the half of the vagina through which the fetus descends gradually dilates satisfactorily. An incomplete septum, however, occasionally interferes with descent of the head or breech, over which the septum may become stretched as a band of varying thickness. **Annular strictures** or bands of congenital origin are unlikely to interfere seriously with delivery. They usually soften as pregnancy advances and yield before the oncoming head, requiring incision only in extreme cases.

Transverse septa are associated with in utero exposure to diethylstilbestrol (Chapter 5). Such a stricture is occasionally mistaken for the upper limit of the vaginal vault, and at the time of labor the opening in the septum is erroneously considered to be an undilated external os.

Vaginal atresias can result from scarring, injury, or inflammation, and the effects of atresia vary greatly. In most cases, the obstruction is gradually overcome by the pressure exerted by the presenting part; less often, manual or hydrostatic dilatation or incisions may become necessary. If, however, the structure is so resistant that spontaneous dilatation appears improbable, cesarean delivery should be performed at the onset of labor.

Among the rare causes of serious dystocia are **vaginal neoplasms,** such as **fibroma, carcinoma,** or **sarcoma,** arising from the vaginal walls or adjacent structures.

CERVICAL ABNORMALITIES

CERVICAL STENOSIS

Cicatricial stenosis of the cervix may follow extensive cauterization or difficult labor associated with infection and considerable destruction of tissue. For example, cervical dystocia may follow treatment of the cervix by conization. Cryotherapy and laser therapy are less likely to produce stenosis.

Ordinarily, because of the softening of the tissues during pregnancy, the stenosis gradually yields during labor. In rare instances, however, cervical stenosis may be so pronounced that dilatation appears improbable, and cesarean delivery should be employed.

CARCINOMA OF THE CERVIX

Dystocia may be a consequence of extensive infiltration of the cervix by carcinoma, since dilatation is likely to be inadequate even when uterine contractions remain forceful.

UTERINE DISPLACEMENTS

ANTEFLEXION OF THE UTERUS

Marked anteflexion of the enlarging pregnant uterus is usually associated with diastasis recti and a pendulous abdomen. Marked improvement may follow maintenance of the uterus in an approximately normal position by means of a properly fitting abdominal binder.

RETROFLEXION OF THE UTERUS

Persistent retroflexion of the pregnant uterus usually is incompatible with advanced pregnancy. If spontaneous or artificial reposition does not occur, the patient either aborts or develops symptoms caused by incarceration of the uterus before the end of the fourth month. In exceptional instances, however, pregnancy may proceed, resulting in uterine sacculation. Spontaneous delivery is impossible, and rupture of the uterus may occur.

UTERINE MYOMAS

A myoma may be **submucous, subserous,** or **intramural.** Intramural myomas may develop significant subserous or submucous (or both) components. Submucous and subserous myomas may at times be attached to the uterus by only a stalk **(pedunculated myoma).**

Myomas during pregnancy or the puerperium occasionally undergo "red" ("carneous") degeneration resulting from **hemorrhagic infarction.** The symptoms and signs are focal pain, with tenderness on palpation and in some cases low-grade fever. Moderate leukocytosis is common. On occasion, the parietal peritoneum overlying the infarcted myoma becomes inflamed and a peritoneal "rub" develops. Infarction is difficult to differentiate at times from appendicitis, placental abruption, ureteral stone, and

pyelonephritis, but the sonographic findings (see below) usually help with diagnosis. Treatment is with analgesics such as codeine. In most cases, the signs and symptoms abate within a few days.

Myomas may become infected during the course of puerperal metritis or septic abortion and are especially likely to do so if the myoma is located immediately adjacent to the placental implantation site or if an instrument such as a sound or curette perforates the myoma.

EFFECTS OF PREGNANCY ON MYOMAS

It has been reported that only about half of myomas changed significantly in size during pregnancy. The importance of this observation is that myoma growth in pregnancy cannot be predicted.

EFFECTS OF MYOMA LOCATION & NUMBER ON PREGNANCY

The probability that cesarean delivery will be required is increased if a myoma is located in the lower uterine segment. Furthermore, the risk of malposition and preterm labor is increased when there are multiple myomas, and the risk of retained placenta is increased when there is a lower uterine segment tumor.

Interestingly, the incidence of abortion, fetal growth retardation, or preterm labor does not appear to be increased substantially unless the placenta is implanted over or adjacent to a myoma. In cases of placental contact with uterine myomas, however, the incidence of uterine bleeding, abortion, preterm labor, and postpartum hemorrhage is increased, compared with cases in which the placenta is not in contact with a myoma.

Myomas in the cervix or lower uterine segment may obstruct labor and may be confused with the fetal head. Decisions regarding method of delivery usually should not be made before the onset of labor.

MYOMECTOMY

This procedure should be limited to those tumors with discrete pedicles that can be easily clamped and ligated. Otherwise, myomas should not be dissected from the uterus during pregnancy or delivery, because bleeding may be profuse and because at times the uterus may have to be sacrificed. Typically, the myomas will undergo remarkable involution after delivery.

OVARIAN TUMORS

BENIGN OVARIAN TUMORS

Ovarian tumors may be serious complications of pregnancy, may undergo torsion, and may pose insuperable obstacles to vaginal delivery. Moreover, even after spontaneous labor and delivery, they may give rise to disturbances during the puerperium.

Although all varieties of ovarian tumors may complicate pregnancy and labor, the most common are cystic, and while such cysts may obstruct delivery, the most serious complication of ovarian cysts during pregnancy is torsion. Torsion is most common in the first trimester. The cyst may rupture and extrude its contents into the peritoneal cavity as a result of torsion, or during spontaneous labor, or during surgical removal. When the tumor blocks the pelvis, it may lead to rupture of the uterus, or the tumor may be forced into the vagina, the rectum, or the intervening rectovaginal septum.

An ovarian tumor complicating pregnancy is often entirely unsuspected. *Careful examination of all pregnant women would eliminate some of these errors.* If an ovarian tumor does not occupy the pelvis, diagnosis through physical examination is difficult. Such abdominal enlargement may be due to a pregnancy more advanced than suggested by menstruation data, to multiple fetuses, or to hydramnios, and the true condition may not be recognized until after labor. Sonography usually provides accurate differentiation between uterine enlargement and an extrauterine cystic mass.

The safest time to perform laparotomy is during the fourth month of gestation, provided the operation can be postponed until that time. When the diagnosis is not made until late in pregnancy, it is usually advisable, except in the case of known or suspected malignant tumors, to delay laparotomy until fetal viability has been achieved. If the ovarian cyst is not impacted, it is usually preferable to permit spontaneous labor and remove the tumor later in the puerperium. If the tumor is impacted in the pelvis, cesarean delivery should be performed followed by resection of the tumor.

CARCINOMA OF THE OVARY

Malignant ovarian neoplasms are rare in pregnancy. If cancer is discovered at the time of laparotomy, the treatment should be the same as for the nonpregnant patient. In some circumstances, it is justifiable to remove the tumor and allow the pregnancy to continue when a few more weeks would assure viability of the delivered infant. Even then, cesarean delivery should be done, with the decision regarding further surgery and chemotherapy based on the results of clinical and histologic examinations.

PELVIC MASSES OF OTHER ORIGINS

Labor may be obstructed by pelvic masses of various origins sufficiently large to render delivery difficult or even impossible. A **distended bladder,** with or without a cystocele, may interfere with delivery. However, a less severely distended bladder does not often delay the normal progress of labor. Tumors of the bladder may impede passage of the fetus, though rarely seriously enough to require operative delivery.

Pelvic ectopic kidney is a rare problem complicating pregnancy. However, a **transplanted kidney** is usually placed in the pelvis and may block the birth canal and sustain injury during passage of the fetus. Most women with an ectopic kidney will deliver vaginally without hazard, but if the kidney is entirely intrapelvic, as is often the case with transplanted kidneys, abdominal delivery is safer.

SUGGESTED READINGS

Dystocia due to soft tissue abnormalities of the reproductive tract. Chapter 22 in: Cunningham FG, MacDonald PC, Gant NF, Leveno KJ, Gilstrap LC (editors): *Williams Obstetrics,* 19th ed. Appleton & Lange, 1993.

Lev-Toaff AS et al: Leiomyomas in pregnancy: Sonography study. Radiology 1987;164:375.

49

Injuries to the Birth Canal & Other Abnormalities of the Third Stage of Labor

INJURIES TO THE PELVIC FLOOR & VAGINA

PERINEAL LACERATIONS

All but the most superficial perineal lacerations are accompanied by varying degrees of injury to the lower portion of the vagina. Such tears may reach sufficient depth to involve the rectal sphincter and may extend to varying depths through the walls of the vagina. Bilateral lacerations into the vagina are usually unequal in length and separated by a tongue-shaped portion of vaginal mucosa. Their repair should form part of every operation for the restoration of a lacerated perineum. Suturing of just the external integument without approximation of underlying perineal and vaginal fascia and muscle will lead to relaxation of the vaginal outlet and may contribute to rectocele and cystocele formation as well as uterine prolapse.

VAGINAL LACERATIONS

Isolated lacerations involving the middle or upper third of the vagina but unassociated with lacerations of the perineum or cervix are less common. Vaginal lacerations in this location are usually longitudinal, resulting from injuries sustained during forceps delivery, though occasionally they accompany spontaneous delivery. Such lacerations frequently extend deep into the underlying tissues and may give rise to copious hemorrhage, which, however, is usually readily controlled by appropriate suturing. They may be overlooked unless thorough inspection of the upper vagina is performed or at least careful attention is paid to bleeding from the genital tract in the presence of a firmly contracted uterus. Bleeding while the uterus is

firmly contracted is strong evidence of genital tract laceration, retained placental fragments, or both.

Lacerations of the anterior vaginal wall in close proximity to the urethra are relatively common. If superficial and not bleeding, repair is not indicated; otherwise, in order to achieve hemostasis, closure is required. If such lacerations are extensive, difficulty in voiding can be anticipated and an indwelling catheter placed.

INJURIES TO THE CERVIX

Traumatic lesions of the upper third of the vagina are uncommon by themselves but are often associated with extensions of deep cervical tears. In rare instances, however, the cervix may be entirely or partially avulsed from the vagina, with colporrhexis in the anterior, posterior, or lateral fornices. Such lesions usually follow difficult forceps deliveries performed through an incompletely dilated cervix with the forceps blades applied over the cervix. The cervical tears may extend to involve the lower uterine segment and uterine artery and its major branches—and even through the peritoneum. Fortunately, such extensive traumatic lesions are rare in modern obstetric practice. They may be totally unsuspected but more often are manifested by excessive external hemorrhage or by the formation of a retroperitoneal hematoma that begins within the leaves of the broad ligaments. These extensive tears of the vaginal vault should be carefully explored. Effective anesthesia, vigorous blood replacement, and assistance are mandatory for a satisfactory outcome.

Cervical lacerations up to 2 cm must be regarded as inevitable in childbirth. Such tears heal rapidly and are rarely the source of any difficulty. In healing, they cause a significant change in the shape of the external os from round before cervical effacement and dilatation to appreciably elongated laterally after delivery and recovery from effacement and dilatation.

Diagnosis

A deep cervical tear should always be suspected in cases of profuse hemorrhage during and after the third stage of labor, particularly if the uterus is firmly contracted. In view of the frequency with which deep tears follow major operative obstetric procedures, the cervix should be inspected routinely at the conclusion of the third stage after all difficult deliveries, even if there is no bleeding. For a definitive diagnosis to be made, however, thorough examination is necessary. Because of the flabbiness of the cervix immediately after delivery, digital examination alone is often unsatisfactory. The extent of the injury can be fully appreciated only after adequate exposure and visual inspection of the cervix. The best exposure is gained by the use of right-angle vaginal retractors by an assistant while the operator grasps the patulous cervix with a ring forceps as shown in Figure 49–1 and described below.

Treatment

Deep cervical tears should be repaired immediately. Treatment varies with the extent of the lesion. When the laceration is limited to the cervix—or even when it extends somewhat into the vaginal fornix—satisfactory results are obtained by suturing the cervix after bringing it into view at the vulva. Visualization is best accomplished when an assistant applies firm downward pressure on the uterus while the operator exerts traction on the lips of the cervix with fenestrated ovum or sponge forceps. The vaginal walls are held apart with retractors manipulated with the aid of the assistant (Figure 49–1). Since bleeding usually comes from the upper angle of the wound, it is advisable to apply the first suture at the angle and suture outward. Associated vaginal lacerations are repaired after the cervical tears. Tamponade with gauze packs will retard hemorrhage from these lesions while cervical lacerations are repaired. Chromic catgut sutures should be employed, since they do not have to be removed. The physician must remember that overzealous suturing to try to restore the normal appearance of the cervix may lead to stenosis during involution of the uterus.

RUPTURE OF THE UTERUS

The incidence of rupture of the uterus varies in different reports from 1:100 deliveries to 1:11,000. Although the frequency of uterine rupture from all causes has probably not decreased remarkably during the past several decades, the causes of rupture have changed and the prognosis has improved.

Uterine rupture may develop as a result of preexisting injury or anomaly, or it may complicate labor in a previously unscarred uterus. Currently, the most common cause of uterine rupture is separation of a previous cesarean scar, and this is increasing with the trend of allowing a trial of labor following one or more prior transverse cesarean deliveries. The National Institute of Child Health and Human Development reported that in 1979 a trial of labor was allowed in 2.1% of women with prior cesarean deliveries, and by 1984 the rate had increased to 8%. The incidence of uterine rupture in these women has been estimated in several studies to be about 0.2–0.5%.

Other common predisposing factors to uterine rupture

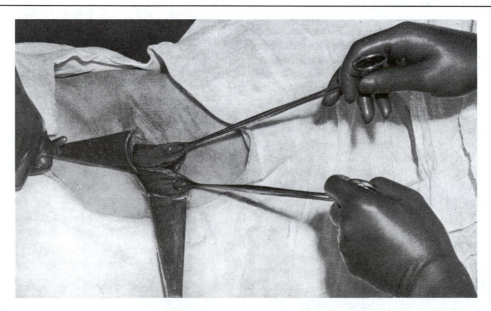

Figure 49–1. Cervical laceration exposed for repair. (Reproduced, with permission, from Cunningham FG, MacDonald PC, Gant NF, Leveno KJ, Gilstrap LC [editors]: *Williams Obstetrics,* 19th ed. Appleton & Lange, 1993.)

are previous traumatizing operations or manipulations such as curettage or perforation. Excessive or inappropriate uterine stimulation with oxytocin—once a common cause—are decreasing. Generally, the previously untraumatized, spontaneously laboring uterus will not persist in contracting so vigorously as to destroy itself.

DEFINITIONS

It is customary to distinguish between **complete** and **incomplete** rupture of the uterus depending on whether the laceration communicates directly with the peritoneal cavity or is separated from it by the visceral peritoneum over the uterus or that of the broad ligament. An incomplete rupture may, of course, become complete at any moment.

It is important to differentiate between **rupture of a cesarean section scar** and **dehiscence of a cesarean section scar.** Rupture refers, at the minimum, to separation of the old uterine incision throughout most of its length, with rupture of the fetal membranes so that the uterine cavity and the peritoneal cavity communicate. In these circumstances, all or part of the fetus is usually extruded into the peritoneal cavity. In addition, there is usually bleeding, often massive, from the edges of the scar or from an extension of the rent into previously uninvolved uterus. By contrast, with dehiscence of a cesarean section scar, the fetal membranes are not ruptured and the fetus is not extruded into the peritoneal cavity. Typically, with dehiscence the separation does not involve all of the previous uterine scar, the peritoneum overlying the defect is intact, and bleeding is absent or minimal. Dehiscence occurs gradually, whereas ruptures are very likely to be symptomatic and, at times, fatal. With labor or intrauterine manipulations, a dehiscence may become a rupture.

COMPARISON OF CLASSIC & LOWER SEGMENT CESAREAN SECTION SCARS

The behavior of a classic scar—ie, a vertical uterine incision through the body of the pregnant uterus rather than the lower uterine segment—in any subsequent pregnancy differs from that of a scar confined to the lower uterine segment. First, the probability of rupture of a classic scar is several times greater than that of a lower segment scar. Second, if a classic scar does rupture, the accident takes place before labor in about one-third of cases. Rupture not infrequently takes place several weeks before term. Therefore, delivery by subsequent cesarean delivery cannot prevent such ruptures. Lower segment scars confined to the noncontractile portion of the uterus rarely, if ever, rupture before labor.

Vertical incisions made lower in the uterus than classic incisions are also liable to undergo separation. An example of the so-called low vertical incision is shown in Figure 49–2. Lower segment scars confined to the noncontractile portion of the uterus rarely, if ever, rupture

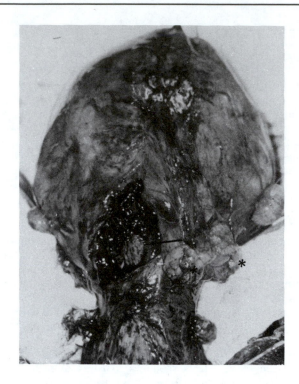

Figure 49–2. Ruptured vertical cesarean scar *(arrow)* identified at time of repeat cesarean delivery early in labor; *asterisks* indicate some of the sites of densely adherent omentum. (Reproduced, with permission, from Cunningham FG, MacDonald PC, Gant NF, Leveno KJ, Gilstrap LC [editors]: *Williams Obstetrics,* 19th ed. Appleton & Lange, 1993.)

before labor. Low-segment incisions invariably are transverse.

Available data are insufficient to permit a precise calculation of the maternal mortality rate associated with rupture of a cesarean section scar. However, rupture following a trial of labor in a woman with a prior transverse incision is not usually associated with maternal death, and perinatal loss is typically very low. In 24 cases of uterine rupture from 1963 to 1983, there was one maternal death and a 46% perinatal loss.

Dehiscence of a lower-segment cesarean section scar is much more frequent than actual rupture, especially if the previous uterine incision was transverse. It is remarkable that these separated scars, covered only by peritoneum, often appear to cause no difficulty in labor or subsequently.

RUPTURE OF A CESAREAN SECTION SCAR

The current trend in obstetric practice is to encourage a trial of labor in anticipation of vaginal delivery in women who have previously been delivered by one transverse cesarean delivery. Even more recently, women with two and even three prior operations have been allowed to go into labor, either spontaneously or with oxytocin stimulation. The main drawback to this plan is that separation of the previous scar complicates about 1:200 trials of labor.

RUPTURE OF THE UNSCARRED UTERUS

TRAUMATIC RUPTURE

Although the uterus is surprisingly resistant to blunt trauma, pregnant women sustaining blunt trauma to the abdomen should be watched carefully for signs of a ruptured uterus. Oxytocin stimulation of labor has been a rather common cause of traumatic rupture, especially in women of high parity. In the past, traumatic rupture during delivery was most often produced by internal podalic version and extraction. Other causes of traumatic rupture include difficult forceps delivery, breech extraction, and unusual fetal enlargement, such as in hydrocephalus. Rupture of the uterus caused by strong pressure on the fundus in an attempt to accomplish vaginal delivery should not occur.

SPONTANEOUS RUPTURE OF THE UTERUS

This catastrophe is more likely to occur in women of high parity. In one study of women para 7 or greater, uterine rupture was 20 times more likely than in women of lower parity. For this reason, oxytocin should rarely be given to undelivered women of high parity. Similarly, in women of high parity, a trial of labor in the presence of cephalopelvic disproportion—or abnormal presentation such as a brow—may prove dangerous not only to the fetus but also to the mother.

Clinical Course

Prior to circulatory collapse from hemorrhage, the symptoms and physical findings may appear bizarre unless the possibility of rupture of the uterus is kept in mind. If the accident occurs during labor, the woman—usually after a period of premonitory signs—at the acme of a uterine contraction suddenly complains of a sharp, shooting pain in the abdomen and may cry out that "something ripped" or "something tore" inside her. Immediately after these symptoms and signs have appeared, there is cessation of uterine contractions, and the woman, until that point in intense agony, suddenly experiences relief. At the same time, there may be external hemorrhage, though it is often slight.

Not all women experience these classic findings of uterine rupture. In some, the appearance is identical to that of placental abruption. In others, rupture is unaccompanied by appreciable pain and tenderness. Furthermore, since most women in labor are given something for discomfort—either narcotics or lumbar epidural analgesia—pain and tenderness may not be readily apparent and the condition becomes evident because of signs of fetal distress or maternal hypovolemia from concealed hemorrhage.

The chances for fetal survival are dismal; the mortality rates found in various studies range between 50% and 75%. However, if the fetus is alive at the time of the accident, the only chance of continued survival is afforded by immediate delivery, most often by laparotomy. Otherwise, hypoxia from both separation of the placenta and maternal hypovolemia is inevitable. Prompt diagnosis, immediate operation, the availability of large amounts of blood, and antibiotic therapy have greatly improved the prognosis for women with rupture of the pregnant uterus.

Immediate Treatment

The patient's life usually depends on the speed and efficiency with which hypovolemia can be corrected and hemorrhage controlled. Whenever rupture of the uterus is diagnosed, it is mandatory that the following procedures be performed immediately and simultaneously: (1) Two large-bore intravenous infusion catheters are established, and crystalloid solution, either lactated Ringer's or saline, is infused vigorously; (2) type-specific whole blood is obtained in large quantities, and rapid infusion is begun as soon as possible; (3) a surgical team, including anesthesia personnel, is assembled and the operating room made ready with instruments necessary to perform cesarean hysterectomy; and (4) pediatric personnel skilled in neonatal resuscitation should be present.

Hysterectomy is usually required, but in highly selected cases suture of the wound may be performed.

SUGGESTED READINGS

American College of Obstetricians and Gynecologists Committee on Maternal and Fetal Medicine: Guidelines for vaginal delivery after a previous cesarean birth. Tech Bull No. 64, October 1988.

Shiono PH et al: Recent trends in cesarean birth and trial of labor rates in the United States. JAMA 1987;257:494.

50

Complications of the Puerperium

PUERPERAL INFECTION

Puerperal infection is bacterial infection of the genital tract after delivery. Less satisfactory older synonyms are puerperal fever, puerperal sepsis, and childbed fever. Along with preeclampsia and obstetric hemorrhage, infection for many decades of this century formed the lethal triad of causes of maternal death in childbirth. In recent years, maternal deaths from infection have become less common.

In general, the likelihood of serious postpartum pelvic infection is related to the following factors:

(1) the length of membrane rupture before delivery,
(2) the number of cervical examinations,
(3) intrauterine manipulation for delivery of the fetus and placenta,
(4) and the size and number of incisions and lacerations.

The most graphic example is cesarean delivery, which increases substantially the puerperal infection rate. It is generally accepted that puerperal infection is much more common in women of lower socioeconomic status compared with middle or upper-class patients.

BACTERIOLOGY

Organisms that invade the placental implantation site, incisions, and lacerations are typically those that normally colonize the cervix, vagina, and perineum. As shown in Table 50–1, most of these bacteria are of relatively low virulence and seldom cause infection in healthy tissues. Antimicrobial treatment directed against the polymicrobial and mixed flora that typically cause these infections is usually effective. Since reliable material for culture often is impractical to obtain, empiric antimicrobial therapy is justified.

EPISIOTOMY INFECTIONS

Infections of perineal wounds, including episiotomy incisions and repaired lacerations, are relatively uncommon considering the degree of bacterial contamination that accompanies delivery. Localized infection of the episiotomy wound is the most common puerperal infection of the external genitalia. The apposing wound edges become red, brawny, and swollen. The sutures often then tear through the edematous tissues, allowing the necrotic wound edges to gape, with the result that serous, serosanguineous, or frankly purulent material exudes. Complete breakdown of the site frequently follows. Local pain and dysuria, with or without urinary retention, are common symptoms. In extreme cases, the entire vulva may become edematous, ulcerated, and covered with exudate. Provided drainage is good, these superficial infections are seldom severe; however, if purulent material is confined within a closed space by suturing, infection may be accompanied by chills and high fever.

Treatment of infected perineal wounds, like that of other infected surgical wounds, is by establishing drainage. Broad-spectrum antimicrobials are also given. Sutures are removed and the infected wound opened—failure to do so may lead not only to extension of the infections into the paracervical and paravaginal connective tissue, but to a worse ultimate anatomic result as well.

METRITIS WITH PELVIC CELLULITIS

Postpartum uterine infection has been known by various terms, including **endometritis, endomyometritis,** and **endoparametritis.** Since the infection actually involves the decidua, myometrium, and parametrial tissues, the term **metritis with pelvic cellulitis** seems more suitable. The pathogenesis of these infections is shown in Figure 50–1. Uterine infections are relatively uncommon following uncomplicated vaginal delivery, but they continue to be a major problem in women delivered by cesarean section.

Although not usually classified as mild or severe, the

Table 50–1. Bacteria commonly responsible for female genital infections.[1]

Aerobes
  Group A, B, and D streptococci
  Enterococci
  Gram-negative bacteria: *Escherichia coli, Klebsiella,* and *Proteus* species
  Staphylococcus aureus
Anaerobes
  Peptococcus species
  Peptostreptococcus species
  Bacteroides bivius, Bacteroides fragilis, Bacteroides disiens
  Clostridium species
  Fusobacterium species
Other
  Mycoplasma hominis
  Chlamydia trachomatis

[1]From the American College of Obstetricians and Gynecologists: Antimicrobial therapy for obstetric patients. Tech Bull No. 117, June 1988.

clinical picture of metritis varies with the extent of the disease, and whenever fever persists postpartum, uterine infection should be suspected. Temperature elevation is probably proportionate to the extent of the infection, and when confined to the endometrium (decidua), the cases are mild and there is minimal fever. More commonly, the temperature is at least 39 °C, if not higher. Chills may accompany fever and suggest bacteremia. The woman usually complains of abdominal pain, and afterpains may be bothersome. There is tenderness on one or both sides of the abdomen, and parametrial tenderness is elicited upon bimanual examination.

Treatment for metritis is with broad-spectrum antimicrobial drugs. For mild cases following vaginal delivery, an oral agent may suffice. For moderately to severely infected women—and this includes those delivered by cesarean section—intravenous therapy is indicated.

In some women—and in almost all cases when metritis follows cesarean delivery—parametrial cellulitis is severe and may form an area of induration termed a **phlegmon** within the leaves of the broad ligament.

Very severe cellulitis of the uterine incision may cause necrosis and separation, with extrusion of purulent material into the peritoneal cavity. The first symptoms of peritonitis are often those of **adynamic ileus,** which usually is absent or mild following uncomplicated cesarean delivery. Puerperal metritis with pelvic cellulitis is typically a retroperitoneal infection, and evidence for peritonitis should alert the physician to the possibility of uterine incisional necrosis with dehiscence or, less commonly, bowel injury or other lesions.

DIFFERENTIAL DIAGNOSIS OF FEVER

Most fevers after childbirth are caused by genital tract infection, especially if the preceding labor was attended by extensive vaginal or uterine manipulation, prolonged membrane rupture, or intrauterine electronic monitoring. Regardless of the cause, every postpartum woman whose temperature rises to 38 °C should be evaluated to rule out extrapelvic causes of fever and to establish the diagnosis of puerperal infection. Common extragenital causes of pu-

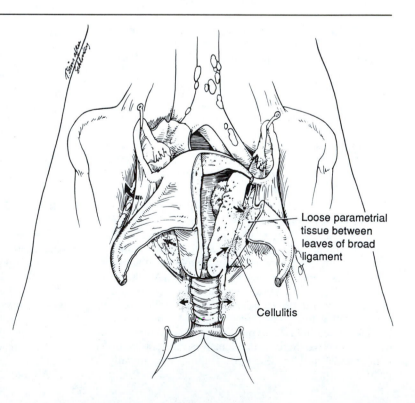

Figure 50–1. Pelvic cellulitis (parametritis) from extension of puerperal infection. Bacteria may enter the parametrial tissue between the leaves of the broad ligament by direct extension or by lymphatic transmission from cervical lacerations or foci of trauma within the uterus, including the site of placental implantation or cesarean section incision. (Reproduced, with permission, from Cunningham FG, MacDonald PC, Gant NF, Leveno KJ, Gilstrap LC [editors]: *Williams Obstetrics,* 19th ed. Appleton & Lange, 1993.)

Loose parametrial tissue between leaves of broad ligament

Cellulitis

erperal fever include respiratory complications, pyelonephritis, severe breast engorgement, bacterial mastitis, thrombophlebitis, and, in cases of laparotomy, wound abscess.

POSTPARTUM HEMORRHAGE

Postpartum hemorrhage has most often been defined as loss of blood in excess of 500 mL during the first 24 hours after delivery. Through quantitative measurements of puerperal blood loss, however, the incongruity of this definition has been clearly demonstrated, as blood loss resulting from vaginal delivery is frequently more than 500 mL. In fact, 5% of women delivering vaginally lose more than 1000 mL of blood. Estimated blood loss commonly is only about half the actual loss.

As a direct factor in maternal fatalities, postpartum hemorrhage is the cause of about one-fourth of the deaths from obstetric hemorrhage—other causes being placenta previa, placental abruption, ectopic pregnancy, hemorrhage from abortion, and rupture of the uterus. The many factors of importance in the genesis of early postpartum hemorrhage are listed in Table 50–2. The two most common causes of immediate hemorrhage are hypotonic myometrium (**uterine atony**) and laceration of the vagina and cervix. Retention of part or all of the placenta, a less common cause, may produce either immediate or delayed hemorrhage (or both). It is uncommon for an episiotomy alone to cause severe postpartum hemorrhage, though blood so lost averages about 200 mL.

Table 50–2. Predisposing factors and causes of immediate postpartum hemorrhage.

Trauma to the genital tract
   Large episiotomy, including extensions
   Lacerations of perineum, vagina, or cervix
   Ruptured uterus
Bleeding from placental implantation site
   Hypotonic myometrium—uterine atony
     Some general anesthetics—halogenated hydrocarbons
     Poorly perfused myometrium—hypotension
     Hemorrhage
     Conduction analgesia
     Overdistended uterus—large fetus, twins, hydramnios
     Following prolonged labor
     Following very rapid labor
     Following oxytocin-induced or augmented labor
     High parity
     Uterine atony in previous pregnancy
     Chorioamnionitis
   Retained placental tissue
     Avulsed cotyledon, succenturiate lobe
     Abnormally adherent—accreta, increta, percreta
Coagulation defects
   Intensify all of the above

Predisposing Factors

In many cases, postpartum hemorrhage can be predicted well in advance of delivery. Examples in which trauma is likely to lead to postpartum hemorrhage include delivery of a large infant, midforceps delivery, forceps rotation, delivery through an incompletely dilated cervix, any intrauterine manipulation, and perhaps vaginal delivery after prior cesarean section or other uterine incisions. Uterine atony causing hemorrhage can be anticipated whenever an anesthetic agent is used that will relax the uterus. Halothane and other halogenated compounds are prominent examples.

The overdistended uterus is liable to be hypotonic after delivery. Thus, the patient with a large fetus, multiple fetuses, or hydramnios is prone to hemorrhage from uterine atony. Blood loss with delivery of twins, for example, averages nearly 1000 mL—or nearly twice that associated with delivery of a singleton—and may be much greater.

The woman whose labor is characterized by uterine activity that is either remarkably vigorous or barely effective is also apt to bleed excessively from uterine atony after delivery. Similarly, labor either initiated or augmented with oxytocin is more likely to be followed by postdelivery uterine atony and hemorrhage. The woman of high parity is at increased risk of hemorrhage from uterine atony.

Clinical Characteristics

Postpartum hemorrhage before delivery of the placenta is called third-stage hemorrhage. Contrary to general opinion, whether bleeding occurs before or after delivery of the placenta or at both times, there may be no sudden massive hemorrhage but rather a steady bleeding that at any given instant appears to be moderate but persists until serious hypovolemia develops. Especially with hemorrhage after delivery of the placenta, the constant seepage may over a period of a few hours lead to enormous loss of blood. The effects of hemorrhage depend to a considerable degree upon the nonpregnant blood volume, the magnitude of pregnancy-induced hypervolemia, and the degree of anemia at the time of delivery. The differentiation between bleeding from uterine atony and from lacerations is tentatively based on the condition of the uterus. If bleeding persists despite a firm, well-contracted uterus, the cause of the hemorrhage most probably is lacerations. Bright red blood also suggests lacerations. To ascertain the role of lacerations as a cause of bleeding, careful inspection of the vagina, cervix, and uterus is essential.

Management After Delivery of the Placenta

Irrespective of the method of delivery of the placenta, the fundus should always be palpated afterward to make certain the uterus is well contracted. If the uterus is not firm, vigorous fundal massage is indicated. Most often, 20 units of oxytocin in 1000 mL of lactated Ringer's injection or normal saline solution intravenously proves effective when administered at approximately 10 mL per min (200 mU of oxytocin per min) concurrently with effective uterine massage. Oxytocin should never be given as an undiluted bolus dose, serious hypotension may follow. The 15-methyl derivative of prostaglandin $F_{2\alpha}$ (carboprost tromethamine) is probably effective for treatment of postpartum hemorrhage from uterine atony when oxytocin fails. The initial recommended dose is 250 µg (0.25 mg) intramuscularly, repeated if necessary at 15- to 90-minute intervals.

If bleeding persists despite these procedures, no time should be lost in haphazard efforts to control hemorrhage, but the following management protocol should be initiated immediately:

(1) Employ bimanual uterine compression. (This procedure will control most hemorrhage.)

(2) Obtain help!

(3) Begin transfusion of blood.

(4) Explore the uterine cavity manually for retained placental fragments or lacerations.

(5) Thoroughly inspect the cervix and vagina after adequate exposure.

PLACENTA ACCRETA, INCRETA, & PERCRETA

Placenta accreta is any implantation of the placenta in which there is abnormally firm adherence to the uterine wall. As a consequence of partial or total absence of the decidua basalis and imperfect development of the fibrinoid layer (**Nitabuch's membrane**), the placental villi are attached to the myometrium (**placenta accreta**), actually invade the myometrium (**placenta increta**), or even penetrate through the myometrium (**placenta percreta**). The abnormal adherence may involve all of the cotyledons (total placenta accreta), a few to several cotyledons (partial placenta accreta), or a single cotyledon (focal placenta accreta).

Abnormal adherence of the placenta is found most often in circumstances where decidual formation was likely to have been defective, eg, implantations in the lower uterine segment, or over a previous cesarean section scar or other previous incisions into the uterine cavity, or after uterine curettage.

Antepartum hemorrhage is common, but in the great majority of cases the antepartum bleeding is the consequence of a coexisting placenta previa. Invasion of the myometrium by placental villi at the site of a previous cesarean section scar may lead to rupture of the uterus during labor or even before. In women whose pregnancies go to term, however, labor is most likely to be normal in the absence of an associated placenta previa or an involved uterine scar.

The problems associated with delivery of the placenta and subsequent developments will vary depending upon the site of implantation, the depth of penetration into the myometrium, and the number of cotyledons involved. With more extensive involvement, however, hemorrhage becomes profuse as delivery of the placenta is attempted. Successful treatment depends upon immediate blood replacement therapy and, nearly always, prompt hysterectomy.

INVERSION OF THE UTERUS

Complete inversion of the uterus after delivery of the infant is almost always the consequence of strong traction on an umbilical cord that is attached to a placenta implanted in the uterine fundus. Contributing to uterine inversion are a tough cord that does not readily break away from the placenta combined with fundal pressure and a relaxed uterus, including the lower segment and cervix. Placenta accreta may be implicated, though uterine inversion can occur without the placenta's being so firmly adherent. At times, the inversion may be incomplete.

Inversion of the uterus following the third stage of labor is most often associated with immediate life-threatening hemorrhage, and without prompt treatment it may be fatal. Delay in treatment increases the mortality rate. Urgent therapy includes blood replacement and repositioning of the uterus.

THROMBOEMBOLIC DISEASE

According to the Consensus Conference sponsored by the National Institutes of Health (1986), the likelihood of venous thromboembolism in normal pregnancy and the puerperium is increased fivefold compared with nonpregnant women of similar age. Venous thrombosis and pulmonary embolism remain a major cause of maternal death in the United States, but venous thromboembolic disease during the puerperium declined in incidence when early ambulation became widely practiced. Until as late as the 1950s, it was common practice after delivery to prohibit ambulation for up to 1 week or more. Stasis is probably the strongest single predisposing cause of deep vein thrombosis.

SUPERFICIAL VENOUS THROMBOSIS

Antepartum or postpartum thrombosis limited strictly to the superficial veins of the saphenous system is treated with analgesia, elastic support, and rest. If it does not soon clear or if deep venous involvement is suspected, heparin is given intravenously, as described below, until the process clears.

DEEP VENOUS THROMBOSIS IN THE LEG

The incidence of combined antepartum and postpartum deep vein thrombosis probably is about 1–2:1000 deliveries. The signs and symptoms involving the lower extremity vary depending on the degree of occlusion and the severity of the inflammatory response. Thus, variable degrees of pain, tenderness, heat, swelling, and discoloration in the leg are encountered. Thrombosis should be confirmed, either by ultrasound, venography, CT scanning, or MRI.

Treatment of deep venous thrombosis consists of heparin given intravenously, bed rest, and analgesia. Most often, the pain is soon relieved by these measures. After the signs and symptoms have completely abated, graded ambulation should be started, with the legs well wrapped in elastic bandages, or, preferably, well-fitting elastic stockings, and the heparin continued. Recovery to this stage usually takes about 7–10 days.

For women who are postpartum and suffering their first attack, who have no obvious chronic vascular disease, and who are observed to be completely asymptomatic while fully ambulatory, anticoagulant therapy may be discontinued. In most cases, signs and symptoms of deep venous thrombosis do not recur. If, however, symptoms and signs do recur, therapy should be promptly restarted and not stopped when relief is obtained. Prolonged anticoagulant therapy is continued on an outpatient basis. After discharge from the hospital, long-term treatment is maintained either with heparin self-administered by subcutaneous injection or with warfarin.

Antepartum thrombosis involving the deep venous system is especially difficult to manage satisfactorily. Confirmation of the clinical diagnosis is imperative; otherwise, the woman will either have to undergo prolonged anticoagulation with its attendant risks or run the risk of pulmonary embolism.

Therapy with intravenous heparin usually soon controls active disease, but thrombosis, perhaps with embolization, may recur antepartum, intrapartum, or postpartum unless anticoagulation is continued throughout those periods. All things considered, the best treatment regimen for prophylaxis against recurrence of deep venous thrombosis is self-administered heparin injected subcutaneously in doses of 5000 units 2 or 3 times a day. With so-called low-dose heparin treatment that provides 10,000–15,000 units/d of heparin subcutaneously, there is some increase in the risk of recurrent thrombosis and perhaps embolism compared to that with larger doses but a much lower risk of hemorrhage. Warfarin is contraindicated during pregnancy because of adverse fetal effects (Chapter 54).

PULMONARY EMBOLISM

The incidence of pulmonary embolism in obstetric patients is about 1:5000 deliveries. In many cases, clinical evidence of deep venous thrombosis of the legs precedes pulmonary embolization. In others—especially those that arise from deep pelvic veins—the woman is usually asymptomatic until symptoms of embolization develop. Chest discomfort, shortness of breath, air hunger, tachypnea, and obvious apprehension should alert the physician to a strong likelihood of pulmonary embolism during the puerperium. Controversy exists with respect to the safest, least invasive technique for diagnosis of pulmonary embolus. To verify the clinical diagnosis, initial evaluation is with chest x-ray, and if this is not suggestive of another diagnosis, a ventilation-perfusion lung scan is performed. A completely normal scan is evidence against embolism and the workup at that point can be considered complete. Conversely, an unequivocally positive result, along with a chest radiograph showing no explicable abnormalities, can be considered diagnostic of embolization and an indication for starting therapy. If the diagnosis is still doubtful after these measures, pulmonary angiography should be performed; a filling defect or vessel cutoff on the angiogram is considered diagnostic of embolization.

VULVAR HEMATOMAS

Vulvar hematomas—particularly those that develop rapidly—may cause excruciating pain, which is often the first symptom (Figure 50–2). Hematomas of moderate size may be absorbed spontaneously. The tissues overlying the hematoma may give way as a result of necrosis

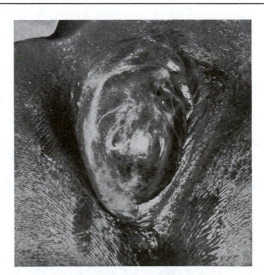

Figure 50–2. Vulvar hematoma bulging into the right vaginal wall. (Reproduced, with permission, from Cunningham FG, MacDonald PC, Gant NF, Leveno KJ, Gilstrap LC [editors]: *Williams Obstetrics,* 19th ed. Appleton & Lange, 1993.)

caused by pressure, and profuse hemorrhage may follow. In other cases, the contents of the hematoma may be discharged in the form of large clots.

A vulvar hematoma is readily diagnosed on the basis of severe perineal pain and the sudden appearance of a tense, fluctuant, and sensitive tumor of varying size covered by discolored skin. When the mass develops adjacent to the vagina, it may temporarily escape detection, but symptoms of pressure—if not pain—and inability to void should soon lead to a vaginal examination and the discovery of a round, fluctuant tumor encroaching on the lumen. When the hematoma extends upward between the folds of the broad ligament, it may escape detection unless a portion of the tumor can be felt on abdominal palpation or unless evidence of anemia or infection appears.

Smaller vulvar hematomas identified after leaving the delivery room may be treated expectantly. If the pain is severe or if the lesion continues to enlarge, the best treatment is prompt incision and evacuation of the blood with ligation of the bleeding points. The cavity can then be obliterated with mattress sutures. With hematomas of the genital tract, blood loss is nearly always greater than the clinical estimate. Hypovolemia and severe anemia should be prevented by adequate blood replacement. Broad-spectrum antibiotics are of value.

DISORDERS OF THE BREASTS

ENGORGEMENT OF THE BREASTS

For the first 24–48 hours after development of the lacteal secretion, it is not unusual for the breasts to become distended, firm, and nodular. This condition, commonly known as engorged breasts, or "caked breasts," often causes considerable pain and may be accompanied by transient fever. The disorder represents an exaggeration of the normal venous and lymphatic engorgement of the breasts, which is a regular precursor of lactation. It is not the result of overdistention of the lacteal system with milk.

Treatment consists of supporting the breasts with a binder or brassiere, applying an ice bag, and, if necessary, orally administering 60 mg of codeine or another analgesic. Pumping of the breasts or manual expression of milk may be necessary at first, but in a few days the condition is usually alleviated and the infant is able to nurse normally.

MASTITIS

Parenchymatous inflammation of the mammary glands is a rare complication antepartum but is occasionally observed during the puerperium and during lactation. The symptoms of suppurative mastitis seldom appear before the end of the first week of the puerperium and, as a rule, not until the third or fourth week. Marked engorgement usually precedes the inflammation, the first sign of which is chills or actual rigor, soon followed by a rise in temperature and an increase in pulse rate. The breast becomes hard and reddened, and the patient complains of pain.

By far the most common offending organism is *Staphylococcus aureus*. The immediate source of the staphylococci that cause this mastitis is nearly always the nursing infant's nose and throat. At the time of nursing, the organism enters the breast through the nipple at the site of a fissure or abrasion, which may be quite small.

Antimicrobials have markedly improved the prognosis of acute puerperal mastitis. Provided that appropriate antibiotic therapy is started before suppuration begins, the infection can usually be cleared within 48 hours. Nursing should be discontinued when a diagnosis of suppurative mastitis is made, since it may be quite painful and the milk is infected; moreover, the infant often harbors the organisms and can therefore cause reinfection.

POSTPARTUM PSYCHOSIS

As discussed in Chapter 41, mild and transient depression, called **postpartum blues,** is common within the first week or so after delivery. Frequently, this does not develop until the patient goes home with the baby, but in any case it is mild and self-limited. Depression thereafter, especially if severe, is not a normal accompaniment of childbearing and requires investigation. There is no evidence that pregnancy per se causes depressive illness or any other psychotic disorder, though its circumstances might certainly precipitate an underlying disease.

SUGGESTED READINGS

American College of Obstetricians and Gynecologists: Antimicrobial therapy for obstetric patients. Tech Bull No. 117, June 1988.

Kaunitz AM et al: Causes of maternal mortality in the United States. Obstet Gynecol 1985;65:605.

National Institutes of Health Consensus Development Conference: Prevention of venous thrombosis and pulmonary embolism. JAMA 1986;256:744.

Operative Obstetrics

51

Forceps Delivery

GENERAL DESIGN OF FORCEPS

Obstetric forceps are designed for extraction of the fetus. Forceps vary widely in size and shape but consist basically of two crossing branches that are introduced separately into the vagina. Each branch is maneuvered into appropriate relationship with the fetal head, and the two branches are then articulated. Each branch has four components: **blade, shank, lock,** and **handle.** Each blade has two curves, cephalic and pelvic. The **cephalic curve** conforms to the shape of the fetal head and the **pelvic curve** with that of the birth canal. The blades are oval to elliptic in outline, and some varieties are fenestrated rather than solid to permit a more firm hold on the fetal head.

The cephalic curve (Figure 51–1) should be of appropriate contour to grasp the fetal head firmly without compression but not so that the instrument slips. The pelvic curve (Figure 51–1) corresponds more or less to the axis of the birth canal but varies considerably among different instruments. The blades are connected to the handles by the shanks, which give the requisite length to the instrument.

DEFINITIONS & CLASSIFICATION

Forceps used to aid in the delivery of a fetus presenting by the vertex are classified according to the level and position of the head in the birth canal at the time the blades are applied. The following classification was revised in 1988 by the American College of Obstetricians and Gynecologists:

(1) **Outlet forceps:** The fetal skull has reached the perineal floor, the scalp is visible between contractions, and the sagittal suture is in the anterior-posterior diameter or in the right or left occiput anterior or posterior position, but not more than 45 degrees from the midline.

(2) **Low forceps:** The leading edge of the skull is station +2 (in centimeters) or more. Rotations are divided into ≤ 45 degrees and ≥ 45 degrees.

(3) **Mid forceps:** The head is engaged, but the leading edge of the skull is above +2 station (in centimeters).

The danger of trauma to the fetus and the mother from low forceps delivery by this definition will vary depending upon the circumstances preceding delivery. It is emphasized that station here is measured in centimeters (0 to +5), rather than by dividing the lower pelvis into thirds (Chapter 48).

FUNCTIONS & CHOICE OF FORCEPS

The forceps may be used as a tractor or a rotator or both. Its most important function is traction, although—particularly in transverse and posterior positions of the occiput—forceps may be employed successfully for rotation. Any properly shaped instrument will give satisfactory results provided it is used intelligently. For general purposes, either Simpson or Tucker-McLane forceps are quite useful.

INDICATIONS FOR THE USE OF FORCEPS

The termination of labor by forceps, provided it can be accomplished without trauma, is indicated in any condition threatening the mother or fetus that is likely to be relieved by delivery. Such maternal indications include heart disease, acute pulmonary edema, intrapartum infection, and exhaustion. Fetal indications include prolapse of the umbilical cord, premature separation of the placenta, and abnormalities in fetal heart rate indicative of fetal jeopardy.

ELECTIVE & OUTLET FORCEPS

The vast majority of forceps operations performed in this country today are elective forceps. Within the past decade, lumbar epidural analgesia for labor and delivery has

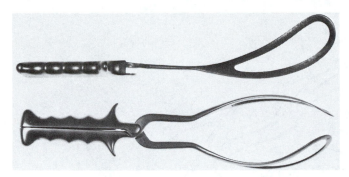

Figure 51–1. Simpson forceps. Note the ample pelvic curve in the single blade above and cephalic curve evident in the articulated blades below. The fenestrated blade and the wide shank in front of the English-style lock characterize the Simpson forceps.

become popular in the United States. Epidural injection of anesthetic agents usually also induces motor blockade sufficient to inhibit maternal expulsive efforts. In order to effect delivery, outlet forceps then are indicated (Chapter 49). The fact that the methods employed to relieve pain frequently necessitate forceps delivery is not an indictment of the procedures provided the obstetrician adheres strictly to the definition of outlet forceps. To maximize safety for mother and fetus, forceps should not be used *electively* until the criteria for outlet forceps are fulfilled.

PREREQUISITES FOR APPLICATION OF FORCEPS

There are at least six prerequisites for the successful application of forceps.

(1) The head must be engaged, and preferably deeply engaged. Even after engagement occurs, the higher the station of the fetal head, the more difficult and traumatic the forceps delivery becomes. Moreover, whenever the blades are applied before the head has reached the perineal floor, it is common to find the head decidedly higher than was believed to be the case from the findings on vaginal examination. This occurs because of extensive caput succedaneum formation and molding. These difficulties of midforceps operation may be encountered even in the presence of a valid maternal indication for forceps delivery. Therefore, forceps should not be used until the station of the head is low enough to ensure a nontraumatic operative procedure.

(2) The fetus must present either by the vertex or by the face with the chin anterior.

(3) The position of the head must be precisely known so that the forceps can be appropriately applied to the fetal head.

(4) The cervix must be completely dilated before the application of forceps. Even a small rim of cervix may offer great resistance when traction is applied, causing extensive cervical lacerations that may reach the lower uterine segment. If prompt delivery becomes imperative before complete dilatation of the cervix, cesarean section is preferable.

(5) Before forceps application, the membranes must be

ruptured to permit a firm grasp of the head by the blades of the forceps.

(6) There should be no disproportion between the size of the head and that of the pelvic inlet, the mid pelvis, or the outlet.

TECHNIQUES OF OUTLET FORCEPS OPERATIONS

PREPARATIONS FOR OPERATION

In the absence of previously instituted adequate continuous conduction analgesia, a decision about the type of analgesia or anesthesia is made based on factors considered in Chapter 44. In many cases, pudendal block will not provide sufficient analgesia for forceps delivery. If spinal analgesia is to be used, the anesthetic agent is introduced before placing the patient in the lithotomy position for delivery. If general anesthesia is to be used, the woman is placed in the lithotomy position, the perineum is cleansed and draped, and the obstetrician is ready to perform the forceps delivery before administering the anesthetic.

The patient's buttocks should be brought to the edge of the delivery table and her legs held in position by appropriate stirrups. She is scrubbed and draped as described in Chapter 44. The bladder should be emptied by catheterization if a midforceps delivery is planned.

APPLICATION OF FORCEPS

Forceps are constructed so that their cephalic curve is closely adapted to the sides of the fetal head (Figure 51–2). The biparietal diameter of the fetal head corresponds to the greatest distance between the appropriately applied blades. Consequently, the head of the fetus is perfectly grasped only when the long axis of the blades corresponds to the occipitomental diameter, with the tips of the blades lying over the cheeks, while the concave margins

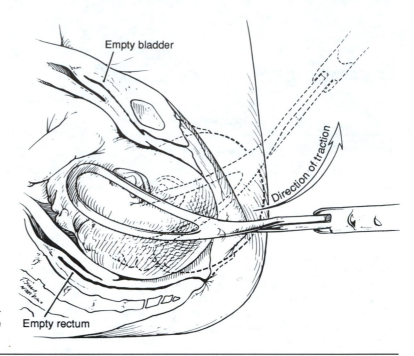

Figure 51–2. Occiput anterior. Delivery by outlet forceps (Simpson). The direction of gentle traction for delivery of the head is indicated.

of the blades are directed toward either the sagittal suture (occiput anterior position) or the face (occiput posterior position). Consideration must be given to the degree of molding. Thus applied, the forceps should not slip, and traction may be applied most advantageously as illustrated in Figure 51–2). When forceps are applied obliquely, however, with one blade over the brow and the other over the opposite mastoid region, the grasp is less secure and the fetal head is exposed to injurious pressure. The forceps must be applied directly to the sides of the head along the **occipitomental diameter,** in what is termed the biparietal or bimalar application.

OUTLET FORCEPS DELIVERY

With the head at the low station required in the definition of outlet forceps, the obstacle to delivery is usually insufficient expulsive forces, appreciable resistance of the perineum, or both. In such circumstances, the sagittal suture occupies the anteroposterior diameter of the pelvic outlet, with the small (posterior) fontanelle directed toward either the symphysis pubis or the concavity of the sacrum. In either event, the forceps, if applied to the sides of the pelvis, grasps the head appropriately. The left blade is introduced by the left hand into the left side of the pelvis, and the right blade is then introduced by the right hand into the right side of the pelvis, as follows: Two fingers of the right hand are introduced inside the left posterior portion of the vulva and into the vagina beside the fetal head. The handle of the left branch is then grasped between the thumb and two fingers of the left hand, as in holding a pen,

and the tip of the blade is gently passed into the vagina between the fetal head and the palmar surface of the fingers of the right hand, which serve as a guide. The handle and branch are held at first almost vertically, but as the blade adapts itself to the fetal head, they are depressed, eventually to a horizontal position. The guiding fingers are then withdrawn, and the handle is left unsupported or held by an assistant. Similarly, two fingers of the left hand are then introduced into the right posterior portion of the vagina to serve as a guide for the right blade, which is held in the right hand and introduced into the vagina. These guiding fingers are then withdrawn and the horizontally positioned branches are articulated, usually without difficulty. Otherwise, first one and then the other blade should be gently maneuvered until the handles are repositioned to effect easy articulation.

Appropriateness of Application

The application is now checked before any traction is applied. For the occiput anterior position, appropriately applied blades are equidistant from the sagittal suture. In the occiput posterior position, the blades are equidistant from the midline of the face and brow. If cervical tissue has been grasped, the forceps should be loosened and, if possible, the incompletely retracted cervix pushed up over the head. Otherwise, labor is allowed to continue or cesarean section is performed.

Traction With Forceps

When it is certain that the blades are placed satisfactorily and the cervix is not entrapped, gentle, intermittent horizontal traction is exerted until the perineum begins to bulge. Traction with forceps is always applied gently and never with excessive force. As the vulva is distended by the occiput, the handles are gradually elevated, eventually pointing almost directly upward as the parietal bones emerge. With the fetal head in the occiput anterior position, this maneuver takes advantage of the smallest diameters of the fetal head and brings the suboccipital region beneath the symphysis. As the handles are raised, the head is extended. Episiotomy is rarely performed immediately prior to application of the blades but most often when forceps traction on the head begins to distend the perineum. During upward traction, the four fingers should grasp the upper surface of the handles and shanks, while the thumb exerts the necessary force upon their lower surface.

During birth of the head, spontaneous delivery should be simulated as closely as possible, employing minimal force. Traction should therefore be intermittent, and the head should be allowed to recede at intervals, as occurs in spontaneous labor. Except when urgently indicated, as in severe fetal distress, delivery should be sufficiently slow, deliberate, and gentle to prevent undue compression of the fetal head. With this in mind, it is preferable to apply traction with each uterine contraction.

After the vulva has been well distended by the head and the brow can be felt through the perineum, delivery may be completed in several ways. Some obstetricians keep the forceps in place in the belief that maximal control of the advance of the head is thus maintained. The thickness of the blades may at times add to the distention of the vulva, however, thus increasing the likelihood of laceration or necessitating a large episiotomy. In such cases, the forceps are removed and delivery is completed by the modified Ritgen maneuver, slowly extending the head by using upward pressure upon the chin through the posterior portion of the perineum while covering the anus with a towel to minimize contamination from the bowel. If the forceps are removed prematurely, the modified Ritgen maneuver may prove to be a tedious and inelegant procedure.

The use of instruments for other than outlet forceps delivery of the occiput anterior vertex is beyond the scope of this book. For descriptions of low forceps and midforceps applications, the reader is referred to Chapter 24 of Cunningham FG, MacDonald PC, Gant NF, Leveno KJ, Gilstrap LC (editors): *Williams Obstetrics,* 19th ed. Appleton & Lange, 1993.

INJURY FROM MIDFORCEPS OPERATIONS

With any midforceps application—and especially those in which rotations are done—serious trauma may result to both fetus and mother unless considerable care is exercised. In most earlier reports, excessive birth trauma has been observed when forceps deliveries were compared with cesarean section. In some more recent reports, however, several investigators found no increased morbidity with midforceps delivery.

There can be no doubt that midforceps delivery performed inappropriately—or by an unsupervised inexperienced operator—can result in considerable maternal as well as fetal trauma. Studies in which these morbid events were reported to be substantially increased were done earlier and at times when cesarean section rates were still around 5%. Moreover, many of these earlier studies undoubtedly included forceps applications that would probably never be attempted today. By contrast, in two of the more recent studies, the authors appropriately emphasize that the majority of midforceps deliveries were done with the fetal vertex at +1 or lower station. ("Station" in these studies divided the pelvis into three measurements from spines to outlet.) It is unlikely that midforceps deliveries included in the Collaborative Perinatal Project during the 1960s were this conservative. Finally, the impact of the popular use of epidural analgesia on the incidence of midforceps deliveries cannot be discounted. The majority of such cases result from inadequate maternal expulsive forces against a relaxed pelvic sling, and thus they are not usually associated with true dystocia. Although it is prudent in these cases to allow a longer second stage of labor, in some women delivery is indicated. Midforceps rotations in such circumstances are likely to be safer than in women with prolonged labors and midpelvic arrest unassociated with conduction analgesia.

VACUUM EXTRACTOR

There have been numerous attempts in the past to attach a traction device by suction to the fetal scalp. The theoretic advantages of the vacuum extractor over forceps include the fact that insertion of space-occupying steel blades within the vagina and positioning the blades precisely over the fetal head—as is required for safe forceps delivery—can be avoided, the fetal head can be rotated without impinging upon maternal soft tissues, and there is great reduction in intracranial pressure during traction. All previously described instruments were unsuccessful until Malmström in 1954 applied a new principle, namely, traction on a metal cap so designed that the suction creates an artificial caput, or *chignon,* within the cup that holds firmly and allows adequate traction. This cup is now replaced by Silastic material; however, high-pressure vacuum generates large amounts of force regardless of the cup used.

In spite of some early enthusiasm in the United States, the vacuum extractor is not used extensively now, partly because of reports of fetal damage, including lacerations and abrasions of the scalp, cephalhematomas, intracranial hemorrhage, and death. In contrast to the American hesitancy, the vacuum extract has had an enthusiastic reception in other parts of the world—although the enthusiasm has waned in at least some foreign institutions.

There have been a few favorable reports from the United States in which the vacuum extractor was used. In one recent study, the authors concluded that vacuum extraction had replaced midforceps deliveries at their institution. It was concluded that vacuum extraction was safer than forceps for the mother and at least as safe as forceps for the fetus. These conclusions were reached despite the fact that two of these studies reported one fetal-neonatal death from cerebral hemorrhage associated with vacuum extraction. The tendency to attempt vacuum deliveries at stations higher than usually attempted with forceps is worrisome. In one study, 3.5% of vacuum deliveries were performed with the vertex above zero station and another 20% were at zero station. If the vacuum instrument is to be used, the same indications for its use should be carefully considered as for any forceps delivery.

SUGGESTED READINGS

American College of Obstetricians and Gynecologists Committee on Maternal and Fetal Medicine: Obstetric Forceps. Tech Bull No. 59, February 1988.

Broekhuizen FF et al: Vacuum extraction versus forceps delivery: Indications and complications, 1979 to 1984. Obstet Gynecol 1987;69:338.

Forceps delivery and related techniques. Chapter 24 in: Cunningham FG, MacDonald PC, Gant NF, Leveno KJ, Gilstrap LC (editors): *Williams Obstetrics,* 19th ed. Appleton & Lange, 1993.

Gilstrap LC et al: Neonatal acidosis and method of delivery. Obstet Gynecol 1984;63:681.

52

Cesarean Delivery

Cesarean delivery is defined as delivery of the fetus through incisions in the abdominal wall (laparotomy) and the uterine wall (hysterotomy). The indications for cesarean delivery are discussed throughout the text wherever the fetal or maternal complications that might necessitate the procedure are presented. In modern obstetric practice, there are virtually no contraindications to cesarean delivery.

The rate for cesarean delivery has been increasing for the past 20 years in the United States and other developed countries. In the USA, the rate increased from 4.5% in 1965 to 23% in 1985. The reasons for this marked increase are not completely understood.

MATERNAL MORTALITY & MORBIDITY RATES

The maternal mortality rate from cesarean delivery is less than 1:1000 procedures. Even this relatively low operative mortality rate must be considered as excessive, because the majority of these deaths occur in young, healthy women undergoing a normal physiologic process.

The major threats to women undergoing cesarean delivery have been anesthesia, severe sepsis, and thromboembolic episodes. Each of these areas has been or will be considered in great detail. It is worth emphasizing, however, that aspiration pneumonia, which had previously been the leading cause of cesarean delivery deaths, has been avoided completely since the routine practice of ingesting 30 mL of milk of magnesia, or more recently a solution of sodium citrate and citric acid (Chapter 44). Despite such efforts to decrease mortality, it is unlikely that deaths from either cesarean or vaginal delivery can be reduced more in severely compromised women who elect, rightly or not, to pursue pregnancies despite their already tenuous medical status.

Even when morbidity and mortality associated with the problem that led to cesarean delivery are excluded, maternal morbidity is more frequent and likely to be more severe following cesarean delivery than following vaginal delivery. The common causes of morbidity from cesarean delivery remain infection, hemorrhage, and injury to the urinary tract.

PERINATAL MORTALITY & MORBIDITY RATES

The frequency of stillbirth and neonatal mortality will depend, of course, on the underlying reason for the cesarean delivery and the gestational age of the fetus.

Birth trauma in general is much less likely with cesarean delivery than with vaginal delivery; however, cesarean delivery is not a guarantee against fetal injury. In fact, the fetus can be wounded during the incision into the uterus.

It is important to emphasize that fetal morbidity has been decreased dramatically with the use of cesarean delivery in instances of certain breech presentations, transverse lie of the fetus, and placenta previa.

TIMING OF REPEAT CESAREAN DELIVERY

The likelihood of rupture of a transverse scar in the lower uterine segment is very low. Unfortunately, a vertical uterine scar may rupture with the onset of labor or even prior to labor.

Iatrogenic Preterm Delivery

Useful guidelines for timing of repeat cesarean delivery can be listed as follows. Note that mandatory amniocentesis to measure the amnionic fluid lecithin/sphingomyelin (L/S) ratio, as recommended by some, is not included. Instead, the following information is used to assess fetal maturity:

(1) Date of onset of the last normal spontaneous menstrual period, if accurately known.
(2) Ultrasonic estimates of fetal age performed in the first trimester or soon thereafter.
(3) Serial measurements of uterine fundal height begun before mid pregnancy.
(4) The time when fetal heart sounds were first heard with an unamplified fetoscope.
(5) Estimated fetal size.

Delivery is carried out after 38 completed weeks of gestation, based on the last normal menstrual period, without measuring the L/S ratio, if (1) the fetal heart was heard at a time when the fundal height was 18–20 cm, if (2) the gestational age at the same time calculated from the normal last menstrual period was 18–20 weeks, or if (3) fetal heart tones have been heard for 20 weeks with a fetoscope—and if (4) the fetus is estimated by two experienced examiners to weigh as much as the previous term infant did, or more than 3000 g when the previous infant was preterm or growth-retarded.

Delivery is postponed if there is discordance that implies a younger gestational age and there are no compelling reasons, maternal or fetal, to effect delivery before the onset of labor—reasons such as a previous vertical incision in the uterus or a strong suspicion of retarded fetal growth.

If the gestational age cannot be absolutely established, pulmonary maturity is established using the L/S ratio, or spontaneous labor is allowed to occur.

VAGINAL DELIVERY SUBSEQUENT TO CESAREAN DELIVERY

Vaginal delivery is usually safe following a previous cesarean delivery. Numerous reports in the past few years confirm this fact.

Guidelines for a Trial of Labor

Specific guidelines for when to permit a trial of spontaneous labor before proceeding with repeat cesarean delivery are set forth by the American College of Obstetricians and Gynecologists (1988). The Committee stresses the importance of availability of personnel to deal appropriately with emergencies that may arise. It is now believed that women who have had one prior transverse cesarean delivery should be counseled to undergo a trial of labor. Those with two prior cesarean deliveries are not discouraged from a trial of labor provided there is no other contraindication. The Committee further concluded that oxytocin induction or augmentation and epidural analgesia are not contraindicated. Unanswered issues include prior low vertical incisions (prior classic incisions contraindicate a trial of labor), twins, breeches, and the singleton fetus with an estimated weight of more than 4000 g.

If a woman is to undergo a trial of labor following a prior cesarean delivery, appropriate technical support must be available in the hospital. There should be an adequate blood bank staffed 24 hours a day with compatible blood promptly available. Electronic fetal heart rate and intrauterine pressure monitoring should be available. There should be adequate facilities and personnel to begin an emergency cesarean delivery within 30 minutes from the time the decision is made.

TECHNIQUE OF CESAREAN DELIVERY

The actual surgical techniques will not be presented in this text. The reader is referred to Chapter 26 of Cunningham FG, MacDonald PC, Gant NF (editors): *Williams Obstetrics,* 19th ed. Appleton & Lange, 1993.

TYPE OF UTERINE INCISION

The classic cesarean incision—a vertical incision into the body of the uterus above the lower uterine segment and reaching the uterine fundus—is seldom used. Almost always, the incision is made in the lower uterine segment transversely or, less often, vertically (Figure 52–1).

The lower segment transverse incision has the advantage of requiring only modest dissection of the bladder from the underlying myometrium. If the incision extends laterally, the laceration may involve large branches of the uterine artery and vein. The low vertical incision may be extended upward so that in circumstances where much more room is needed, the incision can be carried into the body of the uterus; otherwise, it is a less desirable incision. More extensive dissection of the bladder is necessary

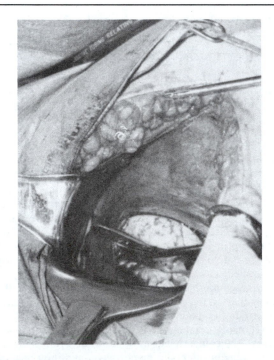

Figure 52–1. A low transverse uterine incision is indicated. (Reproduced, with permission, from Cunningham FG, MacDonald PC, Gant NF, Leveno KJ, Gilstrap LC [editors]: *Williams Obstetrics,* 19th ed. Appleton & Lange, 1993.)

to keep the vertical incision within the lower uterine segment. Moreover, if the vertical incision extends downward, it may tear through the cervix into the vagina and perhaps involve the bladder. If, on the other hand, it is extended upward into the body of the uterus, closure—including satisfactory reperitonealization—is more difficult. It has been the experience of most obstetricians that during the next pregnancy the vertical incision is much more likely to rupture, especially during labor, than is the lower segment transverse incision.

POSTMORTEM CESAREAN DELIVERY

In the case of a postmortem cesarean delivery, a satisfactory outcome for the fetus is dependent upon (1) anticipation of death of the mother, (2) fetal age of more than 28 weeks, (3) personnel and appropriate equipment immediately available, (4) continued postmortem ventilation and cardiac massage for the mother, (5) prompt delivery, and (6) effective resuscitation of the infant. While a few infants have survived after demise of the mother during parturition with no apparent physical or intellectual compromise, others have not been so fortunate. In recent years, the ability of life-support systems to maintain some level of vegetative function for long periods of time and the reluctance of physicians to pronounce a patient dead have decreased further the likelihood of delivering an infant that will survive and thrive following postmortem cesarean delivery.

PERIPARTUM MANAGEMENT

PREOPERATIVE CARE

The woman scheduled for repeat cesarean delivery typically is admitted the day before surgery and evaluated by the obstetrician who will perform surgery and the anesthesiologist who will provide anesthesia. The hematocrit is rechecked, and if the indirect Coombs test is positive, 1000 mL of compatible whole blood or its equivalent in blood fractions is reserved. A sedative such as secobarbital 100 mg may be given at bedtime the night before the operation. In general, no other sedatives, narcotics, or tranquilizers are administered until after the infant is born. Oral intake is stopped at least 8 hours before surgery. An antacid given shortly before the induction of general anesthesia, minimizes the risk of lung destruction from gastric acid should aspiration occur (Chapter 44). This should be done routinely even when regional conduction analgesia will be used; at times it is necessary to switch to—or at least supplement—the regional analgesia with inhalation anesthesia.

INTRAVENOUS FLUIDS

The requirements for intravenous fluids, including blood during and after cesarean delivery, can vary considerably. The woman of average size with a hematocrit of 33% or more and a normally expanded blood volume and extracellular fluid volume most often tolerates an actual blood loss of up to 1500 mL without difficulty. Careful attention must be paid to blood loss so as to avoid both underestimation and overestimation. Unappreciated bleeding through the vagina during the procedure or bleeding concealed in the uterus after its closure commonly lead to underestimation. Blood loss averages about 1 L but is quite variable.

Intravenously administered fluids consist of lactated Ringer's injection or similar solution and 5% dextrose in water. Typically, 1–2 L containing balanced electrolytes is infused during and immediately after the operation. As the shoulders of the infant are delivered, oxytocin, 20 units per L, is added to the infusion, which is then infused for a few minutes at a brisk rate (10 mL per min) until the uterus is well contracted. Throughout the procedure—and subsequently while in the recovery area—the blood pressure and urine flow are monitored closely to ascertain that perfusion of vital organs is satisfactory.

RECOVERY SUITE

In the recovery suite, the amount of bleeding from the vagina must be closely monitored, and the uterine fundus must be identified by palpation frequently to ensure that the uterus is remaining firmly contracted. A thick dressing with an abundance of adhesive tape over the abdomen interferes with fundal palpation and massage and later causes discomfort as the tape and perhaps skin are removed. Deep breathing and coughing are encouraged.

Once the patient is fully awake, bleeding is minimal, blood pressure is satisfactory, and urine flow is at least 30 mL per hour, the patient may be returned to her room.

SUBSEQUENT CARE

Analgesia

For the woman of average size, meperidine, 75 mg—or morphine, 10 mg—is given intramuscularly as often as every 3 hours as needed for discomfort. If she is small, 50 mg, or if large, 100 mg of meperidine is more appropriate. An antiemetic (eg, promethazine, 25 mg) is usually given along with the narcotic. Other analgesic approaches, such as postpartum epidural narcotics or patient-controlled anesthesia, are being evaluated with promising early results.

Vital Signs

Blood pressure, pulse, amount of urine flow, amount of bleeding, and the status of the uterine fundus are checked at least hourly for 4 hours. Abnormalities are reported immediately. Thereafter, for the first 24 hours, these are checked at intervals of 4 hours, along with the temperature.

Fluid Therapy & Diet

Unless there has been pathologic constriction of the extracellular fluid compartment, the puerperium is characterized by excretion of fluid that was retained during pregnancy and became superfluous once delivery was accomplished. Moreover, with the typical cesarean delivery or uncomplicated cesarean hysterectomy, significant sequestration of extracellular fluid in the bowel wall and bowel lumen does not occur unless it was necessary to pack the bowel away from the operative field or unless peritonitis develops. Thus, the woman who undergoes cesarean delivery is rarely a candidate for the development of fluid sequestration in the so-called third space. Large volumes of intravenous fluids during and subsequent to surgery are therefore not needed to replace sequestered extracellular fluid. As a generalization, 3 L of fluid, including lactated Ringer's injection, should prove adequate during surgery and the first 24 hours thereafter. If urine output falls below 30 mL per h, however, the patient should be reevaluated promptly. The cause of the oliguria may range from unrecognized blood loss to an antidiuretic effect from infused oxytocin (Chapter 44). In the absence of extensive intra-abdominal manipulation or sepsis, the woman nearly always should be able to tolerate oral fluids the day after surgery. If she cannot, an intravenous infusion can be continued or restarted. By the second day after surgery, the great majority of women tolerate a general diet.

Bladder & Bowels

The catheter most often can be removed from the bladder by 12 hours after the operation or, more conveniently, the morning after the operation. Subsequent ability to empty the bladder before overdistention develops must be monitored as with a vaginal delivery. Bowel sounds are usually absent on the first day after surgery, faint on the second day, and active on the third day. Gas pains from incoordinate bowel action may be troublesome the second and third postoperative days. A rectal suppository will often provoke defecation; if not, an enema should be given.

Ambulation

In most cases, the patient should get out of bed briefly with assistance at least twice on the day after surgery. Ambulation can be timed so that a recently administered analgesic will minimize the discomfort. With early ambulation, venous thrombosis and pulmonary embolism are uncommon.

Wound Care

The incision is inspected each day. Thus, a relatively light dressing without an abundance of tape is advantageous. Normally the skin sutures (or skin clips) are removed on the fourth day after surgery. By the third postpartum day, shower bathing is not harmful to the incision.

Laboratory Studies

The hematocrit is routinely measured the morning after surgery. It is checked sooner when there was unusual blood loss or when there is oliguria or other evidence to suggest hypovolemia. If the hematocrit is significantly decreased from the preoperative level, it is repeated, and a search is instituted to determine the cause of the decrease. If the lower hematocrit is stable, the mother can ambulate without any difficulty, and if there is little likelihood of further blood loss, hematologic repair in response to iron therapy is preferred to transfusion.

Breast Care

Breast feeding can be initiated by the day after surgery. If the mother elects not to nurse, a breast binder that supports the breasts without marked compression will usually minimize discomfort.

DISCHARGE FROM HOSPITAL

Unless there are complications during the puerperium, the mother may be safely discharged on the fourth or fifth postpartum day. The mother's activities during the following week should be restricted to self-care and care of her baby with assistance. It is advantageous to perform the initial postpartum evaluation during the third week after delivery rather than at the more traditional time of 6 weeks.

PROPHYLACTIC ANTIMICROBIALS

Depalma and colleagues (1982) evaluated therapeutic intervention in a high-risk group of nulliparous women who underwent cesarean delivery because of cephalopelvic disproportion. Since the frequency of pelvic infection was 85% without therapy, they considered administration of antimicrobial drugs to be treatment rather than prophylaxis. They observed that the administration of penicillin plus gentamicin or of cefamandole alone as soon as the cord was clamped—followed by two more doses of the same medications given at intervals of 6 hours—resulted in a dramatic reduction in morbidity from infection. Postoperative metritis, for example, was decreased from 85% to 20%. Associated complications, such as pelvic phlegmons, incisional abscesses, and pelvic thrombophlebitis, also decreased dramatically.

Currently, the author's practice is to administer a single dose of a broad-spectrum antimicrobial such as a cephalosporin or an extended spectrum penicillin. These regimens have been proved equally effective, and the choice of antimicrobial should be based on considerations of patient allergies, local availability, cost, and physician comfort with their individual use.

The woman with clinically diagnosed chorioamnionitis should be given continuous antimicrobial therapy postoperatively until she is afebrile.

SUGGESTED READINGS

American College of Obstetricians and Gynecologists Committee on Maternal and Fetal Medicine: Guidelines for vaginal delivery after a previous cesarean birth. October, 1988.

Cesarean section and cesarean delivery. Chapter 26 in: Cunningham FG, MacDonald PC, Gant NF, Leveno KJ, Gilstrap LG (editors): *Williams Obstetrics,* 19th ed. Appleton & Lange, 1993.

DePalma RT et al: Continuing investigation of women at high risk for infection following cesarean delivery: The three-dose perioperative antimicrobial therapy. Obstet Gynecol 1982; 60:53.

Complications of Pregnancy

Diseases & Abnormalities of the Placenta & Fetal Membranes

ABNORMALITIES OF PLACENTATION

Occasionally, the placenta may be separated into lobes, most frequently two. When the division is incomplete and the vessels of fetal origin extend from one lobe to the other before uniting to form the umbilical cord, the condition is termed **placenta bipartita** or **bilobed placenta** (Figure 53–1).

An important anomaly is **placenta succenturiata,** in which one or more small accessory lobes are developed in the membranes at a distance from the periphery of the main placenta, to which they usually have vascular connections of fetal origin (Figure 53–2). Accessory lobes are common, and their incidence is about 3%. They are of considerable clinical importance because this accessory lobe is sometimes retained in the uterus after expulsion of the main placenta, and when it separates subsequently, it may give rise to serious maternal hemorrhage.

In **extrachorial placenta,** the chorionic plate, which is on the fetal side of the placenta, is smaller than the basal plate, which is located on the maternal side. If the fetal surface of such a placenta presents a central depression surrounded by a thickened, grayish-white ring, which is situated at a varying distance from the margins, it is called a **circumvallate placenta** (Figure 53–3). When the ring coincides with the placental margin, the condition is sometimes described as a marginate or **circummarginate placenta.** While the normal-term placenta weighs on the average about 500 g, in certain diseases, such as syphilis, the placenta may weigh one-fourth, one-third, or even one-half as much as the fetus. The largest placentas are usually encountered in cases of **erythroblastosis fetalis**.

CIRCULATORY DISTURBANCES

The most common placental lesions, though of diverse origin, are referred to collectively as placental infarcts. The principal histopathologic features include fibrinoid degeneration of the trophoblast, calcification, and ischemic infarction from occlusion of spiral arteries. Up to one-fourth of placentas from term uncomplicated pregnancies have infarcts. This incidence is much higher in women with hypertensive diseases. Some examples of placental infarctions are shown in Figure 53–4.

Overclassification of these infarcts has led to unnecessary confusion. Small subchorionic and marginal foci of degeneration are present in every placenta. These lesions are of clinical significance only when they are abundant, in which case they may interfere with the function of a sufficiently large portion of the placenta to seriously interfere with fetal nutrition and on occasion to cause fetal death.

Calcification of the Placenta

Small calcareous nodules or plaques are observed frequently upon the maternal surface of the placenta and are occasionally so abundant that the organ feels like coarse sandpaper. In view of the widespread degenerative changes in the term placenta, calcification is not surprising. In fact, the conditions for calcium deposition in the aging placenta are almost ideal. Moderate degrees of calcification may be detected in at least half of all placentas examined radiographically. Placental calcification is part of normal aging, and the process accelerates in the third trimester. Calcification may be seen using ultrasonography in at least half of placentas by 33 weeks.

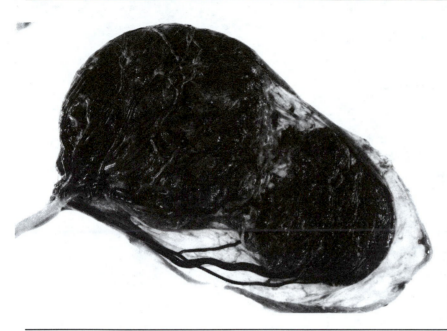

Figure 53–1. Bilobed placenta. Two lobes are present in this placenta. Also shown in this specimen is a marginal and a partial velamentous insertion of the umbilical cord. (Reproduced, with permission, from Cunningham FG, MacDonald PC, Gant NF, Leveno KJ, Gilstrap LC [editors]: *Williams Obstetrics,* 19th ed. Appleton & Lange, 1993.)

ABNORMALITIES OF THE UMBILICAL CORD

Umbilical cord (funis) length varies greatly, with the mean being about 55 cm. Extremes in cord length in abnormal instances range from apparently no cord (achordia) to lengths up to 300 cm. Vascular occlusion by thrombi and true knots are more common in excessively long cords and are more apt to prolapse through the cervix. Rarely, excessively short umbilical cords may be instrumental in abruptio placentae and uterine inversion. They may rupture with intrafunicular hemorrhage, which can cause fetal death from exsanguination.

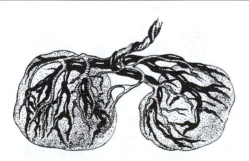

Figure 53–2. Succenturiate lobes. (Reproduced, with permission, from Pernoll ML, Benson RC [editors]: *Current Obstetric & Gynecologic Diagnosis & Treatment,* 6th ed. Appleton & Lange, 1987.)

There is only one umbilical artery in nearly one of every 100 placentas. Nearly 5% of the cords of at least one twin have this malformation. This is important because infants with a single cord artery have greatly increased congenital malformations. In one study, infants with a single-artery cord had an 18% incidence of major malformations, 34% were growth-retarded, and 17% delivered preterm. In another, the mortality rate was very high (14%) among infants with a single umbilical artery; but of those who survived infancy, serious anomalies were not much more common than in the control group.

VELAMENTOUS INSERTION OF CORD

Of considerable practical importance is velamentous insertion of the cord, since the umbilical vessels separate in the membranes at a distance from the placental margin, which they reach surrounded only by a fold of amnion (Figure 53–5). This mode of insertion is noted in a little over 1% of singleton deliveries—but much more frequently with twins, and almost invariably with triplets. With velamentous insertion of the cord, the likelihood of fetal deformity is increased.

VASA PREVIA

In vasa previa, some of the fetal vessels in the membranes with velamentous insertion cross the region of the internal os and occupy a position ahead of the presenting part of the fetus. At times, the careful examiner will be able to palpate a tubular fetal vessel in the membranes overlying the presenting part.

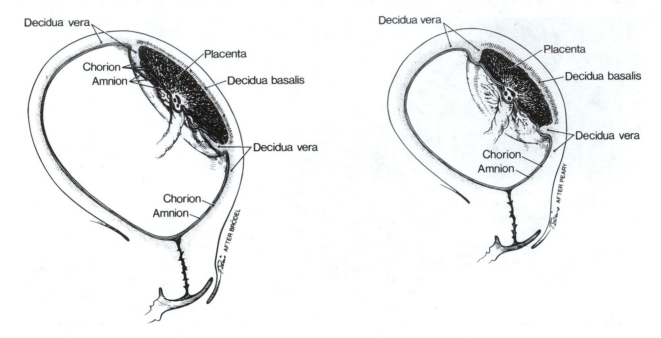

Figure 53–3. Circumvallate *(left)* and marginate *(right)* varieties of extrachorial placentas. (Reproduced, with permission, from Cunningham FG, MacDonald PC, Gant NF, Leveno KJ, Gilstrap LC [editors]: *Williams Obstetrics,* 19th ed. Appleton & Lange, 1993.)

Vasa previa implies considerable danger to the fetus, since rupture of the membranes may be accompanied by rupture of a fetal vessel followed by exsanguination.

CORD ABNORMALITIES CAPABLE OF IMPEDING BLOOD FLOW

Several mechanical and vascular abnormalities of the umbilical cord are capable of impairing fetal-placental blood flow.

False knots, which result from kinking of the vessels to accommodate to the length of the cord, should be distinguished from **true knots,** which result from active movements of the fetus. In nearly 17,000 deliveries in the Collaborative Study on Cerebral Palsy, the incidence of true knots was 1.1%. Perinatal loss was 6.1% in the presence of true knots. The incidence of true knots is especially high in monoamnionic twins.

The cord frequently becomes coiled around portions of the fetus, usually the neck. In 1000 consecutive deliveries in one study, the incidence ranged from one loop around the neck in 21% to three loops in 0.2%. Coiling of the cord around the neck is an uncommon cause of fetal death. Typically, as labor progresses and the fetus descends the birth canal, contractions compress the cord vessels, which causes fetal heart-rate deceleration that persists until the contraction ceases.

DISEASES OF THE AMNION

Brownish-green discoloration of the fetal membranes is characteristic of meconium staining. The amnion may be slippery from mucus discharged in the meconium. Meconium staining of the membranes or fetus was identified in about 10% of 43,000 live-born infants in the Collaborative Study Perinatal Project. The neonatal mortality rate was 3.3% in the group with meconium-stained membranes compared to 1.7% in the nonstained group. Meconium staining of amnionic fluid is more common than meconium staining of membranes and is identified in 20% of all deliveries.

In some cases, amnionitis is a manifestation of an intrauterine infection and is often associated with prolonged membrane rupture and long labors. When mononuclear and polymorphonuclear leukocytes infiltrate the chorion, the resulting microscopic finding is properly designated **chorioamnionitis.** These findings, however, may be nonspecific and are not always associated with other evidence of fetal or maternal infection. When organisms are isolated from amnionic fluid or membranes, they invariably are the same as those that normally colonize in the vagina and cervix.

Clinically occult chorioamnionic infection caused by a wide variety of microorganisms has emerged recently as a possible explanation of many heretofore unexplained

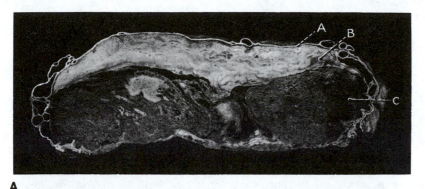

A

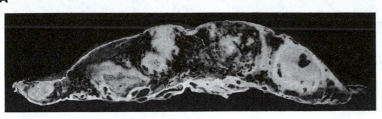

B

Figure 53–4. *A:* Placental infarcts: A, chorioamnionic membrane; B, fibrin deposited locally beneath the chorion; C, normal placental tissue. In this instance, the infarct was unusually extensive, most likely contributing to the death of the fetus. ***B:*** Generalized fibrin deposition with little normal tissue remaining.

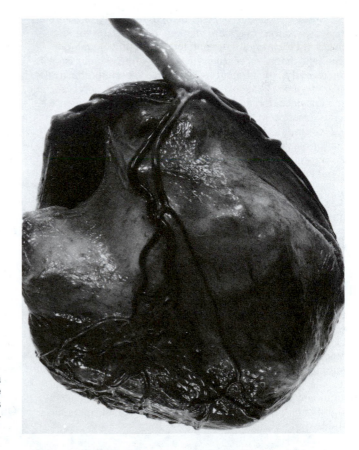

Figure 53–5. Velamentous insertion of cord. The placenta ***(bottom)*** and membranes have been inverted to expose the amnion. Note the large fetal vessels within membranes ***(top)*** and their proximity to the site of rupture of the membranes.

cases of ruptured membranes, preterm labor (Chapter 59), or both.

DISORDERS OF THE AMNIONIC FLUID

HYDRAMNIOS

Hydramnios, sometimes called **polyhydramnios,** is excessive amnionic fluid. Normally, the volume of amnionic fluid increases to about 1 L or somewhat more by 36 weeks but decreases thereafter. Postterm, there may be only a few hundred milliliters or even less. Somewhat arbitrarily, more than 2000 mL of amnionic fluid is considered excessive, or hydramnios. In rare instances, the uterus may contain an enormous quantity of fluid, with reports of as much as 15 L. In most instances, the increase in amnionic fluid is gradual (**chronic hydramnios**). In **acute hydramnios,** the volume increases very suddenly and the uterus may become markedly distended within a few days. The amnionic fluid in hydramnios is usually similar in appearance and composition to the fluid in normal conditions.

Incidence

Minor to moderate degrees of hydramnios (2–3 L) are rather common, but more marked degrees are not. Because of the difficulty of complete collection of amnionic fluid, the diagnosis is usually based on clinical impression or, recently, sonographic estimation. Therefore, the frequency of the diagnosis varies with different observers, and it is not surprising that published data on the incidence have varied from about 1:60 deliveries to 1:750.

Hydramnios is frequently associated with fetal malformations, especially of the central nervous system and gastrointestinal tract. For example, hydramnios accompanies about half of cases of anencephaly and esophageal atresia.

The incidence of hydramnios also is increased in pregnancies complicated by diabetes and in **immune and non-immune hydrops** (Chapter 55). Excessive amnionic fluid in one of the amnionic sacs is common in twin pregnancies and is more frequent and usually more intense in monozygotic than in dizygotic twinning.

Etiology

The volume of amnionic fluid is controlled in a number of ways. Early in pregnancy, the amnionic cavity is filled with fluid similar in composition to extracellular fluid. During the first half of pregnancy, transfer of water and other small molecules takes place not only across the amnion but through the fetal skin. During the second trimester, the fetus begins to urinate, to swallow, and to inspire amnionic fluid. These processes almost certainly have a significant modulating role in the control of amnionic fluid volume.

Symptoms

Symptoms result principally from the pressure upon adjacent organs exerted within and around the overdistended uterus. Excessive distention may cause severe dyspnea, and in extreme cases the mother may be able to breathe only when upright. Edema is common—especially in the lower extremities, the vulva, and the abdominal wall—as a consequence of compression of major venous systems by the very large uterus. Rarely, severe oliguria may result from ureteral obstruction by the very large uterus. With **chronic hydramnios,** the accumulation of fluid takes place gradually and the woman may tolerate abdominal distention with relatively little discomfort. In **acute hydramnios,** however, the distention may lead to distressing symptoms. Acute hydramnios tends to develop earlier in pregnancy than the chronic form—often as early as 16–20 weeks—and it may rapidly expand the hypertonic uterus to enormous size.

Diagnosis

Uterine enlargement in association with difficulty in palpating fetal small parts and in hearing fetal heart tones usually is the main diagnostic sign of hydramnios. In severe cases, the uterine wall may be so tense that it is impossible to palpate any part of the fetus. Such findings call for prompt ultrasonic examination to better quantify amnionic fluid and to identify multiple fetuses or fetal abnormalities.

Treatment

Minor degrees of hydramnios rarely require treatment. Even moderate degrees, including cases in which there is some discomfort, usually can be managed without intervention until labor ensues or until the membranes rupture spontaneously. If there is dyspnea or abdominal pain or if ambulation becomes difficult, hospitalization is necessary.

There is no satisfactory treatment for symptomatic hydramnios other than removal of some of the amnionic fluid. Amniocentesis may be used to relieve maternal distress, and to that end it is successful transiently. At times, amniocentesis appears to initiate labor even though only part of the fluid is removed; hence, relief of distress may not allow continuation of pregnancy. The volume of fluid removed at one time appears to be critical.

OLIGOHYDRAMNIOS

In rare instances, the volume of amnionic fluid may fall far below the normal limits and occasionally be reduced to only a few milliliters of viscid fluid. The cause of this condition is not completely understood. Very small amounts of amnionic fluid may be found relatively often with pregnancies that have continued for weeks beyond term. The risk of cord compression and, in turn, fetal distress is increased as a consequence of the scant volume of fluid. Oligohydramnios is practically always evident when there is either obstruction of the fetal urinary tract or renal agenesis. Therefore, anuria almost certainly has an etiologic role in such cases of oligohydramnios. A chronic leak from a defect in the membranes may reduce the volume of amnionic fluid, but most often labor soon ensues.

Oligohydramnios early in pregnancy is generally associated with poor fetal outcome, owing to its cause as well as its effects. When amnionic fluid is scant, **pulmonary hypoplasia** is very common.

SUGGESTED READINGS

Fox H: *Pathology of the Placenta.* Monograph, Vol 7. Saunders, 1987.

Hankins GDV et al: Nuchal cords and neonatal outcome. Obstet Gynecol 1987;70:687.

Hill LM et al: Polyhydramnios: Ultrasonically detected prevalence and neonatal outcome. Obstet Gynecol 1987;69:21.

Landy JH, Isada NB, Larsen JW: Genetic implications of idiopathic hydramnios. Am J Obstet Gynecol 1987;157:114.

54

Congenital Malformations & Inherited Disorders

Infants commonly are born with obvious structural aberrations, and 3–5% of all newborns have a recognizable anomaly. The causes of these anomalies are myriad and frequently not identifiable. While some are attributed to chromosomal or genetic defects (25%), fetal infections (5%), or maternal illness (5%), the cause of most defects is unknown. Detection of functional congenital aberrations increases with age, and the overall incidence increases to 6–7% in later childhood. The incidence of anomalies is increased in obstetrically abnormal pregnancies, and perhaps 50% of spontaneously aborted fetuses have a chromosomal abnormality (Chapter 9). Preterm and stillborn infants more commonly have major malformations, and performance of routine autopsies increases their detection. Birth defects are the leading cause of infant deaths before age 1, and they account for 20% of such deaths.

Only a few congenital malformations appear to have a major environmental or genetic cause and probably result from interactions between genetic predisposition and subtle factors in the intrauterine environment. Perhaps the most dramatic example in past years of a major environmental cause of human malformation was maternal rubella infection (Chapter 55). When the fetus was infected during the first 8–10 weeks of pregnancy, rubella invariably caused a variety of malformations, including cataracts, cardiac defects, deafness, microcephaly, and mental retardation.

TERATOLOGY

A teratogen is any agent or factor, exposure to which during embryogenesis produces a permanent alteration in form or function of the offspring. When considering whether a given chemical, drug, or physical force may be teratogenic by causing a specific malformation, several crucial factors are involved. Of main importance is the time period in pregnancy during which fetal exposure occurs.

The embryonic period is the most critical with regard to malformations, since it encompasses organogenesis. By way of example, maternal rubella infection results in fetal infection early in pregnancy and frequently causes multiple congenital defects, while chronic but nondebilitating viral shedding less often follows infection late in pregnancy. Alternatively, a drug ingested during late pregnancy cannot cause malformations such as limb reduction defects.

The number of strongly suspected or proven human teratogens is surprisingly small (Table 54–1) and includes androgenic hormones, some antineoplastic drugs, diethylstilbesterol, isotretinoin, most anticonvulsants, some infectious agents, radiation, and maternal alcoholism and diabetes.

DRUGS & MEDICATIONS DURING PREGNANCY

Women commonly ingest medications or drugs while pregnant. The Centers for Disease Control surveyed 492 pregnant women in New York State and found that 90% took either prescription or over-the-counter drugs from 48 different classes. The average woman takes 3.8 different medications during pregnancy. Besides prenatal vitamin and mineral supplements, commonly used drugs include antiemetics, antacids, antihistamines, analgesics, antimicrobials, tranquilizers, hypnotics, and diuretics. With rare exception, any drug that exerts a systemic effect in the mother will cross the placenta to reach the embryo or fetus.

FOOD & DRUG ADMINISTRATION CLASSIFICATION

In 1979, the Food and Drug Administration established five categories for drugs and medications with regard to possible adverse fetal effects (Tables 54–2 and 54–3). This classification has relieved some anxieties for both the

Table 54–1. Strongly suspected or known human teratogens

Drugs and chemicals	Infections
Aminopterin	Cytomegalovirus
Androgenic hormones	Rubella virus
Busulfan	Syphillis
Chlorbiphenyls	Toxoplasmosis
Coumarins	Venezuelan equine virus
Cyclophosphamide	**Maternal disorders**
Diethylstilbesterol	Alcoholism
Goitrogens (antithyroid drugs)	Connective tissue diseases
Isoretinoin	Diabetes
Lithium	Endemic cretinism
Organic mercury	Hyperthermia
Penicillamine	Virilizing tumors
Phenytoin	**Radiation**
Tetracyclines	Atomic weapons
Thalidomide	Radioiodine
Trimethadione	Radiotherapy
Valproic acid	

(Adapted from Shepard: *Adv Pediatr* 33:225, 1986.)

patient and the physician concerning drug prescription during pregnancy.

ENVIRONMENTAL TERATOGENS

A variety of environmental hazards are associated with teratogenicity and include some viral, bacterial, and protozoal infections as well as ionizing radiation and some chemicals. Several viruses and bacteria that cause fetal in-

Table 54–2. FDA categories for drug use in pregnant women[1]

A (Safest)	Controlled studies in women fail to demonstrate a risk to the fetus in the first trimester, and the possibility of fetal harm seems remote.
B	Studies in animals do not indicate a risk to the fetus, and there are no controlled studies in humans *or* Studies in animals do show an adverse effect on the fetus, but well-controlled studies in pregnant women have failed to demonstrate a risk to the fetus.
C	Studies in animals have shown the drug to have teratogenic or embryocidal effects, but there are no controlled studies in women *or* No studies in either animals or women are available.
D	Positive evidence of human fetal risk exists, but benefits in certain situations (eg, life-threatening situations or diseases for which safer drugs cannot be used or are ineffective) may make use of the drug acceptable despite its risks.
X (Least safe)	Studies in animals or humans have demonstrated fetal abnormalities or there is evidence of fetal risk based on human experience (or both), and the risk clearly outweighs any possible benefit.

[1]Regardless of the designated category or presumed safety of the drug, no drug should be administered during pregnancy unless it is clearly needed. (Modified and reproduced from *FDA Drug Bulletin* 1982;12:24.)

fections result in morphologic and functional derangements and are considered in Chapter 55.

INHERITED DISORDERS

At least 20–25% of congenital malformations are the result of chromosomal abnormalities or single-gene defects. The majority (perhaps 65–75%) of birth defects are due to unidentifiable causes; however, because of their patterns of inheritance, they are presumed to result from a complex interaction between genetic predisposition and intrauterine environmental factors.

CHROMOSOMAL ABNORMALITIES

The incidence of chromosomal abnormalities in liveborn infants is between 1:200 and 1:50 and averages 1:178. The frequency among stillbirths and infants who die during the neonatal period is 6–7%. As pointed out in Chapter 9, *chromosomal abnormalities are identified in at least 50% of early spontaneous abortions.*

Whether the involved chromosome is an autosome or a sex chromosome, the pathogenetic mechanism seems to be the same. During meiotic division in the gonad, a chromosome may "drop out" of the dividing cell (anaphase lagging) and thus be lost. Fertilization of such a gamete results in a zygote with one chromosome too few. In trisomies, one of the explanations of a chromosomal gain is **nondisjunction,** or failure of the gamete to split equally at meiotic division. If the cell with the extra chromosome is fertilized, the zygote becomes **trisomic.** These errors of meiotic division produce individuals whose cells are chromosomally equal but with an abnormal increase in chromosomal number.

AUTOSOMAL TRISOMIES (Down Syndrome)

Down syndrome is the most common chromosomal defect reliably detected by amniocentesis early in the second trimester. In the past, it was referred to as mongolism, and affected individuals were termed mongoloid. Most cases of Down syndrome result from an extra chromosome, and the most common trisomy is that of chromosome 21, which is identified in approximately 1:800 liveborns. Trisomies of chromosomes 13 and 18 are less common but more lethal than trisomy 21. Also less common is a chromosomal **translocation,** ie, the transfer of a segment of one chromosome to a different site on the same chromosome or to a different chromosome.

Whereas in mothers up to the age of 30 the risk of birth of a liveborn infant with Down syndrome is less than

Table 54–3. Classification by indication of some drugs and medications used during pregnancy

Asthma	Cardiovascular disease	Hormones	Miscellaneous	Pain and inflammation
Albuterol C	β-blockers C	Clomiphene X	Antihistamines	Acetaminophen B
Corticosteroids B,C,D	Coumarins D/X	Contraceptives X	Barbituates D	Aspirin C/D
Cromolyn B	Digoxin B/C	Estrogens X	Cocaine C	Codeine C/D
Ephedrine C	Furosemide C	Progestins D	Dextroamphetamine D/C	Ibuprofen B/D
Epinephrine C	Heparin B		Ethanol D/X	Indomethacin B/D
Metaproterenol C	Hydrochlorothiazide D	**Infections**	Guaifenesin C	Meperidine B/D
Terbutaline B	MethyldopaC	Acyclovir C	Heroin B/D	Morphine B/D
Theophylline C	Procainamide C	Amphotericin B	Insulin B	
	Quinidine C	Cephalosporins B	Isoretinoin X	**Psychiatric disorders**
Cancer	Verapamil C	Chloroquine X	Thioureas D	Amitriptyline D
Azathioprine D		Erythromycin B		Chlordiazepoxide D
Chlorambucil D		Lindane B		Diazepam D
Cisplatin D	**Convulsive disorders**	Metronidazole B	**Nausea and vomiting**	Imipramine D
Cyclophosphamide D	Carbamazepine C	Miconazole B	Chlorpromazine	Lithium D
Fluorouracil D	Phenobarbital D/X	Nitrofurantoin B	Cyclizine B	Nortriptyline D
Melphalan D	Phenytoin D	Nystatin B	Meclizine B	Phenothiazines C
Methotrexate D	Trimethadione D/X	Penicillins B	Promethazine C	
Procarbazine D	Valproic acid D/X	Quinine D	Trimethobenzamide C	
Vincristine D		Sulfonamides B		
		Tetracyclines D		
		Trimethoprim C		
		Zidovudine C		

Categories according to Food and Drug Administration guidelines, either by manufacturer or according to Briggs, Freeman and Yaffee: Drugs in Pregnancy and Lactations, 2nd ed. Baltimore, Williams & Wilkins, 1986.

1:800, this risk increases to about 1:100 by age 40 and to 1:32 by age 45.

SEX CHROMOSOMAL ANOMALIES

Abnormalities of the sex chromosomes are relatively common and may result from either monosomies or polysomies. McKusick (1986) lists 124 X-linked defects.

1. TURNER SYNDROME (45,X)

Most sex monosomies result in early pregnancy loss, and nearly 20% of early spontaneous abortions are sex monosomies. Loss of the long arm of the X chromosome results in streaked ovaries and amenorrhea. In 70% of cases, the paternal X is missing. The short arm of X controls height, and phenotypic females with 45,X monosomy have normal intelligence and gonadal dysgenesis along with short stature and other physical stigmas, including a high incidence of cardiac and renal anomalies.

2. KLINEFELTER SYNDROME (47,XXY)

Additional X chromosomes to the normal male XY karyotype are relatively common polysomies and are seen in 1: 1000 male infants. Males with 47,XXY represent the most frequent abnormality of sexual differentiation and, except for some mosaics, are invariably infertile. They have testicular atrophy, azoospermia, and elevated gonadotropins; usually there are associated somatic abnormalities, especially gynecomastia and obesity. Mild mental de-

ficiency is common, and in syndromes caused by more than two X chromosomes these abnormalities are greatly magnified.

3. FRAGILE X SYNDROME

This X chromosome abnormality is the most commonly inherited cause of mental impairment and is second only to Down syndrome as a chromosomal cause of retardation. The prevalence in the general population is estimated at 1:2000 males, with a heterozygous prevalence in females of 1:1000. The prevalence in severely mentally retarded populations varies from 2% to 6%.

SINGLE-GENE DEFECTS

Single-gene mutations cause defects that are manifest clinically by mendelian inheritance patterns that cause phenotypic abnormalities in 1% of all newborns. Individual disorders are rare, but the number so far catalogued— nearly 4000—underscores the complexity of these mutations. As with any mendelian inheritance, their clinical presentation can be classified into autosomal dominant, autosomal recessive, or X-linked.

MULTIFACTORIAL OR POLYGENIC INHERITANCE

Genetic variability is the result of the combined actions of a number of genes with small individual effects. The great range of effects so produced is thought to be responsible for the continuous variation seen among normal human beings, as expressed in stature, intelligence, blood pressure, and, quite likely, susceptibility to a number of common diseases.

Many of the more common congenital malformations have a genetic factor in their causation. In multifactorial genetic diseases, there is a **polygenic** component, ie, a series of genes interacting to produce a cumulative effect. The increased incidence in relatives compared to the incidence in the general population is difficult to explain in terms of any known environmental factors. Common congenital malformations with an incidence at birth of at least 1:1000—such as cleft lip, pyloric stenosis, talipes equinovarus, congenital hip dislocations, spina bifida, anencephaly, and congenital heart defects—are polygenically inherited with varying degrees of environmental modification. Overall, these abnormalities are identified in about 1% of newborn infants.

NEURAL TUBE DEFECTS

Neural tube defects result from the tube's failure to close by days 26–28. This produces a spectrum of cranial and spinal canal defects that range from anencephaly to very slight defects of the vertebra.

ANENCEPHALY

Anencephaly is characterized by absence of the skull and by cerebral hemispheres that are either rudimentary or absent (Figure 54–1). The pituitary gland is usually either absent or markedly hypoplastic. Absence of the cranial vault renders the face very prominent and somewhat extended; the eyes often bulge from their sockets; and the tongue hangs from the mouth. About 70% of anencephalic fetuses are females.

In addition to the virtual absence of brain tissue in anencephalic fetuses, typically there is extreme diminution in the size of the adrenal glands. The duration of anencephalic pregnancies, especially in the absence of hydramnios, may be remarkably long and can exceed that reported in any other form of gestation with a living fetus.

Elevated levels of α-fetoprotein in amnionic fluid or maternal serum reliably predict the majority of cases of larger open neural tube defects, including anencephaly. Closed or very small open neural tube abnormalities may not be detected.

SPINA BIFIDA & MENINGOMYELOCELE

Spina bifida consists of a hiatus—usually in the lumbosacral vertebrae—through which a meningeal sac may protrude, forming a **meningocele.** If the sac contains the spinal cord as well, the anomaly is called **meningomyelocele.**

HYDROCEPHALY

Because of the clinical importance of hydrocephaly as a cause of dystocia and rupture of the uterus and the difficulties in decision making concerning route of delivery, this malformation is considered also in Chapter 46 along with other fetal causes of dystocia.

The characteristic ultrasonic finding is dilatation of the lateral ventricles. Associated anomalies, including spina bifida, are fairly common. Hydrocephaly is seldom identified at or before mid pregnancy, but if it should be recognized, pregnancy termination is an option.

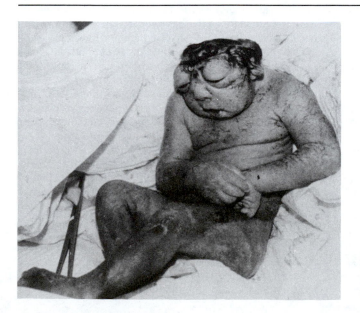

Figure 54–1. Anencephalic infant. (Reproduced, with permission, from Cunningham FG, MacDonald PC, Gant NF, Leveno KJ, Gilstrap LC [editors]: *Williams Obstetrics,* 19th ed. Appleton & Lange, 1993.)

CONGENITAL HEART DISEASE

Because of the inconsistency with which cases of congenital heart disease are reported, the frequency of these malformations cannot be stated precisely, but they are among the more common abnormalities. Cardiac malformations include such conditions as patent ductus arteriosus, coarctation of the aorta, septal defects, pulmonary stenosis, and tetralogy of Fallot. Cardiac anomalies also commonly occur as parts of other syndromes.

CLEFT LIP & CLEFT PALATE

A cleft in the lip, either unilateral or bilateral, may or may not be associated with a cleft in the alveolar arch—ie, a cleft palate. Cleft lip is one of the most frequent congenital deformities, with an incidence of 1.3:1000 births.

ABDOMINAL-WALL DEFECTS

Omphalocele and gastroschisis are relatively common ventral wall defects that may be confused on ultrasonic examination. While antepartum detection has increased, these defects commonly still are overlooked. An omphalocele is a defect in the umbilical ring from which protrudes a sac—covered with amnion and peritoneum—and into which abdominal contents have typically herniated. It is the more common of the two and is seen in about 1:4000 live births. Gastroschisis is intestinal herniation through a defect in the anterior abdominal wall, usually to the right of the umbilicus. There is no sac, and the intestines are covered with a thickened inflammatory exudate. This anomaly is identified in perhaps 1:10,000 births.

Associated congenital anomalies contribute to a high mortality rate for either condition. Chromosomal aberrations also are common. Omphalocele is associated with other anomalies in up to 70% of cases and gastroschisis in 10–30%.

GENETIC COUNSELING

Birth of an affected child or disease in a near relative often calls attention to a genetic disorder. In other cases, couples may be unaware that a condition is genetically transmitted. Thus, forecasting the probability of an inherited disorder is an important step, but it requires a precise medical history. In addition to the routine history obtained from all pregnant women, specific questions should be asked to help identify the expectant mother whose fetus is at unusual risk of having or subsequently acquiring a serious disability.

In prospective counseling, advice is provided to possible carriers of recessive genes before birth or, ideally, before conception. First, there is identification of heterozygotes by population screening procedures. The individual then is advised of the risk of an affected child if conception is with another carrier. Finally, the heterozygote couple is counseled concerning the possibility of pregnancy interruption if the disease can be diagnosed in utero.

SCREENING PROGRAMS

There are screening programs to identify some of the more common autosomal recessive disorders—examples include sickle cell anemia, Tay-Sachs disease, thalassemia major, and more recently, some forms of cystic fibrosis. These programs raise many social, ethical, economic, and legal questions, not to mention the possible psychologic stigma of carrying "bad genes." Equally important to the success of such screening programs is an intensive education program for persons undergoing testing, and this, unfortunately, is where many programs typically have failed.

Because of problems inherent with testing the entire population, several screening programs have been developed for the pregnant woman. Examples discussed below include maternal serum α-fetoprotein screening for neural tube defects and cytogenetic studies on fetal cells obtained by amniocentesis or chorionic villus sampling in women over 35.

PRENATAL DIAGNOSIS

No other area in clinical obstetrics has experienced more rapid practical application of technologic advances than prenatal diagnosis. In the past 20 years, techniques have been developed that permit early and accurate diagnosis of many fetal disorders. Beginning with simple cytogenetic techniques to determine gross chromosomal abnormalities, there are now methods that permit rapid detection using minute quantities of fetally derived DNA obtained by direct sampling of chorionic tissue. This, coupled with the techniques of molecular genetics, allows detection of a large number of inherited conditions. The number of these conditions increases almost daily.

Ultrasound plays a major role in detection of fetal anomalies. Moreover, its value as a guide to obtaining fetal tissue for analysis has become indispensable as older and less precise fetoscopic techniques have been replaced by sonar-directed chorionic villus sampling, amniocentesis, and fetal blood and tissue sampling.

Easy and safe accessibility of amnionic fluid undoubtedly has greatly influenced obstetric care. Amniocentesis allows access to fetal somatic cells and fluid that can be used to identify the cytogenetic constitution of the fetus or to assess a variety of abnormal biochemical processes.

To identify several genetic disorders in the fetus, chromosomal or other laboratory analysis can be employed. It is most often of value in the following circumstances:

(1) Pregnancies in women 35 years of age or older.

(2) A previous pregnancy that resulted in the birth of a chromosomally abnormal offspring.

(3) Chromosomal abnormality in either parent.

(4) Down syndrome or other chromosomal abnormality in a close relative.

(5) Biochemical studies in pregnancies at risk of a serious autosomal or X-linked recessive disorder.

(6) A previous child or a parent with a neural tube defect or an abnormally low or high maternal serum α-fetoprotein level obtained during routine screening.

(7) An abnormal fetus identified by sonographic examination (not always done).

(8) A previous infant with multiple major malformations in whom no cytogenetic study was performed (not always done).

(9) Fetal sex determination in pregnancies at risk of a serious X-linked hereditary disorder (better accomplished using DNA techniques to identify Y chromosomal material).

A great variety of inheritable disorders have been detected by appropriate study of amnionic fluid contents. About 75 recessively inherited X-linked or autosomal metabolic disorders are now detectable in tissue culture systems and therefore are approachable in the fetus through amniocentesis or chorionic villus sampling. It is emphasized that this list is expanding rapidly. The risk of an autosomal recessive disorder in the fetus may have become apparent from the previous birth of an affected infant, from screening of the parents for the carrier state, or from the family history.

ELEVATED α-FETOPROTEIN

The value of measurement of α-fetoprotein in amnionic fluid between 16 and 20 weeks' gestation to detect fetal abnormalities—especially open neural tube defects—is now established.

The site of production of most, if not all, of the increased α-fetoprotein is the fetus. It is the major protein in the serum of the embryo and early fetus. Initially, it is produced in the yolk sac, but by the end of the first trimester it is nearly all of hepatic origin. In both fetal serum and amnionic fluid, the concentration of α-fetoprotein is highest around the 13th week of gestation. The concentration in fetal serum is about 150 times that in amnionic fluid. The normal source of the protein in amnionic fluid is fetal urine. Some of that protein, in turn, crosses the fetal membranes to enter the maternal circulation. The concentration of α-fetoprotein levels in maternal serum are only 0.001–0.01 those of fetal serum. After 13 weeks, the levels in both fetal serum and amnionic fluid normally decrease rapidly in essentially parallel fashion, while those in ma-

ternal serum continue to rise until late in pregnancy. Since fetal serum and amnionic fluid levels decrease sharply, correct interpretation of its concentration requires precise knowledge of gestational age. Some conditions associated with abnormally elevated or low levels of α-fetoprotein in maternal serum and amnionic fluid are shown in Table 54–4.

MATERNAL SERUM α-FETOPROTEIN SCREENING

Routine screening for neural tube defects by measuring α-fetoprotein levels in maternal serum currently is now widely employed in the United States, as it has been for some time in many European countries. Indeed, some states mandate that such screening be made available to all prenatal patients. After initial controversy surrounding its implementation—primarily because of technical problems—the American College of Obstetricians and Gynecologists (1986) now recommends that such screening programs be established but only within a coordinated system that includes quality control, counseling, follow-up, and high-level sonographic facilities.

If the procedure is accepted after informed consent is obtained, initial serum screening is done at 16–18 weeks of gestation. About 5% of all women will have abnormally high levels, defined by most as greater than 2.5 multiples of the median determined for the population under study. Repeat serum testing eliminates 2% of the total, and ultrasound evaluation is performed for the remaining 3%.

Table 54–4. Some conditions associated with abnormal maternal serum α-fetoprotein concentrations.[1]

High levels
  Neural tube defects
  Pilonidal cysts
  Esophageal or intestinal obstructions
  Liver necrosis
  Cystic hygroma
  Sacrococcygeal teratoma
  Abdominal wall defects—omphalocele, gastroschisis
  Urinary obstruction
  Renal anomalies—polycystic or absent kidneys
  Congenital nephrosis
  Osteogenesis imperfecta
  Congenital skin defects
  Cloacal exstrophy
  Low birthweight
  Oligohydramnios
  Multifetal gestation
  Decreased maternal weight
  Underestimated gestational age
Low levels
  Chromosomal trisomies
  Gestational trophoblastic disease
  Fetal death
  Increased maternal weight
  Overestimated gestational age

[1]Reproduced, with permission, from Cunningham FG, MacDonald PC, Gant NF, Leveno KJ, Gilstrap LC: *Williams Obstetrics*, 19th ed. Appleton & Lange, 1993.

In 1% of the total, multiple gestation, inaccurate gestational age estimation, or missed abortion are identified. Thus, 2% of all women screened will need to undergo amniocentesis so that amnionic fluid α-fetoprotein concentration can be measured as described above—and only a small fraction of these will be found to have abnormally elevated levels.

It is important to emphasize that a growing number of conditions other than neural tube defects have been recognized as associated with both abnormally elevated and low serum α-fetoprotein concentrations. Some of these are shown in Table 54–4.

CHORIONIC VILLUS BIOPSY

Since its development beginning in the early 1970s, biopsy or sampling of the chorion, either transvaginally or transabdominally, has become a widely accepted first-trimester alternative to amniocentesis for prenatal diagnosis. The chorion is of fetal origin, and cells obtained by villus biopsy can thus be examined using the same techniques as for amniocytes obtained by amniocentesis. The primary difference is that amniocentesis must be used for assays for which amnionic fluid is integral, an example being α-fetoprotein concentration. The major advantage of villus biopsy is that fetal cells are obtained earlier and lengthy culture procedures are unnecessary, since chorion cells divide rapidly. Thus, a diagnosis is made earlier and pregnancy can be terminated sooner and with greater safety. The major disadvantage is that the risk of subsequent abortion is slightly increased over that for genetic amniocentesis.

SUGGESTED READINGS

American College of Obstetricians and Gynecologists: Antenatal diagnosis of genetic disorders. Tech Bull No. 108, September 1987.

American College of Obstetricians and Gynecologists: Prenatal detection of neural tube defects. Tech Bull No. 99, December 1986.

Beckman DA, Brent RL: Mechanism of known environmental teratogens: Drugs and chemicals. Clin Perinatol 1986;13:649.

Briggs GG, Freeman RK, Yaffe SJ: *Drugs in Pregnancy and Lactation,* 2nd ed. Williams & Wilkins, 1986.

Goldstein JC, Brown MS: Genetics aspects of disease. Page 285 in: *Harrison's Principles of Internal Medicine,* 11th ed. Braunwald E et al (editors). McGraw-Hill, 1987.

McKusick VA: *Mendelian Inheritance in Man: Catalogs of Autosomal Dominant, Autosomal Recessive, and X-linked Phenotypes,* 7th ed. Johns Hopkins Univ Press, 1986.

Shepard TH: Human teratogenicity. Adv Pediatr 1986;33:225.

Wilson JG: Experimental studies on congenital malformations. J Chron Dis 1959;10:111.

55

Diseases, Infections, & Injuries of the Fetus & Newborn

The fetus and newborn infant are subject to a great variety of diseases, some of which are the direct consequence of maternal diseases and are taken up along with those sections elsewhere in this book and especially in Chapter 60. This chapter provides an introduction to other fetal and neonatal diseases and injuries of major clinical importance. Congenital malformations are considered in Chapter 54.

DISEASES OF THE FETUS & NEWBORN

HYALINE MEMBRANE DISEASE
(Idiopathic Respiratory Distress Syndrome)

To provide prompt blood gas exchange after birth, the infant must rapidly fill its lungs with air while clearing them of fluid and at the same time greatly increase the volume of blood perfusing the lungs. Some of the fluid usually is expressed as the chest is compressed during vaginal delivery and the remainder is absorbed, especially through the pulmonary lymphatics. Of great importance is the presence of appropriate surfactant synthesized by the type II pneumonocytes to stabilize the air-expanded alveoli by lowering surface tension and in that way preventing lung collapse during expiration.

About two decades ago, the development of idiopathic respiratory distress syndrome—also termed hyaline membrane disease—was found to be due to deficiency of pulmonary surfactant. If the alveoli cannot be maintained in an expanded state because of inappropriate surfactant action, obvious respiratory distress develops that is characterized by the formation of hyaline membranes in the distal bronchioles and alveoli, considerable cardiopulmonary shunting of blood, and the likelihood of death from hypoxemia and acidosis unless treatment is given promptly.

In severe cases, mechanical ventilation may be lifesaving. Such measures allow for decreased oxygen concentrations to be given, thus avoiding some problems from oxygen toxicity. In some studies, the use of aerosolized surfactant has reduced the morbidity rate from the disease.

Diagnosis

The atelectatic lungs are stiff, with substantively decreased compliance, and thus the work of breathing is increased. Progressive shunting of blood through nonventilated areas of the lung contributes to the hypoxemia and to both metabolic and respiratory acidosis. Clinically these infants exhibit an increased respiratory rate accompanied by severe retraction of the chest wall during inspiration. Expiration is often accompanied by a whimper and grunt. Grunting is common in the newborn whenever there is uneven expansion of the lungs or lower airway obstruction. Finally, poor peripheral circulation and systemic hypotension may be evident.

Other forms of respiratory insufficiency may be confused with idiopathic respiratory distress syndrome. These include respiratory insufficiency as the consequence of sepsis, pneumonia, aspiration, pneumothorax, diaphragmatic hernia, and heart failure. In case of idiopathic respiratory distress, the chest x-ray shows a diffuse reticulogranular infiltrate throughout the lung fields with an air-filled tracheobronchial tree (air bronchogram).

Treatment

The establishment of appropriately staffed and equipped neonatal intensive care units has served to reduce dramatically the number of deaths from idiopathic respiratory distress, even in very small infants. Similarly, advances in respiratory therapy and ventilatory support have been crucial. An arterial Po_2 below 40 mm Hg is indicative of the need for effective oxygen therapy.

Oxygen therapy is not innocuous. Persistent hypoxia in

itself is likely to injure the lung, especially the alveoli and capillaries. If hyperoxemia is produced, the infant is at risk of developing **retrolental fibroplasia.** Therefore, the concentration of oxygen administered must be reduced appropriately as the arterial Po_2 rises. Endotracheal tubes after prolonged use cause erosion and serious infection of the upper airway, and they must be removed as soon as possible. **Bronchopulmonary dysplasia,** or oxygen toxicity lung disease, may develop in infants treated for severe respiratory distress with high concentrations of oxygen at high pressures. This is a chronic lung condition characterized by hypoxia, hypercapnia, and oxygen dependence as the consequence of alveolar and bronchiolar epithelial damage followed by peribronchial and interstitial fibrosis.

MECONIUM ASPIRATION

The aspiration of some amnionic fluid before birth is most likely a physiologic event. Unfortunately, this normal process can be the cause of inhalation by the fetus of amnionic fluid containing thick meconium, which in some cases leads to subsequent respiratory distress and hypoxia with many complications as described above. On the other hand, some neonates inhale meconium at birth. Thus, meconium aspiration syndrome may follow delivery in otherwise normal labor, but it more often is encountered in postterm pregnancy or in those complicated by fetal growth retardation. The common feature of these pregnancy complications appears to be reduced amnionic fluid volume into which the fetus defecates copious amounts of meconium.

Aspiration of meconium is likely to cause both mechanical obstruction of the airways and chemical pneumonitis. Atelectasis, consolidation, and pneumothorax and pneumomediastinum may prove rapidly fatal unless vigorously treated. Even with prompt and appropriate therapy, seriously affected infants frequently die. Vigorous suctioning of the mouth and nares before delivery of the shoulders, as well as tracheal suction after delivery, may prevent further aspiration. These practices have been questioned, and recently it was reported that tracheal suctioning of meconium did not reduce the incidence or severity of respiratory distress from aspiration.

INTRAVENTRICULAR HEMORRHAGE

Intraventricular hemorrhage—bleeding into the germinal matrix tissues, which then may extend into the ventricular system and brain parenchyma—is a common problem in preterm neonates. While these lesions are usually seen in infants born at less than 34 weeks, they may develop later and even are seen in term neonates. Most hemorrhages will develop within 72 hours after birth; however, they have been observed as late as 24 days. While external perinatal and postnatal influences undoubtedly alter the incidence and severity of these lesions, the greatest impact is that of prematurity. Unfortunately, since their onset is usually within 3 days after delivery, their origin often is erroneously attributed to birth events.

The incidence undoubtedly depends upon the level of immaturity; about half of all neonates born before 34 weeks will have evidence of some hemorrhage. Interestingly, 4% of asymptomatic term neonates have sonographic evidence of subependymal hemorrhage. Very low birth weight infants have the earliest onset of hemorrhage, the greatest likelihood for progression into parenchymal tissue, and the highest mortality rate. The severity of intraventricular hemorrhage can be assessed by ultrasound and CT scan, and various grading schemes are used to quantify the extent of the lesion.

BRAIN DISORDERS

In 1862, a London orthopedist, William Little, described 47 children with spastic rigidity. He concluded that virtually nothing other than abnormalities of birth could cause this clinical picture. Although others have suggested that prenatal events may be causal factors, the *presumed* birth-injury etiology of cerebral palsy has endured and has influenced the opinions and practice of countless obstetricians and pediatricians. This presumption probably accounts in part for the high malpractice premiums among those who deliver and care for newborns.

CEREBRAL PALSY

A National Institutes of Health panel has defined cerebral palsy as a nonprogressive motor disorder with onset in early infancy, involving one or more limbs, with resulting muscular spasticity or paralysis. It affects at least 1:500 school-age children. While affected children may have associated mental retardation or epilepsy, many often have neither, and 70% of cerebral palsy victims are of normal intelligence.

In many cases, cerebral palsy is erroneously attributed to perinatal events. Contrary to earlier teachings, perinatal asphyxia—another poorly defined term—is identified in only about one-third of cases of cerebral palsy.

Findings from the Collaborative Perinatal Project of the National Institute of Child Health and Human Development indicate that maternal mental retardation, birth weight less than 2000 g, and fetal malformations were leading predictors of cerebral palsy, while obstetric complications were not strongly predictive. Only 21% of affected children had markers for perinatal asphyxia, and over half of these had associated congenital malformations, low birth weight, microcephaly, or another explanation for the brain disorder. *They concluded that the causes of most cases of cerebral palsy are unknown.*

MENTAL RETARDATION

Severe mental retardation has a prevalence of 3:1000 children. In a National Institutes of Health report, the panel ascertained that isolated mental retardation—ie, mental retardation not associated with epilepsy or cerebral palsy—was associated with perinatal hypoxia in only 5% of cases. Alternatively, mental retardation coincidental with cerebral palsy is strongly associated with evidence of perinatal asphyxia or hypoxia.

FETAL-TO-MATERNAL HEMORRHAGE

The presence of fetal red cells in the maternal circulation may be identified by use of the acid elution principle first described by Kleihauer, Brown, and Betke or any of its several modifications. Very small volumes of red cells commonly escape from the fetal intravascular compartment across the generally intact placental barrier into the maternal intervillous space. Large bleeds are uncommon, and in 500 cases, only six women had fetal hemorrhage at delivery exceeding 30 mL. Although the bleed is usually small, it may incite maternal isoimmunization, as discussed later.

ISOIMMUNIZATION
(Hemolytic Disease of the Newborn)

Any person who lacks a specific red cell antigen can potentially produce an antibody when exposed to that antigen. The antibody may prove harmful to the individual in case of a blood transfusion or to a fetus when a woman conceives. The vast majority of humans have at least one such factor inherited from their father and lacking in their mother. In these cases, the mother could be sensitized if enough erythrocytes from the fetus were to reach her circulation to elicit an immune response.

A D-negative woman delivered of a D-positive, ABO-compatible infant has a likelihood of isoimmunization of 16%.

Common Causes of Isoimmunization

A. CDE (Rhesus) Blood Group System: The CDE, or rhesus, blood group system has clinical importance because most individuals who lack its major antigenic determinant—D or Rh—become immunized after a single exposure to erythrocyte antigen. Rhesus antigens other than D have low immunogenicity and are typically ignored unless the pregnant woman has already formed an antibody to them, which in turn is detected by an antibody screening test. All pregnant women should be routinely tested for the presence or absence of D (Rho) antigen on their erythrocytes and for other irregular antibodies in their serum. The possibility of hemolytic disease from rarer blood groups may be suspected from the results of the indirect Coombs test done to screen for abnormal antibodies in maternal serum.

Major causes of clinically significant isoimmunization other than anti-D include anti-E, anti-c, anti-C, and anti-Kell.

B. ABO Blood Group System: The major blood group antigens A and B are the most common but not the most serious cause of hemolytic disease of the newborn. For example, group 0 women may from early life have anti-A and anti-B isoagglutinins, which may be augmented by pregnancy, particularly if the fetus is a secretor. Although about 20% of all infants have an ABO maternal blood group incompatibility, only 5% show overt signs of hemolytic disease. Moreover, when they do, the disease is usually much milder than what is seen with D isoimmunization. Unlike Rh hemolytic disease, the incidence of stillbirths among ABO incompatible pregnancies is not increased.

D antigen incompatibility and ABO heterospecificity account for approximately 98% of all cases of hemolytic disease.

Pathologic Changes

Maternal antibodies gain access to the fetal circulation. In D-positive fetuses, such antibodies are both adsorbed to the D-positive erythrocytes and exist unbound in fetal serum. The adsorbed antibodies act as hemolysins, leading to an accelerated rate of red cell destruction. The earlier this process begins in utero and the greater its intensity, the more severe will be the effects upon the fetus.

The pathologic changes in the organs of the fetus and newborn infant vary with the severity of the process. The severely affected fetus or infant may show considerable subcutaneous edema as well as effusion into the serous cavities (**hydrops fetalis).** At times, the edema is so severe that the diagnosis can be easily identified using sonography. In these cases, the placenta also is markedly edematous, enlarged, and boggy, with prominent cotyledons and edematous villi. The ascites and, to a lesser degree, hepatomegaly and splenomegaly, may be so massive as to lead to severe dystocia owing to the greatly enlarged abdomen. Hydrothorax may be so severe as to compromise respirations after birth.

Fetuses with hydrops may die in utero from profound anemia and circulatory failure (Figure 55–1). A sign of severe anemia and impending death is a **sinusoidal fetal heart rate** pattern. The liveborn hydropic infant appears pale, edematous, and limp at birth, often requiring resuscitation. The spleen and liver are enlarged, and there may be widespread ecchymoses or scattered petechiae. Dyspnea and circulatory collapse are common. Death may occur within a few hours in spite of transfusions.

Less severely affected infants may appear well at birth, only to become jaundiced within a few hours. Marked hyperbilirubinemia, if untreated, may lead to central nervous system damage—especially to the basal ganglia—or to **kernicterus.**

Prevention

The incidence of hemolytic disease of the fetus and newborn from D isoimmunization has become much

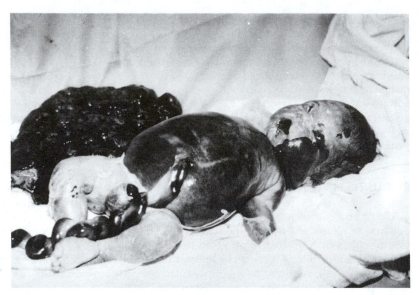

Figure 55–1. Severe erythroblastosis fetalis. Hydropic macerated stillborn infant and characteristically large placenta.

lower because of passive immunization of D-negative women delivered of D-positive infants. Anti-D immune globulin is a 7S immune globulin G extracted by cold alcohol fractionation from plasma containing high-titer D antibody. Each dose provides not less than 300 μg of D antibody as determined by radioimmunoassay. Although the administration of D immune globulin to the apparently nonsensitized mother within the first 72 hours after delivery of an D-positive infant has decreased dramatically the risk of maternal isoimmunization, the problem has not been eliminated.

The failure rate of 2% is due to spontaneous silent fetal-maternal bleeds before delivery and before the administration postpartum of D immune globulin. Therefore, to try to avoid isoimmunization from fetal-maternal bleeds remote from term, 300 μg of antibody is now routinely administered intramuscularly to all nonsensitized D-negative women at 28 weeks as well as at the time of amniocentesis or uterine bleeding. If the infant was D-positive, a third dose of the immunoglobulin is administered to the mother after delivery. This reduces the incidence of D isoimmunization during pregnancy from 1.8% to 0.07%.

Treatment

The management of isoimmunization—except for ABO incompatibility—is similar regardless of the inciting antigen. Since D isoimmunization is the most common type, general management for this clinical situation is discussed.

An antibody titer no higher than 1:16 as measured using the indirect Coombs test almost always means that the fetus will not die in utero from hemolytic disease and that with appropriate care after birth it will survive. A titer higher than this indicates the *possibility* of severe hemolytic disease.

Whenever the antibody titer is sufficiently elevated to be clinically significant, fetal evaluation is warranted. In most institutions, this critical titer is considered to be 1:16 or greater; however, in some laboratories, if the titer remains below 1:32, a good fetal outcome is anticipated.

If use of intrauterine transfusion is being considered, amniocentesis may be initiated at as early as 22 weeks of gestation. The absorbance of breakdown pigments, mostly bilirubin, in the supernatant of amnionic fluid, when measured in a continuously recording spectrophotometer, is demonstrable as a hump with maximum absorbance at 450 nm (ΔOD_{450}). The magnitude of the increase in optical density above baseline at 450 nm usually correlates well for any gestational age with the intensity of the hemolytic disease.

Some have concluded that the only reliable means of determining severity in the second trimester is direct measurement of fetal hemoglobin by cordocentesis. Most recommend that transfusions be started when the hemoglobin deficit exceeds 2 g/dL from the mean for normal fetuses of corresponding gestational age.

The severely affected fetus is transfused with packed erythrocytes cross-matched against maternal blood. Using sonography, blood is placed in the peritoneal cavity or directly into an umbilical cord vessel.

In many circumstances, as alluded to above, delivery before term is advantageous. Obviously, when it is considered necessary to utilize fetal transfusions, delivery rather than further attempts at fetal transfusion is desirable once sufficient maturity has been achieved to ensure a good chance of survival.

HYPERBILIRUBINEMIA

The great concern over unconjugated hyperbilirubinemia in the newborn is its association with **kernicterus.** This complication occurs with greater frequency in preterm infants. The yellow staining of the basal ganglia and hippocampus is indicative of profound degeneration in these regions. Surviving infants show spasticity, muscular incoordination, and varying degrees of mental retardation. There is a positive correlation between kernicterus and unconjugated bilirubin levels above 18–20 mg per dL, though kernicterus may develop at lower concentrations, especially in very premature infants.

By far the most common form of unconjugated nonhemolytic jaundice is so-called **physiologic jaundice of the newborn.** In the mature infant, the serum bilirubin increases for 3–4 days to achieve serum levels up to 10 mg per dL or so and then falls rapidly. In preterm infants, the rise is more prolonged and may be greater.

NONIMMUNE HYDROPS FETALIS

Hydrops fetalis need not always have an immunologic basis, and nonimmune hydrops has become more common in recent years than that from isoimmunization. Undoubtedly, hydrops is identified in utero much more frequently since high-resolution sonography has become available, and these cases most often come under scrutiny because of increased intrauterine volume, almost always associated with hydramnios.

The formation and the accumulation of serous fluid in body cavities and subcutaneous edema have been attributed to a great variety of causes. Cardiac abnormalities, either structural or rhythm-related, or both, are associated with 20–45% of cases of nonimmune hydrops. About 35% are due to chromosomal anomalies or other malformations, and 10% are associated with twin-twin transfusions. Those cases previously labeled idiopathic are less common.

The mortality rate of nonimmune hydrops depends on the cause, but in general the prognosis is poor. Less than 10–20% of affected fetuses survive.

Ultrasonic evaluation is the most useful means of evaluating pregnancy complicated by fetal hydrops; however, there are other noninvasive steps that may be taken. After immunologic hydrops has been excluded, hematologic, chemical, and serologic studies are done to look for maternal causes such as severe anemia, diabetes, or syphilis. A Kleihauer-Betke stain of maternal blood may disclose evidence of significant fetomaternal hemorrhage. If these and detailed sonar evaluation fail to disclose the apparent cause, then fetal echocardiography is done to search again for cardiac abnormalities. If still no cause is found, some recommend amniocentesis or sonographically directed fetal blood sampling for karyotyping or other tests appropriate for investigation of the specific cause.

HEMORRHAGIC DISEASE OF THE NEWBORN

Hemorrhagic disease of the newborn is a syndrome characterized by spontaneous internal or external bleeding accompanied by hypoprothrombinemia and very low lev-

els of other vitamin K-dependent coagulation factors (V, VII, IX, and X). Bleeding may begin any time after birth but typically is delayed for a day or two. The infant may be mature and healthy in appearance, though a greater incidence of the disease has been noted in preterm infants. The prothrombin and partial thromboplastin times are greatly prolonged.

Hypoprothrombinemia in the neonate appears to be the consequence of poor placental transport of vitamin K_1 to the fetus. Plasma vitamin K_1 levels are somewhat lower in pregnant women than in nonpregnant adults, and the vitamin is undetectable in cord plasma.

As prophylaxis against hemorrhagic disease of the newborn, the infant should receive 1 mg of phytonadione (vitamin K_1) intramuscularly within 1 hour after delivery. Although controversial in other countries, this practice is almost universal in the United States.

THROMBOCYTOPENIA

A number of diseases or conditions are associated with neonatal thrombocytopenia of varying degrees. It tends to be more severe in preterm fetuses, especially those with respiratory distress and hypoxia or sepsis.

Antiplatelet IgG antibody transferred from mother to fetus and causing thrombocytopenia in the fetus-neonate can be suspected when the mother has thrombocytopenia from an autoimmune disease, especially **immunologic thrombocytopenic purpura.** Avoidance of traumatic delivery and appropriate corticosteroid therapy to try to improve hemostasis are important to a successful outcome.

Isoimmune thrombocytopenia may develop in a manner similar to D antigen isoimmunization. In this condition, thrombocytopenia follows maternal isoimmunization against fetal platelet antigens, usually PL_{A1}, which is found in 98% of the population. Thus, the mother lacks the common platelet antigen and becomes immunized when exposed to the antigen by fetal platelets that enter the maternal circulation.

INFECTIONS OF THE FETUS & NEWBORN

The active immunologic capacity of the fetus and neonate is compromised in comparison with that of older children and adults. Passive immunity is provided by the mother principally by IgG transferred across the placenta; however, the degree of passive immunity is much lower in preterm infants. Infection, especially in its early stages, may be difficult to diagnose because of the newborn's failure to respond in classic fashion. The signs of infection can be vague, nonspecific, and certainly not dramatic until the infant becomes moribund. If infection occurred in utero, the infant may have been depressed and acidotic at birth for no apparent reason. It may suck poorly, vomit, or develop abdominal distention—or may develop respiratory insufficiency which is similar in many ways to idiopathic respiratory distress syndrome. It may be lethargic or jittery. Any infant who appears ill should be suspected of having an infection.

GROUP B STREPTOCOCCUS INFECTION

Neonatal infections with group B β-hemolytic streptococci are almost as prevalent as those from coliform organisms, which are the most common pathogens that cause neonatal septicemia. It is clear that intrapartum transmission to the fetus of group B streptococci from a colonized maternal genital tract may lead to severe sepsis in the infant soon after birth. Depending on the population studied, as many as 10–40% of women during late pregnancy are colonized with group B streptococci in the lower genital tract, and half of newborn infants exposed become colonized. Maternally transmitted antibodies protect most of these infants; however, 1–2% develop clinical disease. Preterm or low-birth-weight infants are at highest risk, but more than half of cases of neonatal streptococcal sepsis are in term neonates. For infants with infection, the mortality rate is nearly 25%. With septicemia from group B streptococci that characterizes early onset disease, signs of serious illness usually develop within 48 hours after birth. The signs of early onset infection include respiratory distress, apnea, and shock.

RUBELLA (German Measles)

Rubella—a disease usually of minor importance except when it occurs during pregnancy—has been directly responsible for untold numbers of fetal deaths and severe congenital malformations. Although large epidemics of rubella have virtually disappeared in the United States because of immunization, sporadic cases still occur. It is advised that rubella vaccination be avoided shortly before or during pregnancy, since the vaccine is an attenuated live virus.

The diagnosis of rubella is at times difficult. Not only are the clinical features of other illnesses quite similar, but subclinical cases with viremia and infection of the embryo and fetus do occur. Absence of rubella antibody indicates lack of immunity. The presence of antibody denotes an immune response to rubella viremia that may have been acquired anywhere from a few weeks to many years earlier. If maternal rubella antibody is demonstrated at the time of exposure to rubella or before, the mother can be assured that it is exceedingly unlikely her fetus will be affected.

The nonimmune person who acquires rubella viremia demonstrates peak antibody titers 1– 2 weeks after the onset of the rash or 2–3 weeks after the onset of viremia, since viremia precedes clinically evident disease by about 1 week. The promptness of the antibody response, therefore, may complicate serodiagnosis unless serum is collected initially within a very few days after the onset of the rash.

With rubella—as with any fetal infection—the concept of an infected versus an affected infant must be understood. Rubella is a potent teratogen, and 80% of women with rubella infection and a rash during the first 12 weeks have a fetus with congenital infection. At 13–14 weeks, this incidence was 54%, and it was 25% at the end of the second trimester. As the duration of pregnancy increases, infections are less likely to cause congenital malformations. For example, rubella-induced defects were seen in all infants with evidence of intrauterine infections before 11 weeks but in only 35% of those infected at 13–16 weeks.

The syndrome of congenital rubella includes one or more of the following abnormalities:

(1) Eye lesions, including cataracts, glaucoma, microphthalmia, and various other abnormalities.
(2) Heart disease, including patent ductus arteriosus, septal defects, and pulmonary artery stenosis.
(3) Neural auditory defects.
(4) Central nervous system defects including meningoencephalitis.
(5) Retarded fetal growth.
(6) Thrombocytopenia and anemia.
(7) Hepatosplenomegaly and jaundice.
(8) Chronic diffuse interstitial pneumonitis.
(9) Osseous changes.
(10) Chromosomal abnormalities.

Infants born with congenital rubella may shed the virus for many months and thus be a threat to other infants as well as to susceptible adults who come in contact with them.

CYTOMEGALOVIRUS INFECTION

Cytomegalovirus is an ubiquitous organism that eventually infects the majority of humans, and evidence for fetal infection is found in 0.5–2% of all neonates. Following primary infection, which is usually asymptomatic, the virus becomes latent and there is periodic reactivation with viral shedding despite the presence of serum antibody.

The risk of seroconversion among susceptible women during pregnancy is 1–4%. Immunity from previous infection can be demonstrated in up to 85% of pregnant women from lower socioeconomic backgrounds, whereas the seropositivity rate for women in higher income groups is only about 50%. Women who are not immune at conception constitute the major reservoir of those who give birth to infants with clinically apparent infection. Thus, primary infection, which is transmitted to the fetus in approximately 40% of cases, is more often associated with severe morbidity. Unfortunately, there is no effective therapeutic agent that can be used to treat this organism.

Congenital cytomegalovirus infection, called **cytomegalic inclusion disease,** causes a syndrome that includes low birth weight, microcephaly, intracranial calcifications, chorioretinitis, mental and motor retardation, sensorineural deficits, hepatosplenomegaly, jaundice, hemolytic anemia, and thrombocytopenic purpura. Fortunately, of the estimated 33,000 infants born infected in the United States each year, only about 10% demonstrate this syndrome, which, as discussed above, is more prevalent in neonates born to women with primary infection during the first half of pregnancy. The mortality rate among these congenitally infected infants may be as high as 20–30%, and more than 90% of the survivors have mental retardation, hearing loss, impaired psychomotor development, seizures, or other central nervous system impairment.

SYPHILIS

In the past, syphilis accounted for nearly one-third of stillbirths—indeed, delivery of a macerated fetus was considered diagnostic of infection with *Treponema pallidum.* Today, syphilis has a persistent but lesser role as a cause of fetal deaths.

Half of the mothers of infants so affected have had inadequate prenatal care, with the result that infection was not diagnosed. Half of congenitally infected infants were born to women who received prenatal care but in whom serologic screening was not done, which meant that maternal syphilis was not treated. Predictably, the rise in congenital infection paralleled a similar increase in adult primary and secondary syphilis.

Syphilis is a chronic infection, and the spirochete causes lesions in the internal organs that include interstitial changes in the lungs (**pneumonia alba of Virchow**), liver (**hypertrophic cirrhosis**), spleen, and pancreas. It causes **osteochondritis** in the long bones, which is most readily recognizable radiographically at the lower ends of the femur, tibia, and radius. Under the influence of syphilitic infection, the placenta becomes large and pale.

Maternal treatment for syphilis is described in Chapter 60. There is concern that despite recommended treatment during pregnancy, almost 20% of newborns have obvious clinical stigmas of congenital syphilis.

CHLAMYDIAL INFECTIONS

Chlamydia trachomatis is an obligate intracellular bacterium considered to be the most prevalent cause of sexually transmitted disease in the United States. There are several serovars (serotypes), but those important in neonatal infection are the same as those that cause cervical infection near delivery. Maternal infections with chlamydiae are considered in Chapter 60. Depending upon epidemiologic variables, the prevalence of maternal cervical carriage ranges from 3% to 26%.

Seldom is the fetus infected despite the fact that neonatal disease is acquired by contact with the infected cervix at delivery. About 10% of infants born through an infected cervix develop chlamydial pneumonitis within 1–3 months. These infections are characteristic of chlamydiae by their long latency periods and indolence.

Ophthalmic chlamydial infections are one of the most common causes of preventable blindness in undeveloped countries. Inclusion conjunctivitis develops in as many as one-third of neonates born to mothers with cervical infection, and there is some preliminary evidence that erythromycin ointment applied topically for gonococcal ophthalmia may substantively decrease this attack rate.

Oral erythromycin is given for both conjunctivitis and pneumonitis. Treatment of maternal cervical infection at 36 weeks with erythromycin ethylsuccinate, 400 mg 4 times daily for 7 days, eradicated cervical chlamydiae in 92% of women. In infants of treated women, there was a substantially decreased incidence of neonatal chlamydial infections, compared with infants born to women with untreated infection (7% versus 50%).

TOXOPLASMOSIS

Toxoplasmosis is a protozoal infection caused by *Toxoplasma gondii.* Infection is transmitted through encysted organisms by eating infected raw or undercooked meat or through contact with infected cat feces, or it can be congenitally acquired by transfer across the placenta. Maternal immunity appears to protect against intrauterine transmission of the parasite; therefore, for congenital toxoplasmosis to develop, the mother must have acquired the infection during pregnancy. About a third of American women acquire protective antibody before pregnancy, and this is higher in those keeping cats as pets.

Fatigue, muscle pains, and lymphadenopathy may be identified in the infected mother, but most often the maternal infection is subclinical. Infection in pregnancy may cause abortion or may result in a liveborn infant with evidence of disease. The risk of infection increases with duration of pregnancy and is approximately 15%, 30%, and 60% in the first, second, and third trimesters.

Virulence of fetal infection is greatest when maternal infection is acquired early in pregnancy—fortunately, the time when transplacental infection is least common. Less than 10% of newborns with congenital toxoplasmosis have signs of clinical illness at birth. Affected infants usually have evidence of generalized disease, with low birth weight, hepatosplenomegaly, icterus, and anemia. Some infants have primarily neurologic disease, with convulsions, intracranial calcifications, and hydrocephaly or microcephaly. Both groups of infants eventually develop chorioretinitis.

INJURIES OF THE FETUS & NEWBORN

INTRACRANIAL HEMORRHAGE

Hemorrhage within the head of the fetus-infant may be located at any of several sites: subdural, subarachnoid, cortical, white matter, cerebellar, intraventricular, and periventricular. Intraventricular hemorrhage into the germinal matrix is the most common type.

Birth trauma may cause intracranial hemorrhage, but it is no longer a common cause. The head of the fetus may undergo appreciable molding during passage through the birth canal. The skull bones, the dura mater, and the brain itself permit considerable alteration in the shape of the fetal head without untoward results. The dimensions of the head are changed, with lengthening especially of the occipitofrontal diameter of the skull. Bridging veins from the cerebral cortex to the sagittal sinus may tear as a consequence of severe molding and marked overlap of the parietal bones or of difficult forceps delivery.

Infants with intracranial hemorrhage from mechanical injury are commonly born depressed but appear to improve until about 12 hours of age, whereupon drowsiness, apathy, feeble cry, pallor, failure to nurse, dyspnea, cyanosis, vomiting, and convulsions may become evident. Atelectasis, hypoxia, acidosis, meconium aspiration, and forceps trauma may be associated findings. In recent years, head scanning using sonography and computed tomography not only has proved of diagnostic value but has contributed also to our understanding of the cause of some forms of intracranial hemorrhage and the frequency with which they occur. For example, periventricular and intraventricular hemorrhages occur often in infants born quite preterm, and these hemorrhages usually develop without birth trauma.

CEPHALOHEMATOMA

Cephalohematoma is usually caused by injury to the periosteum of the skull during labor and delivery, though it may develop in the absence of birth trauma when hemostasis is defective. The reported incidence is about 2.5%.

Subperiosteal hemorrhages may develop over one or both parietal bones. The periosteal limitations with definite palpable edges differentiate cephalohematoma from **caput succedaneum.** The latter lesion consists of a focal swelling of the scalp from edema fluid that overlies the periosteum. Furthermore, a cephalohematoma may not appear for hours after delivery, often growing larger and disappearing only after weeks or even months. In contrast, caput succedaneum is maximal at birth, grows smaller, and disappears usually within a few hours if small and within a few days even when very large.

BRACHIAL PLEXUS INJURY

Brachial plexus injuries are common and encountered in nearly 1:500 term births. The injury usually follows a difficult delivery, but in rare cases after an apparently easy one the infant is born with a partially or fully paralyzed arm. **Duchenne,** or **Erb, paralysis** involves paralysis of the deltoid and infraspinatus muscles, as well as the flexor muscles of the forearm, causing the entire arm to fall limply close to the side of the body with the forearm extended and internally rotated. The function of the fingers is usually retained.

The lesion results from stretching or tearing of the upper roots of the brachial plexus, which is readily subjected to extreme tension as a result of pulling laterally upon the head, thus sharply flexing it toward one of the shoulders. Since traction in this direction is employed frequently to effect delivery of the shoulders in normal vertex presentations, Erb paralysis may result without what seems to be a difficult delivery. In extracting the shoulders, therefore, care should be taken not to cause excessive lateral flexion of the neck. Most often, in the case of cephalic presentations, the afflicted fetus is unusually large, typically weighing 4000 g or more. Other risk factors are prolonged labor, forceps delivery, and shoulder dystocia.

SUGGESTED READINGS

American College of Obstetricians and Gynecologists: Committee Statement—Use and misuse of the Apgar score. November 1986.

American College of Obstetricians and Gynecologists: Management of isoimmunization in pregnancy. Tech Bull No. 90, January 1986.

Diseases, infections, and injuries of the fetus and newborn infant. Chapter 44 in: *Williams Obstetrics,* 19th ed. Cunningham FG, MacDonald PC, Gant NF, Leveno KJ, Gilstrap LC (editors). Appleton & Lange, 1993.

Freeman J (editor): Prenatal and perinatal factors associated with brain disorders. US Department of Health and Human Services, Public Health Service, National Institutes of Health, NIH Publication No. 85-1149, 1985.

Nelson KB, Ellenberg JH: Obstetric complications as risk factors for cerebral palsy or seizure disorders. JAMA 1984;251:1843.

56
Multifetal Pregnancy

Morbidity and mortality rates are increased appreciably in pregnancies with multiple fetuses. It is not an overstatement, therefore, to consider a pregnancy with multiple fetuses to be a complicated one. Many of the complications that occur more commonly with multiple fetuses are listed in Table 56–1.

ETIOLOGY OF MULTIPLE FETUSES

Twin fetuses more commonly result from fertilization of two separate ova (double-ovum, dizygotic, or "fraternal" twins). About one-third as often, twins arise from a single fertilized ovum that subsequently divides into two similar structures, each with the potential for developing into a separate individual (single-ovum, monozygotic, or "identical" twins). Either or both processes may be involved in the formation of higher numbers of fetuses. Quadruplets, for example, may arise from one, two, three, or four ova.

FRATERNAL VERSUS IDENTICAL TWINS

Dizygotic (fraternal) twins are not in a strict sense true twins, since they result from the maturation and fertilization of two ova during a single ovulatory cycle. Furthermore, **monozygotic (identical) twins** are not always identical. As is pointed out below, the process of division of one fertilized zygote into two does not necessarily result in equal sharing of protoplasmic materials. In fact, dizygotic twins of the same sex may appear more nearly identical at birth than do monozygotic twins; growth of monozygotic twin fetuses may be discordant, at times dramatically so.

The frequency of monozygotic twinning is relatively constant worldwide at approximately one set per 250 births and is largely independent of race, heredity, age, and parity. The incidence of delivery of dizygotic twins is influenced greatly by race, heredity, maternal age, parity, and, especially, the use of fertility-enhancing drugs.

It is now apparent through the use of ultrasound early in pregnancy that the incidence of twin conceptions is much higher than indicated by figures based on the delivery of two fetuses. Undoubtedly, some "threatened" abortions have resulted in actual abortion of one embryo from an unrecognized twin gestation while the other embryo continued its growth and development.

CONJOINED TWINS

In the United States, united or conjoined twins are commonly referred to as Siamese twins, after Chang and Eng Bunker of Siam (Thailand), who were displayed worldwide by P.T. Barnum. If twinning is initiated after the embryonic disk and the rudimentary amnionic sac have been formed—and if division of the embryonic disk is incomplete—conjoined twins result. When each of the joined twins is nearly complete, the commonly shared body site may be anterior **(thoracopagus),** posterior **(pyopagus),** cephalic **(craniopagus),** or caudal **(ischiopagus).**

VASCULAR COMMUNICATIONS BETWEEN FETUSES

Frequently demonstrable in monochorionic placentas are vascular anastomoses, either artery-to-artery, artery-to-vein, or vein-to-vein. The most troublesome interfetal vascular connection is artery-to-vein. Anastomoses are rarely demonstrable in dichorionic placentas. As a result of such anastomoses, blood is pumped from artery to vein, out of one fetus into the other. The effects of arteriovenous anastomoses can be profound. One monozygous twin may be much smaller than the other as a result of chronic intrauterine malnutrition; and in monozygotic twins with anastomosed circulations, the hemoglobin concentration may be 8 g per dL or less in the hypoperfused twin and as much as 27 g per dL in the other. Hypotension, microcardia, and generalized runting characterize the overtly affected hypovolemic "identical" donor twin, in contrast to hypertension and cardiac hypertrophy in the hypertransfused twin. Hydramnios—perhaps the consequence of increased renal perfusion and, in turn, increased urine formation—may accompany the hypervolemia and polycythemia in the typically larger recipient twin. At the same time, amnionic fluid may be scant to absent in the other sac, perhaps as a result of marked oliguria in the underperfused donor twin.

Table 56–1. Pregnancy complications associated with multiple fetuses.

1. Abortion
2. Perinatal death
3. Low birthweight
   Preterm delivery
   Fetal growth retardation
4. Malformations
5. Fetal-fetal hemorrhage
   Hypovolemia and anemia
   Hypervolemia and hyperviscosity
   Central nervous system abnormalities
6. Pregnancy-induced or -aggravated hypertension
7. Maternal anemia
   Acute blood loss
   Iron deficiency
   Folate deficiency
8. Placental accidents
   Placental abruption
   Placenta previa
9. Uterine atony
10. Cord accidents
    Prolapse
    Entwinement
    Vasa previa
11. Hydramnios
12. Complicated labor
    Preterm labor
    Ineffective labor
13. Abnormal fetal presentation

DIAGNOSIS OF MULTIPLE FETUSES

It is unfortunate that the diagnosis of twins often is not made until late in pregnancy, perhaps as late as the time of parturition. A family history of twins by itself provides only a weak clue, but recent administration of either clomiphene or pituitary gonadotropin raises a strong likelihood that twinning may occur.

Physical examination with accurate measurement of fundal height, as described in Chapter 42, is essential. During the second trimester, a discrepancy develops between gestational age determined from menstrual data and that from uterine size. The uterus that contains two or more fetuses clearly becomes larger than one with a single fetus!

A variety of techniques are utilized to identify a multifetal pregnancy. Before the third trimester, it is difficult to diagnose twins by palpation of fetal parts. Even late in pregnancy, it may not always be possible to identify twins by transabdominal palpation, especially if one twin overlies the other, if the woman is obese, or if hydramnios is present. Late in the first trimester, fetal heart action may be detected with Doppler ultrasonic equipment. Sometime thereafter, it becomes possible to identify the separate contractions of two fetal hearts if their rates are clearly distinct from each other as well as from that of the mother. It is possible by careful examination to identify fetal heart sounds with the usual aural fetal stethoscopes at 18–20 weeks of gestation.

By careful ultrasonic examination, separate gestational sacs can be identified very early in twin pregnancy. Sub-

sequently, the identification of each fetal head should be made in two perpendicular planes so as not to mistake a cross section of the fetal trunk for a second fetal head. A cross section of the fetal head remains nearly round in both planes, whereas the trunk does not. Carefully performed sonographic scanning should detect practically all sets of twins.

PREGNANCY OUTCOMES

ABORTION

Abortion is more likely to occur with multiple fetuses than with a single fetus. The demonstration sonographically of two gestational sacs with the subsequent disappearance of one or even both sacs is evidence of silent early abortion or resorption of one embryo. Both spontaneous abortion and surgically induced abortion have on occasion served to remove one embryo or fetus, with the pregnancy nevertheless continuing until the birth of another fetus who survives.

It sometimes happens that one fetus succumbs remote from term but the pregnancy continues with one living fetus. At delivery, the dead fetus with placenta and membranes may be readily identified but may be appreciably compressed (**fetus compressus**) or may be remarkably flattened through loss of fluid and most of the soft tissue except skin (**fetus papyraceus**). The dead fetus may undergo complete resorption even though the conceptus had advanced well beyond the status of an embryo before succumbing.

PERINATAL MORTALITY

The perinatal mortality rate for pregnancies complicated by twin fetuses has been remarkably higher than for single fetuses. Perinatal loss with twins at many centers in the United States commonly has in the recent past ranged from 10% to 15%.

The perinatal death rate for monozygotic twins is 2.5 times that for dizygotic twins. There is an extremely high fetal death rate with the relatively rare variety of monozygous twinning in which both fetuses occupy the same amnionic sac—ie, **monoamnionic twins.** A common cause of death is intertwining of their umbilical cords, which has been estimated to complicate 50% or more of cases.

DURATION OF GESTATION

As the number of fetuses increases, the duration of gestation and birthweight decrease. Up to one-half of twin infants are born weighing less than 2500 g. Retarded fetal growth, as well as preterm delivery, is important in the genesis of low birth weight in multifetal gestations. After the second trimester, growth of the multiple fetuses, as determined either by sonographic measurements or by birthweight, is likely to be impaired compared with that of the singleton fetus. In general, the larger the number of fetuses, the greater the degree of growth retardation. Marked discordance in size may also complicate pregnancies in which each fetus arose from a separate ovum (Figure 56–1). In one such example, dizygotic twins weighed 2300 g and 785 g at birth. Both survived, but one remains appreciably smaller than the other.

MALFORMATIONS

The frequency of malformations is nearly twice as great in each twin as in singletons. Malformations are more common among monozygotic than dizygotic twins. Persistent or chronic hydramnios is more likely to be associated with fetal anomalies of one or both twins. Monochorionic twinning is associated especially with central nervous system abnormalities that appear to arise as a result of placental vascular anastomoses that cause impaired cerebral blood flow.

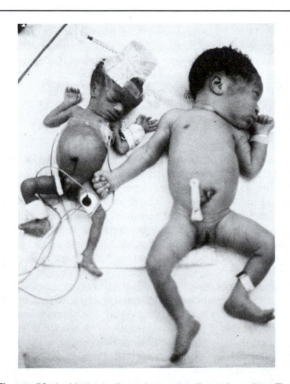

Figure 56–1. Marked discordance in dizygotic twins. The larger infant weighed 2300 g, appropriate for gestational age. The markedly growth-retarded smaller infant weighed only 785 g. Both thrived.

MANAGEMENT OF PREGNANCIES WITH MULTIPLE FETUSES

Perinatal mortality and morbidity rates are significantly reduced in pregnancies complicated by twins when the following objectives are achieved: (1) when delivery of markedly preterm infants is prevented; (2) when failure of one or both fetuses to thrive is identified so that fetuses so afflicted can be delivered before they become moribund; (3) when fetal trauma during labor and delivery is minimized; and (4) when expert neonatal care is provided continuously from the time of birth. The first major step in fulfilling these goals is early identification of the pregnancy complicated by multiple fetuses. As soon as multiple fetuses (or embryos) are identified, meaningful efforts should be directed toward providing the fetuses with the best intrauterine environment possible.

MATERNAL HYPERTENSION

Pregnancy-induced or pregnancy-aggravated hypertension is much more likely to develop when there are multiple fetuses (Chapter 57). Hypertension not only develops more often but tends to develop earlier and to be more severe. In singleton pregnancies, pregnancy-induced hypertension occurs less commonly in parous than in nulliparous women. This is not true, however, in multifetal pregnancies.

ANTEPARTUM SURVEILLANCE OF FETAL GROWTH

Fetal growth is slower in multifetal pregnancies. An important aspect of ultrasonic assessment of fetal growth is to identify **discordance** between twin pairs. This most often is defined by using the larger twin as the index. When a 15% difference in birth weight is used as a criterion, 25% of twins are discordant. The perinatal mortality rate with discordance of this magnitude was 97:1000 compared to 37:1000 for nondiscordant twin pairs.

PREVENTION OF PRETERM DELIVERY

Techniques to prolong gestation in multifetal pregnancy include protracted bed rest, especially through hospitalization; prophylactic administration of beta-mimetic drugs; prophylactic cervical cerclage; and repeated injections of progestins. Several authors have claimed bed rest to be beneficial to twin fetuses presumably by enhancing uterine perfusion and perhaps by reducing the physical forces that might act deleteriously on the cervix to hasten effacement and dilation. However, the benefits from bed rest are difficult to evaluate.

DELIVERY OF MULTIPLE FETUSES

LABOR

Many complications of labor and delivery—including preterm labor, uterine dysfunction, abnormal presentations, prolapse of the umbilical cord, premature separation of the placenta, and immediate postpartum hemorrhage—are encountered much more often with multiple fetuses. Therefore, the conduct of labor and delivery in such cases calls upon the highest skills of the obstetric team.

It is not always feasible to safely arrest established preterm labor. Pulmonary edema associated with the use of beta-mimetic agents—eg, ritodrine—has been observed much more frequently in twin gestations. Bed rest should be instituted if not already in force.

As soon as it is apparent that labor has been established, an obstetric attendant should be assigned to remain with the mother throughout labor. The fetal heart rates should be monitored frequently. Continuous external electronic monitoring or—if the membranes are ruptured and the cervix dilated—evaluation of both fetuses by simultaneous internal and external electronic monitoring may prove satisfactory.

Two obstetricians must be immediately available for the delivery. At least one should be skilled in intrauterine identification of fetal parts and intrauterine manipulation of the fetus. An anesthesiologist should be immediately available in case intrauterine manipulation or cesarean section is necessary. For each fetus, two people, one of whom is skilled in resuscitation and care of newborn infants, should be appropriately informed about the case and remain immediately available.

Presentation & Position

With twins, all possible combinations of fetal positions may be encountered. Either or both fetuses may present by the vertex, breech, or shoulder. Compound, face, brow, and footling breech presentation are relatively common, especially when the fetuses are quite small or there is excess amnionic fluid or when maternal parity is high. Prolapse of the cord is fairly common in these circumstances.

Analgesia & Anesthesia

During labor and delivery of multiple fetuses, deciding what to use for analgesia and for anesthesia is difficult because of problems imposed by (1) prematurity, (2) maternal hypertension, (3) desultory labor, (4) need for intrauterine manipulation, and (5) uterine atony and hemorrhage after delivery.

When intrauterine manipulation is necessary, as with

internal podalic version, uterine relaxation is probably best accomplished with halothane or one of the other halogenated hydrocarbons. Although halothane provides effective relaxation for intrauterine manipulation, it also commonly leads to an increase in blood loss during the third stage of labor until the uterus regains its ability to contract.

VAGINAL DELIVERY

Cephalic presentation of the first twin will occur in about three-fourths of multifetal gestations. Seldom with cephalic presentations are there unusual problems with delivery of the first infant. After appropriate episiotomy, spontaneous delivery—or delivery assisted by outlet forceps—usually proves to be satisfactory.

When the first fetus presents as a breech, major problems are most likely to develop if (1) the fetus is unusually large and the aftercoming head taxes the capacity of the birth canal; (2) the fetus is quite small, so that the extremities and trunk are delivered through a cervix inadequately effaced and dilated for the head to escape easily; or (3) the umbilical cord prolapses. When these problems are anticipated or identified, cesarean section will often be the better way to effect delivery, except when the fetuses are so immature that they will not survive. Otherwise, breech delivery may be accomplished as described in Chapter 46.

The safety of vaginal delivery for the second nonvertex twin has been reported by several investigators. They all stress that vaginal delivery for the second twin presenting as breech and weighing less than 1500 g has not been studied adequately to warrant its routine application. Unfortunately, cesarean section does not guarantee an atraumatic delivery.

DELIVERY OF SECOND TWIN

Delivery of the second twin demands experience that includes in some cases manual dexterity inside the uterus. As soon as the first twin has been delivered, the presenting part of the second twin, its size, and its orientation in the birth canal are quickly determined by careful combined abdominal, vaginal, and at times intrauterine examination. Intrapartum real-time sonography has proved quite valuable in some cases. If the vertex or the breech is fixed in the birth canal, moderate fundal pressure is applied and the membranes are ruptured. Immediately afterward, the examination is repeated to identify prolapse of the cord or other abnormality. Labor is allowed to resume while the fetal heart rate is monitored closely. With reestablishment of labor, there is no need to hasten delivery unless there is ominous deceleration of the fetal heart rate, or persistent bradycardia, or bleeding from the uterus. The latter indicates placental separation, which can be deleterious to both the fetus and the mother. If contractions do not resume within 10 minutes or so, dilute oxytocin may be used to stimulate appropriate myometrial activity, which will

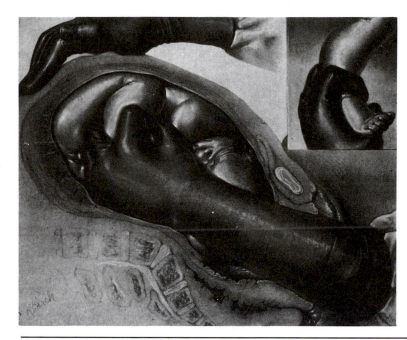

Figure 56–2. Internal podalic version. Note the use of the long version gloves, which are not currently available.

lead to spontaneous delivery or delivery assisted by outlet forceps.

If the occiput or breech presents immediately over the pelvic inlet but is not fixed in the birth canal, the presenting part can often be guided into the pelvis with the vaginal hand while a hand on the uterine fundus exerts moderate pressure. More recently, intrapartum external version of the nonvertex second twin has become popular.

If the occiput or the breech is not over the pelvic inlet and cannot be so positioned by gentle pressure on the presenting part—or if appreciable uterine bleeding develops—the problem of delivery of the second twin assumes serious dimensions. To take maximum advantage of the very recently dilated cervix before the uterus contracts and the cervix retracts, procrastination must be avoided. An obstetrician skilled in intrauterine manipulation of the fetus and an anesthesiologist skilled in providing anesthesia that will effectively relax the uterus are essential for vaginal delivery with a favorable outcome. Prompt delivery of the second fetus by cesarean section is the better choice if no one present is skilled in the performance of internal podalic version (Figure 56–2) or if anesthesia that will provide effective uterine relaxation is not immediately available.

CESAREAN SECTION

There has been a trend recently for delivery of multiple fetuses by cesarean section. The most common indication may be presentation other than cephalic by one or both fetuses. Other major indications are hypotonic uterine dysfunction, hypertension induced or aggravated by the pregnancy, fetal distress, gross discordance in the size of the fetuses—with the smaller fetus the first candidate for vaginal delivery—and prolapsed cord.

SUGGESTED READINGS

Blickstein I et al: Vaginal delivery of the second twin in breech presentation. Obstet Gynecol 1987;68:774.

Gilstrap LC III et al: Twins: Prophylactic hospitalization and ward rest at early gestational age. Obstet Gynecol 1987; 69:578.

Leveno KJ et al: Sonar cephalometry in twins: A table of bipari-etal diameters for normal twin fetuses and a comparison with singletons. Am J Obstet Gynecol 1979;135:727.

Rabinovici J et al: Randomized management of the second non-vertex twin: Vaginal delivery or cesarean section. Am J Obstet Gynecol 1987;156:52.

57

Hypertensive Disorders in Pregnancy

Pregnancy may induce hypertension in previously normotensive women or may aggravate the disorder in women who have underlying hypertensive disease. The cause in either case is unknown. Generalized edema, proteinuria, or both often accompany hypertension induced or aggravated by pregnancy. Convulsions may develop in association with hypertension, especially if ignored. Hypertensive disorders complicating pregnancy are common and form one element of the triad—along with hemorrhage and infection—that continues to be responsible for a large number of maternal deaths in the United States. Most adverse pregnancy outcomes related to hypertension can be prevented with good prenatal supervision and treatment when necessary.

PREGNANCY-INDUCED HYPERTENSION

As shown in Table 57–1, pregnancy-induced hypertension is divided into three categories: (1) hypertension alone, (2) preeclampsia, and (3) eclampsia. The diagnosis of **preeclampsia** is based on the development of hypertension plus proteinuria or of edema that is generalized and overt, or both. **Eclampsia** is characterized typically by those same abnormalities with the addition of convulsions that are precipitated by the pregnancy-induced hypertension. Only rarely does preeclampsia develop earlier than 20 weeks of gestation, and then usually in cases of hydatidiform mole or appreciable molar degeneration (Chapter 32). Preeclampsia without underlying chronic hypertension is almost exclusively a disease of nulliparous women. Although it more commonly affects females at the extremes of reproductive age—ie, teenagers or those older than 35 years—preeclampsia in the latter (older) group usually reflects pregnancy-aggravated hypertension. Pregnancy-induced hypertension is occasionally seen in the multipara with multifetal pregnancy or fetal hydrops. Pregnancy-aggravated hypertension is common in multiparas with vascular disease, including chronic essential hypertension and diabetes mellitus, or those with coexisting renal disease.

The diagnosis of pregnancy-induced hypertension is usually straightforward and made when the blood pressure is 140/90 mm Hg or higher. Although it has been accepted in the past that an increase over baseline values of 30 mm Hg systolic or 15 mm Hg diastolic on at least two occasions 6 or more hours apart be considered as possibly diagnostic for pregnancy-induced hypertension, these vague criteria have little clinical value.

Although the diagnosis of preeclampsia has traditionally required the identification of pregnancy-induced hypertension plus proteinuria or generalized edema, many authorities agree that edema, even of the hands and face, is such a common finding in pregnant women that its presence should not confirm the diagnosis of preeclampsia any more than its absence should rule out the diagnosis.

Proteinuria is an important sign of preeclampsia. Proteinuria is defined as 300 mg or more of urinary protein during a 24-hour period or 30–100 mg per dL (1–2+) or more in at least two random urine specimens collected 6 hours or more apart. The degree of proteinuria may fluctuate widely over any 24-hour period even in severe cases. Therefore, a single random sample may fail to detect significant proteinuria.

When the blood pressure rises appreciably during the latter half of pregnancy, it is dangerous—to the fetus especially—not to take action simply because proteinuria has not yet developed. Ten percent of eclamptic seizures develop before overt proteinuria. Thus, from pathophysiologic and epidemiologic perspectives, it is clear that hypertension is the sine qua non of preeclampsia and that from the moment blood pressure begins to rise, both mother and fetus are at increased risk. Once the blood pressure exceeds 140/90 mm Hg, the diagnosis of pregnancy-induced hypertension is established and treatment should be given accordingly. Proteinuria is a sign of worsening hypertensive disease—specifically preeclampsia—and when it is overt and persistent, the maternal and fetal risks are increased even more.

The severity of pregnancy-induced hypertension is as-

Table 57–1. Classification of hypertensive disorders complicating pregnancy.

Pregnancy-induced hypertension
Hypertension that develops as a consequence of pregnancy and regresses postpartum
1. Hypertension without proteinuria or pathologic edema
2. Preeclampsia—with proteinuria or pathologic edema (or both)
    a. Mild
    b. Severe
3. Eclampsia—proteinuria or pathologic edema (or both) along with convulsions

Pregnancy-aggravated hypertension
Underlying hypertension worsened by pregnancy
1. Superimposed preeclampsia
2. Superimposed eclampsia

Coincidental hypertension
Chronic underlying hypertension that precedes pregnancy or persists postpartum

---

sessed by the frequency and intensity of the abnormalities listed in Table 57–2. Many women have clinical syndromes falling between those two "mild or severe" extremes. Furthermore, apparently mild disease may rapidly become severe.

Blood pressure alone is not always a dependable indicator of severity. For example, an adolescent patient may have 3+ proteinuria and convulsions while her blood pressure is 140/85 mm Hg, whereas most women with blood pressures as high as 180/120 mm Hg do not have seizures. Convulsions usually are preceded by an unrelenting severe headache or visual disturbances; thus, these symptoms are considered ominous.

Proteinuria is an important indicator of severity, since it usually develops late in the course of the disease. Certainly, persistent proteinuria of 2+ or more—or 24-hour urinary excretion of 4 g or more—is indicative of severe preeclampsia. With severe renal involvement, glomerular filtration may be impaired and the plasma creatinine concentration may become abnormally high, or it may begin to rise. Epigastric or right upper quadrant pain is presumed to result from hepatocellular necrosis and edema that stretches Glisson's capsule. Thrombocytopenia is

Table 57–2. Indicators of severity of pregnancy-induced hypertension.

Abnormality	Mild	Severe
Diastolic blood pressure	< 100 mm Hg	110 mm Hg or higher
Proteinuria	Trace to 1 +	Persistent 2+ or more
Headache	Absent	Present
Visual disturbances	Absent	Present
Upper abdominal pain	Absent	Present
Oliguria	Absent	Present
Convulsions	Absent	Present
Serum creatinine	Normal	Elevated
Thrombocytopenia	Absent	Present
Hyperbilirubinemia	Absent	Present
Liver enzyme elevation	Minimal	Marked
Fetal growth retardation	Absent	Obvious
Pulmonary edema	Absent	Present

characteristic of worsening preeclampsia and is probably caused by microangiopathic hemolysis engendered by severe vasospasm. The more profound the frequency and intensity of these aberrations, the more severe the disease and the greater the need for pregnancy termination.

In neglected or, less often, fulminant cases of pregnancy-induced hypertension, eclampsia may develop. The seizures are grand mal and may appear for the first time before labor, during labor, or postpartum. Any seizure that develops more than 48 hours postpartum is more likely to be due to some other lesion of the central nervous system.

Pathophysiology

Vasospasm is basic to the pathophysiology of preeclampsia-eclampsia. Vascular constriction causes a resistance to blood flow and accounts for the development of arterial hypertension. The vascular changes, together with local hypoxia of the surrounding tissues, presumably lead to hemorrhage, necrosis, and other end-organ disturbances that have been observed at times with severe preeclampsia.

Hemoconcentration is common in women with severe preeclampsia and eclampsia. The woman of average size can be expected to have a blood volume of nearly 5000 mL during the last several weeks of a normal pregnancy, compared to about 3500 mL when nonpregnant. With eclampsia, however, much or all of the added 1500 mL of blood normally present late in pregnancy can be anticipated to be missing. The woman with eclampsia, therefore, is unduly sensitive to vigorous fluid therapy given in an attempt to expand the contracted blood volume to normal pregnancy levels. She is sensitive as well to even normal blood loss at delivery.

PREECLAMPSIA

The two principal features of preeclampsia—hypertension and proteinuria—are abnormalities of which the pregnant woman is usually unaware. By the time symptoms such as headache, visual disturbances, or epigastric pain develop, the disorder is most always severe. Hence, the importance of prenatal care in the early detection and management of preeclampsia becomes obvious.

Clinical Findings

A. Symptoms and Signs:

1. Hypertension–The basic derangement in preeclampsia is arteriolar vasospasm, and it is not surprising, therefore, that the most dependable warning sign is an increase in blood pressure. The diastolic pressure is probably a more reliable prognostic sign than the systolic pressure, and any diastolic pressure of 90 mm Hg or more that persists is abnormal. The fifth Korotkoff sound is used as the measuring level.

2. Weight gain–A sudden increase in weight may precede the development of preeclampsia—indeed, excessive weight gain in some women is the first sign. Weight increase of about 1 pound per week is normal, but when weight gain exceeds much more than 2 pounds in any given week or 6 pounds in a month, developing preeclampsia must be suspected. Characteristic of preeclampsia is the suddenness of the excessive weight gain rather than an increase distributed throughout gestation. Sudden and excessive weight gain is attributable almost entirely to abnormal fluid retention and is demonstrable, as a rule, before visible signs of nondependent edema, such as swollen eyelids and puffiness of the fingers. In cases of fulminating preeclampsia or eclampsia, fluid retention may be extreme, and in such women a weight gain of 10 pounds or more within a week is not unusual.

3. Headache–Headache is unusual in milder cases but frequent in more severe disease. It is often frontal but may be occipital, and it is resistant to relief from ordinary analgesics. In women who develop eclampsia, severe headache almost invariably precedes the first convulsion.

4. Abdominal pain–Epigastric or right upper quadrant pain often is a symptom of severe preeclampsia and may be indicative of imminent convulsions. It may be the result of stretching of the hepatic capsule, possibly by edema and hemorrhage.

5. Visual disturbances–A spectrum of visual disturbances, ranging from slight blurring of vision to scotomas to partial or complete blindness, may accompany preeclampsia. These develop as a result of vasospasm, ischemia, and petechial hemorrhages within the occipital cortex. In some women, visual symptoms may arise from retinal arteriolar spasm, ischemia, and edema, and in rare cases, retinal detachment.

B. Laboratory Findings: The degree of proteinuria varies greatly in preeclampsia, not only from case to case but also in the same woman from hour to hour. The variability points to a functional (vasospasm) rather than an organic cause. In early preeclampsia, proteinuria may be minimal or absent. In the most severe forms, proteinuria is usually demonstrable and may be as much as 10 g per 24 h. Proteinuria almost always develops later than hypertension and usually later than excessive weight gain.

Treatment: Mild to Moderate Preeclampsia

The basic management objectives for *any pregnancy* complicated by pregnancy-induced hypertension are (1) termination of the pregnancy with the least possible trauma to the mother and the fetus; (2) birth of an infant who subsequently thrives; and (3) complete restoration of the health of the mother. In certain cases of preeclampsia, especially in women at or near term, these three objectives may be served equally well by careful induction of labor. Therefore, the most important piece of information for the successful management of any pregnancy—but especially pregnancy complicated by hypertension—is the age of the fetus.

A. Bed Rest: Ambulatory treatment has no place in the management of pregnancy-induced or pregnancy-aggravated hypertension; bed rest throughout the greater part of the day is essential. Moreover, these women should be examined at least twice weekly and should be instructed in detail about reporting symptoms. With minor

elevations of blood pressure, the response to this regimen is often immediate, but the patient must be cooperative and the obstetrician wary.

B. Hospitalization: The indication for hospitalization of women with pregnancy-induced hypertension is a sustained elevation in systolic blood pressure of 140 mm Hg or above or a diastolic pressure of 90 mm Hg or above. For continuing appraisal of the severity of the disease, upon admittance to the hospital, a systematic study should be instituted that includes the following:

1. An appropriate history and general physical examination followed by daily search for the development of signs and symptoms such as headache, visual disturbances, epigastric pain, and rapid weight gain.

2. Weight measurement on admittance and every 2 days thereafter.

3. Urine test for protein on admittance and subsequently at least every 2 days.

4. Blood pressure readings with an appropriate-sized cuff every 4 hours except between midnight and morning (unless the midnight pressure has increased).

5. Measurements of plasma creatinine, hematocrit, platelets, and serum liver enzymes, the frequency to be determined by the severity of hypertension.

6. Frequent evaluation of fetal size and amnionic fluid volume by the same experienced examiner and by serial sonography if remote from term.

C. Obstetric Management: The further management of a pregnancy complicated by preeclampsia will depend upon (1) its severity, determined by the presence or absence of the conditions cited in Table 57–2, (2) the duration of gestation, and (3) the condition of the cervix. Fortunately, many cases prove to be sufficiently mild and near enough to term that they can be managed conservatively until labor commences spontaneously or until the cervix becomes favorable for labor induction. Complete abatement of all signs and symptoms, however, is uncommon until after delivery. *Almost certainly, the underlying disease persists until after delivery!*

Treatment: Severe Preeclampsia

Occasionally, fulminant or neglected preeclampsia is encountered, with blood pressure recordings in excess of 160/110 mm Hg, edema, and proteinuria. Headache, visual disturbances, or epigastric pain are indicative that convulsions are imminent, and oliguria is another ominous sign.

Severe preeclampsia demands anticonvulsant and usually antihypertensive therapy followed by delivery. Treatment is identical to that described below for eclampsia. The prime objectives are to forestall convulsions, to prevent intracranial hemorrhage and serious damage to other vital organs, and to deliver a healthy infant.

ECLAMPSIA

Eclampsia is characterized by generalized tonic-clonic convulsions that develop in some women with hypertension induced or aggravated by pregnancy. Depending on whether convulsions first appear before labor, during labor, or in the puerperium, eclampsia is designated as antepartum, intrapartum, or postpartum.

Eclampsia is most common in the last trimester and becomes increasingly more frequent as term approaches. Nearly all cases of postpartum eclampsia develop within 24 hours after delivery. Certainly, in women in whom the convulsions first appear more than 48 hours postpartum, another diagnosis should be considered.

Clinical Findings

Almost without exception, preeclampsia precedes the onset of eclamptic convulsions. Headache, visual disturbances, and epigastric or right upper quadrant pain are symptoms that should incite grave concern.

The first convulsion is usually the forerunner of other convulsions, which may vary in number from one or two in mild cases to 10, 20, or even 100 or more in untreated severe cases. In rare instances, they follow one another so rapidly that the woman appears to be in a prolonged, almost continuous convulsion.

The duration of coma after a convulsion is variable. When the convulsions are infrequent, the patient usually recovers some degree of consciousness after each attack. As she arouses, a semiconscious combative state may ensue.

In antepartum eclampsia, labor may begin spontaneously shortly after the onset of convulsions. If the attack occurs during labor, the contractions may increase in frequency and intensity and the duration of labor may be shortened. Because of maternal hypoxemia and lactic acidosis caused by convulsions, it is not unusual for fetal bradycardia to follow a seizure. The heart rate usually recovers within 3–5 minutes; if bradycardia persists more than 10 minutes, another cause must be considered (eg, rapid labor or placental abruption).

In some women with eclampsia, sudden death occurs synchronously with a convulsion or follows shortly thereafter as a result of a massive cerebral hemorrhage (Figure 57–1). Hemiplegia may result from sublethal hemorrhage. Cerebral hemorrhages are more apt to occur in older women with underlying chronic hypertension; less commonly, they may be due to a ruptured berry aneurysm or arteriovenous malformation. Rarely, coma or substantively altered consciousness follows a seizure or may even accompany preeclampsia without convulsions.

Differential Diagnosis

Eclampsia is more apt to be diagnosed too frequently rather than overlooked, because epilepsy, encephalitis, meningitis, cerebral tumor, ruptured cerebral aneurysm, and even hysteria during late pregnancy and the puerperium may simulate it. Consequently, such conditions

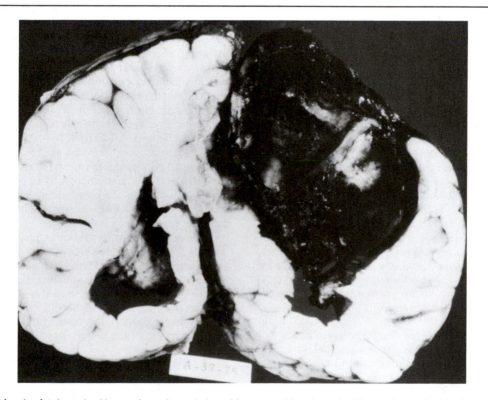

Figure 57–1. Massive fetal cerebral hemorrhage in a primigravid woman with eclampsia. Magnesium sulfate had been given appropriately, but diastolic blood pressures of 120 mm Hg were not treated. (Courtesy of K Leveno.)

should be borne in mind whenever convulsions or coma develop during pregnancy, labor, or the puerperium and should be excluded before a tentative diagnosis of eclampsia is confirmed. Until other causes are excluded, all pregnant women with convulsions should be considered to have eclampsia.

Treatment

The treatment of eclampsia should be in accordance with a hospital protocol whose features should include the following: (1) control of convulsions with magnesium sulfate, using an intravenously administered loading dose and periodic intramuscular or intravenous injections standardized in the amount injected and the frequency of injections; (2) control of severe hypertension with intermittent intravenous injections of hydralazine to lower the blood pressure whenever the diastolic pressure is 110 mm Hg or higher; (3) avoidance of diuretics and hyperosmotic agents; (4) limitation of intravenous fluid administration unless fluid loss is excessive; and (5) initiation of steps to effect delivery.

A. Magnesium Sulfate: Magnesium sulfate is used to arrest and prevent the convulsions of eclampsia without producing generalized central nervous system depression in either the mother or the fetus-infant. Magnesium sulfate may be given intramuscularly or by continuous intravenous infusion. Magnesium sulfate is not given to treat hypertension. The drug probably exerts a specific anticonvulsant action on the cerebral cortex. Typically, the mother stops convulsing after the initial administration of magnesium sulfate, and within an hour or so regains consciousness sufficiently to be oriented as to place and time.

B. Hydralazine: At the time that this treatment regime for eclampsia was formulated, it was appreciated that severe acute hypertension increased the maternal risk of intracranial hemorrhage (Figure 57–1). From the outset the regimen provided for intravenous injections of hydralazine whenever the diastolic blood pressure was 110 mm Hg or higher, to be administered in 5- to 10-mg doses at 15- to 20-minute intervals until a satisfactory response was achieved. A satisfactory response antepartum or intrapartum was defined as a decrease in diastolic blood pressure to 90 to 100 mm Hg, but not much lower lest placental perfusion be compromised. Hydralazine so administered has proved effective, and cerebral hemorrhage has been avoided.

A variety of other agents—nitroglycerin, prazosin, nifedipine, beta-blockers, and others—have been used for acute hypertension control. Their use in place of hydralazine will depend upon local experience and further studies as they appear in the literature.

C. Fluid Therapy: Fluid—primarily lactated Ringer's containing 5% dextrose—should be given at a rate of 60–125 mL per h intravenously (not faster) unless there is unusual fluid loss from vomiting, diarrhea, diaphoresis, or, more likely, excessive blood loss at delivery. Oliguria is common in severe preeclampsia and eclampsia, making it tempting to administer intravenous fluids more vigorously. However, the infusion of large volumes of fluid enhances the maldistribution of extracellular fluid and in that way increases the risk of pulmonary and cerebral edema.

Hemoconcentration, or lack of normal pregnancy-induced hypervolemia, is an almost predictable feature of severe preeclampsia. The woman with severe preeclampsia or eclampsia who consequently lacks normal pregnancy hypervolemia is much less tolerant to blood loss than is the normally pregnant woman.

D. Delivery: Delivery is the only known "cure" for preeclampsia-eclampsia. Because women with severe disease may be quite ill, one should try to achieve vaginal delivery. Cesarean delivery should be performed according to the criteria set forth in Chapter 52.

COINCIDENTAL CHRONIC HYPERTENSION

Hypertension that antedates pregnancy is one of the most common medical complications encountered during pregnancy. Its variable incidence and severity, along with the well-known tendency for pregnancy to induce or aggravate hypertension, has caused much confusion concerning the management of the pregnant hypertensive woman. For example, most pregnant women with underlying chronic hypertension demonstrate improved blood pressure control and have largely uneventful pregnancies. However, about 15–20% experience dangerous worsening of hypertension that frequently is accompanied by proteinuria, pathologic edema, and convulsions, and—except that chronic hypertension antedated pregnancy—they are indistinguishable from an otherwise healthy young nullipara with severe preeclampsia-eclampsia.

In most women with chronic hypertensive vascular disease, increased blood pressure is the only demonstrable finding. A few women, however, have complications that are often grave in relation not only to pregnancy but also to life expectancy. These include hypertensive heart disease, ischemic heart disease, renal insufficiency, and retinal hemorrhages and exudates.

Hypertensive vascular disease in pregnancy is encountered more frequently in older women. Obesity is another important predisposing factor. As perhaps may be expected in these older and commonly obese women, diabetes is also prevalent. Finally, heredity—which includes racial factors—has an important role in the development of chronic hypertension; it is more common in blacks, and many members of the patient's family may be hypertensive.

In most women with chronic hypertension the blood pressure falls by the second trimester, but the decrement is usually temporary. Blood pressure usually rises during the third trimester to levels somewhat above those in early pregnancy. Adverse outcomes in these women are largely dependent on whether superimposed preeclampsia develops. The incidence of pregnancy-aggravated hypertension or superimposed preeclampsia averages about 15–25%, and estimates are influenced largely by criteria used in making the diagnosis. Other factors that impact on its incidence are the severity of underlying disease, whether there is renal involvement, and whether other conditions coexist, notably diabetes and obesity. Although adverse pregnancy outcomes are more likely in chronically hypertensive women who develop superimposed preeclampsia, they also are increased in those who remain normotensive throughout pregnancy. Some of the more common complications include hypertensive encephalopathy, heart failure, worsening of renal insufficiency, placental abruption, fetal growth retardation, and fetal death.

Treatment During Pregnancy

The value of continued administration of antihypertensive drugs to pregnant women with chronic hypertension is debated. For example, though it may be of benefit to the hypertensive mother to lower her blood pressure, the lower pressure may reduce uteroplacental perfusion and thereby jeopardize the fetus. A number of investigators reported that superimposed preeclampsia or pregnancy-aggravated hypertension was a bad complication. Importantly, most pregnancy outcomes were good for these women with chronic hypertension, whether or not antihypertensive treatment was given. The uncorrected perinatal mortality rates were acceptable unless superimposed preeclampsia developed.

PREGNANCY-AGGRAVATED HYPERTENSION

The most common hazard faced by pregnant women with chronic hypertensive vascular disease is the superimposition of preeclampsia. The frequency of pregnancy-aggravated hypertension is difficult to specify precisely, since the incidence varies with the diagnostic criteria employed. It typically becomes manifest by a sudden rise in blood pressure that almost always is eventually complicated by substantive proteinuria. In neglected cases especially, extreme hypertension (systolic pressure > 200 mm Hg and diastolic pressure of ≥ 130 mm Hg), oliguria, and impaired renal clearance may rapidly ensue; the retina may contain extensive hemorrhages and cotton wool exudates; and convulsions and coma are likely. Therefore, in its most severe form, the resultant syndrome is similar to hypertensive encephalopathy. With the development of superimposed preeclampsia or eclampsia, the outlook for both the infant and the mother is grave unless the pregnancy is rapidly terminated. The frequency of fetal growth retardation and preterm delivery is increased appreciably because of its relatively early onset in pregnancy as well as the severity of the process itself.

SUGGESTED READINGS

American College of Obstetricians and Gynecologists: Management of preeclampsia. Tech Bull No. 91, February 1986.

Cunningham FG, Pritchard JA: How should hypertension during pregnancy be managed? Experience at Parkland Memorial Hospital. Med Clin North Am 1984;68:505.

Gilstrap LC, Cunningham FG, Whalley PJ: Management of pregnancy-induced hypertension in the nulliparous patient remote from term. Semin Perinatol 1978;2:73.

Mabie WC et al: A comparative trial of labetalol and hydralazine in the acute management of severe hypertension complicating pregnancy. Obstet Gynecol 1987;70:328.

Pritchard JA, Cunningham FG, Pritchard SA: The Parkland Memorial Hospital protocol for treatment of eclampsia: Evaluation of 245 cases. Am J Obstet Gynecol 1984;148:951.

Sibai BM et al: A comparison of no medication versus methyldopa or labetalol in chronic hypertension during pregnancy. Am J Obstet Gynecol 1990;162:960.

United States Department of Health and Human Services: *Working Group Report on High Blood Pressure in Pregnancy.* NIH Publication No. 90–3029, August, 1990.

58

Hemorrhage

Obstetrics is "bloody business." Even though the maternal mortality rate has been reduced dramatically by hospitalization for delivery and the availability of blood for transfusion, death from hemorrhage remains prominent in the majority of mortality reports. Obstetric hemorrhage is most likely to be fatal to the mother in circumstances in which whole blood or blood components are not immediately available. The establishment and maintenance of facilities that allow prompt administration of blood are absolute requirements for acceptable obstetric care.

Postpartum hemorrhage has traditionally been defined as loss of 500 mL or more of blood after completion of the third stage of labor. Almost half of all women who are delivered vaginally and virtually all who undergo cesarean delivery shed that amount or more when measurements are accurate.

Pregnancy hypervolemia normally increases the blood volume by 30–60%, or about 1000–2000 mL for an woman of average size. This means that blood loss in that range during delivery can be tolerated physiologically and without any great decrease in hematocrit postpartum.

Listed in Table 58–1 are the many clinical circumstances in which risk of obstetric hemorrhage is appreciably increased. It is apparent that severe obstetric hemorrhage may occur at any time throughout pregnancy and the puerperium. Moreover, more than one of the conditions listed may contribute either simultaneously or in sequence to continuation of hemorrhage.

Etiology

Obstetric hemorrhage is the consequence of excessive bleeding from the placental implantation site or trauma to the genital tract and adjacent structures, or both.

A. Bleeding From Placental Site: Near term, it is estimated that about 600 mL per min of blood flows through the intervillous spaces that make up the maternal blood compartment of the placenta. With separation of the placenta, the many arteries and veins of the uterus that carry blood to and from the maternal compartment of the placenta are severed abruptly. Effective hemostasis demands that the patency of these vessels be quickly obliterated.

Elsewhere in the body, hemostasis in the absence of surgical ligation depends upon intrinsic vasospasm and formation of blood clots locally. At the placental implan-

tation site, contraction and retraction of the myometrium to compress the vessels and obliterate their lumens are most important for achieving hemostasis. Adherent pieces of placenta or large blood clots—and especially a hypotonic myometrium—will prevent effective contraction and retraction of the myometrium and in that way impair hemostasis at the implantation site. In fact, the most frequent cause of postpartum hemorrhage is a hypotonic myometrium. Fatal postpartum hemorrhage can occur from a hypotonic uterus while the maternal blood coagulation mechanism is quite normal. Conversely, if the myometrium at and adjacent to the denuded implantation site contracts and retracts vigorously, fatal hemorrhage from the placental implantation site is unlikely even though the coagulation mechanism may be severely impaired.

B. Bleeding From Sites of Trauma: Lacerated or incised blood vessels in the reproductive tract other than those in the body of the uterus lack the unique mechanism for obliterating vessel patency that is provided by a vigorously contracting and retracting myometrium. Consequently, oxytocic drugs and uterine massage to stimulate vigorous myometrial contractions are ineffective in controlling hemorrhage if the hemorrhage is not of uterine origin. Therefore, following delivery of an intact placenta, hemorrhage from the genital tract that persists with the uterus firmly contracted and retracted is almost certainly indicative of bleeding from lacerations of the genital tract.

C. Consumption Coagulopathy: Gross derangement of the coagulation mechanism as direct consequence of a variety of obstetric accidents or, less commonly, coincidental disease may incite or enhance obstetric hemorrhage. The observation that extensive placental abruption and other accidents of pregnancy were frequently associated with hypofibrinogenemia stimulated interest in this disorder, which is also called **disseminated intravascular coagulation.**

Consumption coagulopathy almost always is seen as a complication of an identifiable underlying pathologic process requiring treatment to reverse defibrination. With pathologic activation of procoagulants that trigger disseminated intravascular coagulation, there is consumption of platelets and coagulation factors in variable quantities, probably dictated by the degree of the stimulus.

The likelihood of life-threatening hemorrhage in obstetric situations complicated by defective coagulation will

Table 58–1. Conditions that predispose to or worsen obstetric hemorrhage.

Abnormal placentation
  Placenta previa
  Abruptio placentae
  Placenta accreta
  Ectopic pregnancy
  Hydatidiform mole
 	
Trauma during labor and delivery
  Complicated vaginal delivery
  Cesarean section or hysterectomy
  Uterine rupture; risk increased by:
    1. Previously scarred uterus
    2. High parity
    3. Hyperstimulation
    4. Obstructed labor
    5. Intrauterine manipulation
 	
Small maternal blood volume
  Small woman
  Pregnancy hypervolemia not yet maximal
  Pregnancy hypervolemia constricted
    1. Severe preeclampsia
    2. Eclampsia
	Uterine atony
	  Overdistended uterus
	    1. Multiple fetuses
	    2. Hydramnios
	    3. Distention with clots
	  Anesthesia or analgesia
	    1. Halogenated agents
	    2. Conduction analgesia with hypertension
	  Exhausted myometrium
	    1. Rapid labor
	    2. Prolonged labor
	    3. Oxytocin or prostaglandin stimulation
	  Previous uterine atony
	
	Coagulation defects–intensifies other causes
	  Placental abruption
	  Prolonged retention of dead fetus
	  Amnionic fluid embolism
	  Saline-induced abortion
	  Sepsis with endotoxemia
	  Severe intravascular hemolysis
	  Massive transfusions
	  Severe preeclampsia and eclampsia
	  Congenital coagulopathies

depend not only on the extent of the coagulation defects but—of great importance—on whether or not the vasculature is intact or disrupted and, when it is disrupted, the magnitude of the disruption. With gross derangement of blood coagulation, there may be fatal hemorrhage when vascular integrity is disrupted yet no hemorrhage as long as all blood vessels remain intact.

Management of Hemorrhage

Irrespective of the apparent cause, whenever there is any suggestion at delivery or postpartum of excessive blood loss from the genital tract, immediate steps must be taken to identify the presence of uterine atony, retained placental fragments, and trauma. At least one or, in the presence of frank hemorrhage, two intravenous infusion systems of large caliber must be established right away to permit rapid administration of aqueous electrolyte solutions and blood as needed. An operating room and a surgical team, including an anesthesiologist, must be immediately available.

Treatment of serious hemorrhage demands prompt refilling of the intravascular compartment. Two general guidelines have proved to be valuable for determining what fluids that are needed: Lactated Ringer's injection and whole blood are given in such amounts and in such proportions that (1) urine flow is at least 30 mL per h and ideally approaches 60 mL per h and (2) the hematocrit is maintained at 30%.

Fresh compatible whole blood rather than stored blood would appear to be preferable for treatment of hypovolemia from serious acute hemorrhage. Because many blood banks practice fractionation of donor units to provide component therapy, the availability of whole blood has diminished remarkably in the past decade. Fresh-frozen plasma and packed red cells are not adequate substitutes for whole blood in obstetric practice.

PLACENTAL ABRUPTION

Separation of the placenta from its site of implantation in the uterus before delivery of the fetus has been called variously placental abruption, abruptio placentae, ablatio placentae, accidental hemorrhage, and premature separation of the normally implanted placenta. Separation may be partial or total, and the incidence is about 1:150 deliveries. The cause is unknown, but hypertension is identified in half of women with placental abruption.

Some of the bleeding of placental abruption usually insinuates itself between the membranes and uterus, then escapes through the cervix and appears externally, causing **external hemorrhage** (Figure 58–1). Less often, the blood does not escape externally but is retained between the detached placenta and uterus, leading to **concealed hemorrhage.**

Clinical Findings

A. Symptoms and Signs: The signs and symptoms can vary considerably. External bleeding can be profuse even though placental separation is not extensive enough to compromise the fetus directly, or there may be no external bleeding but the placenta is completely sheared off and the fetus dead. Common findings are vaginal bleeding, uterine tenderness, back pain, fetal distress, uterine hypertonus or high-frequency contractions, idiopathic preterm labor, and a dead fetus.

Severe placental abruption is usually marked by such classic signs and symptoms that the diagnosis is obvious, but the more common milder forms are difficult to recognize and the diagnosis is often made by exclusion. Therefore, with vaginal bleeding in the last trimester, it often becomes necessary to rule out placenta previa and other causes of bleeding by clinical inspection and ultrasound evaluation.

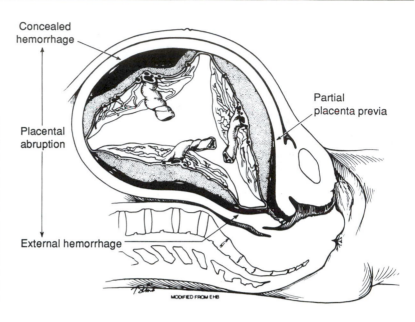

Figure 58–1. Hemorrhage from premature placental separation. **Upper left:** Extensive placental abruption but with the periphery of the placenta and the membranes still adherent, resulting in completely concealed hemorrhage. **Lower:** Placental abruption with the placenta detached peripherally and with the membranes between the placenta and cervical canal stripped from underlying decidua, allowing external hemorrhage. **Right:** Partial placenta previa with placental separation and external hemorrhage. (Reproduced, with permission, from Cunningham FG, MacDonald PC, Gant NF, Leveno KJ, Gilstrap LC [editors]: *Williams Obstetrics,* 19th ed. Appleton & Lange, 1993.)

B. Laboratory Findings: The most common cause of consumptive coagulopathy in pregnancy is placental abruption. Overt hypofibrinogenemia (< 150 mg per dL of plasma) along with elevated concentrations of fibrinogen-fibrin degradation products and variable decreases in other coagulation factors can be demonstrated in about 30% of women with placental abruption severe enough to kill the fetus. Such coagulation defects may be found but are uncommon in cases in which the fetus survives.

Treatment

Treatment depends upon the status of the mother and of fetus. With the development of massive external bleeding, whole blood plus electrolyte solution and prompt delivery to try to control hemorrhage are life-saving for the mother and may rescue the fetus as well.

If blood loss is occurring at a much slower rate, management will be influenced by the status of the fetus. If the fetus is alive and there is no evidence of fetal distress (persistent bradycardia, ominous decelerations, or a sinusoidal heart rate pattern), and if maternal hemorrhage is not causing serious hypovolemia or anemia, observation is warranted as long as facilities for immediate intervention are maintained in a ready state. This plan of treatment is likely to prove most beneficial when the fetus is immature.

If the degree of separation is extensive, ominous decelerations in fetal heart rate are liable to occur, especially when the myometrium contracts. Absence of this sign of fetal distress, however, does not guarantee the safety of the intrauterine environment. The placenta may separate further at any instant and will soon seriously compromise or even kill the fetus unless delivery is performed immediately.

If the fetus is alive but cesarean delivery is not performed promptly, the fetus must be monitored closely for evidence of distress and be delivered immediately whenever distress is detected. Therefore, appropriate facilities and staff for cesarean section must be continuously available whenever placental abruption is suspected.

If the separation is so severe that there is no evidence of fetal life, vaginal delivery is preferred unless hemorrhage is so brisk that it cannot be successfully managed even by vigorous blood replacement or there are other obstetric complications that prevent vaginal delivery.

To treat hypovolemia from hemorrhage, whole blood must be available in large quantities. Coagulation defects are not treated if the woman is delivered vaginally, but if cesarean section is performed when consumptive coagulopathy is identified, fibrinogen replacement with cryoprecipitate is given. Platelet transfusion may also be necessary.

PLACENTA PREVIA

In placenta previa, the placenta, instead of being implanted in the body of the uterus well away from the cervical internal os, is located over or very near the internal os. Four degrees of the abnormality have been recognized:

(1) **Total placenta previa:** The cervical internal os is completely covered by placenta (Figure 58–2).

(2) **Partial placenta previa:** The internal os is partially covered by placenta.

(3) **Marginal placenta previa:** The edge of the placenta is at the margin of the internal os.

(4) **Low-lying placenta:** The placenta is implanted in the lower uterine segment so that the placental edge does

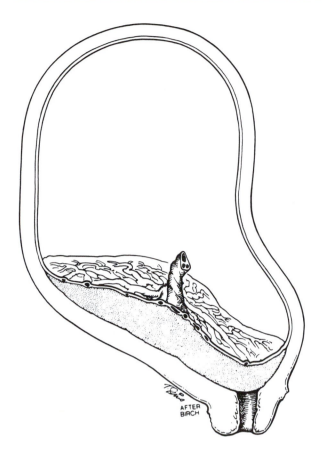

Figure 58–2. Total placental previa. Even with the modest cervical dilatation illustrated, copious hemorrhage would be anticipated. (Reproduced, with permission, from Cunningham FG, MacDonald PC, Gant NF, Leveno KJ, Gilstrap LC [editors]: *Williams Obstetrics,* 19th ed. Appleton & Lange, 1993.)

not actually reach the internal os but is in close proximity to it.

The degree of placenta previa will depend in large measure on the degree of cervical dilatation at the time of examination. For example, a low-lying placenta at 2 cm dilatation may become a partial placenta previa at 8 cm dilatation because the dilating cervix has uncovered placenta. Conversely, a placenta previa that appears to be total before cervical dilatation may become partial at 4 cm dilatation because the cervix dilates beyond the edge of the placenta. One should be aware that digital palpation to try to ascertain these changing relations between the edge of the placenta and the internal os as the cervix dilates can incite severe hemorrhage.

When the placenta is located over the internal os, the formation of the lower uterine segment and the dilatation of the internal os inevitably cause tearing of placental attachments, followed by hemorrhage from the uterine vessels. Bleeding is augmented by inability of the myometrial fibers of the lower uterine segment to contract and retract

and thus compress the torn vessels, as occurs normally when the placenta separates from the otherwise empty uterus during the third stage of labor.

Clinical Findings & Diagnosis

A. Symptoms and Signs: The most characteristic event in placenta previa is **painless hemorrhage,** which usually does not appear until near the end of the second trimester or after. Hemorrhage from placenta previa often occurs without warning in a pregnant woman in previous good health. Occasionally, it makes its first appearance while she is asleep—on awakening, she is surprised to find herself in a pool of blood. Fortunately, the initial bleeding is rarely lethal. It usually ceases spontaneously, only to recur. In some cases, particularly when the placenta is implanted near but not over the cervical os, bleeding does not occur until the onset of labor, when it may vary from slight to profuse.

In women with uterine bleeding during the latter half of pregnancy, placenta previa or abruptio placentae should always be suspected. The possibility of placenta previa should not be dismissed until appropriate evaluation, including sonography, has clearly demonstrated its absence, in which case placental abruption must be considered. The diagnosis of placenta previa seldom can be firmly established by clinical examination unless a finger is passed through the cervix and the placenta is palpated. Such examination of the cervix is never permissible unless the woman is in an operating room with all preparations made for immediate cesarean section, since even the gentlest examination of this sort can cause torrential hemorrhage.

B. Imaging Studies: The simplest, most precise, and safest method of placental localization is **sonography,** which can locate the placenta with up to 98% accuracy. False-positive results probably are due to bladder distention. Therefore, ultrasonic scans in apparently positive cases should be repeated after nearly emptying the bladder. An uncommon source of error has been identification of abundant placenta implanted in the uterine fundus without realizing that the placenta was large and extended downward all the way to the internal cervical os.

Management of Pregnancy

Women with placenta previa may be assigned to the following groups: (1) those in whom the fetus is preterm but there is no pressing need for delivery, (2) those in whom the fetus is within 3 weeks of term, (3) those in whom labor is in progress, and (4) those in whom hemorrhage is so severe as to necessitate delivery despite the immaturity of the fetus.

Management of the pregnancy known to be complicated by placenta previa and a preterm fetus—but with no active bleeding—consists of procrastination in an environment that provides the greatest safety for both mother and fetus. Hospitalization which provides close observation, a sedentary life-style, avoidance of intravaginal manipulation, and immediate availability of appropriate therapy if needed, ie, intravenous electrolyte solution, blood, cesarean delivery, and expert neonatal care from the time of delivery. However, for practical and economic reasons, ideal care in the hospital cannot always be provided for these patients. In such cases, the mother and her family must fully appreciate the problems of placenta previa and be prepared to proceed to the hospital immediately where, in turn, her problem must be recognized immediately by the hospital staff.

Cesarean section is the preferred method of delivery in virtually all cases. In justifying cesarean section in the presence of a dead fetus, it is again necessary to understand that abdominal delivery is done for the welfare of the mother.

FETAL DEATH & DELAYED DELIVERY

If labor does not ensue after fetal death, consumptive coagulapathy may develop. This is unusual, however, and after 1 month only about 25% of women develop significant changes in the coagulation mechanism. Thus, the old wives' tale that the dead baby would poison the mother, although scoffed at by physicians for many generations, proved to be true. It is now clearly established that consumptive coagulopathy, presumably mediated by thromboplastin from the dead products of conception, is operational in these cases.

Treatment consists of termination of pregnancy. Near term, intravenously administered oxytocin usually is effective when given in a dose that stimulates uterine activity, though induction may have to be repeated. Remote from term, however, oxytocin is less likely to prove effective unless given in high concentration and on more than one occasion. One or more laminaria tents placed in the cervical canal before the use of oxytocin may enhance expulsion of the dead products. The magnitude of risk of infection from the use of laminaria in the presence of dead products of conception has not yet been quantified.

Dinoprostone (prostaglandin E_2) given as a 20-mg vaginal suppository to induce labor in pregnancy complicated by fetal death is one option. Since after 28 weeks there is a greater likelihood of hyperstimulation, the possibility of uterine rupture increases and special cautions must be used. These are presumed to include careful clinical monitoring of the woman in labor. Almost all women develop nausea, vomiting, and diarrhea after prostaglandin suppositories are inserted intravaginally; fever is also common.

AMNIONIC FLUID EMBOLISM

Entry of amnionic fluid into the maternal circulation in some circumstances may prove fatal. Essential to the development of amnionic fluid embolism are (1) a rent through the amnion and chorion, (2) opened uterine or endocervical veins, and (3) a pressure gradient sufficient to force the fluid into the venous circulation. Marginal separation of the placenta or laceration of the uterus or cervix serves to create an opening into the maternal circulation. Vigorous labor, including that induced with overdosage of oxytocin, is more likely to provide the pressure. These events may also distress the fetus, leading to defecation of meconium in utero, thereby markedly potentiating the toxic nature of amnionic fluid if it should enter the maternal circulation.

In the typical case of amnionic fluid embolism, the woman is laboring vigorously—or has just completed labor—and is in the process of being delivered when she develops varying degrees of respiratory distress, circulatory collapse, and occasionally, convulsions. If she does not die immediately, serious hemorrhage with severe coagulation defects are soon evident from the genital tract and all other sites of trauma.

The lethality of intravenously infused amnionic fluid varies greatly depending upon the amount of particulate matter it contains, especially thick meconium. Particulate matter previously shed into the amnionic fluid or contained in meconium—including fetal squamous cells (squames), fetal hairs (lanugo), vernix caseosa, and mucin—is pumped by a vigorous contraction into a vein. Severe pulmonary vascular obstruction from the particulate matter and possibly from fibrin formed intravascularly leads to **acute cor pulmonale.**

Hypoxia and reduced cardiac output develop abruptly, and if they are not immediately fatal, hemorrhage from coagulation defects is soon evident from disrupted blood vessels.

Treatment

Prompt treatment is mandatory and usually consists of mechanical ventilation and blood replacement. The patient with cor pulmonale, however, tolerates any deficit or excess in blood volume very poorly.

With lesser degrees of meconium contamination—and probably to some extent with large amounts of mucus-containing but clear amnionic fluid—the pulmonary insult is subacute, resulting in oxygen desaturation, which is amenable to treatment. Simultaneously, intravascular coagulation is incited and may cause death from hemorrhage, but survival may follow if bleeding is arrested and subsequent infection promptly treated.

SUGGESTED READINGS

American College of Obstetricians and Gynecologists: Diagnosis and management of fetal death. Tech Bull No. 98, November 1986.

Chattopadhyay SK, Deb Roy B, Edrees YB: Surgical control of obstetric hemorrhage: Hypogastric artery ligation or hysterectomy? Int J Gynaecol Obstet 1990;32(4):345.

Consensus Conference: Fresh-frozen plasma: Indications and risks. JAMA 1985;253:551.

Hurd WW et al: Selective management of abruptio placentae: A prospective study. Obstet Gynecol 1983;61:467.

Jimenez JM, Pritchard JA: Pathogenesis and treatment of coagulation defects resulting from fetal death. Obstet Gynecol 1968;32:449.

Pritchard JA: Changes in the blood volume during pregnancy and delivery. Anesthesiology 1965;26:393.

59

Preterm & Postterm Pregnancy & Inappropriate Fetal Growth

A fetus or newborn infant whose weight is significantly above or below normal is at increased risk of dying or, if it survives, at risk for physical and intellectual impairment. These increased risks are related to gestational age and fetal growth rate. A low-birth-weight neonate may be of early gestational age or may have failed to maintain a normal fetal growth rate. A large neonate may be of older gestational time or may have surpassed the normal fetal growth rate. In any pregnancy, it is essential to have precise information about gestational age of the fetus; this knowledge is even more important when the pregnancy is complicated. Gestational age must be known before any diagnosis of inappropriate fetal growth can be made.

The fetus or newborn infant is referred to as a **fetus at term** or **infant at term** during the interval from the 38th to the 42nd weeks after the onset of a menstrual period that was followed 2 weeks later by ovulation. The critical date for determining the age of the fetus is the date of ovulation or of fertilization. The date of onset of the last normal menstrual period is of clinical importance for determining fetal age because it is usually known rather precisely; when menstrual bleeding is spontaneous and regular, it most often is followed by ovulation and fertilization 2 weeks later. Before the 38th week, the word **preterm** is used to categorize the fetus and the pregnancy; at 42 completed weeks and thereafter, **postterm** is the appropriate term. Gestational (menstrual) age should always be cited in weeks rather than months or trimesters.

With respect to gestational age, a fetus or infant may be preterm, term, or postterm. With respect to size, the fetus or infant may be normally grown or **appropriate for gestational age (AGA),** small in size or **small for gestational age (SGA),** or overgrown and consequently **large for gestational age (LGA).** The term SGA has been widely used to categorize an infant whose birth weight is clearly below average and usually below the 10th percentile for its gestational age. The infant whose birth weight is above the 90th percentile has been categorized as LGA,

and the infant whose weight is between the 10th and 90th percentiles is designated AGA (Figure 59–1).

PRETERM BIRTH

Obstetric approaches to preterm labor and delivery are guided in large part by the obstetrician's expectations for survival of the premature or immature neonate as well as the therapeutic alternatives available for management of labor. That some very small infants do survive after prolonged and very expensive special care has created problems in decision-making for the obstetrician. The obstetrician faces the challenge of effecting delivery that will optimize the status of the fetus-infant at birth in the event that intensive care will be applied. The neonatologist in turn must decide how best to dispense the finite resources for medical care provided by the insurance carrier, the family, government agencies, the hospital, and the health care team.

Aside from survival, one must consider the quality of life achieved by immature infants of very low birth weight, many of whom must endure physical and intellectual deficits as children and adults. Given these concerns, a question arises about when during gestation obstetric intervention is appropriate. Although it is impossible to make precise judgments about the earliest limit for neonatal survival, we do know that many factors inevitably have an impact on the clinical decision-making process. Several of these factors are discussed throughout the remainder of this chapter—including preterm delivery and fetal maturity and size—along with their management.

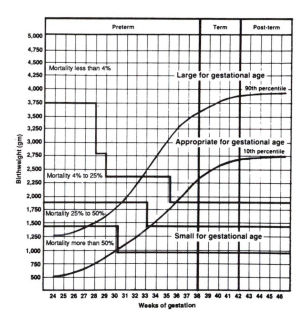

Figure 59–1. Perinatal mortality in relation to birth weight plotted as a function of gestational age. A significant increase in mortality rate is observed in growth-retarded fetuses below 1500 g. (Reproduced, with permission, from Queenan JT: How to diagnose IUGR. Contemp Ob/Gyn 1982;19:195.)

CAUSES OF PRETERM LABOR

The causes of preterm labor are usually not known. Listed below are some conditions that predispose to preterm labor and delivery:

(1) Amnionic fluid infection.
(2) Spontaneous rupture of membranes.
(3) Anomalies of conception.
(4) Previous preterm delivery or late abortion.
(5) Overdistended uterus.
(6) Fetal death.
(7) Cervical incompetency.
(8) Uterine anomalies.
(9) Faulty placentation.
(10) Retained intrauterine device.
(11) Serious maternal disease.
(12) Medically indicated labor induction.
(13) Unknown causes.

Chorioamnionic infection caused by a variety of microorganisms has emerged as a possible explanation for many heretofore unexplained cases of ruptured membranes or preterm labor. In one series of women with preterm labor and intact membranes, bacterial colonization of amnionic fluid was identified without clinical evidence of infection in 25%. Women with infected fluid almost always delivered within 48 hours despite tocolysis, in contrast to those with sterile amnionic fluids.

Rupture of the membranes remote from term is better referred to as *preterm* rather than premature rupture. Preterm rupture (before 38 weeks) is an important cause of maternal and perinatal morbidity and mortality. If there is no fever, current management before 34 weeks consists of observation. However, preterm rupture is associated with other obstetric complications that influence perinatal outcome, including multifetal gestation, breech presentation, chorioamnionitis, and fetal distress in labor. Extrapolating from a major study of such women, it can be estimated that as a consequence of these complications, cesarean deliveries are done in nearly 40% of women. The most striking finding is the apparent inevitability of labor within a short time following membrane rupture. At admission, 76% of the women are already in labor, 5% are delivered for other complications, and another 11% are delivered following spontaneous labor within 48 hours. Thus, in only 7% is delivery delayed 48 hours or more after membrane rupture.

MANAGEMENT OF PRETERM LABOR & DELIVERY

In general, the more immature the fetus, the greater the risks from labor and delivery. This is well established for breech delivery, which is a common presentation for the preterm fetus and undoubtedly also is true to some degree for all immature fetuses regardless of presentation.

If labor is induced, it must not be unduly forceful (Chapter 45). Whether labor is induced or spontaneous, abnormalities of fetal heart rate and uterine contractions should be looked for, preferably by continuous electronic monitoring. If the fetal heart rate is not monitored continuously, it must be evaluated at brief intervals (Chapter 45). *Tachycardia, especially in the presence of ruptured membranes, is suggestive of sepsis.* Periodic decelerations imply cord compression, which is rather common with preterm rupture of membranes and loss of amnionic fluid, but late decelerations may also occur and are suggestive of placental insufficiency.

In the absence of a relaxed vaginal outlet, a liberal episiotomy for delivery is advantageous once the fetal head reaches the perineum. The use of outlet forceps of appropriate size may be of aid when conduction analgesia is used and voluntary expulsion efforts are obtunded. Forceps should not be employed to pull the fetus through a vagina that is resistant to dilation or over a firm perineum.

A physician proficient in resuscitative techniques who has been fully informed about the specific problems of the case should be present at delivery. The principles of resuscitation described in Chapter 40 are applicable, including prompt tracheal intubation and ventilation.

METHODS USED TO ARREST PRETERM LABOR

Before an attempt is made to arrest preterm labor, one must consider whether further intrauterine stay is more likely to benefit or to harm the fetus. For example, retarded fetal growth may be confused with a preterm fetus, and the malnourished fetus may be left in a hostile uterine environment rather than the more salubrious one provided by the nursery. Thus, one should not delay delivery in all cases of presumed preterm labor. The decision to attempt arrest of labor is made much easier if the gestational age is precisely known.

The usual treatment is bed rest with the mother lying comfortably on her side.

Intravenous **magnesium sulfate** is used by many to arrest preterm labor. The patient must be monitored closely for evidence of hypermagnesemia that might prove toxic to her and to her fetus-infant. Magnesium promptly crosses the placenta to produce concentrations in fetal plasma comparable to those in the mother. If magnesium intoxication is to be avoided, the patellar reflex should be present and respirations should not be depressed.

Several compounds capable of reacting predominantly with β-adrenergic receptors have been investigated. Some are used extensively in obstetrics, but only ritodrine hydrochloride has been approved by the Food and Drug Administration for use in the treatment of preterm labor.

Antiprostaglandins have been the subject of considerable interest since it became known that prostaglandins are intimately involved in the myometrial contractions that characterize labor. Antiprostaglandin agents may act by inhibiting the synthesis of prostaglandins or by blocking the action of prostaglandins on target organs.

Unfortunately, none of the agents are completely satisfactory, and complications occur with all of them. If β-adrenergic agonists are to be used, certain precautions must be taken to avoid misuse. The woman considered to be in preterm labor must be carefully evaluated for pregnancy complications that may not be readily apparent, eg, placental abruption or intrauterine sepsis. The possibility of underlying maternal disease that would contraindicate the use of tocolytics must be considered. These diseases include many forms of heart disease, diabetes, pregnancy-induced or pregnancy-aggravated hypertension, hyperthyroidism, and severe anemia. The status of the fetus must also be considered, and unless the intrauterine environment is normal, its interests may be served better by prompt delivery. This is true for the overtly growth-retarded fetus or when there is intrauterine infection. Finally, if the fetus has achieved reasonable maturity, delivery is more advantageous than are attempts at pharmacologic intervention.

POSTTERM PREGNANCY

A postterm pregnancy is one that persists for 42 weeks or more from the onset of a menstrual period that was followed by ovulation 2 weeks later. Although this includes perhaps 10% of pregnancies, some may not be actually postterm but rather the result of an error in the estimation of gestational age.

Once again the value of precise knowledge of the duration of gestation is evident, since in general the longer the truly postterm fetus stays in utero, the greater the risk of a severely compromised fetus and newborn infant.

The postterm fetus may continue to gain weight in utero and thus be an unusually large infant at birth or may gain weight postterm and be LGA (Figure 59–2). The fact that the fetus continues to grow serves as an indication of uncompromised placental function, with the implication that it should be able to tolerate the rigors of normal labor without difficulty. This, however, may not be the result. For example, continued growth may have created a worrisome degree of fetopelvic disproportion, and labor may therefore not progress normally. Moreover, as discussed below, oligohydramnios commonly develops as pregnancy advances past 42 weeks, and decreased amnionic fluid is associated with cord compression, which leads to fetal distress, including defecation and aspiration of thick meconium.

ANTEPARTUM MANAGEMENT OF POSTTERM PREGNANCY

Even in the absence of any recognizable maternal complication, there is little doubt that some fetuses who stay in utero much beyond 42 weeks are in increasing danger of sustaining serious morbidity or even death. Therefore, it is advantageous to effect delivery by 42 weeks.

If gestational age is known, most obstetricians agree that delivery should be induced after 42 weeks regardless of the condition of the cervix. If induction fails, many favor cesarean delivery. There is no agreement about the best method of fetal surveillance between 42 and 44 weeks in those pregnancies in which induction of labor is not done.

In many institutions, management between 42 and 44 weeks consists of serial evaluations directed especially at identifying fetal jeopardy while awaiting the onset of spontaneous labor. With documented or suspected fetal distress, the infant is delivered either by labor induction or by cesarean, depending on obstetric indications.

In many medical centers, if gestational age is unknown, clinical, electronic, or biochemical surveillance techniques (Chapter 43) are used after the best estimate of the 42nd week, and delivery is not induced unless there is evidence of fetal jeopardy. In these studies, because delivery dates most often are miscalculated, there is generally a favorable outcome.

There is no doubt that when amnionic fluid is decreased in a postterm pregnancy—or, for that matter, any pregnancy—the fetus is at increased risk. Besides fetal mortality, which is not common, there is significant morbidity with oligohydramnios. For example, the incidence of meconium-stained amnionic fluid and the need for cesarean delivery are greatly increased if oligohydramnios is iden-

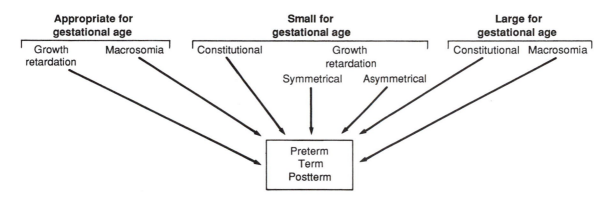

Figure 59–2. Fetal-neonatal age compared to birth weight and functional growth. "Preterm" denotes a neonate delivered prior to 38 weeks of gestation, and "postterm" after 42 weeks. A "term" neonate is one delivered between 38 and 42 weeks. A small for gestational age fetus-neonate is below the 10th percentile for weight, while a large for gestational age fetus-neonate is above the 90th percentile. An appropriate for gestational age fetus-neonate is between the 10th and 90th percentiles. A fetus-neonate destined to be either large or small may be described as constitutionally large or small—ie, normal growth potential was reached for that infant. A pathologic process results in a growth-retarded or macrosomic fetus-neonate.

tified. In this instance, fetal jeopardy from significant umbilical cord compression is more common during labor.

INTRAPARTUM MANAGEMENT OF POSTTERM PREGNANCY

Labor is a particularly dangerous time for the postterm fetus. Therefore, it is important that women whose pregnancies are known or suspected to be postterm come to the hospital as soon as they suspect they are in labor. Upon arrival, while being observed for possible labor, electronic fetal heart rate and uterine contractions should be closely monitored for rate variations consistent with fetal distress.

Identification of **thick meconium** in amnionic fluid is evidence of recent fetal distress that may or may not persist. Meconium aspiration may cause severe pulmonary dysfunction and death during the newborn period (Chapter 55). This may be minimized but not eliminated by effective suctioning of the pharynx as soon as the head is delivered but before the thorax is delivered.

At times, the continued growth of the fetus postterm will result in a postterm and LGA infant, and shoulder dystocia may develop following delivery of the head. Therefore, an obstetrician experienced in managing shoulder dystocia should be available to effect delivery (Chapter 46).

INAPPROPRIATE FETAL GROWTH

Inappropriate fetal growth occurs whenever the fetus is either too large or too small for its age. The problems associated with macrosomic or constitutionally large fetuses are addressed in other chapters, especially along with discussions of shoulder dystocia (Chapter 46), postterm pregnancy (above), and diabetes (Chapter 60). This section is devoted to the problem of the fetus too small for its gestational age.

The actual number of growth-retarded neonates is unknown. In fact, it was not until 25 years ago that physicians first recognized that **runting,** or fetal growth retardation, was a human as well as an animal phenomenon.

A typical fetal-infant growth curve is shown in Figure 59–1.

CLASSIFICATION OF SMALL FOR GESTATIONAL AGE FETUSES

Small for gestational age infants are those whose weights are below the 10th percentile for gestational age. Large (LGA) infants have weights above the 90th percentile, and infants between the 10th and 90th percentiles are classified as appropriate for gestational age (AGA). SGA infants, whether preterm or term, have significantly increased perinatal mortality rates.

As illustrated in Figure 59–2, a fetus may be SGA due to a genetically predetermined reason (constitutionally small) or due to a pathologic process (fetal growth retardation). Because fetal growth retardation may be caused by many diseases and conditions, there is no obvious way to avoid that outcome. Advances have been made, however, in ways to arrive at etiologic diagnoses, screening techniques for early recognition of the problem, management, and follow-up of this complication. It is emphasized again that before recognition and management of fetal growth retardation can be accomplished, gestational age must be established accurately.

There are two types of fetal growth retardation: **type I,**

or symmetric;, and **type II, or asymmetric.** These two types are likely to be the consequence of different times of onset and duration of the events that caused the retarded growth.

Type I, symmetric growth retardation, probably results from early noxious influences, ie, at a time when fetal growth is predominantly from hyperplasia. Injuries to the fetus at this time might be expected to produce profound effects. This is borne out clinically, because symmetric forms of growth retardation most often are caused by structural or chromosomal abnormalities or early congenital infections, such as rubella. This type of growth retardation is thus intrinsic. Perhaps 20% of cases of retarded fetal growth are symmetric.

Type II (asymmetric) growth retardation usually results from adverse effects during the phase of cellular hypertrophy, ie, during later gestation. Thus, most asymmetrically growth-retarded fetuses have the appropriate number of cells but the cells are smaller than normal. Fetal injury at this time would not be expected to cause damage as severe as an earlier insult, and this indeed has been observed clinically.

The cause of asymmetric growth retardation cannot be explained merely by a reduction in the size of all cells; it is probably the consequence also of sparing of selected cells, eg, those of the central nervous system. The pathologic processes that most often result in asymmetric growth retardation are maternal diseases extrinsic to the fetus. These diseases may alter fetal size by reducing uteroplacental blood flow, as in the case of hypertensive disorders; or by restricting oxygen and nutrient transfer, as with sickle cell disease; or by reducing placental size, as with infarcts. A combination of events may be seen with twins, when blood supply and placental size both are reduced late in pregnancy as a consequence of "sharing."

ANTEPARTUM IDENTIFICATION OF FETAL GROWTH RETARDATION

The challenge remains primarily with the obstetrician to identify the fetus who is growing inappropriately in utero. This difficulty is underscored by the fact that such identification is not always possible even in the nursery. Even so, certain clinical techniques and sophisticated equipment may prove useful in helping to screen and perhaps diagnose fetal growth retardation.

Serial uterine fundal height measurements throughout gestation are a simple, safe, inexpensive, and reasonably accurate screening method that may be used to detect many SGA fetuses. The principal problem is a high false-positive predictive value and the inability to differentiate between symmetrically or asymmetrically growth-retarded fetuses. These measurements are not applicable, however, in multifetal pregnancies or hydramnios or for fetuses in a transverse lie.

Evaluation and measurement by sonar for screening, diagnosis, and management of inappropriate fetal growth has become indispensable. Several techniques are used,

and it is emphasized again that accurate information about gestational age is of paramount importance.

MANAGEMENT OF FETAL GROWTH RETARDATION

Clinical screening using carefully obtained gestational age and serial uterine fundal height measurements will identify many SGA fetuses. Carefully obtained serial ultrasonic measurements done in high-risk groups such as women with chronic hypertension, diabetes, or those with renal or autoimmune diseases will identify even more fetuses at risk. *Even with intensive screening, not all fetuses can be identified.* Once an SGA fetus is suspected, however, intensive efforts should be made to determine if growth retardation is present and, if so, the type of growth retardation and the cause. The physician should ensure delivery, when possible, of an infant who will subsequently thrive and grow to its normal potential. Finally, this must be done at the least cost to the patient in terms both of money and of physical risk to herself and the fetus.

If a fetus is suspected of being growth-retarded, a sonographic survey should be done to look for structural abnormalities. Anthropometric measurements should include head and abdominal circumferences, biparietal diameter, femur length, and the ratio of head circumference to abdominal girth. Amnionic fluid volume should be assessed clinically and by ultrasound. The gestational age is confirmed or (if not already known) established if possible. When the status of the cervix is assessed, a decision can be made about whether to deliver the fetus. Prompt delivery achieves the best outcome for the fetus suspected of being growth-retarded at or near term.

If the fetus is symmetrically growth-retarded, a meticulous search should be made for fetal anomalies, and consideration should be given to obtaining umbilical blood for karyotyping, especially if a chromosomal anomaly is suspected (Chapter 54). Umbilical venous blood can be obtained by ultrasonically directed percutaneous umbilical blood sampling (Chapter 43). Some authorities recommend screening for toxoplasmosis, rubella, cytomegalovirus, herpes, and other viral agents, the so-called TORCH organisms, but the clinical yield in this situation is usually not rewarding.

Having excluded as nearly as possible structural and chromosomal abnormalities and congenital infection, the patient with a growth-retarded fetus should be hospitalized and placed at decreased physical activity with an adequate diet. Fetal surveillance is then started, including at a minimum fetal movement charts and clinical and sonographic assessment of fetal growth and amnionic fluid volume. Many also recommend a battery of fetal surveillance tests, including nonstress tests, contraction stress tests, biophysical profiles, and serial Doppler velocity waveform measurements.

The preterm patient whose fetus shows asymmetric growth retardation should be hospitalized, and fetal surveillance should be started as described above. Since a number of asymmetrically growth-retarded fetuses are the consequence of abnormalities in uteroplacental perfusion, many obstetricians choose to monitor these pregnancies with Doppler velocimetry. In most such reports, the fetus is already severely ill and often acidotic when the tests become ominous.

In most instances of fetal growth retardation remote from term, there is no specific treatment that can be given. A very sedentary activity status that approaches full-time bed rest may favorably influence fetal growth and perhaps reduce the risk of preterm labor. Occasionally, the overtly growth-retarded fetus is in serious jeopardy irrespective of whether it remains in utero or is delivered. For the fetus that is severely growth-retarded but remote from term, the decision to proceed with delivery becomes a matter of trying to ascertain the degree of risk from further uterine stay compared with the risks from preterm delivery. The presence of maternal disease that is worsening as a consequence of the pregnancy and thus threatening the well-being of the mother as well as the fetus certainly should influence the decision to deliver the severely growth-retarded fetus. Almost any maternal disease falls into this category when it involves the vascular system or kidneys, and the decision for delivery is further reinforced if preeclampsia supervenes (Chapter 57). With prompt delivery, fetal and neonatal salvage is likely to be improved compared to unduly delayed delivery even though the L/S ratio is considered immature.

SUGGESTED READINGS

Battaglia FC, Lubchenco LO: A practical classification of newborn infants by weight and gestational age. J Pediatr 1967;71:159.

Benedetti TJ, Easterling T: Antepartum testing in postterm pregnancy. J Reprod Med 1988;33:252.

Cox S, Williams ML, Leveno KJ: The natural history of preterm ruptured membranes: What to expect of expectant management. Obstet Gynecol 1988;71:558.

Gilstrap LC et al: Survival and short-term morbidity of the premature neonate. Obstet Gynecol 1985;65:37.

Leveno KJ et al: Prolonged pregnancy: I. Observations concerning the causes of fetal distress. Am J Obstet Gynecol 1984;150:465.

Lubchenco LO et al: Intrauterine growth as estimated from liveborn birth-weight data at 24 to 42 weeks of gestation. Pediatrics 1963;32:793.

Small JL et al: An active management approach to the postdate fetus with a reactive nonstress test and fetal heart rate decelerations. Obstet Gynecol 1987;70:636.

Walker D-JB et al: Cost-benefit analysis of neonatal intensive care for infants weighing less than 1,000 grams at birth. Pediatrics 1984;74:20.

60

Medical & Surgical Illnesses Complicating Pregnancy

Almost any disease that affects a nonpregnant woman of childbearing age may complicate pregnancy, and most diseases that occur in young women do not prevent conception. For many systemic illnesses, the physiologic and anatomic changes inherent in normal pregnancy influence the symptoms, signs, and laboratory values to a considerable degree. As a consequence, the physician who is not aware of these normal pregnancy-induced changes may fail to recognize a disease or may diagnose incorrectly some other disease, to the jeopardy of the mother and her fetus. Throughout this chapter, emphasis has been placed on the effect of interaction between the disease and the pregnancy as well as on the diagnostic and therapeutic problems pregnancy may give rise to. In practically all instances, the following questions are pertinent:

(1) Is pregnancy apt to make the disease more serious, and if so, how?

(2) Does the disease jeopardize the pregnancy, and if so, how and to what degree?

(3) Should the pregnancy be terminated because of serious risk to the mother or a likelihood of grave damage to the fetus?

(4) Should the pregnancy be allowed to continue under a carefully defined regimen of therapy?

(5) If the disease exists before pregnancy, is pregnancy contraindicated? If so, what steps should be taken to protect the woman from pregnancy?

A woman should never be penalized because she is pregnant. Put differently—if a treatment regimen usually given a nonpregnant woman is altered because of pregnancy, there must be strong justification for the modification. This approach allows individualization of care for most disorders that complicate pregnancy and should always be remembered, especially when dealing with the medical and surgical consultants who often are asked to see such patients.

HEMATOLOGIC DISORDERS

Anemia probably exists in women residing at lower altitudes if the hemoglobin is much below 12 g per dL in the nonpregnant state or less than 10 g per dL during pregnancy or the puerperium. However, early in pregnancy and again near term, the hemoglobin level of most healthy iron-sufficient women is usually 11 g per dL or higher. During the puerperium, the hemoglobin concentration, in the absence of excessive blood loss, is not appreciably lower than the predelivery level. The observed differences between hemoglobin concentrations in pregnant and nonpregnant women, coupled with the well-recognized phenomenon of hypervolemia induced by normal pregnancy, have led to the use of the term "physiologic anemia"—a poor term for normal process, and one that should be discarded since there is virtually no anemia during normal pregnancy if anemia is defined as a decrease in hemoglobin mass.

IRON-DEFICIENCY ANEMIA

The two most common causes of anemia during pregnancy and the puerperium are iron deficiency and acute blood loss. The two are often intimately related, since excessive blood loss with its concomitant loss of hemoglobin iron and exhaustion of iron stores in one pregnancy can be an important cause of iron-deficiency anemia in the next pregnancy.

The iron requirements of pregnancy are considerable, and most American women have small stores. In a typical gestation with a single fetus, the maternal need for iron induced by pregnancy averages close to 800 mg, of which about 300 mg go to the fetus and placenta whereas about

500 mg, if available, is used to expand the maternal hemoglobin mass. About 200 mg more are shed through the gut, urine, and skin. This total amount—1000 mg—greatly exceeds the iron stores of most women. Unless the difference between the amount of stored iron available and the iron requirements of normal pregnancy is compensated for by absorption of iron from the gastrointestinal tract, iron deficiency anemia develops.

For treatment, oral iron preparations are preferred if the patient understands the importance of taking the medication regularly. If she cannot be relied on to take the oral doses, parenteral iron therapy is an alternative.

MEGALOBLASTIC ANEMIA

The prevalence of megaloblastic anemia during pregnancy varies considerably throughout the world, and the disorder is rare in the United States. In this country, megaloblastic anemia beginning during pregnancy almost always results from folic acid deficiency—and in the past was referred to as **pernicious anemia of pregnancy.** Folate requirements are increased substantially during pregnancy, and folate deficiency is usually found in pregnant women who consume neither fresh vegetables—especially uncooked green leafy vegetables—nor foods with a high content of animal protein.

The treatment of megaloblastic anemia induced by pregnancy should include folic acid, a nutritious diet, and iron. As little as 1 mg of folic acid administered orally once a day produces a striking hematologic response.

SICKLE CELL HEMOGLOBINOPATHIES

Sickle cell anemia (SS disease), sickle cell-hemoglobin C disease (SC disease), and sickle cell-β-thalassemia disease (S-β-thalassemia disease) are the most common of the sickle hemoglobinopathies. Maternal morbidity and mortality rates, the abortion rate, and the perinatal mortality rate are variably increased with each of these diseases (Table 60–1).

Pregnancy is a serious burden to the woman with SS disease, for the anemia often becomes more intense, vaso-occlusive episodes with severe pain—so-called sickle cell crises—usually become more frequent, and infections and pulmonary complications are more common. Maternal mortality rates are high, and nearly one-half of pregnancies have terminated in abortion, stillbirth, or neonatal death.

Adequate care of women with sickle cell anemia or other sickle cell hemoglobinopathies in pregnancy necessitates close observation, with careful evaluation of all symptoms, physical findings, and laboratory studies. The term sickle cell crisis, if used, should be accepted only after all other possible causes of pain or reduction in hemoglobin concentration have been excluded. Anemia is moderate, and rarely is the hemoglobin concentration less than 7 g per dL. Pyelonephritis and pneumonia are common infections and may worsen the anemia, so that red cell transfusions are required. Many workers recommend prophylactic transfusions to prevent morbidity associated with the sickle syndromes.

For severe pain, use of potent analgesics—eg, meperidine or morphine administered parenterally—is indicated. Red cell transfusions administered after the onset of severe pain have no dramatic effect on the intensity or duration of the attack of pain, whereas prophylactic red cell transfusions have almost eliminated pain by preventing these vaso-occlusive episodes.

THALASSEMIAS

The thalassemias are a group of genetically determined hematologic disorders characterized by an impaired rate of production of one or more of the peptide chains that are normal components of globin. **Thalassemia minor** is characterized by mild hypochromic microcystic anemia unresponsive to iron therapy. The various forms of thalassemia are classified according to the globin chain which is deficient in amount compared to its partner chain. The two major forms of thalassemias involve either impaired production of alpha peptide chains, causing α-thalassemia, or of beta chains, causing β-thalassemia.

THROMBOCYTOPENIAS

Thrombocytopenia may appear clinically to be idiopathic or, more often, to be associated with one of the following disorders: acquired hemolytic anemia, severe preeclampsia or eclampsia, severe obstetric hemorrhage with blood transfusions, consumptive coagulopathy from placental abruption or similar hypofibrinogenemic states, septicemia, lupus erythematosus, antiphospholipid antibodies, megaloblastic anemia caused by severe folate deficiency, drug toxicity, viral infections, allergies, aplastic anemia, or excessive irradiation.

The entity referred to as **immune thrombocytopenic purpura (ITP)** is the consequence most often of an immune process in which antibodies against platelets are the culprits. Antibody-coated platelets are destroyed prematurely in the reticuloendothelial system, especially the spleen. The mechanism of production of antibodies is not known, but an antibody is thought to be responsible.

There is no strong contraindication to the use of corticosteroids such as prednisone during pregnancy. Large doses may be required for improvement, and treatment will probably have to be continued for the duration of the pregnancy. IgG antibodies are formed in immune

Table 60–1. Pregnancy outcomes in women with sickle hemoglobinopathies.

	Maternal Deaths	Perinatal Deaths
Sickle cell (SS) disease	2.7%	191:1000
SC disease	2.3%	75:1000

thrombocytopenia, and these can cross the placenta and cause thrombocytopenia in the fetus and neonate. The severely thrombocytopenic fetus is at increased risk of serious hemorrhage, especially intracranial hemorrhage, as the consequence of labor and delivery. To prevent complications, most obstetricians advocate fetal platelet estimation, using either blood obtained by ultrasonically guided umbilical vessel sampling or scalp blood taken transvaginally after labor ensues. If severe thrombocytopenia is identified in the fetus, cesarean delivery is indicated to avoid birth trauma.

CARDIOVASCULAR DISEASE

Heart disease probably complicates about 1% of pregnancies. The likelihood of a favorable outcome for the mother with heart disease and her baby depends upon (1) the functional capacity of her heart, (2) the likelihood of other complications that increase further the cardiac load during pregnancy and the puerperium, (3) the quality of medical care provided, and (4) the psychologic and socioeconomic resources of the expectant mother, her family, and the community health system.

Many of the physiologic changes of normal pregnancy tend to make the diagnosis of heart disease more difficult than in the nonpregnant state. For example, in normal pregnancy, functional systolic heart murmurs are quite common. Some widely accepted criteria used to confirm the diagnosis of heart disease in pregnancy are as follows: (1) a diastolic, presystolic, or continuous heart murmur; (2) unequivocal cardiac enlargement; (3) a loud, harsh systolic murmur, especially if associated with a thrill; or (4) serious arrhythmias. Pregnant women who have none of these findings rarely have serious heart disease.

CLINICAL CLASSIFICATION OF HEART DISEASE

There is no clinically applicable test for measuring functional capacity of the heart. A helpful clinical classification provided by the New York Heart Association is based on past and present disability and is uninfluenced by the presence or absence of physical signs:

Class I. Uncompromised—Patients with cardiac disease and no limitation of physical activity. These patients do not have symptoms of cardiac insufficiency, nor do they experience anginal pain.

Class II: Slightly compromised—Patients with cardiac disease and slight limitation of physical activity. These women are comfortable at rest, but if ordinary physical activity is undertaken, discomfort results in the form of excessive fatigue, palpitation, dyspnea, or anginal pain.

Class III: Markedly compromised—Patients with cardiac disease and marked limitation of physical activity. These women are comfortable at rest, but less than ordinary activity causes discomfort in the form of excessive fatigue, palpitation, dyspnea, or anginal pain.

Class IV: Patients with cardiac disease and inability to perform any physical activity without discomfort. Symptoms of cardiac insufficiency or of anginal syndrome may develop even at rest, and if any physical activity is undertaken, discomfort is increased.

GENERAL MANAGEMENT OF HEART DISEASE

The treatment of heart disease in pregnancy is dictated by the functional capacity of the heart. In all pregnant women, but especially those with cardiac disease, excessive weight gain, abnormal fluid retention, and anemia should be prevented. Increased bodily bulk increases the cardiac work, and anemia with its compensatory rise in cardiac output also predisposes to cardiac failure. The development of pregnancy-induced hypertension is hazardous. At the same time, hypotension is undesirable, especially in women with septal defects or patent ductus arteriosus. Infection increases cardiac workload appreciably and should be prevented if possible and treated vigorously if it develops.

With rare exceptions, all women with class I and most with class II heart disease are allowed to go through pregnancy. Throughout pregnancy and the puerperium, special attention should be directed toward both prevention and early recognition of heart failure. A sedentary life-style is recommended, and foods rich in sodium must be avoided.

Admission remote from delivery of women with class II cardiac disease should be considered. Delivery should be accomplished vaginally unless there are obstetric indications for cesarean section. In spite of the physical effort inherent in labor and vaginal delivery, lower rates of morbidity and mortality have been recorded when such a delivery has been accomplished. Relief from pain and apprehension without undue depression of the infant or the mother are especially important during labor and delivery.

Women who have shown little or no evidence of cardiac distress during pregnancy, labor, or delivery sometimes decompensate after delivery. Therefore, it is important that the same meticulous care provided during the antepartum and intrapartum periods be continued into the puerperium. Postpartum hemorrhage, infection, and thromboembolism are much more serious complications of pregnancy in the woman with heart disease.

Women whose cardiac function is so seriously diminished as to be placed in class III present difficult problems that demand expert medical care. Maternal mortality rates for classes III and IV have been reported to be about 5%. About a third of class III cardiac patients will decompensate during pregnancy unless preventive measures are taken. When such a woman is seen in the first trimester, the question of therapeutic abortion inevitably arises.

CYANOTIC HEART DISEASE

Women with cyanotic heart disease do poorly during pregnancy. If the hematocrit is very high, spontaneous early abortion usually follows conception. With somewhat lesser degrees of polycythemia, there is still an increased incidence of abortion and low birth weight infants.

PULMONARY HYPERTENSION

Pulmonary hypertension is usually secondary to cardiac or pulmonary disease. Primary pulmonary hypertension is idiopathic, and pregnancy should be avoided since the maternal mortality rate has been as high as 50%. These reports describe women with severe primary pulmonary hypertension, but milder degrees of secondary pulmonary hypertension probably go unnoticed.

INFECTIVE ENDOCARDITIS

Acute or subacute bacterial endocarditis is uncommon during pregnancy and the puerperium, but it may cause occasional maternal deaths in women who take illicit drugs intravenously. Most obstetricians recommend that antimicrobial agents be given prophylactically during labor in order to minimize the risk of bacterial endocarditis and arteritis in pregnant women with valvar prostheses or mitral valve prolapse or those with aortic abnormalities such as patent ductus arteriosus or coarctation.

PULMONARY DISORDERS

Pregnancy induces a number of changes in the respiratory system. Uterine enlargement causes the diaphragm to rise, the transverse thoracic diameter to increase, the vertical chest diameter to decrease, and the residual lung volume to be reduced. In response to the modest hyperventilation that is normal for pregnancy, the tidal volume is increased somewhat and the plasma carbon dioxide is lowered slightly. During the latter part of pregnancy, oxygen consumption is increased 15–25% above that of normal nonpregnant women.

PNEUMONIA

Pneumonitis causing an appreciable loss of ventilatory capacity is tolerated less well by women during pregnancy. This generalization seems to hold true regardless of whether the cause of the pneumonia is bacterial, viral, or chemical. Moreover, hypoxia and acidosis are poorly tolerated by the fetus and frequently lead to preterm labor after mid pregnancy. Therefore, it is important to the pregnant woman and her fetus that pneumonia be diagnosed as soon as possible and that she be promptly hospitalized so that the disease can be treated effectively. Any pregnant woman suspected of having pneumonia should have anteroposterior and lateral chest x-rays. Bacterial pneumonias are most common, and pneumococcal infections predominate. Mycoplasmal pneumonia, influenza A, and other causes must be considered as well.

ASTHMA

This rather common respiratory illness is encountered relatively often in pregnant women. With active but otherwise uncomplicated asthma, indices of expiratory air flow are reduced while diffusing capacity is normal. A low P_{CO_2} indicates hyperventilation and an elevated P_{CO_2} is ominous evidence of carbon dioxide retention. Pregnancy does not seem to exert any consistent predictable effect on bronchial asthma. Treatment is the same as for nonpregnant patients except for the use of iodine-containing medications.

ADULT RESPIRATORY DISTRESS SYNDROME

Respiratory failure is either caused by or is associated with a growing number of illnesses or injuries, and it is now widely recognized that these are often nonpulmonary in origin. Adult respiratory distress syndrome is characterized by lung injury with increased capillary membrane permeability, pulmonary edema, and reduced lung compliance. The injury also causes loss of surfactant, followed by alveolar collapse and worsening of hypoxia. A number of conditions may lead to the syndrome, but in obstetrics, the most common predisposing causes are viral or bacterial pneumonias; severe acute hemorrhage with ectopic pregnancy (Chapter 8), placenta previa, or placental abruption (Chapter 44); aspiration of gastric acid contents (Chapter 58); or septicemia, most commonly complicating acute pyelonephritis, septic abortion, or postpartum metritis (Chapter 50). Moreover, if plasma colloid oncotic pressure is decreased further than in normal pregnancy, such as is common with severe preeclampsia (Chapter 57), pulmonary edema is made worse. Survival is dependent upon the cause, the duration, and, of course, the effectiveness of the therapy.

DISEASES OF THE KIDNEY & URINARY TRACT

URINARY TRACT INFECTIONS

Infections of the urinary tract are the most common bacterial infections encountered during pregnancy. Symptomatic infection may involve the lower tract to cause cystitis, or it may involve the renal calices, pelvis, and parenchyma to cause pyelonephritis. Most symptomatic urinary infections are acute and are characterized by a high frequency of recurrence, especially during pregnancy.

Organisms that cause urinary infections are those from the normal perineal flora, which in most cases have gained urinary tract access before pregnancy. Pregnancy does not seem to enhance virulence factors, but urinary stasis and diminished ureteral tone and peristalsis caused by ureteral compression of the enlarging uterus—and to a lesser extent by the smooth muscle relaxant effects of progesterone—predispose to symptomatic urinary infections.

The reported prevalence of **asymptomatic bacteriuria** during pregnancy varies from 2% to 12% depending on parity, race, and socioeconomic status. The highest incidence has been reported in black multiparas with sickle cell trait and the lowest incidence in affluent white women of low parity.

If asymptomatic bacteriuria is not treated, about 25% of infected women subsequently develop acute symptomatic infection during that pregnancy. Fortunately, eradication of bacteriuria with antimicrobial agents prevents most of these clinically evident infections. Treatment is discussed in Chapter 16.

Typically, **cystitis** is characterized by dysuria, particularly at the end of urination, as well as urgency and frequency. Women with bacterial cystitis respond readily to any of several regimens discussed in Chapter 16.

Acute pyelonephritis is one of the most common serious medical complications of pregnancy. Pyelonephritis is more common after mid pregnancy and is unilateral and right-sided in more than half of cases and bilateral in one-fourth. In most cases, renal parenchymal infection is caused by bacteria that ascend from the lower tract. Pregnant women with acute pyelonephritis should be hospitalized for prompt treatment. Intravenous hydration to ensure adequate urinary output is essential. During the first few days of therapy, these women should be watched carefully to detect symptoms of bacterial shock or its sequelae. Initial therapy is usually ampicillin while awaiting culture and sensitivity reports.

URINARY CALCULI

Renal and ureteral lithiasis are uncommon complications of pregnancy. Since pregnancy is associated with two of the cardinal prerequisites for stone formation—urinary stasis and infection—the incidence might be expected to be higher were it not for the relatively short duration of pregnancy. Urinary tract dilatation may also predispose to fewer symptoms. Women with a history of renal stones are at greater risk, though pregnancy does not increase that risk. Those with stones have a greater frequency of urinary tract infections. Calculi seldom cause severe symptomatic obstruction during pregnancy. Persistent pyelonephritis despite adequate antimicrobial therapy should prompt a search for renal obstruction, which is most frequently due to nephrolithiasis.

CHRONIC RENAL DISEASE

Chronic renal disease is a global term that denotes either underlying renal insufficiency or proteinuria or, in many cases, both. As described above, a number of primary renal disorders as well as multisystem diseases affect the kidneys. In many cases, renal biopsy is necessary to determine the cause of underlying renal disease; however, most defer this procedure until pregnancy is completed. The degree of renal insufficiency is more important than the type of lesion in determining pregnancy outcome. Accompanying preexisting hypertension also is predictive of pregnancy outcome. However, even if renal function is normal and the woman normotensive, pregnancy outcome is still not always good. Common complications include chronic hypertension, anemia, preeclampsia, fetal growth retardation, and preterm birth.

ENDOCRINE DISORDERS

DIABETES MELLITUS

Women whose pregnancies are complicated by diabetes can be separated into those who were known to have diabetes before pregnancy and those who develop gestational diabetes. Shown in Table 60–2 is the classification proposed by the American College of Obstetricians and Gynecologists (1986). Its salient features are that the duration of diabetes relates to the severity of end-organ derangement, especially the eyes, kidneys, and cardiovascular system.

The diabetogenic effects of pregnancy are evidenced by the fact that some women who have no evidence of diabetes when not pregnant develop during pregnancy distinct abnormalities of glucose tolerance and, at times, clinically overt diabetes. These changes are usually reversible. After

Table 60–2. Classification of diabetes complicating pregnancy.[1]

Class	Age at Onset		Duration (Yr)	Vascular Disease	Therapy
	Pregestational Diabetes				
A	Any		Any	None	A–1, diet only
B	Over 20		< 10	None	Insulin
C	10–19	or	10–19	None	Insulin
D	< 10	or	> 20	Benign retinopathy	Insulin
F	Any		Any	Nephropathy	Insulin
R	Any		Any	Proliferative retinopathy	Insulin
H	Any		Any	Heart disease	Insulin

Class	Fasting Plasma Glucose		Postprandial Plasma Glucose
	Gestational Diabetes		
A–1	< 105 mg per dL	and	< 120 mg per dL
A–2	> 105 mg per dL	and/or	> 120 mg per dL

[1]From The American College of Obstetricians and Gynecologists: Tech Bull No. 92, May 1986.

delivery, evidence of onset or worsening of diabetes usually disappears rapidly, and the patient's ability to metabolize carbohydrate returns to the prepregnancy status. As discussed in Chapter 36, physiologic pregnancy alterations impair peripheral insulin action. Insulin antagonism during pregnancy is probably due to the actions of placental lactogen, which is secreted in enormous quantities, and to lesser degrees the actions of estrogens and progesterone.

Diabetes may be deleterious to pregnancy in a number of ways. Adverse **maternal effects** include the following:

(1) The likelihood of preeclampsia-eclampsia is increased about fourfold.

(2) Some infections are more common and more severe in women with diabetes.

(3) The fetus can be much larger, and its size may lead to difficult delivery with injury to the birth canal.

(4) Because of substantively increased perinatal jeopardy as well as the possibility of dystocia, the rate of cesarean delivery is increased.

(5) Hydramnios is common.

(6) Postpartum hemorrhage is more common than in the general obstetric population.

Maternal diabetes adversely affects the **fetus and newborn infant** in the following ways:

(1) In the absence of good management of diabetes and pregnancy, the perinatal death rate is elevated.

(2) Major anomalies are increased threefold.

(3) Morbidity is common in the newborn. In some instances, morbidity results from birth injury as a consequence of fetal macrosomia. In other instances, it takes the form of severe respiratory distress and metabolic derangements, including hypoglycemia and hypocalcemia.

(4) The infant may inherit at least a predisposition to diabetes.

THYROID DISEASES

The vast majority of cases of **thyrotoxicosis** in pregnancy are caused by Graves' disease. Hyperthyroidism nearly always can be controlled by thioamide drugs, so that the disease need not be a serious threat to the mother. However, medical treatment has the potential for causing fetal complications. Propylthiouracil and methimazole readily cross the placenta and may induce fetal hypothyroidism and goiter.

Hypothyroidism is diagnosed if the expected rise during pregnancy in the level of circulating thyroxine fails to take place and the level of thyrotropin is elevated. In most women, a history of surgical or radioiodine treatment, usually for Graves' thyrotoxicosis, will be elicited. Overt hypothyroidism complicating pregnancy is rare and is often associated with infertility. Hypothyroid women who do become pregnant have a high incidence of preeclampsia and placental abruption with a correspondingly inordinate number of low-birth-weight and stillborn infants.

PHEOCHROMOCYTOMA

Pheochromocytoma is a rare but dangerous complication of pregnancy. Maternal morbidity may be as high as 50%. Maternal death from hypertensive crisis is much more common if the tumor is not diagnosed antepartum. Using CT scanning and MRI, tumor localization is now possible. In some women, surgery may be performed during pregnancy, but in all cases, medical management with phenoxybenzamine or a similar drug is imperative. Favorable outcomes have been described more recently for women in whom the diagnosis was made late in pregnancy and whose blood pressure was controlled pharmacologically during cesarean section and tumor resection.

DISEASES OF THE LIVER & GALLBLADDER

INTRAHEPATIC CHOLESTASIS OF PREGNANCY

This syndrome is also called recurrent jaundice of pregnancy, idiopathic cholestasis of pregnancy, cholestatic hepatosis, and icterus gravidarum. It is characterized clinically by pruritus, icterus, or both. The major histologic lesion is intrahepatic cholestasis with centrilobular bile staining without inflammatory cells or proliferation of mesenchymal cells. Its cause is unknown, but it appears to be stimulated in susceptible persons by high estrogen concentrations.

Bile acids are incompletely cleared by the liver and accumulate in the plasma of women with cholestasis. Levels typically are much higher than in normal pregnancy, and total bile acids may be elevated 30-fold. Modest hyperbilirubinemia results predominantly from retention of conjugated pigment. Serum aspartate aminotransferase activity is usually mildly to moderately elevated. Pruritus associated with elevated plasma bile salts may be intense. Cholestyramine has been reported to provide relief, but experience has not been uniformly favorable.

ACUTE FATTY LIVER OF PREGNANCY

Acute liver failure may occur with fulminant viral hepatitis, drug-induced hepatic toxicity, or acute fatty liver of pregnancy. The latter is fortunately a rare complication of pregnancy that often has proved to be fatal for both mother and fetus. The chief histologic abnormality consists of swollen hepatocytes in which the cytoplasm is filled with microvesicular fat, with central nuclei and periportal sparing, and minimal hepatocellular necrosis. The mechanism by which pregnancy incites fatty liver changes is not known. Acute fatty liver of pregnancy almost always develops in late pregnancy. It is probably more common with multifetal gestation. Typically, there is rapid onset of malaise, anorexia, nausea and vomiting, upper abdominal pain, and progressive jaundice. In many women there is also hypertension, proteinuria, and edema—all signs suggestive of preeclampsia.

The coagulopathy that complicates fatty liver of pregnancy almost certainly results from increased consumption of procoagulants and their impaired production by the liver. Since spontaneous resolution usually follows delivery, many assume that delivery is essential for cure.

LIVER INVOLVEMENT IN PREECLAMPSIA-ECLAMPSIA

The liver may be involved in women with severe preeclampsia and eclampsia. Both the degree of dysfunction and the histologic changes that develop can vary considerably. Typically, upper abdominal pain—epigastric or right upper quadrant—signals potentially dangerous liver involvement. Intrahepatic and subcapsular hemorrhage may develop and become so intense as to rupture the liver and produce extensive and even fatal hemorrhage. Hepatic dysfunction from preeclampsia and eclampsia is considered in Chapter 57.

HYPEREMESIS GRAVIDARUM

Nausea and vomiting of moderate intensity are especially common complaints from early pregnancy until about 16 weeks (Chapter 42). Fortunately, vomiting severe enough to produce weight loss, dehydration, acidosis from starvation, alkalosis from loss of hydrochloric acid in vomitus, and hypokalemia have become quite rare. Hyperemesis may lead to some elevation in serum transaminases and slight jaundice, which return to normal with hydration and feeding. Appropriate steps should be taken to detect other diseases, eg, gastroenteritis, cholecystitis, pancreatitis, hepatitis, peptic ulcer, and pyelonephritis. In many instances, social and psychologic factors contribute to the illness.

VIRAL HEPATITIS

Hepatitis is the most common liver disease that afflicts pregnant women. The effects of **hepatitis A** on pregnancy and vice versa are not dramatic in developed countries. However, at least in some underprivileged populations, both perinatal and maternal deaths are substantially increased. Treatment consists of a well-balanced diet and sedentary activity status. All pregnant women with suspected hepatitis should be hospitalized until it is clear that they are able to eat and drink and that liver function is improving, or at least not continuing to deteriorate.

Hepatitis B disease is found most often among intravenous drug abusers, homosexuals, health care personnel, and individuals who have been treated often with blood products, eg, hemophiliacs. It is transmitted usually in infected blood or blood products but also in saliva, vaginal secretions, and semen—thus, it is a sexually transmitted disease. The course of hepatitis B infection in the mother does not seem to be altered by pregnancy, at least in developed countries. As with hepatitis A, the likelihood of preterm delivery is increased. Treatment is supportive. Transplacental transfer of the virus from the mother to the fetus (except at delivery) is thought to be rare. Infection of the fetus-infant is by ingestion of infected material during delivery or exposure subsequent to birth. The infant may obtain the virus through breast feeding. Some infected infants are asymptomatic, but others develop fulminant disease and succumb. The majority—nearly 85%—become chronic carriers who can infect others. They are also at appreciable risk for later development of hepatocellular carcinoma or cirrhosis.

Infection of the newborn infant whose mother chronically carries the virus usually can be prevented by the administration of hepatitis B immune globulin very soon after birth followed promptly by hepatitis B vaccine.

CHOLELITHIASIS & CHOLECYSTITIS

Acute cholecystitis during pregnancy or the puerperium is managed in somewhat the same way as in nonpregnant women. For uncomplicated cases, most obstetricians prefer medical therapy with nasogastric suction and intravenous hydration and antimicrobials. Some favor cholecystectomy for uncomplicated disease. If cholecystectomy is to be performed during pregnancy, the second trimester is the optimal time since the risk of spontaneous abortion or preterm labor and delivery is reduced and the uterus is not yet large enough to impinge on the field of operation. When surgery is indicated, procrastination is not warranted.

GASTROINTESTINAL DISORDERS

APPENDICITIS

Pregnancy does not predispose to appendicitis, but its occurrence in about 1:2000 pregnancies reflects the general prevalence of the disease. Pregnancy often makes diagnosis of appendicitis more difficult for the following reasons: (1) Anorexia, nausea, and vomiting that accompany normal pregnancy are fairly common symptoms of appendicitis; (2) as the uterus enlarges, the appendix commonly moves upward and outward toward the flank, so that pain and tenderness may not be prominent in the right lower quadrant; (3) some degree of leukocytosis is the rule during normal pregnancy; and (4) during pregnancy, other diseases may be more readily confused with appendicitis, such as pyelonephritis, renal colic caused by a stone or kinking of a ureter, placental abruption, and red (carneous) degeneration of a myoma.

Appendicitis increases the likelihood of abortion or preterm labor, especially if there is peritonitis. If appendicitis is suspected, then treatment, regardless of the stage of gestation, is immediate surgical exploration. Even though diagnostic errors sometimes lead to removal of a normal appendix, it is better to operate unnecessarily than to postpone intervention until generalized peritonitis has developed.

PANCREATITIS

Pancreatitis complicating pregnancy is uncommon. Unlike nonpregnant patients, women with pancreatitis during pregnancy seldom have associated alcoholism. Serial determinations of serum amylase and lipase activity remain the best means of confirming the clinical diagnosis. Amylase values do not correlate with the severity of disease. Associated cholelithiasis is common, as may be demonstrated by ultrasonic or radiologic examination, including endoscopic retrograde cholangiopancreatography (ERCP). The principles of therapy are the same as for nonpregnant patients, and if the diagnosis is secure, medical treatment is indicated. Nasogastric suction is begun and intravenous fluids given to ensure adequate blood volume as indicated by urine output. Careful monitoring for severely ill women is essential, and bad prognostic signs include respiratory insufficiency, hypotension, a need for massive fluid replacement, and hypocalcemia.

INTESTINAL OBSTRUCTION

Intestinal obstruction is a grave complication of pregnancy and results most frequently from pressure of the growing uterus on intestinal adhesions that were formed after previous abdominal surgical procedures. The mortality rate can be very high, principally because of errors in diagnosis, late diagnosis, reluctance to operate on a pregnant woman, and inadequate preparation for surgery. Limited x-ray examinations, including plain abdominal films and those following administration of soluble contrast medium, either orally or by enema, should be done if indicated.

INFLAMMATORY BOWEL DISEASE

Chronic inflammatory bowel disease—ulcerative colitis or Crohn disease—is relatively common in women of childbearing age, and thus may complicate pregnancy. In general, pregnancy does not exacerbate either disease. Women with active disease at conception frequently do not improve or worsen during pregnancy. Treatment is given as if the woman were not pregnant, and surgery is performed if indicated. Diagnostic evaluations, including radiologic studies, are postponed unless their results would alter management substantively.

OBESITY

Marked obesity is a hazard to the pregnant woman and her fetus. As shown in Table 60–3, a number of pregnancy complications are increased. Management of obesity during pregnancy is a challenge. A program of weight reduction utilizing a diet restricted in calories but providing all essential nutrients commonly has been recommended for obese pregnant women. It seems unrealistic that weight

Table 60–3. Percentage of complications that were significantly increased in 588 obese (> 250 lb) women compared with 588 nonobese (< 200 lb) controls.[1]

Complication	Obese	Nonobese
Diabetes		
All types	10	2
Gestational	8	0.7
Hypertension	28	3
Postterm pregnancy	15	4
Oxytocin induction	23	8
Oxytocin augmentation	17	8
Macrosomic infant	24	7
Shoulder dystocia	5	0.6
Primary cesarean section	13	6
Wound infection	38	10
Excessive blood loss	38	14

[1]Modified from Johnson SR et al: Maternal obesity and pregnancy. Surg Gynecol Obstet 1987;164:431.

reduction will be substantial, but if such a regimen is chosen, the quality of the diet must be monitored closely and ketosis must be avoided.

CONNECTIVE TISSUE DISORDERS

SYSTEMIC LUPUS ERYTHEMATOSUS

Nearly a half million individuals in the United States have lupus, the great majority of them women. Pregnancy does not greatly exacerbate the disease, but about one-fourth will have modest exacerbations. The perinatal mortality rate is increased, especially in women with lupus nephritis. Treatment during pregnancy is not different from that given nonpregnant women.

The **lupus anticoagulant** is either an IgG or IgM immunoglobulin that has been identified in some patients with systemic lupus erythematosus and in others with no apparent evidence of lupus. In vitro, the lupus anticoagulant is characterized by a prolonged partial thromboplastin time. The anticoagulant, paradoxically, can incite thrombosis. The interest of obstetricians in this entity stems from the association of lupus anticoagulant with decidual vasculopathy, placental infarction, fetal growth retardation, and recurrent abortion and fetal death. The anticoagulant is associated also with a high incidence of venous and arterial thromboses, hypertension, hemolytic anemia, and biologically false-positive tests for syphilis.

RHEUMATOID ARTHRITIS

Although a number of humoral and cellular immunologic abnormalities have been identified, the cause of rheumatoid arthritis is unknown. Like lupus erythematosus, rheumatoid disease is more common in women than men. For unknown reasons, rheumatoid disease usually improves during pregnancy—not true of lupus. Exacerbations are treated with aspirin, and adrenal corticosteroids are given if needed. Severe hip deformities due to rheumatoid arthritis may preclude vaginal delivery.

DISEASES OF THE SKIN

ALOPECIA

During pregnancy, hair growth is stimulated; however, postpartum, hair reenters the resting phase and the numbers of hairs shed within 3–6 months may increase considerably. Thinning of the hair, or **telogen effluvium,** ceases gradually. The mother can be reassured that the phenomenon is not ominous and that she can anticipate full recovery.

PRURITIC URTICARIAL PAPULES & PLAQUES OF PREGNANCY

This is the most common pruritic dermatosis of pregnancy and is an intensely pruritic cutaneous eruption of late pregnancy. Erythematous urticarial papules and plaques (Figure 60–1) first develop on the abdomen, usually in the periumbilical area, and spread to the thighs and extremities. Typically, the face is spared, and excoriation seldom occurs. The disease is more common in nulliparas and seldom recurs in subsequent pregnancies. It may resemble herpes gestationis, but there are no vesicles or bullae. Furthermore, immunofluorescent staining of skin shows no immunoglobulin or complement deposition. Rather, there is a mild nonspecific lymphohistiocytic perivasculitis. Topical corticosteroid preparations usually provide relief, and oral prednisone is occasionally given for intense pruritus. There is no evidence that perinatal morbidity is increased.

HERPES GESTATIONIS

Herpes gestationis is a serious but rare dermatologic disease peculiar to pregnancy. Although the matter is in dispute, the perinatal mortality rate may be increased. In spite of its name, it is not a viral disease. This blistering disease of pregnancy usually presents as an extremely pruritic widespread eruption with lesions that vary from ery-

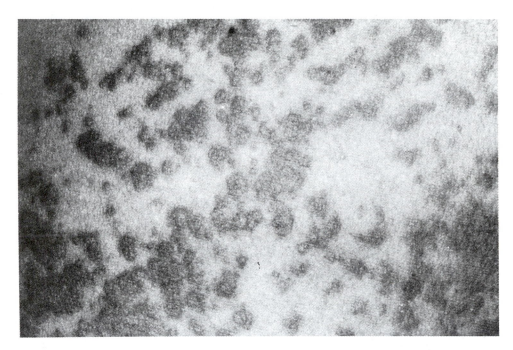

Figure 60–1. Pruritic urticarial papules and plaques of pregnancy. Numerous edematous and erythematous papular lesions are present on the lower trunk. (From Yancey KB, Hall RP, Lawley TJ: Pruritic urticarial papules and plaques of pregnancy: Clinical experience in 25 patients. J Am Acad Dermatol 1984;10:473.)

thematous and edematous papules to large, tense bullae. Common sites of involvement are the abdomen and the extremities. Immunofluorescent techniques applied to a skin biopsy are of value for confirming the diagnosis, and both IgG and C3 are deposited along the basement membrane zone. Prednisone in doses of 40–60 mg daily usually brings relief promptly and inhibits the formation of new lesions.

NEUROLOGIC DISORDERS

SEIZURE DISORDERS

The effect of pregnancy on the frequency of epileptic seizures has been argued for more than 100 years. It appears that if seizures are well controlled before pregnancy, there is little risk of increased frequency during pregnancy. If seizures are poorly controlled before pregnancy, however, there is a likelihood that even further deterioration may occur during pregnancy. The therapeutic goal for the treatment of epilepsy during pregnancy is to administer to the mother the least amount of drug likely to affect her fetus adversely yet effectively control her convulsions.

Women with epilepsy who take anticonvulsant medications have a two- to threefold increased risk for giving birth to infants with congenital anomalies. It is not clear whether epilepsy per se or anticonvulsant drug teratogenicity is responsible (see Chapter 54). The fetal phenytoin syndrome includes craniofacial anomalies, distal limb dysmorphosis, and mental deficiency. Use of phenytoin has been accompanied also by increased frequencies of cleft lip and cleft palate and of congenital heart lesions.

CEREBROVASCULAR DISEASES (Stroke)

While distinctly uncommon in young women, disorders of the cerebral circulation have continued to be the third or fourth leading cause of maternal deaths in the United States. Because of the low incidence of strokes in young women, the exact contribution of cerebral thrombosis as a cause of stroke during pregnancy is uncertain, but it probably is not more common than stroke from cerebral embolism or intracranial hemorrhage. In all cases, a vigorous search should be made to determine the cause.

Several lesions may cause serious intracranial hemorrhage. Intracerebral hemorrhage from hypertension is uncommon during pregnancy but may complicate chronic essential hypertension with superimposed preeclampsia.

Lesions that cause subarachnoid hemorrhage are more likely to be associated with otherwise normal pregnancy and include ruptured saccular aneurysms and bleeding arteriovenous malformations that complicate about 1:15,000 pregnancies.

PSEUDOTUMOR CEREBRI

Benign intracranial hypertension (pseudotumor cerebri) is characterized by headache, visual disturbances, and papilledema from increased intracranial pressure in an otherwise healthy individual. Criteria for diagnosis include elevated pressure of cerebrospinal fluid of normal composition along with normal cranial CT scans. Pregnancy is said to be an inciting factor.

BELL PALSY

Isolated facial nerve palsy (Bell palsy) is relatively common. Pregnancy seems to be complicated by a disparate number of these cases, which typically develop in late gestation. Pregnancy does not seem to alter the overall good prognosis for spontaneous recovery, and nearly 90% of affected women will recover function within a few weeks to months. Treatment with corticosteroids remains controversial, but the bulk of evidence suggests that these drugs do not hasten resolution.

CARPAL TUNNEL SYNDROME

The median nerve is vulnerable to compression within the carpal tunnel at the wrist. Symptoms of nerve compression are common during pregnancy, and as many as 25% of women may complain of these symptoms. Typically, the woman awakens with burning, numbness, or tingling in the thenar half of one or both hands. The fingers otherwise feel numb and useless. A splint applied to the very slightly flexed wrist and worn during sleep usually provides relief. The signs and symptoms most often regress after delivery.

INFECTIONS DURING PREGNANCY

VARICELLA

Most adults have acquired chickenpox during childhood and are immune. For adults who do become infected, varicella tends to be much more severe than in children. This is especially so during pregnancy, and about 10% of infected women develop pneumonitis. Maternal chickenpox during the first trimester has been implicated as a cause of congenital malformations from transplacental infection.

About 10% of maternal infections result in clinical evidence of fetal infection, and this risk is the same for all trimesters. Infection early in pregnancy resulted in severe congenital malformations, including chorioretinitis, cerebral cortical atrophy, hydronephrosis, and cutaneous and bony leg defects. Exposure of the fetus to the virus just before or during delivery—and therefore before it has received antibody from the mother—poses a serious threat to the newborn. In some instances, the infant will develop disseminated visceral and central nervous system disease which in the past, at least, were likely to be fatal. Varicella-zoster immune globulin (VZIG) or zoster immune globulin (ZIG) should be administered to the neonate whenever the onset of maternal clinical disease was within 5 days before delivery or 2 days postpartum.

LISTERIOSIS

Listeria monocytogenes is an uncommon but probably underdiagnosed cause of neonatal sepsis. From 1% to 5% of adults have listeriae in their feces, and outbreaks of listeriosis have been reported from contaminated cabbage, pasteurized milk, and fresh Mexican-style cheese. Listeriosis during pregnancy may be asymptomatic or may cause a febrile illness that is mistaken for influenza or pyelonephritis, and the diagnosis is not apparent until the blood culture is reported as positive. Maternal listeremia causes fetal infection that produces characteristically disseminated granulomatous lesions with microabscesses. There is evidence that maternal antimicrobial treatment may also be effective for fetal infection.

SYPHILIS

An unusually critical time to detect and treat syphilis is during pregnancy, not only to protect the mother and her sexual partner from the numerous complications of syphilis but also to protect the fetus from the extensive pathologic changes that characterize congenital syphilis (Chapter 55). Of the many congenital infections, syphilis is not only the most readily prevented but also is one of the most susceptible to therapy. Unfortunately, therapy does not reverse the anatomic defects already caused by the infection.

Penicillin remains the treatment of choice. The recommendations for treatment provided by the Centers for Disease Control are set forth in Chapter 7.

GONORRHEA

The greatly increased prevalence of gonorrhea in recent years has not spared pregnant women, and many public obstetric clinics have reported gonococcal infections of the lower genitourinary tract to be common. The pregnant woman may have asymptomatic local infection involving— singly or in combination—the lower genital tract, lower urinary tract, rectum, or pharynx. Without adequate treatment, persistence of the infection may allow the mother to infect her sexual partner; to develop gonococcal arthritis or other disseminated disease; to infect her infant at the time of delivery, thereby causing gonorrheal ophthalmia; or to develop an ascending genital infection postpartum. Consequently, even asymptomatic disease during pregnancy should be identified and eradicated. Ideally, all pregnant women should have an endocervical culture made to detect gonorrhea at the time of their first visit.

Sexual partners exposed to gonorrhea should be examined, diagnosed by culture if urethral discharge is present, and treated at once if the results are positive. Individuals treated for gonorrhea should be followed up with repeat cultures 5–7 days after completion of the treatment.

All adults treated for gonorrhea should be treated for coexistent chlamydial infection. Recommended treatment regimens are given in Chapter 7.

CHLAMYDIAL INFECTIONS

Chlamydia trachomatis is an obligate intracellular bacterial organism thought to be the most prevalent cause of sexually transmitted disease in the United States. Chlamydial infections are characterized by their indolence, often associated with a paucity of clinical findings. Lower genital tract infections generally are minimally symptomatic. They are manifested most often by mucopurulent cervicitis characterized by cervical erythema and edema with cloudy or white "mucopus" that contains abundant polymorphonuclear leukocytes. It is difficult to distinguish normal cervical eversion and erythema of pregnancy from chlamydial cervicitis.

Verification of these infections has been made easier by the use of a direct-slide fluorescence-tagged chlamydial monoclonal antibody test considered by many to be almost as accurate as culture. When these tests confirm maternal genital chlamydial infection, treatment is given with either erythromycin base, 500 mg, or erythromycin ethylsuccinate, 800 mg, 4 times daily for 7 days.

HERPES SIMPLEX VIRUS INFECTIONS

Two types of herpesvirus—types 1 and 2—have been distinguished, and type 2 virus is recovered almost exclusively from the genital tract and is transmitted in the great majority of instances by sexual contact. Almost always, the fetus becomes infected by virus shed from the cervix or lower genital tract. The virus then either invades the uterus following rupture of the membranes or contacts the fetus at delivery. Newborn infection takes on one of three forms: (1) disseminated, with involvement of major viscera; (2) localized, with involvement confined to the central nervous system, eyes, skin, or mucosa; or (3) asymptomatic. Nearly half of neonates infected with herpesvirus are preterm, and their risk of infection correlates with whether there is primary or recurrent maternal infection.

Neonatal infection is associated with a mortality rate of at least 60%, and serious ophthalmic and central nervous system damage has been identified in at least half of survivors. In general, treatment of the neonate has been disappointing; therefore, considerable emphasis is placed upon prevention of contact between fetus and virus during delivery.

Because of the severity of neonatal herpesvirus infection, cesarean delivery has been used widely in instances when genital herpetic lesions are suspected. It is certainly prudent to choose cesarean delivery if there is a reasonable chance that virus is being shed. In many cases, however, this is difficult to prove with currently available technology.

ACQUIRED IMMUNODEFICIENCY SYNDROME

The prevalence of asymptomatic HIV infection in the United States is estimated at 1–1.5 million persons. During 1991, almost 150,000 person were diagnosed with AIDS, and it is estimated that another 50,000 per year will develop AIDS. The exact incubation period is unknown; however, it may be as short as 2 months or as long as 5 years. The mortality rate of AIDS is extremely high, and 60–80% of persons who develop the syndrome die within 2 years.

The rate of perinatal transmission of human immunodeficiency virus is unknown, but available data suggest that it is about 40%. Perinatal transmission is by transplacental infection, and almost all women who are delivered of infants who subsequently develop AIDS have been asymptomatic during pregnancy. The possibility exists that during pregnancy clinical illness is more likely to follow asymptomatic infection, presumably because of suppressed cell-mediated immunity.

At present, the issue of screening for HIV is mired in the legal processes of each state. Because of the uncertain state of these laws and regulations, physicians must seek out for themselves the current status of screening programs in their own communities and hospitals.

HUMAN PAPILLOMAVIRUS INFECTION

Several types of human papillomaviruses cause mucocutaneous warts. Condylomata acuminata (genital warts, venereal warts) are usually caused by types 6 and 11. Viral types 16, 18, 31, 33, and 35 have been implicated in the cause of cervical intraepithelial neoplasia and possibly invasive cancer, as well as other female genital cancers. The virus also can cause laryngeal papillomatosis in children, and evidence is consistent that types 6 and 11 in some cases may be transmitted by aspiration of infected material at delivery. For unknown reasons, in some women the growth of genital warts is stimulated during pregnancy (Figure 60–2). Certainly the constant mucorrhea throughout pregnancy provides ideal moist conditions for their growth. Treatment may be very unsatisfactory, but it is usual for these lesions to clear rapidly following delivery.

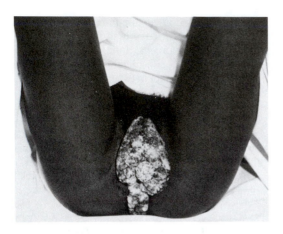

Figure 60–2. Condylomata acuminata. (Reproduced, with permission, from Cunningham FG, MacDonald PC, Gant NF [editors]: *Williams Obstetrics,* 18th ed. Appleton & Lange, 1989.)

NEOPLASTIC DISEASES

BREAST CARCINOMA

Breast carcinoma is the most common cancer of women, and it is not surprising that it is encountered with some frequency during pregnancy. Its exact incidence is not known, but it has been estimated to be about 1:10,000–1:3000 pregnancies.

Pregnancy does not appear to exert much influence on the course of mammary cancer, and therapeutic abortion does not improve its prognosis. Thus, results to be anticipated will be comparable to the survival rates expected with the same stage of the disease in nonpregnant women.

Unfortunately, pregnant women as a group have more advanced stages of cancer at diagnosis, and thus their prognosis is worse. These results can best be explained by delayed diagnosis because of confusion between tumor growth with normal breast growth during pregnancy. It has been hypothesized that increased breast vascularity may accelerate cancer spread. Any suspicious breast mass found in the pregnant woman should set in motion an aggressive plan to determine its cause, whether by fine-needle aspiration, mammography, or excisional biopsy.

SUGGESTED READINGS

American College of Obstetricians and Gynecologists: Human immune deficiency virus infections. Tech Bull No. 123, 1988.

American College of Obstetricians and Gynecologists: Management of diabetes mellitus in pregnancy. Tech Bull No. 92, 1986.

American College of Obstetricians and Gynecologists: Perinatal herpes simplex virus infections. Tech Bull No. 122, 1988.

Centers for Disease Control: Recommendations of the Immunization Practices Advisory Committee: Prevention of perinatal transmission of hepatitis B virus: Prenatal screening of all pregnant women for hepatitis B surface antigen. MMWR 1988;37:341.

Cunningham FG: Urinary tract infections complicating pregnancy. Clin Obstet Gynecol 1988;1:891.

Donaldson RM: Management of medical problems in pregnancy—inflammatory bowel disease. N Engl J Med 1985; 312:1618.

Gabbe SG: Management of diabetes mellitus in pregnancy. Am J Obstet Gynecol 1985;153:824.

Landers D et al: Acute cholecystitis in pregnancy. Obstet Gynecol 1987;69:131.

Riely CA: Acute fatty liver of pregnancy. Semin Liver Dis 1987;7:47.

Index